The Cambridge Textbook of Bioethics

Medicine and healthcare generate many bioethical problems and dilemmas that are of great academic, professional and public interest. This comprehensive resource is designed as a succinct yet authoritative text and reference for clinicians, researchers, bioethicists, and students seeking a better understanding of the ethical problems in the healthcare setting. Each chapter illustrates an ethical problem that might be encountered in everyday practice; defines the concepts at issue; examines their implications from the perspectives of ethics, law, and policy; and then provides a practical resolution. There are 10 key sections presenting the most vital topics and clinically relevant areas of modern bioethics. International, interdisciplinary authorship and cross-cultural orientation ensure suitability for a worldwide audience. This book will assist all clinicians in making well-reasoned and defensible decisions by developing their awareness of ethical considerations and teaching the analytical skills to deal with them effectively.

Peter A. Singer is Director Emeritus, University of Toronto Joint Centre for Bioethics; Senior Scientist, McLaughlin-Rotman Centre for Global Health, University Health Network, University of Toronto; Sun Life Financial Chair in Bioethics and Professor of Medicine, University of Toronto.

A. M. Viens is a Senior Scholar at Hertford College, Oxford, a Doctoral Student in the Faculty of Philosophy at the University of Oxford and a member of the Joint Centre for Bioethics, University of Toronto.

The Cambridge Textbook of Bioethics

Editor-in-Chief

Peter A. Singer

University of Toronto and University
Health Network, Canada

Executive Editor

A. M. Viens

Hertford College, Oxford, UK

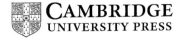

CAMBRIDGE UNIVERSITY PRESS
Cambridge, New York, Melbourne, Madrid, Cape Town, Singapore, São Paulo

Cambridge University Press
The Edinburgh Building, Cambridge CB2 8RU, UK

Published in the United States of America by Cambridge University Press, New York

www.cambridge.org
Information on this title: www.cambridge.org/9780521872843

© Cambridge University Press 2008

First published 2008

Printed in the United Kingdom at the University Press, Cambridge

A catalogue record for this publication is available from the British Library

ISBN 978-0-521-87284-3 hardback
ISBN 978-0-521-69443-8 paperback

Contents

Section VI Health systems and institutions

Section VII Using clinical ethics to make an impact in healthcare

Section VIII Global health ethics

Contributors

Editor-in-Chief   Peter A. Singer

Executive Editor   A. M. Viens

Section Editors   Richard E. Ashcroft, Solomon R.
  Benatar, Joseph M. Boyle, Jr., Abdallah S. Daar,
  John Lantos, Susan K. MacRae, David Novak,
  Anne Slowther, James A. Tulsky, Ross Upshur,
  and A. M. Viens.

James Andrews
School of Medicine, Stanford University, Palo Alto,
CA, USA

Kyle W. Anstey
Bioethicist, University Health Network, Toronto,
Canada

Robert Arnold
Leo H. Criep Chair in Patient Care, Institute to
Enhance Palliative Care, Section of Palliative Care and
Medical Ethics, University of Pittsburgh, Pittsburgh,
USA

Richard E. Ashcroft
Professor of Bioethics, School of Law, Queen Mary,
University of London, UK

Tarif Bakdash
Pediatric Neurologist; Lecturer, Damascus University,
Syria

Françoise Baylis
Professor and Canada Research Chair in Bioethics and Philosophy, Department of Bioethics, Faculty of Medicine, Dalhousie University, Halifax, Canada

David Benatar
Professor, Department of Philosophy, University of Cape Town, South Africa

Solomon R. Benatar
Professor of Medicine and Founding Director of the University of Cape Town's Bioethics Centre, South Africa; Joint Centre for Bioethics, University of Toronto, Canada

Sidney Bloch
Professor, Department of Psychiatry and Adjunct Professor, Center for Health and Society, University of Melbourne, Australia

Kerry W. Bowman
Bioethicist, Mount Sinai Hospital and Assistant Professor, Department of Family and Community Medicine, University of Toronto, Canada

Joseph M. Boyle, Jr.
Professor, Department of Philosophy, University of Toronto, Canada

Barry F. Brown
Professor Emeritus, Department of Philosophy, University of Toronto, Canada

Ruth Chadwick
Distinguished Research Professor and Director, Centre for Economic and Social Aspects of Genomics, Cardiff Law School, Cardiff University, UK

Julie Chalmers
Consultant General Adult Psychiatrist, OBMH Partnership NHS Trust Oxford and Honorary Senior Clinical Lecturer, University of Oxford, UK

Larry R. Churchill
Ann Geddes Stahlman Professor of Medical Ethics, Vanderbilt University Medical Center, Vanderbilt, USA

Jillian Clare Cohen-Kohler
Assistant Professor, Leslie Dan Faculty of Pharmacy, University of Toronto, Canada

Michael H. Cohen
Assistant Professor, Department of Health Policy and Management, Harvard School of Public Health, Harvard University, Cambridge, USA

Eoin Connolly
Bioethicist, Centre for Clinical Ethics (a shared service of Providence Healthcare, St. Joseph's Health Centre, & St. Michael's Hospital), Toronto, Canada

Harold Coward
Professor of History and Former Director, Centre for Studies in Religion and Society, University of Victoria, Canada

Abdallah S. Daar
Senior Scientist and Co-director, Program on Life Sciences, Ethics and Policy, McLaughlin–Rotman Centre for Global Health, University Health Network and University of Toronto and Professor of Public Health Sciences and Surgery, University of Toronto, Canada

Lori d'Agincourt-Canning
Clinical Ethicist, Children's and Women's Health Centre, Vancouver, Canada

Kate Dewhirst
Corporate Counsel to the Centre for Addiction and Mental Health, Toronto, Canada

Bernard M. Dickens
Professor Emeritus, Faculty of Law and Faculty of Medicine; Joint Centre for Bioethics, University of Toronto, Canada

Jocelyn Downie
Director, Health Law Institute School of Law,
Dalhousie University, Halifax, Canada

Mary Jane Dykeman
Barrister and Solicitor; Adjunct Professor (Mental
Health), Osgoode Hall Law School, York University,
Toronto, Canada

Margaret L. Eaton
Lecturer in Management, Graduate School of
Business, Stanford University, Palo Alto, USA

Jonathan H. Ellerby
Spiritual Program Director, Canyon Ranch Health
Resort, Tucson, USA

Linda L. Emanuel
Professor, Division of General Internal Medicine,
Feinberg School of Medicine, Northwestern
University, Chicago, USA

Halley S. Faust
Board of Regents and Secretary-Treasurer, American
College of Preventive Medicine; Managing Director,
Jerome Capital, LLC, Santa Fe, USA

Ellen Fox
Director, National Center for Ethics in Health Care, US
Department of Veterans Affairs, Washington DC, USA

Linda Ganzini
Professor of Psychiatry and Medicine; Senior Scholar,
Center for Ethics in Health Care, Oregon Health and
Science University, Portland, USA

Jennifer L. Gibson
Assistant Professor, Department of Health Policy,
Management and Evaluation and Director,
Partnerships and Strategy, Joint Centre for Bioethics,
University of Toronto, Canada

Kathleen C. Glass
Director, Biomedical Ethics Unit and Associate
Professor, Departments of Human Genetics and

Pediatrics, McGill University; Clinical Ethicist, The
Montréal Children's Hospital, Montréal, Canada

M. Dianne Godkin
Clinical Ethicist and Manager, Centre for Clinical
Ethics (a shared service of Providence Healthcare,
St. Joseph's Health Centre, and St. Michael's Hospital),
Toronto, Canada

Gary Goldsand
Clinical Ethicist, Royal Alexandra Hospital, Edmonton,
Canada

Susan Dorr Goold
Associate Professor of Internal Medicine and Director,
Bioethics Program, University of Michigan, Ann Arbor
USA

Michael Gordon
Vice President Medical Services and Head of Geriatrics
and Internal Medicine, Baycrest Centre for Geriatric
Care; Professor, Faculty of Medicine, University of
Toronto, Canada

Ronald M. Green
Eunice & Julian Cohen Professor for the Study of
Ethics and Human Values and Director of the Ethics
Institute, Dartmouth University, Hanover, USA

Stephen A. Green
Clinical Professor, Department of Psychiatry,
Georgetown University Hospital, Washington DC, USA

Heather L. Greenwood
Program on Life Sciences, Ethics and Policy,
McLaughlin–Rotman Centre for Global Health and
University Health Network, University of Toronto,
Canada

Christine Harrison
Director of the Bioethics Department, The Hospital for
Sick Children; Joint Centre for Bioethics and Associate
Professor, Department of Paediatrics, University of
Toronto, Canada

Philip C. Hébert
Bioethicist and Director of the Clinical Ethics Centre, Sunnybrook Health Sciences Centre; Joint Centre for Bioethics and Associate Professor, Department of Family and Community Medicine, University of Toronto, Canada

Barry Hoffmaster
Professor, Department of Philosophy, University of Western Ontario, London, Canada

Mark Hughes
Assistant Professor, Division of General Internal Medicine, School of Medicine; Berman Institute of Bioethics, Johns Hopkins University, Baltimore, USA

Edwin C. Hui
Professor of Medical Ethics, Lee Ka Shing Faculty of Medicine, University of Hong Kong, China

Roger C. Hutchinson
Professor Emeritus of Church and Society, Emmanuel College of Victoria University in the University of Toronto, Canada

Judy Illes
Director of the Program in Neuroethics, Stanford Center for Biomedical Ethics, Stanford University, Palo Alto, USA

Patricia Illingsworth
Associate Professor, Department of Philosophy and Religions, Northeastern University, Boston, USA

Jay A. Jacobson
Chief of the Division of Medical Ethics and Humanities; LDS Hospital and the University of Utah School of Medicine, Salt Lake City, USA

Carolyn Johnston
Adviser in Medical Law and Ethics, School of Medicine, King's College London, UK

Harvey Kayman
Public Health Medical Officer III, Bioterrorism and Pandemic Influenza Planning and Preparedness Section, Immunization Branch, California Department of Public Health, USA

Nuala Kenny
Professor, Departments of Bioethics and Pediatrics, Faculty of Medicine, Dalhousie University, Halifax, Canada

Damien Keown
Professor of Buddhist Ethics, Department of History, Goldsmiths College, University of London, UK

Ahmed B. Khitamy
Department of Microbiology, Sultan Qaboos University Hospital, Oman

Nancy M. P. King
Professor, Department of Social Sciences and Health Policy; Wake Forest University School of Medicine, Winston-Salem, USA

Irwin Kleinman
Department of Psychiatry, Faculty of Medicine, University of Toronto, and Mount Sinai Hospital, Toronto, Canada

Bartha Maria Knoppers
Canada Research Chair in Law and Medicine and Professor, Faculté de Droit, Université de Montréal, and Researcher, Centre de Recherche en Droit Public, Université de Montréal, Canada

Jacob C. Langer
Chief, Department of General Surgery, Hospital for Sick Children and Professor, Department of Surgery, University of Toronto, Canada

John Lantos
John B. Francis Chair in Bioethics, Center for Practical Bioethics and Associate Director, MacLean Center for Clinical Medical Ethics, University of Chicago, USA

Neil Lazar
Site Director, Medical Surgical ICU, Toronto General Hospital; Associate Professor of Medicine and Member of the Joint Centre for Bioethics, University of Toronto, Canada

Trudo Lemmens
Associate Professor, Faculty of Law, University of Toronto, Canada

Benjamin H. Levi
Associate Professor, Departments of Humanities and Pediatrics, Penn State University, University Park, USA

Alex V. Levin
Associate Professor, Departments of Paediatrics, Genetics and Ophthalmology and Vision Sciences, and Director, Postgraduate Bioethics Education, Faculty of Medicine, University of Toronto, Canada

Phillip D. Levin
Attending Physician, Department of Anesthesiology and Critical Care Medicine, Hadassah Hebrew University Hospital, Jerusalem, Israel

Lori Luther
Faculty of Law, University of Toronto, Canada

Neil MacDonald
Director, McGill Cancer Nutrition and Rehabilitation Programme, Department of Oncology, McGill University, Canada

Susan K. MacRae
Deputy Director and the Director of the Clinical Ethics Fellowship, Joint Centre for Bioethics, University of Toronto, Canada

Hazel J. Markwell
Bioethicist and Director of the Centre for Clinical Ethics (shared service of Providence Healthcare, St. Joseph's Health Centre, and St. Michael's Hospital); Joint Centre for Bioethics and Assistant Professor, Department of Anaesthesia, University of Toronto, Canada

Douglas K. Martin
Associate Professor, Department of Health Policy, Management and Evaluation, and Joint Centre for Bioethics, University of Toronto, Canada

Martin F. McKneally
Professor Emeritus, Department of Surgery, University of Toronto, Canada

Eric M. Meslin
Director, Indiana University Center for Bioethics, Associate Dean for Bioethics, School of Medicine and Professor of Medicine, Medical and Molecular Genetics, and Philosophy, Indiana University, Indianapolis, USA

Margaret Moon
Assistant Professor, Division of Pediatrics and Adolescent Medicine, School of Medicine; Berman Institute of Bioethics, Johns Hopkins University, Baltimore, USA

Osamu Muramoto
Regional Ethics Council and Department of Neurology, Kaiser Permanente Northwest Division, Portland, USA

Roxanne Mykitiuk
Associate Professor, Osgoode Hall Law School, York University, Toronto, Canada

William A. Nelson
Associate Professor of Psychiatry, Department of Community and Family Medicine, Dartmouth Medical School, Hanover, USA

Jeff Nisker
Professor, Departments of Obstetrics–Gynaecology and Oncology and Coordinator of Health Ethics and Humanities, Schulich School of Medicine and Dentistry, University of Western Ontario, London, Canada

David Novak
J. Richard and Dorothy Shiff Chair of Jewish Studies, Department of Religious Studies, University of Toronto, Canada

Merril Pauls
Director of Medical Humanities and Member of the
Section of Emergency Medicine, Faculty of Medicine,
University of Manitoba, Winnpeg, Canada

Robert A. Pearlman
Department of Medicine, and Department of
Medical History and Ethics, University of
Washington, Seattle, USA

Eric Racine
Director, Neuroethics Research Unit, Institut de
recherches cliniques de Montréal, Montréal, Canada

Howard Radest
Adjunct Professor, Department of Philosophy,
University of South Carolina at Beaufort, USA

Jason Scott Robert
Assistant Professor, School of Life Sciences, Arizona
State University, Tempe, USA

Gerald Robertson
Faculty of Law, University of Alberta, Edmonton,
Canada

Sanda Rodgers
Shirley E. Greenberg Professor of Women and the
Legal Profession, Faculty of Law, University of
Ottawa, Canada

Zahava R. S. Rosenberg-Yunger
Joint Centre for Bioethics, University of Toronto,
Canada

Kelley Ross
Joint Centre for Bioethics, University of Toronto,
Canada

Lainie Friedman Ross
Carolyn and Matthew Bucksbaum Professor of Clinical
Ethics and Professor of the Departments of Pediatrics
and Medicine, University of Chicago, USA

Madelaine Saginur
Research Associate, Centre de Recherche en Droit
Public, Université de Montréal, Canada

Arthur B. Sanders
Professor, Emergency Medicine, College of Medicine,
University of Arizona, Tucson, USA

Jared M. Schmidek
Center for the Evaluative Clinical Sciences,
Dartmouth Medical School, Hanover, USA

Sam D. Shemie
Division of Pediatric Critical Care, Montréal Children's
Hospital, McGill University and the Bertram Loeb
Chair in Organ and Tissue Donation, University of
Ottawa, Canada

Robert Sibbald
Clinical Ethicist, London Health Sciences Centre,
London, Canada

Tejinder Sidhu
Family Physician, Victoria, British
Columbia, Canada

Peter A. Singer
Director Emeritus, Joint Centre for Bioethics,
University of Toronto, Senior Scientist,
McLaughlin–Rotman Centre for Global Health,
University Health Network and University of Toronto,
and Professor of Medicine, and Sun Life Chair in
Bioethics, University of Toronto, Canada

Jerome Amir Singh
Howard College School of Law; CAPRISA, University of
KwaZulu-Natal; Adjunct Professor, Department of
Public Health Sciences; Joint Centre for Bioethics,
University of Toronto

Anne Slowther
Senior Lecturer in Clinical Ethics, University of
Warwick Medical School, Coventry, UK

Ann Sommerville
Head of Ethics Department, British Medical
Association, London, UK

Charles L. Sprung
Professor of Medicine and Critical Care Medicine,
Department of Anesthesiology and Critical Care
Medicine, Hadassah Hebrew University Hospital,
Jerusalem, Israel

Gopal Sreenivasan
Canada Research Chair and Associate Professor,
Department of Philosophy; Joint Centre for Bioethics,
University of Toronto, Canada

Jeremy Sugarman
Harvey M. Meyerhoff Professor of Bioethics and
Medicine and Deputy Director for Medicine, Berman
Institute of Bioethics, Johns Hopkins University,
Baltimore, USA

C. Shawn Tracy
Research Associate, Primary Care Research Unit,
Sunnybrook Health Sciences Centre; Joint Centre for
Bioethics, University of Toronto, Canada

James A. Tulsky
Professor of Medicine and Director of the Center for
Palliative Care, Duke University and the Durham VA
Medical Center, Durham, USA

Ross d Upshur
Director, Joint Centre for Bioethics, Canada Research
Chair in Primary Care Research and Associate
Professor, Departments of Family and Community
Medicine and Public Health Sciences, University of
Toronto, Canada

Gail A. Van Norman
Clinical Associate Professor of Anesthesiology and
Affiliate Associate Professor of Medical History and
Ethics, University of Washington, Seattle, USA

A. M. Viens
Senior Scholar, Hertford College, Oxford; Doctoral
Student, Faculty of Philosophy, University of Oxford,
UK; Joint Centre for Bioethics, University of Toronto,
Canada

Frank Wagner
Bioethicist, Toronto Central Community Care Access
Centre; Joint Centre For Bioethics and Assistant
Professor, Department of Family and Community
Medicine, University of Toronto, Canada

Sally Webb
Associate Professor of Pediatrics and Emergency/
Critical Care Medicine, Medical University of South
Carolina, Charleston, USA

Brent C. Williams
Associate Professor, Department of Internal Medicine,
University of Michigan, Ann Arbor, USA

John R. Williams
Adjunct Professor, Faculty of Medicine, University of
Ottawa, Canada

Linda Wright
Senior Bioethicist, University Health Network, Joint
Centre for Bioethics, University of Toronto, Canada

David Young
Professor and Head, Department of Obstetrics and
Gynaecology, Faculty of Medicine, Dalhousie
University, Halifax, Canada

Larry Zaroff
Senior Research Scholar, Center for Biomedical Ethics,
Stanford University, Palo Alto, USA

Randi Zlotnik Shaul
Bioethicist, The Hospital for Sick Children; Joint
Centre for Bioethics, University of Toronto, Canada

Acknowledgements

We would like to extend our appreciation and warmest thanks to all that made this project possible. We are both grateful to the University of Toronto Joint Centre for Bioethics, truly one of the world's great bioethics centres, for providing the support to make this book become a reality. In particular, the Deputy Director, Sue MacRae, and the Centre's great new Director, Ross Upshur, was instrumental in creating this book. The Joint Centre is filled with wonderful colleagues, many of whom you will meet as authors of chapters in this book. We would also like to thank Richard Barling, Dan Dunlavey, Nicholas Dunton, Rachael Lazenby, Jane Ward and Richard Marley from Cambridge University Press, and especially all of the section editors and contributors.

A. M. Viens would like to acknowledge the family, friends, and colleagues who provided help and support over the course of this project. In particular, Jeffrey Bibbee, Melanie Bigold, Eoin Connolly, Roger Crisp, Markus Kohl, James Morauta, Mary Rowell, Julian Savulescu, Peter A. Singer, Eli Tyshynski, and especially Louise Viens. He would also like to thank the Joint Centre for Bioethics at the University of Toronto for awarding him an Ethics Fellowship that allowed him to complete this project.

Peter A. Singer would like to express his thanks to those who have mentored and supported his career in bioethics: Mark Siegler, the late Alvan R. Feinstein, Frederick H. Lowy, Arnie Aberman, C. David Naylor, Catharine Whiteside, Michael Baker, Wendy Levinson, Bob Bell, and Joseph L. Rotman. His close friends Abdallah Daar and James G. Wright have served as constant sounding boards. But his greatest thanks and love go to his family. His children – David, Erin, and Rebecca – provide a very special motivation. His wife, Heather, was a constant companion, steadfast support, and great friend.

Introduction

A. M. Viens and Peter A. Singer

You probably faced a clinical issue today with an ethical component. Did you recognize it? Did you know how to address it? Did you have an organized framework? Did you know what to say to the patient and their family? Did you know what to do? Did you feel comfortable and confident in this aspect of your clinical practice? This book seeks to address how greater recognition of ethical issues and their resolution can improve patient care, research practices, and institutional arrangements.

What is bioethics?

Bioethics, while a modern term, is as old as medicine itself. The Code of Hammurabi and the Hippocratic Oath, for instance, include provisions concerning the importance of ethical considerations to clinical practice. In addition to its initial focus on ethical issues relevant to clinical care, bioethics concerns the moral, legal, political, and social issues raised by medicine, biomedical research, and life sciences technologies.

While bioethical considerations will remain a central aspect of medicine, it can do so at different levels. One can distinguish between three broad spheres of bioethics. The first is academic bioethics, a sphere primarily focused on how theoretical and practical aspects of medicine affect considerations such as special obligations or responsibilities of clinicians, what is valuable, good, right, etc. in the biomedical context and how one might go about

providing systematic accounts of such considerations. The second is public policy and law bioethics, where concerns lies in how legal and extra-legal institutions can and should be involved in the regulation of clinical and research practices. The final sphere is clinical ethics, and its focus is directly related to how the incorporation of bioethics into clinical practice can help to improve patient care. Indeed, as a multidisciplinary field, these spheres are often interconnected, and scholars and clinicians can work across multiple spheres. This book seeks to incorporate the best of all three spheres, with primary attention paid to clinical ethics.

Audience of the book

This book has been written with practicing clinicians (e.g., physicians, surgeons, nurses, dentists, physical/occupational/respiratory therapists, etc.) and allied health professionals (e.g., social workers, bioethicists, healthcare managers/executives, etc.) in mind, but it can also be invaluable to educators teaching bioethics in medical schools, residency programs, and continuing medical education programs. Additionally, this book will also be relevant for researchers and students in non-clinical disciplines interested in bioethics (e.g., philosophy, law, religious studies, health policy, public health, health administration/management, etc.) as illustrative of how the recognition and management of ethical issues at the clinical interface relates to theoretical considerations and organizational structures. As such, we also expect that the book will serve as a textbook for courses in bioethics. Finally, since bioethics has moved very much to the public arena, we also anticipate that the book will be of interest to patients and the public. Its case-based approach makes it particularly accessible.

Aims of the book

Firstly, the book is meant to be *practical*. In particular, the practical aims of the book are *pedagogical* and *clinical*. The goal is to support performance (i.e., what clinicians actually do) by helping to develop awareness and skills in the analysis of normative considerations that affect clinical and research practices. All of the chapters provide guidance on applying bioethical concepts in daily practice and serve to show how the integration of such bioethical knowledge into clinical practice facilitates the ability to make well-reasoned and defensible decisions. Almost 30 years ago, Mark Siegler (1978; cf. Siegler *et al.*, 1990) emphasized that the goal of teaching bioethics is to improve the quality of patient care by identifying, analyzing, and attempting to resolve the ethical problems that arise in the practice of clinical medicine. Today, virtually all medical schools incorporate bioethics into their curricula and most regulatory authorities require the teaching of bioethics as a condition of accrediting residency programs. Clinicians desire and actively seek help with how to deal with ethical issues in clinical practice. For instance, the British Medical Association (BMA) receives several thousand enquiries about ethical issues from clinicians – indeed, in just one week, the BMA's online ethics guidance was accessed by more than 1400 visitors (BBC, 2003).

Secondly, the book is meant to be *versatile*. Each chapter provides a focused and detailed examination of bioethical issues, which can be read sequentially, used as a reference when particular problems arise, and used as a set text in group teaching or open learning environments. While some readers will want to read all of the chapters, the book is structured in thematic sections that provide an easy and accessible way of concentrating on how ethical issues surrounding a particular topic are connected. Professional performance with respect to bioethical matters depends on many factors, including the clinician's values, beliefs, knowledge of ethical and legal constructs, ability to recognize and analyze ethical problems, and interpersonal and communications skills. Although this book cannot address every aspect of bioethics in medical practice, the contributors hope that it will provide a helpful starting point for clinicians, and its versatility will also serve to complement educational and training initiatives. In many cases, the relevant chapter will be all a busy clinician needs to read for help in dealing with an ethical issue faced in patient care.

Thirdly, the book is meant to be *comprehensive*. The book is comprehensive in terms of the *breadth and substance* of the over 60 chapters that are organized under 10 key sections presenting the most vital topics and clinically relevant areas in bioethics: (I) Information problems, (II) End of life-care, (III) Pregnant women and children, (IV) Genetics and biotechnology, (V) Research ethics, (VI) Health systems and institutions, (VII) Using clinical ethics to make an impact on healthcare, (VIII) Global health bioethics, (IX) Religious and cultural perspectives in bioethics, and (X) Specialty bioethics. The book is also comprehensive in terms of its *interdisciplinarity*. Chapter contributors have trained and practiced in a wide spectrum of clinical specialities and academic disciplines (e.g., medicine, surgery, pharmacy, physical medicine, law, philosophy, theology). This interdisciplinary approach will help to ensure that concepts are described faithfully with respect to their empirical context in medicine and with an understanding of their theoretic roots in ethics and law. Finally, it is comprehensive in terms of its *internationalism*; in virtue of both having expert contributors from a number of different countries (e.g., Australia, Canada, China, Israel, Oman, South Africa, Syria, UK, and USA) and ensuring that the material is internationally applicable. Clinicians become involved in healthcare choices as facilitators of the patient's decision-making process. As such, they need an awareness of the cultural and religious background that may influence their view of the patient's situation, as well as familiarity with religious and culturally based values different from their own. Although understanding and accommodating the unique cultural and religious views of patients – especially in relation to the ethical aspects of practice – is a critical determinant of quality of care, guidance for clinicians on how to do so is not easy to locate in the medical literature.

Structure of the book

Each chapter begins with one or more clinical cases highlighting the issue under discussion and ends with suggested approaches to these cases. The cases reflect the authors' experience and are not intended to refer to any particular patient. We have included clincial cases as a way of presenting ethical dilemmas within a specific, plausible context and providing a means of contextualizing the relevant ethical issues in terms of how they related to clinical practice (also cf. Kimball, 1995; Davis, 1999). These cases illustrate that bioethics is not an esoteric pursuit removed from the exigencies of everyday practice; rather, bioethics is in the background of every encounter between clinicians, researchers, administrators, patients, and their families. All clinicians understand why the chapters begin and end with cases – cases are how we learn medicine. As the great Canadian physician Sir William Osler (1906) said: " . . . the student begins with the patient, continues with the patient, and ends his studies with the patient, using books and lectures as tools, as means to an end."

Each chapter aims to answer three basic questions about the bioethical issue at hand. Firstly, *what is it?* – i.e., how the concept/issue so defined is to be understood in the context to be discussed and why it has relevance to clinical practice. Secondly, *why is it important?* – i.e., how the concept/issue has clinical relevance from the perspectives of ethics, law, policy, and empirical studies. Thirdly, *how should it be approached in practice?* – i.e., how

the concept/issue under consideration is applied and/or can be used in clinical practice to improve patient care. The chapter concludes by discussing the resolution of the case(s) introduced at the beginning of the chapter.

The book is based on the very popular 28-part series, *Bioethics for Clinicians*, published in the *Canadian Medical Association Journal* between 1996 and 2002 and edited by Peter A. Singer. These frequently downloaded articles have been used by clinicians throughout the world and have been translated into several languages. This collection, however, provides a far more comprehensive and up-to-date resource, but with the same spirit of improving clinical practice. Therefore, our goal in writing this book is to provide clinicians with the knowledge and tools they need to provide better care to patients and research subjects.

Bioethical methodologies and our approach

There are a number of different bioethical methodologies that have been advanced for the incorporation of bioethics into clinical practice. Broadly speaking, there are four such approaches (Agich, 2005).

The first is practical or applied ethics, or even an applied philosophy of medicine. This approach addresses ethical issues that arise in practice through the application of aspects of particular ethical theories, or specific notions/concepts (e.g., double effect, treatment versus enhancement distinction, etc.), to concrete clinical or research cases. The focus is not on providing a decision procedure for how to solve ethical issues but to provide theoretical framework concerning, for instance, what considerations would make an action good or a policy right. For more on this approach, see Caplan (1983), Beauchamp (1984), and Young (1986).

The second is principlism. This approach seeks to provide ethical guidance in clinical practice through a specified number of moral principles. By applying general principles to ethical problems, it is argued that such principles do a better job of obtaining the right answer concerning what one morally ought to do compared to trying to reason through what to do in each instance. The most famous versions of bioethical principlism are articulated by Beauchamp and Childress (2001), with the principles of autonomy, beneficence, non-malfeasance, and justice, or, for instance, some catholic healthcare institutions, which adopt a theologically based form of principlism. While principlism has been notably criticized for being too blunt an instrument in trying to apply a few ethical principles to all problems in all circumstances, and thus being too insensitive to the complexities and tensions inherent in morality, some forms of this approach are more multifaceted and responsive to the intricacies of moral considerations related to medicine. For more on this approach, see Clouser and Gert (1990), Daniels (1996), Richardson (2000), and Beauchamp and Childress (2001).

The third is casuistry. This case-based approach addresses ethical problems by guiding clinicians through specific issues via paradigm cases that have come up in clinical education or practice – something analogous to the use of case-based reasoning in the process of differential diagnosis. As opposed to theory-laden or top-down approaches, which apply general frameworks or concepts to particular issues when they arise, casuistry provides a bottom-up approach where clinicians use case-based reasoning to identify the morally relevant features of a situation and relate it to the specific circumstances of a previous case and its resolution. Given the prominent use of cases in clinical practice (e.g., case reports in journals, case conferences and rounds, etc.), clinicians may find this approach an appealing way to deal with ethical problems (for some of the reasons we have highlighted in the previous section). However, as a standalone bioethical methodology, the approach has been criticized for not providing a clear method for working through ethical issues. For more on this approach, see Jonsen (1991), Kopelman (1994), and Jonsen and Toulmin (1998).

The fourth is combination of techniques for identifying and resolving ethical conflicts, disagreements, and related problems. This approach treats the ethical issues that arise in clinical practice as those similar to inter-personal issues alleviated through techniques such as conflict resolution, mediation, negotiation, and arbitration. This approach has been criticized by some on the basis that, in treating ethical issues as just another set of considerations that can cause disagreement, it fails to adequately address the source of moral conflict or why we have good reasons to act one way as opposed to another in favor of securing consensus amongst participants. Admittedly, compromise plays an important role in clinical practice; however, achieving agreement for its own sake fails to appreciate sufficiently what is distinctive about moral considerations and how greater attention to resolving ethical issues can improve clinical practice. For more on this approach, see West and Gibson (1992), Dubler and Marcus (1994), and Reynolds (1994).

We believe none of these methodologies gets everything right. Since the aim of the book is not to argue for which methodology, or combinations of methodologies, is correct, we recommend that clinicians will most benefit from borrowing the best of each methodology in an effort to better recognize and resolve ethical issues in practice. Each chapter in this book contains elements of all these approaches. The chapters start and end with clinical cases, and this most resembles casuistry. In the section on why a particular topic is important, the ethics subsection will often emphasize principles and often expands this into a practical ethics approach. However, we recognize that the sources of knowledge and frameworks required by clinicians are not limited to ethics, so the chapters also review and apply relevant legal and policy frameworks to the topic. Moreover, empirical research also helps to illuminate how clinicians can effectively approach a clinical ethics problem, so we include a section on empirical studies too. The section on how a clinician should approach a particular problem in practice emphasizes the techniques and tools a clinician can use to resolve the particular ethical challenge. Therefore, the methodology in this book can be described as a "mixed methodology" that is focused on the goal of optimally supporting clinicians in identifying and attempting to resolve ethical problems they face in actual clinical practice.

Coda: a personal reflection

One of us (PAS) has been working in the field of bioethics for almost 30 years, a pathway initiated in the following way. I finally decided to make a career of bioethics when many years ago as an intern I was caring for a young woman with disseminated cancer. She also happened to have a low phosphorus level in her blood. I realized that I could rattle off 20 causes of low phosphorus, but when it came to whether or not we were going to resuscitate this young woman when her heart stopped, we wrote that order in pencil on the nurses' notes and rubbed it out afterwards. I thought at the time that, even if the scientific problem of low phosphorus and the bioethical issue of end of life care were equally important, the rigor with which we approached the bioethical issue was disproportionately low. In caring for many patients, I also realized that there is no "one size fits all" framework for approaching clinical problems. Clinicians have a heuristic for approaching abdominal pain and another for approaching chest pain. That is why we do not offer a single set of principles, or a decision-making rubric, to address all clinical problems. Context matters in medicine. These clinical insights and experiences have shaped a framework to approaching bioethics problems that over the years has evolved into this book.

The approach herein has also been shaped by working with my colleagues Mark Siegler and Edmund Pellegrino on a review of bioethics every 10 years. The writings of Mark and Ed are the best of class and have stood the test of time in relation to emphasizing a clinically based approach to bioethics, and how bioethics is at the moral center of the clinician's work. As Mark used to emphasize, the bull looks different from the stands than it does from the bullring. Another close colleague and mentor, the late Alvan R. Feinstein, emphasized this very same theme in another field – clinical epidemiology – although he was also deeply interested in the "softer" side of medicine and humanistic care. For Mark, and Ed, and Alvan, the clinical experience is everything, and they are right. This insight is infused throughout this book.

In closing, every clinician knows why bioethics is important. What is often missing is how best to approach bioethics problems in a practical way. Although a textbook can only take us so far, and dialogue, role modeling, experience, attitude, and character take us the rest of the way, we have tried herein to provide an effective textbook platform for improvements in patient care related to bioethics. If, in the course of caring for patients, you consult one of these chapters, and your care and the patient's experience is improved as a result, we have reached our true objective in writing this book.

REFERENCES

Agich, G. J. (2005). What kind of doing is clinical ethics? *Theor Med* **26**: 7–24.

Beauchamp, T. L. (1984). On eliminating the distinction between applied ethics and ethical theory. *Monist* **67**: 514–31.

Beauchamp, T. L. and Childress, J. F. (2001). *The Principles of Biomedical Ethics*, 5th edn, Oxford: Oxford University Press.

BBC (2003). Doctors make medical ethics plea. *BBC News* 2 December (http://news.bbc.co.uk/1/hi/health/3253786.stm) accessed 1 November 2006.

Caplan, A. L. (1983). Can applied ethics be effective in healthcare and should it strive to be? *Ethics* **93**: 311–19.

Clouser, K. D. and Gert, B. (1990). A critique of principlism. *J Med Philos* **15**: 219–36.

Daniels, N. (1996). *Justice and Justification: Reflective Equilibrium in Theory and Practice*. Cambridge: Cambridge University Press.

Davis, M. (1999). Case method. In *Ethics and the University*. London: Routledge, pp. 143–74.

Dubler, N. N. and Marcus, L. J. (1994). *Mediating Bioethics Disputes: A Practical Guide*. New York: United Hospital Fund of New York.

Jonsen, A. R. (1991). Casuistry as methodology in clinical ethics. *Theor Med* **12**: 295–307.

Jonsen, A. R. and Toulmin, S. (1998). *The Abuse of Casuistry: A History of Moral Reasoning*. Berkeley, CA: University of California Press.

Kimball, B. A. (1995). *The Emergence of Case Method Teaching, 1872–1990s: A Search for Legitimate Pedagogy*. Bloomington, IN: The Poynter Center for the Study of Ethics and American Institutions at Indiana University.

Kopelman, L. M. (1994). Case method and casuistry: the problem of bias. *Theor Med* **15**: 21–37.

Osler, W. (1906). The hospital as a college. In *Aequanimitas, With Other Addresses to Medical Students, Nurses and Practitioners of Medicine*. Philadelphia, PA: P. Blakiston, pp. 327–42.

Reynolds, D. F. (1994). Consultectonics: ethics committee case consultation as mediation. *Bioethics Forum* 10, **4**: 54–60.

Richardson, H. S. (2000). Specifying, balancing and interpreting bioethical principles. *J Med Philos* **25**: 285–307.

Siegler, M. (1978). A legacy of Osler: teaching clinical ethics at the bedside. *JAMA* **239**: 951–6.

Siegler, M., Pellegrino, E. D., and Singer, P. A. (1990). Clinical medical ethics. *J Clin Ethics* **1**: 5–9.

West, M. B. and Gibson, J. M. (1992). Facilitating medical ethics case review: what ethics committees can learn from mediation and facilitation techniques. *Camb Q Healthc Ethics* **1**: 63–74.

Young, J. O. (1986). The immortality of applied ethics. *The Int J App Ethics* **3**: 37–43.

SECTION I

Information problems

Introduction

Anne Slowther

Clinicians have many different roles in the provision of healthcare, including individual patient care, public health delivery, health services management, and policy development. Each of these roles involves complex decisions and interactions that require ethical reflection. However, for the majority of clinicians, those who provide day-to-day care in hospitals, clinics, and patients' homes, it is the relationship with individual patients that forms the professional and ethical core of their work. It is this relationship that initially attracted attention from ethicists as the field of clinical ethics developed, and which has been the main focus of regulatory guidance from professional organizations. This section focuses on three key concepts that define this relationship, namely consent, confidentiality, and truth telling.

A common thread that runs through these three aspects of the patient–clinician relationship is the importance and use of information. Patients provide information to their clinicians about their symptoms, their concerns, and their expectations of what the clinician can do to help them. Clinicians take this information, and then seek further information to develop a differential diagnosis of the patient's problem, select appropriate investigations, and identify possible treatments or management plans. Clinicians provide information to their patients about diagnoses, investigations, treatment options, progress, and outcomes. The therapeutic relationship is thus founded on sharing of information. The way in which information is used by both patient and clinician within this relationship is explored in the following chapters.

The first four chapters in this section describe in detail the concept of consent, which forms the cornerstone of clinical practice. Chapter 2 provides an overview of consent, relating it to the underlying ethical principle of respect for autonomy and pointing out that consent is not simply about acceptance of a suggested treatment but about choice between a range of options, including the option of refusing treatment. The three elements of a valid consent, capacity, information, and voluntariness, are each addressed in the subsequent chapters. Chalmers in Ch. 3 describes the ethical and legal importance of capacity as the key to determining the clinician's approach to treatment decisions. Determination of capacity is not always straightforward and this chapter leads the reader through some of the difficulties and idiosyncrasies in this process. Strategies for optimizing capacity in the clinical setting are suggested and two approaches to formal assessment are described. A key component of these assessments includes the provision of relevant information to ascertain whether the patient is able to understand and evaluate the information necessary to make a treatment decision. The importance of disclosure and the legal requirements governing its provision are discussed by d'Agincourt-Canning and Johnston in Ch. 4. They document the change in standards relating to the degree of information required that has taken place in since the 1980s, reflecting an increasing emphasis on individual patient autonomy within both the healthcare and legal systems. However, access to relevant and comprehensive information is not sufficient for a patient to make an autonomous decision about his or her healthcare. Freedom to make a specific choice is also required. The concept of voluntariness and what this means in the context of a patient's relationship with both an individual clinician and the wider healthcare system is considered by Dykeman and Dewhirst in Ch. 5.

The ethical requirement to provide patients with information is not restricted to situations where consent to treatment is necessary. Patients have a right to know what is wrong with them, and keeping such information from them demonstrates a lack of respect, as well as potentially causing them harm. But bad news can cause distress and some patients may not want to hear it. So can it ever be ethically justified to withhold information from a patient, or even to lie to them? Chapter 6 explores the nature of truth telling in the patient–clinician relationship and its correlation with respect for persons and maintenance of trust. The authors emphasize the importance of communication skills in sharing information with patients. It is not only *what* information is provided but *how* it is provided that is crucial to good clinical practice. In the final chapter in this section, Ch. 7, we move from concerns about sharing information with patients to the issue of sharing information about patients with others. Slowther and Kleinman discuss the concept of confidentiality in the increasingly complex field of healthcare, acknowledging new and diverse challenges including the increased use of electronic information systems and the impact of genetic technology.

The chapters in this section summarize specific aspects of information sharing within the patient–clinician relationship, providing an overview of the legal and ethical principles involved. The ethical concepts of respect for persons, individual autonomy, and trust, considered here in the context of individual clinical care, are threads that run through all aspects of information sharing in healthcare. Consequently, the discussions in this section will be of wider relevance to clinicians as they reflect on the ethical issues that they face in their professional practice.

2

Consent

John R. Williams

Mrs. A is an 85-year-old woman living at home with her husband, who has moderately severe Alzheimer disease and for whom she provides daily care. She has an 8.5 cm abdominal aortic aneurysm. Three months ago she consulted a vascular surgeon, who recommended surgical repair of her aneurysm. However, another physician told Mrs. A that she "would never survive the operation." Mrs. A decided to "take her chances" and refused surgery, primarily because of her wish to provide uninterrupted care for her husband; however, she agreed to discuss the decision further with the surgeon at a future visit. Before such a visit can take place, however, Mrs. A is taken to the emergency department after collapsing at home with abdominal pain. Physical examination reveals a systolic blood pressure of 50 mmHg and a tender pulsatile abdominal mass. Mrs. A is moaning and barely conscious. The surgeon diagnoses a ruptured aortic aneurysm and believes that Mrs. A will die without emergency surgery.

Mr. B is a 25-year-old man affected by extensive muscular atrophy resulting from Guillain–Barré syndrome. For two years he has been dependent on a ventilator and his prognosis indicates no chance of recovery. One day he announces that he wants the ventilator support withdrawn and that he be allowed to die because he considers his life intolerable. Those caring for him disagree with his decision and the reasons for it because he is not terminally ill and because others with his condition have meaningful and fulfilling lives. Their arguments do not convince Mr. B and he demands that the ventilator be withdrawn.

What is consent?

Consent can be defined as the "autonomous authorization of a medical intervention ... by individual patients" (Beauchamp and Faden, 2004, p. 1279). There is a widespread consensus in both ethics and law that patients have the right to make decisions about their medical care and to be given all available information relevant to such decisions. Obtaining consent is not a discrete event; rather, it is a process that should occur throughout the relationship between clinician and patient (Arnold and Lidz, 2004). Although the term "consent" implies acceptance of a suggested treatment, the concept of consent applies also to choice among alternative treatments and to refusal of treatment.

Consent has three components: disclosure, capacity, and voluntariness. Disclosure refers to the communication of relevant information by the clinician and its comprehension by the patient. Capacity refers to the patient's ability to understand the information and to appreciate those consequences of his or her decision that might reasonably be foreseen. Voluntariness refers to the patient's right to come to a decision freely, without force, coercion, or manipulation.

Consent may be explicit or implied. Explicit consent can be given orally or in writing. Consent is implied when the patient indicates a willingness to

An earlier version of this chapter has appeared: Etchells, E., Sharpe, G., Walsh, P., Williams, J. R. and Singer, P. A. (1996). Consent. *CMAJ* **155**: 177–80.

undergo a certain procedure or treatment by his or her behavior. For example, consent for venipuncture is implied by the action of rolling up one's sleeve and presenting one's arm. For treatments that entail risk or involve more than mild discomfort, it is preferable to obtain explicit rather than implied consent.

A signed consent form documents but does not replace the consent process. There are no universal rules as to when a signed consent form is required. Some hospitals may require that patients sign a consent form for surgical procedures but not for other equally risky interventions. If a signed consent form is not required, and the treatment carries risk, clinicians should write a note in the patient's chart to document that consent has been given.

This chapter will discuss the concept of patient consent and exceptions to the requirement to obtain consent. Subsequent chapters will provide detailed discussions of disclosure, capacity, voluntariness, and truth telling, as well as consent for incapable patients, requirements for consent to participation in medical research, and involving children in medical decisions.

Why is consent important?

Ethics

The notion of consent is grounded in the fundamental ethical principles of patient autonomy and respect for persons. Autonomy refers to the patient's right to make free decisions about his or her healthcare. Respect for persons requires that healthcare professionals foster patients' control over their own lives and refrain from carrying out unwanted interventions.

Fully informed consent is an ethical ideal that is seldom realized in practice. Obstacles include diagnostic uncertainty, the complexity of medical information, linguistic and cultural differences between clinicians and patients, overworked medical personnel, and psychological barriers to rational decision making. However, given the fundamental importance of patient autonomy and

respect for persons, clinicians have an ethical obligation to seek the highest degree of informed consent that can be reasonably achieved in the specific situation.

There are two exceptions to the requirement for informed consent by competent patients.

- Situations where patients voluntarily waive or give over their decision-making authority to the clinician or to a third party. Because of the complexity of the matter or because the patient has complete confidence in the clinician's judgement, the patient may tell the clinician, "Do what you think is best." Clinicians should not be eager to act on such requests but should provide patients with basic information about the treatment options and encourage them to make their own decisions. However, if after such encouragement the patient still wants the clinician to decide, the clinician should do so according to the best interests of the patient.

- Instances where the disclosure of information would cause harm to the patient. The traditional concept of "therapeutic privilege" is invoked in such cases; it allows clinicians to withhold medical information if disclosure would be likely to result in serious physical, psychological, or emotional harm to the patient, for example, if the patient would be likely to commit suicide if the diagnosis indicates a terminal illness. This privilege is open to great abuse, and clinicians should make use of it only in extreme circumstances. They should start with the expectation that all patients are able to cope with the facts and reserve non-disclosure for cases in which they are convinced that more harm will result from telling the truth than from not telling it.

Law

In many jurisdictions, obtaining the patient's consent to medical care is a legal requirement. Under UK common law, treating a patient without his or her consent constitutes battery, whereas treating a patient on the basis of inadequately informed consent constitutes negligence. The Council of Europe's (1997) *Convention on Human Rights and Biomedicine* states:

An intervention in the health field may only be carried out after the person concerned has given free and informed consent to it. This person shall beforehand be given appropriate information as to the purpose and nature of the intervention as well as on its consequences and risks. The person concerned may freely withdraw consent at any time.

In most jurisdictions, law recognizes that the emergency treatment of incapable persons is an exception to the requirement for consent. An emergency exists when immediate treatment is required in order to save the life or preserve the health of the patient. The rationale for this exception is that a reasonable person would consent to the treatment and that a delay in treatment would lead to death or serious harm.

The emergency exception to the requirement to obtain consent has important limitations. Clinicians should not administer emergency treatment without consent if they have reason to believe that the patient would refuse such treatment if he or she were capable. A signed and dated advance directive ("living will") can provide evidence of such a decision.

A patient's incapacity does not necessarily exempt the clinician from the requirement to obtain consent. In some jurisdictions, if a patient is mentally incapable of making medical decisions, the clinician must obtain consent from a substitute decision maker.

Some jurisdictions permit non-consensual treatment in specific circumstances, such as the involuntary admission of psychiatric patients and the treatment of irresponsible patients with communicable disease. Non-consensual treatment will be discussed in the chapter on voluntariness.

There are other potential legal exceptions to the requirement to obtain consent. As noted above, "therapeutic privilege" refers to the physician's withholding of certain information in the consent process in the belief that disclosure of this information would harm or cause suffering to the patient; however, the scope of therapeutic privilege has become smaller over the years in many jurisdictions. "Waiver" refers to a patient's voluntary request to forgo one or more elements of disclosure.

Policy

The requirement to obtain patient consent is affirmed by most international and national health professional organizations. For example, the World Medical Association's (2005) *Declaration on the Rights of the Patient* states:

The patient has the right to self-determination, to make free decisions regarding himself/herself. The physician will inform the patient of the consequences of his/her decisions. A mentally competent adult patient has the right to give or withhold consent to any diagnostic procedure or therapy. The patient has the right to the information necessary to make his/her decisions. The patient should understand clearly what is the purpose of any test or treatment, what the results would imply, and what would be the implications of withholding consent.

In the UK, both the General Medical Council (1998) and the British Medical Association (2003) have issued guidance documents on consent, and the codes of ethics of most, if not all, national medical associations contain provisions on consent.

Empirical studies

Several meta-analyses and reviews have suggested that the process of obtaining consent can be an important component of a successful physician–patient relationship. One review (Stewart, 1995) found that effective physician–patient communication improved emotional health, symptom resolution, level of function, results of physiological measures, and pain control. A review of informed consent in psychotherapy concluded that its benefits include fostering a positive treatment outcome through enhancing patient autonomy, responsibility, and self-therapeutic activity; lessening the risks of regressive effects and therapist liability; and helping the practice of psychotherapy extend beyond particular parochialisms by providing checks and balances on therapist judgements (Beahrs and Gutheil, 2001). A meta-analysis by Suls and Wan (1989) showed that providing information about what the patient would feel and what would be done in the course of stressful and painful medical procedures consistently reduced negative feelings, pain, and distress. Another demonstrated that information giving by physicians was associated with small to moderate increases in patient satisfaction and compliance with treatment (Hall *et al.*, 1988).

Other empirical studies have shown that many, but by no means all, patients expect the physician to assume the role of problem solver rather than decision maker (Siminoff and Fetting, 1991; Deber, 1994; Janz *et al.*, 2004; Mazur *et al.*, 2005). Problem solving involves identifying the patient's presenting problem and developing a list of treatment options. Numerous studies have shown that patients' desire for decision-making responsibility, which involves choosing from the treatment options, is variable (Ende *et al.*, 1989; Larsson *et al.*, 1990; Lerman *et al.*, 1990; Mark and Spiro, 1990; Waterworth and Luker, 1990; Cohen and Britten, 2003; Ford *et al.*, 2003; Hagerty *et al.*, 2004). Even patients who actively seek information do not necessarily wish to make the decision about which treatment option to follow. Some, particularly those who are elderly or acutely ill, are predisposed to follow the physician's recommendation (Emanuel and Emanuel, 1992; Pinquart and Duberstein, 2004; Levinson *et al.*, 2005).

How should I approach consent in practice?

Obtaining valid consent requires that patients participate in problem solving as much as they wish. Patients should be free to ask questions and receive answers about treatment options not discussed by the clinician. The consent process also

requires that patients actively participate in decision making and authorize the decision. Even if the patient is predisposed to follow the clinician's recommendation, the clinician should actively engage the patient in the consent process.

Ethical and legal exceptions to the requirement to obtain consent for medical interventions are noted above. There may also be cultural differences in how this requirement is understood. In some cultures, it is widely held that the physician's obligation to provide information to the patient does not apply when the diagnosis is a terminal illness. It is felt that such information would cause the patient to despair and would make the remaining days of life much more miserable than if there were hope of recovery. Throughout the world, it is not uncommon for family members of patients to plead with physicians not to tell the patients that they are dying. Physicians do have to be sensitive to cultural, as well as personal, factors when communicating bad news, especially of impending death. Nevertheless, the patient's right to consent is becoming increasingly widely accepted, and the physician has a primary duty to help patients to exercise this right.

The principle of informed consent incorporates the patient's right to choose from among the options presented by the physician. To what extent patients have a right to services not recommended by physicians is becoming a major topic of controversy in ethics, law, and professional policy. Until this matter is decided by governments, medical insurance providers, and/or professional organizations, individual physicians will have to decide for themselves whether they should agree to requests for inappropriate treatments.

The cases

Mrs. A's physician must decide whether to perform surgical repair of the aneurysm. Mrs. A is now an incapable person in a medical emergency. In such a circumstance, the surgeon may proceed without the patient's consent unless a clear wish to the contrary has been expressed earlier. Should the surgeon proceed, given that Mrs. A had previously refused elective repair of the aneurysm? Mrs. A's refusal of elective surgery was based on her wish to continue caring for her husband. She would likely want to undergo emergency surgery because it would give her the best chance of continuing to care for her husband. Therefore, the surgeon may proceed without the patient's consent. If Mrs. A had previously considered and refused emergency surgery, the surgeon would not be entitled to proceed.

If Mr. B is competent to make decisions about his medical treatment, his caregivers should respect this decision, even if refusing consent to the continued use of his ventilator will result in his death. In carrying out his wishes, they should provide appropriate palliative care.

REFERENCES

Arnold, R. M. and Lidz, C. W. (2004). Clinical aspects of consent in healthcare. In *Encyclopedia of Bioethics*, 3rd edn, Vol. 3, ed. S. G. Post, New York: Macmillan Reference USA, pp. 1293–5.

Beauchamp, T. L. and Faden, R. R. (2004). Informed consent: II. Meaning and elements of informed consent. In *Encyclopedia of Bioethics*, 3rd edn, Vol. 3, ed. S. G. Post, New York: Macmillan Reference USA, pp. 1277–80.

Beahrs, J. O. and Gutheil, T. G. (2001). Informed consent in psychotherapy. *Am J Psychiatry* **158**: 4–10.

British Medical Association (2003). *Consent Tool Kit*. London: British Medical Association (http://www.bma.org.uk/ap.nsf/Content/consenttk2).

Cohen, H. and Britten, N. (2003). Who decides about prostate cancer treatment? A qualitative study. *Fam Pract* **20**: 724–9.

Council of Europe (1997). *Convention on Human Rights and Biomedicine*. Brussels: Council of Europe (http://conventions.coe.int/Treaty/EN/WhatYouWant.asp?NT=164&CM=7&DF=).

Deber, R. B. (1994). Physicians in health care management: 8. The patient–physician partnership: decision making, problem solving and the desire to participate. *CMAJ* **151**: 423–7.

Emanuel, E. J. and Emanuel, L. L. (1992). Four models of the physician–patient relationship. *JAMA* **267**: 2221–6.

Ende, J., Kazis, L., Ash, A., *et al.* (1989). Measuring patients' desire for autonomy: decision making and information-seeking preferences among medical patients. *J Gen Intern Med* **4**: 23–30.

Ford, S., Schofield, T., and Hope, T. (2003). What are the ingredients for a successful evidence-based patient choice consultation? A qualitative study. *Soc Sci Med* **56**: 589–602.

Hagerty, R. G., Butow, P. N., Ellis, P. A., *et al.* (2004). Cancer patient preferences for communication of prognosis in the metastatic setting. *J Clin Oncol* **22**: 1721–30.

Hall, J. A., Roter, D. L., and Katz, N. R. (1988). Meta-analysis of correlates of provider behavior in medical encounters. *Med Care* **26**: 657–75.

Janz, N. K., Wren, P. A., Copeland, L. A., *et al.* (2004). Patient–physician concordance: preferences, perceptions, and factors influencing the breast cancer surgical decision. *J Clin Oncol* **22**: 3091–8.

Larsson, U. S., Svardsudd, K., Wedel, H., *et al.* (1990). Patient involvement in decision-making in surgical and orthopaedic practice: the Project Perioperative Risk. *Soc Sci Med* **28**: 829–35.

Lerman, C. E., Brody, D. S., Caputo, G. C., *et al.* (1990). Patients' perceived involvement in care scale: relationship to attitudes about illness and medical care. *J Gen Intern Med* **5**: 29–33.

Levinson, W., Kao, A., Kuby, A., *et al.* (2005). Not all patients want to participate in decision making. A national study of public preferences. *J Gen Intern Med* **20**: 531–5.

Mark, J. S. and Spiro, H. (1990). Informed consent for colonoscopy. *Arch Intern Med* **150**: 777–80.

Mazur, D. J., Hickam, D. H., Mazur, M. D., *et al.* (2005). The role of doctor's opinion in shared decision making: what does shared decision making really mean when considering invasive medical procedures? *Health Expect* **8**: 97–102.

Pinquart, M. and Duberstein, P. R. (2004). Information needs and decision-making processes in older cancer patients. *Crit Rev Oncol Hematol* **51**: 69–80.

Siminoff, L. A. and Fetting, J. H. (1991). Factors affecting treatment decisions for a life-threatening illness: the case of medical treatment of breast cancer. *Soc Sci Med* **32**: 813–18.

Stewart, M. A. (1995). Effective physician–patient communication and health outcomes: a review. *CMAJ* **152**: 1423–33.

Suls, J. and Wan, C. K. (1989). Effects of sensory and procedural information on coping with stressful medical procedures and pain: a meta analysis. *J Consult Clin Psychol* **57**: 372–9.

UK General Medical Council (1998). *Seeking Patients' Consent: The Ethical Considerations*. London: General Medical Council.

Waterworth, S. and Luker, K. A. (1990). Reluctant collaborators: do patients want to be involved in decisions concerning care? *J Adv Nurs* **15**: 971–6.

World Medical Association (2005). *Declaration of Lisbon on the Rights of the Patient*. Ferney-Voltaire, France: World Medical Association (www.wma.net/e/policy/l4.htm).

3

Capacity

Julie Chalmers

Ms. C is a 22-year-old woman with unstable insulin-dependent diabetes who has suffered an intrauterine death at 36 weeks of gestation. She is refusing medical induction of labor, which has been recommended to avoid the risk of potentially life-threatening sepsis. She insists that the birth must be "natural" and becomes extremely distressed when attempts are made to discuss this further. In the past, she has had repeated admissions to hospital as a result of poor diabetic control and, consequently, is well known to staff. Although the current clinical state is stable, the medical team have become extremely anxious about the possible consequences of her refusal of treatment and they have requested an assessment of capacity. Ms. C refuses to discuss her decision and turns her back to the interviewer. A further attempt to discuss this is met with a similar response.

What is capacity?

Capacity is a complex construct that refers to the presence of a particular set of "functional abilities" that a person needs to possess in order to make a specific decision (Grisso and Applebaum, 1998). These abilities include being able to understand the relevant information needed to make the decision and to appreciate the relatively foreseeable consequences of the various options available. In the medical setting, the key decision to be made is whether to give or withhold consent to investigation or treatment.

The term "competence" is often used, sometimes interchangeably with capacity. These are equivalent terms and their use depends on the context in which the issue is discussed. In the UK, capacity is used in the legal context and the term competence in medical settings. In other countries, this may be reversed. In this chapter, the term capacity will be preferred.

Why is capacity important?

Ethics

The possession of capacity has been described as the "gateway" to the exercise of autonomy (Gunn, 1994). Autonomy, literally meaning self-rule, has been defined as the capacity to think, decide, and act on the basis of such thought and decision, freely and independently (Gillon, 1986).

On occasions, a patient may express an autonomous choice to refuse treatment that the doctor thinks is essential. In such situations, there will be a tension between respect for the patient's autonomy and the beneficence arising from the medical intervention. In Western society, the liberal tradition emphasizes the importance of liberty and freedom for the individual and, in particular, freedom from the interference of others (Hope *et al.*, 2003). Based on this tradition, the exercise of autonomy will trump beneficence.

An earlier version of this chapter has appeared: Etchells, E., Sharpe, G., Elliott, C., and Singer, P. A. (1996). Capacity. *CMAJ* **155**: 657–61.

Law

The presence of decision-making capacity is an essential, although not sufficient, element of valid consent. The law relating to consent is founded upon the patient's autonomy and there are clear legal consequences if the clinician acts in its absence.

This was clearly articulated in the well-known statement by Judge Cardozo in *Schloendorff* v. *Society of New York Hospitals* (1914): "Every adult person of sound mind has a right to determine what shall be done with his own body; and a surgeon who performs an operation without his patient's consent commits an assault, for which he is liable in damages."

Most jurisdictions approach capacity from the starting point that all adults have the capacity to make their own decisions. The legal position with regard to children is more complicated. Whether or not they may be presumed to have capacity, and the approach to assessment, will depend on the particular jurisdiction in which the clinician practices.

The law has also acknowledged that the threshold for a finding of capacity may vary. A senior English judge, Lord Donaldson, stated this very simply when he said: "The more serious the decision, the greater the capacity required" (*Re T* [*Adult Refusal of Treatment*], 1992).

As identified by Roth *et al.* (1977) the threshold may also depend on whether the patient is consenting or refusing treatment. For example, a high-benefit/low-risk procedure will require a lower threshold for consent and a higher one for refusal. If the benefit is low and risks high, then there will be a high threshold for consent and a low one for refusal. Thresholds may also differ as different judicial standards may be applied to the same fact situation (Grisso and Applebaum, 1995a).

This ambiguity in where the threshold is set is problematical but, as has been observed, this "is inevitable as individuals and societies hold different views about the balance between the respect for autonomy and the protection of vulnerable people from harm" (Wong *et al.*, 1999, p. 439).

Identifying a lack of decision-making capacity is also legally important, as treatment will then need to be given under a different legal framework – or under the framework of substitute decision making (see Ch. 9 for more information). Incapacity often fails to be identified in day-to-day practice, particularly when the patient passively accepts the treatment offered (Raymont *et al.*, 2004).

Depending on jurisdiction, treatment of the incapacitated person may require clinicians to act in the person's best interests, follow a valid and applicable advance directive, or call upon substitute decision makers.

Policy

Capacity, as one of the cornerstones of valid consent, is considered in policies concerning consent to medical treatment. The functional approach to capacity assessment is widely accepted, although other details regarding the consent process may differ depending on jurisdiction.

Such policies have been produced by central and local government and by the professional bodies that regulate and guide medical practice. Hospitals will also have a local policy, which should reflect national guidance, and all clinicians must ensure that they are familiar with those policies that apply to their place of work and area of specialization.

Capacity or, more specifically, lack of capacity is also discussed in policy documents that consider the approach to the treatment of those who lack the capacity to decide for themselves. Again, the approach to capacity assessment contained in such documents is a functional one.

Empirical studies

Studies have suggested that in situations where capacity is questionable general impressions can be misleading (Etchells *et al.*, 1999); therefore, a structured approach to assessment is likely to yield more accurate results.

A number of studies have focused on an examination of the decision-making abilities of people who fall within certain diagnostic groups (Grisso and Applebaum, 1995b; Wong et al., 2000). Grisso and Applebaum (1998, p. 18) have noted that while impairments can be identified it does not invariably follow that decision-making capacity is lost: "A patient may be psychotic, seriously depressed, or in a moderately advance state of dementia, yet still be found competent to make some or all decisions."

Some associations between impaired decision-making capacity and specific symptoms have been identified. For example, cognitive impairment has been shown to be a predictor of incapacity in medical patients (Raymont et al., 2004) and scores of between 0 and 16 on the standardized Mini-Mental State Examination have been found to increase significantly the likelihood of a finding of incapacity (Etchells et al., 1999).

There is evidence to suggest that simple interventions such as breaking up the information into bite-size pieces (Grisso and Applebaum, 1995b) or, for some patients, presenting material visually (Wong et al., 2000) can improve decision-making capacity.

How should I approach capacity in practice?

In routine clinical practice, capacity is not usually considered explicitly until consent is required from a person whose membership of a particular diagnostic group may suggest that their capacity may be impaired, or if a patient refuses a treatment that the clinician strongly endorses.

A decision about the presence or absence of capacity based solely on the membership of a particular group, referred to as a status approach to capacity determination, has been widely rejected (Presidents Commission, 1982; Law Commission, 1995).

Unusual decisions, such as a refusal of treatment, particularly if this will have life-threatening consequences, may lead to the conclusion that capacity is lacking. This has been called an outcomes approach to capacity determination.

For example, in a well-known case that came before the British court, refusal of a caesarean section required to prevent the death of both the pregnant woman and her baby was viewed by the treating clinicians as clear evidence of incapacity. This was rejected by the judge, who found, on applying the legal criteria for capacity, that the woman had the ability to refuse treatment and had based her decision on long-standing views about natural delivery (St George's Healthcare NHS Trust v. S, 1998).

In general, the assessment of capacity that is now broadly endorsed by clinicians (Roth et al., 1977; Grisso and Applebaum, 1998), lawyers (Presidents Commission, 1982; Law Commission, 1995), and ethicists (Buchanan and Brock, 1989) adopts an approach that focuses on the quality of the decision making, often referred to as a functional approach to capacity assessment.

Grisso and Applebaum (1998) have proposed that the abilities needed to make a decision about treatment include the ability to *understand* the information necessary to come to a treatment decision, the ability to *appreciate* the relevance of the information to the person's individual situation, and the ability to process the information in a logical manner (*reasoning*). Finally, the person must be able to *express a choice*.

The nature of appreciation is an area that has given rise to theoretical debate and can give rise to particular difficulty in assessment. Grisso and Applebaum (1998) viewed appreciation as the ability to believe the information and to accept its relevance to the person's situation while others (Charland, 1998) have highlighted the importance of the person's values and emotional responses in understanding this concept.

Problems may arise when the beliefs that are held by the patient are very different from those of the clinician. Some beliefs, although not necessarily shared by the clinician, are, however, legitimized by society, for example certain religious beliefs. However, some alternative lifestyle choices and belief systems can give rise to conflict. In such a situation, it is essential that clinicians be aware of their own views or prejudices and the impact, sometimes subtle, that these may have on the assessment of capacity (Kopelman, 1990). When such a possibility is identified, it may be helpful to discuss the situation with a colleague.

Further difficulties can arise when it is suspected that a patient's beliefs have been influenced by the presence of mental illness. It is relatively straightforward when a person has a symptom of illness, such as a delusion, that clearly impacts on decision making. However, particular difficulties arise when the ideas held by the person fall short of delusions but are nevertheless unusual, for example the distortions in body image that occur in anorexia nervosa. Put simply, the question is as follows: "Is it the person or the illness talking?" These can be exquisitely difficult judgements.

Buchanan and Brock (1989, p. 24) suggest that a necessary element of capacity is that the person must have a "set of values or conception of the good." This set of values must be "at least minimally consistent, stable, and affirmed as his or her own. This is needed in order to evaluate particular outcomes as benefits or harms, goods or evils, and to assign different relative weight or importance to them." Such a value system may be viewed as a unique sieve through which the elements of decision making are filtered.

Who should do it?

Clinicians seek consent to treatment on a day-to-day basis; therefore, the ability to assess capacity is a basic skill that all clinicians should possess. However, there are situations when those with specialist skills may be required and, depending on the nature of the putative impairment, the assessment of decision-making capacity may be delegated to psychologists or psychiatrists. In a few academic centers, there may be specialist teams or, if time permits, the clinician may discuss any areas of difficulty with the hospital bioethicist or clinical ethics committee. It should, however, be remembered that the final decision regarding capacity is a legal one.

General approach

It is important to remember some underlying considerations concerning capacity. Firstly, capacity is decision specific. Secondly, there is a presumption in favor of capacity. Finally, there must be a commitment to enhance decision-making capacity as much as possible. The interview process has an enabling function as well as one of assessment.

Enabling strategies

Enabling strategies might include treatment of an underlying mental illness, reducing the impact of prescribed medication, or, in the case of fluctuating capacity, waiting to assess during a more lucid period. The use of an aide-mémoire or the presentation of information in diagrammatic form may aid those with cognitive difficulties. Families may assist by providing support and reassurance by their presence or may assist in presenting material in the most effective way. Sometimes a person simply needs some time to take in and process bad news. Finally, attention to environmental factors may be helpful to minimize distraction and reduce anxiety.

Information

It is essential that those undertaking the assessment should be fully briefed about the nature of the illness, proposed treatment, alternatives, and the risks of refusing treatment. In addition to this clinical information, it will also be necessary to have an awareness of the legal test for capacity applicable to the relevant jurisdiction. An understanding of what has led to the request for an assessment of capacity is helpful as it may prepare the clinician for potential problems in undertaking the assessment, such as hostility from the patient.

The formal assessment interview

It is important to be open regarding the purpose of assessment. This can be introduced by indicating that some concerns have been raised by others about the person's decision-making ability and that you wish to discuss their thoughts about the proposed treatment in more detail. Where a patient is hostile, it may be helpful to be clear that the ability to exercise the important right to give or refuse treatment may hinge on the outcome of the interview.

There are two broad approaches to assessment: a directed clinical interview or use of a structured instrument and rating procedure, such as the MacArthur Competence Assessment Tool-Treatment (MacCAT-T).

Directed clinical interview

The assessment should begin with a discussion of the person's understanding of the disorder for which they are being offered treatment. This is then followed by a discussion of the recommended treatment, its benefits, the risks of refusing this treatment, and any available alternatives. Patients may be able to provide information in these domains in response to open questions; however, the relevant information may need to be disclosed and re-disclosed as the assessment progresses. While a structured approach is recommended, the clinician will need to be flexible and responsive to the presenting problems of the patient.

The Aid to Capacity Evaluation (ACE) is a semi-structured method for capacity assessment that covers the same areas as those assessed during the clinical interview. It may act as a useful prompt, and the form provides space to document responses. The ACE is easily accessible via the website of the University of Toronto Joint Centre for Bioethics (http://www.utoronto.ca/jcb).

This sequence of questions can be easily adapted to cover other types of decision that a person may face as a result of being in a medical setting, for example the decision to go into residential accommodation.

As the interview progresses, the clinician may gain pointers to any abnormalities in mental state, such as the presence of psychotic or mood disorder, and this should prompt a more detailed mental state examination. Assessment of cognitive function will also be required. It may also be important to gain an appreciation of the values underpinning the decision-making process and to explore these in context of the person's life history. On occasions third-party information may be helpful.

Formal assessment tools

The MacCAT-T is a well validated, semistructured interview that assesses and rates abilities in four domains: understanding of the disorder and its treatment, appreciation, reasoning, and ability to express a choice. The interview follows a fixed sequence of topics in the order outlined above. The assessor discusses the essential information and requires the patient to respond to specifically worded questions. The responses are then rated using a standard format. It should be noted that the scores generated do not translate directly into determination of capacity or incapacity and need to be understood in a broader clinical context and in relation to the nature of the decision to be made.

Documentation

It is essential to document the capacity assessment, not only for clinical but also for legal purposes. If there is a possibility that the case will come before the courts, there should be reference to the relevant legal standards. A brief summary of the questions asked and the patient's responses should be recorded. If a formal tool was used, then a copy should be retained in the notes.

There should be a well-reasoned decision supporting the conclusion regarding capacity. Grisso and Applebaum (1998, p. 146) suggested that a statement regarding the outcome of the capacity assessment should begin: "In my opinion the courts would be likely to find ... " in recognition that this is ultimately a legal, not medical, judgement. The assessment should make it clear that a finding of incapacity relates to a specific decision, otherwise there is a potential risk is that person will be labeled as being globally incompetent.

Suggestions for interventions that may allow a patient to regain capacity should also be documented.

The case

Ms. C presents a difficult problem in assessing capacity, as she is not cooperative with formal assessment. Given her lack of engagement with the formal process, a decision is made to utilize, with expert support, the clinical team with whom she has a good relationship and to guide them through the assessment process. The clinical team decide that she clearly understands the issues, including the potential risks, and she is able to express a choice. However, further discussion with the team reveals very little attention has been paid to acknowledging the emotional impact of the loss, and she should be assisted in this by seeing a specialist bereavement nurse.

It emerges that Ms. C is overwhelmed with grief and holds herself responsible for the baby's death. She accepts that others may have a different perspective, but she feels that unless she gives birth without medical intervention she will have failed completely as a mother. She will not shift from this view despite careful explanation.

As there are potentially life-threatening consequences of refusing treatment, the threshold for a finding of capacity must be high. Her grief appears to be impairing her ability to make use of the information about the proposed treatment. As the clinical situation is currently stable, it is agreed that further grief work should be undertaken. Plans are made to name the baby and for there to

be a funeral. With these plans in place, Ms. C agrees to medical induction of labor.

REFERENCES

Buchanan, A. E. and Brock, D. W. (1989). *Deciding for Others: The Ethics of Surrogate Decision Making*, Cambridge: Cambridge University Press.

Charland, L. C. (1998), Appreciation and emotion: theoretical reflections on the MacArthur Treatment Competence Study. *Kennedy Inst Ethics J* **8**: 359–76.

Etchells, E., Darzins, P., Silberfeld, M., *et al.* (1999). Assessment of patient capacity to consent to treatment. *J Gen Intern Med* **14**: 27–34.

Gillon, R. (1986). *Philosophical Medical Ethics*. Chichester, UK: John Wiley and Sons.

Grisso, A. and Applebaum, P. S. (1995a). Comparison of standards for assessing patients' capacities to make treatment decisions. *Am J Psychiatry* **152**: 1033–7.

Grisso, A. and Applebaum, P. S. (1995b). The MacArthur Treatment Competence Study III. Abilities of patients to consent to psychiatric and medical treatments. *Law Hum Behav* **19**: 149–73.

Grisso, A. and Applebaum, P. S. (1998). *Assessing Competence to Consent to Medical Treatment, A Guide for Physicians and Other Health Professionals.* New York: Oxford University Press.

Gunn, M. (1994). The meaning of incapacity. *Med Law Rev* **2**: 8–29.

Hope, T., Savulescu, J., and Henrick, J. (2003). *Medical Ethics and the Law, The Core Curriculum*. Edinburgh: Churchill Livingstone.

Kopelman, L. M. (1990). On the evaluative nature of competency and capacity judgements. *Int J Law Psychiatry* **13**: 309–29.

Law Commission (1995). *Law Commission Report 231: Mental Incapacity*. London: HMSO.

President's Commission for the Study of Ethical Problems in Medicine and Biomedical and Behavioral Research (1982). *Making Healthcare Decisions*. Washington, DC: US Government Printing Office.

Raymont, V., Bingley, W., Buchanan, A., *et al.* (2004). Prevalence of mental incapacity in medical inpatients and associated risk factors: cross sectional study. *Lancet* **364**: 1421–7.

Re T (Adult Refusal of Treatment) [1992] 4 All ER 649.

Roth, L. H., Meisel, A., and Lidz, C. W. (1977). Tests of competency to consent to treatment. *Am J Psychiatry* **134**: 279–84.

Schloendorff v. *Society of New York Hospitals* (1914) 211 NY 125.

St George's Healthcare NHS Trust v. *S* [1998] 3 All ER 673.

Wong, J. G., Clare, I. C. H., Gunn, M. J., and Holland, A. J. (1999). Capacity to make healthcare decisions: its importance in clinical practice. *Psychol Med* **29**: 437–46.

Wong, J. G., Clare, I. C. H., Holland, A. J., Watson, P. C., and Gunn, M. (2000). The capacity of people with a ''mental disability'' to make a healthcare decision. *Psychol Med* **30**: 295–306.

4

Disclosure

Lori d'Agincourt-Canning and Carolyn Johnston

Mrs. D is 75 years old and lives at home with her husband. She has a remote history of gastric ulcers and has mild renal insufficiency as a consequence of hypertension. She visits her family physician because of acute worsening of chronic arthritis in her right shoulder. She is having trouble lifting and carrying objects. Her family physician is considering treating Mrs. D with a non-steroidal anti-inflammatory drug.

Mrs. E is 80 years old and lives alone in an apartment. She is fully independent and has never had a serious illness. She prefers not to see doctors. She is admitted to hospital after falling on the stairs and suffering a fracture of the femoral neck. A consultant in internal medicine diagnoses critical aortic stenosis; this is confirmed by echocardiography. The anesthetist visits Mrs. E to discuss the proposed surgery and anesthesia. When he says that serious risks are associated with the surgery, Mrs. E says she does not want to know about them. She wants her hip fixed because she simply cannot live with reduced mobility. The anesthetist feels that he has a duty to disclose the risks of anesthesia.

What is disclosure?

Disclosure refers to the process during which physicians provide information about a proposed medical investigation or treatment to the patient. Disclosure, along with capacity, understanding, voluntariness, and consent, makes up the main elements of informed consent (Beauchamp and Childress, 2001).

Why is disclosure important?

Ethics

The justification for disclosure related to proposed diagnostic tests and treatments is the same as that for consent generally. The patient has a right to decide about available treatment options grounded in respect for autonomy (Snyder and Leffler, 2005). Physicians have a duty to inform patients about their illness and available treatment options and to help patients to decide which of the options is best for them based on the patient's goal and values. In these ways, physicians show respect for the patient and moreover, show "they see and care about the person not solely as a patient but more importantly, as a unique person" (Anderson, 2000, p. 6). In addition to respect for autonomy, disclosure is also grounded in beneficence and the physician's primary obligation of service to their patients (Royal College of Physicians and Surgeons of Canada, 2006). Further, consistent disclosure is necessary for developing a continuing and trusting relationship between the patient and his or her physician (Parascandola *et al.*, 2002).

Law

Legal standards of disclosure concerning informed consent differ in different jurisdictions (Doyal, 2001).

An earlier version of this chapter has appeared: Etchells, E., Sharpe, G., Burgess, M. M., and Singer, P. A. (1996). Disclosure. *CMAJ* **155**: 387–91.

For example, the legal right of patients to information about their healthcare is stronger in North America than in the UK, Europe, and other parts of the world (Doyal, 2001; Miyata *et al.*, 2005). However, laws are constantly evolving and the trend in ethical and legal thinking has led to increased information disclosure and involvement of patients in healthcare decision making. Three general aspects can be identified: the elements of disclosure, the standards of disclosure to maintain, and the consequences of a failure in disclosure (causation).

Elements of disclosure

A valid consent given for a medical treatment or procedure provides a defense to the tort of battery. In order for consent to be valid, the patient must be informed in "broad terms" of the nature of the procedure. This is a fairly basic level of information, but nevertheless it highlights the significance of bodily integrity of the patient.

In addition, the patient must also be informed about the inherent risks, alternatives, and consequences of the proposed treatment. This is a higher level of information than that which is necessary to make the patient's consent valid. It is referred to as "informed consent" and underscores the need to respect the autonomous choice of the patient – whether or not to undergo the treatment or procedure, based on his/her assessment of whether the risks are worth taking. Benefits flowing from disclosure to the patient, thus enabling an exchange of information, include the establishment of trust, the cooperation of the patient in proposed treatment options, and the empowerment of the patient in what is essentially an unequal relationship.

Certain risks are considered so "obvious" that the patient is taken to be aware of them and need not specifically be informed of them. However, this will depend on current practice. In 1985, in the important English House of Lords decision of *Sidaway* v. *Board of Governors*, Lord Keith said that it was "generally accepted that there is no need to warn of the risks inherent in all surgery under general anaesthesia ... on the ground that the patient may be expected to be aware of such risks or that they are relatively remote." A patient leaflet produced by the UK Royal College of Anaesthetists, 21 years later (2006), gives the statistical risks of death and brain damage during surgery and states "your surgeon and anaesthetist will be able to tell you more about your individual risks and then you can decide whether you want to go ahead with the operation." Disclosure generally "has tended to a greater degree of frankness over the years, with more respect being given to patient autonomy" (*Chester* v. *Afshar*, 2005).

Standards of disclosure

Failure to provide the patient with treatment information may give rise to a claim in negligence, but only if disclosure has fallen below the required standard. The standard could be what the medical profession considers appropriate (the "reasonable doctor" standard), or what a reasonable person in the patient's position would want to know (the "prudent patient" standard). In *Sidaway*, the judges considered that primarily the standard of disclosure should be set on the basis of medical evidence, in other words what is the practice of disclosure of a "responsible body of medical opinion"? However, the House of Lords did recognize that there may be some risks that the patient should always be informed about those risks which are "so obviously necessary to an informed choice on the part of the patient," regardless of the medical view. The English courts have considered both the seriousness of the risk and the likelihood of it eventuating in deciding whether such a risk should be disclosed. An inherent 10% risk of a stroke from an operation should be disclosed (*Sidaway* v. *Board of Governors*, 1985), so too should a 1–2% risk of paralysis (*Chester* v. *Afshar*, 2005).

But the "reasonable doctor" standard fails to acknowledge the importance to a particular patient of information that may be highly relevant to his/her choice. Certainly the courts in Canada (*Reibl* v. *Hughes*, 1980) and Australia have adopted a patient-led standard of disclosure. In *Rogers* v. *Whitaker* (1992) the Australian High Court held that the doctor's duty was to "warn a patient of a material risk inherent in the proposed treatment; a risk is material if, in the circumstances of the particular case, a reasonable person in the patient's position if warned of the risk, would be likely to attach significance to it." This approach increasingly appears to find favor in the English courts. In *Pearce* v. *United Bristol Healthcare N.H.S. Trust* (1999) the Court of Appeal said that "if there is a significant risk which would affect the judgment of the reasonable patient, then in the normal course it is the responsibility of a doctor to inform the patient of that significant risk."

Causation

To succeed in an action alleging that the healthcare professional negligently failed to disclose information, the claimant must prove that a duty to disclose was owed (this is part of the general duty of care), that the duty to disclose was breached (i.e., the healthcare professional did not meet the standard of disclosure), and also that, if the claimant had been properly informed, he would not have consented to the operation or procedure. In the case of *Chester* v. *Afshar* (2005) the House of Lords extended the boundaries of causation and allowed the claimant to succeed by showing that, if she had properly been informed of the risks, she would have sought further advice and would not have agreed to undergo that operation on that particular day.

Policy

The importance of patient-focused consent procedures is highlighted by guidance from professional bodies. In the UK, the General Medical Council (GMC) maintains that doctors "must take appropriate steps to find out what patients want to know and ought to know about their condition and its treatment" (paragraph 3) and that "existing case law gives a guide to what can be considered minimum requirements of good practice in seeking

informed consent from patients" (paragraph 2) (General Medical Council, 1998).

Information should not be withheld from patients. The few legal exceptions to this obligation include (i) an emergency situation; (ii) waiver, where the patient expresses directly to that physician he/she does not want the offered information (however, such decisions should be documented along with the patient's consent to go forward without detailed information); and (iii) incompetency (Beauchamp and Childress, 2001; National Health and Medical Research Council, 2004).

In addition, therapeutic privilege has been recognized by the courts (*Canterbury* v. *Spence*, 1972; *Sidaway* v. *Board of Governors*, 1985) in some countries as an exception to the usual standard of disclosure: "'Therapeutic privilege' refers to the withholding of information by the clinician during the consent process in the belief that disclosure of this information would lead to the harm or suffering of the patient" (Etchells *et al.*, 1996, p. 388). The deliberate withholding of information, and the resulting reduction in the exercise of autonomous choice, is based on the justification of patient welfare. GMC guidance (paragraph 10) also recognizes the doctrine: "You should not withhold information necessary for decision making unless you judge that disclosure of some relevant information would cause the patient serious harm. In this context serious harm does not mean the patient would become upset, or decide to refuse treatment." Although therapeutic privilege may have legal recognition, it is arguable whether the deliberate withholding of information from a competent patient can be ethically justified. Johnston and Holt (2006, p. 150) commented: "There are only a limited number of clinical situations where providing specific information to a patient under certain circumstances can arguably be expected to cause foreseeable and preventable serious harm to him or her."

Empirical studies

Evidence continues to show that most patients value candidness about their medical situation and wish to be given the appropriate information necessary to making an informed choice (Edwards *et al.*, 2001). Even in Japan, where the trend toward disclosure of information (e.g., cancer diagnosis) has been slow to gain acceptance by the medical profession, a population survey revealed that full disclosure was preferred by 86.1% of respondents, while only 2.7% wanted non-disclosure (Miyata *et al.*, 2005). Similarly, some studies suggest that patients want more detailed information than they currently receive and that physicians may overestimate how much they provide (Ende *et al.*, 1989; Fallowfield *et al.*, 1995; Makoul *et al.*, 1995; Butow *et al.*, 1997; Jenkins *et al.*, 2001).

A qualitative study in the palliative care setting revealed that information disclosure serves several important purposes. Patients in such a situation described information as important not only to meaningful involvement in decision making but also for keeping a sense of control (Kirk *et al.*, 2004). It was also seen as necessary for family communication and involvement (Clarke *et al.*, 2004; Kirk *et al.*, 2004). In contrast, a perception of insufficient information was reported to add stress, frustration, and uncertainty. It implied powerlessness and a lack of control (Thorne *et al.*, 2006).

Interestingly, this study also revealed that the process of disclosure was equally as important as the content. The timing, management, and delivery of the information, and the perceived attitude of physicians, were crucial to the process. This applied to information sharing and disclosure at all stages of the illness. The importance of process in effective communication and information disclosure has been described elsewhere (Edwards *et al.*, 2001; Weiner *et al.*, 2005).

While most patients value disclosure and candidness about their illness, research also indicates that a small percentage prefers not to engage actively in decision making nor wishes to know about the risk of treatment (Farnill and Inglis, 1993; Dawes and Davison, 1994; Miyata *et al.*, 2005). Moreover, many of those who value information may not do so in all situations and may prefer to let the physician take the lead at different stages of their illness (Towle and Godolphin, 1999; Edwards *et al.*, 2001; Parascandola *et al.*, 2002). In such cases, respect for autonomy does not mean forced patient involvement but rather accepting each person's preferences for information and involvement in decision making. Understanding how best to assess patients' information needs or determine their preferences, however, is difficult. While further research is needed in this area, a few tools exploring patients' preferences and information needs have been developed (Sayers *et al.*, 2001; Murtagh and Thorns, 2006).

How should I approach disclosure in practice?

The goal of disclosure is to ensure that patients have appropriate information to make an informed choice about their healthcare. While information disclosure needs to be individualized to each situation (Towle and Godolphin, 1999; Kirk *et al.*, 2004), it should include the following elements (Dickens, 1985):

- description of the patient's condition or illness; prognosis and consequences if the patient remains untreated or there is a delay in treatment
- reasonable treatment options, their benefits and special risks, and the likelihood of achieving the desired goal taking into account patient's values, expectations, and personal situation
- side effects, both reversible and irreversible, and expected discomforts of treatment options and the chance of these side effects occurring whether treatment is successful or not
- the extent of uncertainty and/or limited medical knowledge surrounding the prognosis and recommended treatment options
- information that the patient specifically asks about
- physician's opinion regarding which treatments should be undertaken in view of relevant patient's goals, values, and expectations.

Effective disclosure requires open and balanced communication. In the medical consultation, the clinicians must decide what ought to be communicated and the patient must integrate that information into their medical and social life experiences. Thus, communication is not a morally neutral dispensation of information but, rather, a highly complex ethical situation (Edwards and Elwyn, 2001) Good patient–physician communication can dispel the uncertainty and fear and improve patient satisfaction (Snyder and Leffler, 2005). While a full discussion of communication skills is beyond the scope of this article, a few "principles" are important when providing information to the patient (Anderson, 2000):

- make it clear; avoid jargon and technical language
- use language appropriate to the patient's level of understanding in a language of their fluency; provide professional interpreter if necessary
- pause and observe the patient's reactions after providing information
- invite questions from the patient and check understanding
- invite the patient to share concerns, fears, hopes, and expectations
- watch for patient's emotional responses: verbal and non-verbal cues
- show empathy and compassion
- check the patient's need for more time or information
- summarize the imparted information
- provide contact information.

The physician has an ethical and legal obligation to make reasonable efforts to ensure understanding. Supplementing verbal information with written material might be helpful as it enables the patient to read or review the information if desired. Educational video or computer programs may assist patients who face a complicated decision (Jonsen et al., 1998; Woolf et al., 2005).

Disclosure should be seen as a process, not an event (Etchells et al., 1996). Each patient is different and may wish for varying amounts of information at different times. Further, if therapy is given over a prolonged period, it is important that the disclosure process continues. The physician should regularly seek feedback from patients about their treatment and desire for more information. Similarly, disclosure about new information or relevant uncertainties concerning treatment will contribute to long-term trust between physicians and patients (Parascandola et al., 2002).

Patients bring their cultural, religious, and ideological beliefs with them as they enter into a relationship with the physician (Kagawa-Singer and Blackhall, 2001). Occasionally, these beliefs may challenge or conflict with the physician's professional duty to disclose. For example, autonomy is a principle highly valued in European and North American cultures, and thus it is expected that the person experiencing the illness is the best person to whom to disclose pertinent medical information. However, many non-Western cultures do not support the idea of full disclosure when it comes to illness, while others hold the family or community responsible for receiving and disclosing information, and for making decisions about patient care (Kagawa-Singer and Blackhall, 2001). In order to provide ethical cross-cultural care, applying the concept of autonomy will mean negotiating and accepting each person's terms of preference for information and decision making. In situations in which the family demands that the patient not be told, one strategy is to offer to provide the information to the patient, allowing the patient "informed refusal" (Kagawa-Singer and Blackhall, 2001). If the patient designates someone else be given the task of decision making, this preference should be documented in the patient's chart. The impact of cultural differences on bioethics is explored in greater depth in Section IX.

The cases

Mrs. D has no questions about the "arthritis pill" because she trusts her physician, whom she has known for many years. The physician initiates a discussion of the risks – in particular, gastro-intestinal bleeding and renal insufficiency. Mrs. D appears concerned, and the clinician invites her to discuss this concern. Mrs. D explains that the shoulder pain must be relieved so that she can care for her young granddaughter, who will be visiting next month. The physician mentions that acet-aminophen (paracetamol) may also be effective and has a lower risk of side effects. Although pain relief is a high priority, Mrs. D would prefer to avoid side effects, particularly because she was once admitted to hospital because of her gastric ulcer. She agrees to try acetaminophen therapy for two weeks and, if there is no effect, then to try the non-steroidal anti-inflammatory drug. The phys-ician makes a note of their discussion and arranges a follow-up appointment for two weeks hence.

Mrs. E has asked the anesthetist not to disclose further the risks associated with hip surgery. She says that her goal is to be able to walk and that further suffering from pain and immobility is not acceptable to her. She tells the anesthetist that any further discussion of risks will not change her mind but might upset her. The anesthetist respects Mrs. E's request but tells her that she can change her mind regarding the discussion of risks at any time. He also asks her if there are family members whom Mrs. E would like to involve in the decision-making process. Mrs. E wants her daughters to participate in the decision, and so the proposed surgery and its possible risks are disclosed to them. The entire discussion is documented, including Mrs. E's reasons for waiving further disclosure of the risks of surgery. Mrs. E undergoes uncompli-cated repair of her hip fracture and returns home to live independently.

REFERENCES

Anderson, I. (2000). *Continuing Education Program in End of Life Care*, Module 5: *Communication with Patients and Families*. Toronto: University of Toronto (http://www.cme.utoronto.ca/endoflife/). Accessed 21 July 2006.

Beauchamp, T. L. and Childress, J. F. (2001). *The Principles of Biomedical Ethics*, 5th edn, Oxford: Oxford University Press.

Butow, P., Maclean, M., Dunn, S., Tattersall, M., and Boyer, M. (1997). The dynamics of change: cancer patients' preferences for information, involvement and support. *Ann Oncol* **8**: 857–63.

Canterbury v. *Spence* (1972) 464 F. 2d 772 D.C. Cir.1972.

Chester v. *Afshar* [2005] 1 A.C. 134.

Clarke, G., Hall, R., and Rosencrance, G. (2004). Physician–patient relations: no more models. *Am J Bioethics* **4**: W16–W19.

Dawes, P. J. D. and Davison, P. (1994). Informed consent: what do patients want to know? *J R Soc Med* **87**: 149–52.

Dickens, B. (1985). The doctrine of "informed consent": informed choice in medical care. *Justice Beyond Orwell*, ed. R. Abella and M. Rothman. Montreal: Editions Yvon Blais, pp. 243–63.

Doyal, L. (2001). Informed consent: moral necessity or illusion? *Qual Health Care* **10**(Suppl I): i29–i33.

Edwards, A. and Elwyn, G. (2001). Understanding risk and lessons for clinical risk communication about treat-ment preferences. *Qual Health Care* **10**(Suppl. 1): i19–i13.

Edwards, A., Elwyn, G., Smith, C., Williams, S., and Thornton, H. (2001). Consumers' views of quality in the consultation and their relevance to "shared decision-making approaches." *Health Expect* **4**: 151–61.

Ende, J., Kazis, L., Ash, A., and Moskowitz, M. A. (1989). Measuring patients' desire for autonomy: decision making and information–seeking preferences among medical patients. *J Gen Intern Med* **4**: 23–30.

Etchells, E. E., Sharpe, G., Burgess, M., and Singer, P. A. (1996). Bioethics for clinicians. 2. Disclosure *CMAJ* **155**: 387–91.

Fallowfield, L., Ford, S., and Lewis, S. (1995). No news is not good news: information preferences of patients with cancer. *Psychooncology* **4**: 197–202.

Farnill, D. and Inglis, S. (1993). Patients' desire for information about anaesthesia: Australian attitudes. *Anaesthesia* **48**: 162–4.

General Medical Council (1998). *Seeking Patients' Consent: The Ethical Considerations*. London: General Medical Council.

Jenkins, V., Fallowfield, L., and Saul, J. (2001). Information needs of patients with cancer: results from a large study in UK cancer centres. *Br J Cancer* **84**: 48–51.

Johnston, C. and Holt, G. (2006). The legal and ethical implications of therapeutic privilege: is it ever justified to withhold treatment information from a competent patient?' *Clin Ethics* **1**: 146–51.

Jonsen, A., Siegler, M., and Winslade, W. (1998). *Clinical Ethics*, 4th edn, New York: McGraw–Hill Health Professions Division.

Kagawa-Singer, M. and Blackhall, L (2001). Negotiating cross-cultural issues at the end of life. *JAMA* **286**: 2993–3002.

Kirk, P., Kirk, I., and Kristjanson, L. (2004). What do patients receiving palliative care for cancer and their families want to be told? A Canadian and Australian qualitative study. *BMJ* **328**: 1343.

Makoul, G., Arntson, P., and Schofield, T. (1995). Health promotion in primary care: physician–patient communication and decision–making about prescription medications. *Soc Sci Med* **41**: 1241–4.

Miyata, H., Takahashi, M., Saito, T., Tachimori, H., and Kai, I. (2005). Disclosure preferences regarding cancer diagnosis and prognosis: to tell or not to tell? *J Med Ethics* **31**: 447–51.

Murtagh, F. and Thorns, A. (2006). Evaluation and ethical review of a tool to explore patient preferences for information and involvement in decision making. *J Med Ethics* **32**: 311–15.

National Health and Medical Research Council (2004). *Communicating with Patients: Advice for Medical Practitioners*. Melbourne: Commonwealth of Australia, NHMRC Publications.

Parascandola, M., Hawkins, J., and Danis, M. (2002). Patient autonomy and the challenge of clinical uncertainty. *Kennedy Inst Ethics J* **12**: 245–64.

Pearce v. *United Bristol Healthcare N.H.S. Trust* [1999] E.C.C. 167.

Reibl v. *Hughes* (1980) 114 D.L.R. (3d) 1 (S.C.C.).

Rogers v. *Whitaker* (1992) 67 ALJR 47.

Royal College of Anaesthetists (2006). *Risks Associated with your anaesthetic*, Section 14: *Death or Brain Damage*. London: Royal College of Anaesthetists.

Royal College of Physicians and Surgeons of Canada (2006). *Bioethics Education Project Surgery Curriculum*: *Module Disclosure*. Ottawa: Royal College of Physicians and Surgeons in Canada (http://rcpsc.medical.org/bioethics/index.php). Accessed 21 July 2006.

Sidaway v. *Board of Governors of the Bethlem Royal Hospital and the Maudsley Hospital* [1985] AC 871.

Sayers, G. M., Barratt, D., Gothard, C., *et al.* (2001). The value of taking an ''ethics'' history. *J Med Ethics* **27**: 114–117.

Snyder, L. and Leffler, C. (2005). Ethics manual, 5th edn, *Ann Intern Med* **142**: 560–582.

Thorne, S., Hislop, G., Kuo, M., and Armstrong, E. A. (2006). Hope and probability: patient perspectives of the meaning of numerical information in cancer communication. *Qual Health Res* **16**: 318–336.

Towle, A. and Godolphin, W. (1999). Framework for teaching and learning informed consent decision making. *BMJ* **319**: 766–71.

Weiner, S., Bernet, B., Cheng, T., and Daaeman, T. (2005). Processes for effective communication in primary care. *Ann Intern Med* **142**: 709–14.

Woolf, S., Chan, E., Harris, R., *et al.* (2005). Promoting informed choice: transforming healthcare to dispense knowledge for decision making. *Ann Intern Med* **143**: 293–300.

5

Voluntariness

Mary Jane Dykeman and Kate Dewhirst

Mr. F is a 59-year-old taxi driver who has been admitted to hospital with severe iron-deficiency anemia. After his condition is stabilized by means of a blood transfusion, and an endoscopy is ordered, the attending physician tells Mr. F that he will "have a test" because "he must be bleeding from the bowel." As he is being wheeled down the hall to the endoscopy suite, the physician calls out: "You have to have this test before you can go home." The endoscopist arrives at the same time as Mr. F.

Ms. G is a 38-year-old mother of two young children. She is an outpatient at a mental health facility where she is finishing up a program for an addiction to painkillers. She is in the midst of a bitter custody battle with her former husband, who is insisting that she sign a consent form to release her health records to him for the purpose of the custody hearing. She is scared that her husband may try to use the information against her, and that she will lose her children. Nevertheless, her social worker has told her she needs to accept responsibility for her addiction and the only way to do that is to share all details of her treatment with her husband.

What is voluntariness?

In the context of consent, "voluntariness" refers to a patient's right to make treatment decisions and decisions about his or her personal information free of any undue influence. A patient's freedom to decide can be impinged upon by internal factors arising from the patient's condition or by external factors. External factors, which are the focus of this article, include the ability of others to exert control over a patient by force, coercion, or manipulation. Force involves the use of physical restraint or sedation to enable a treatment to be given. Coercion involves the use of explicit or implicit threats to ensure that a treatment is accepted (e.g., "If you don't let us do these tests, then we will discharge you from the hospital!"). Manipulation involves the deliberate distortion or omission of information in an attempt to induce the patient to accept a treatment or make a certain decision (Faden and Beauchamp, 1986; Kuczewski and McCruden, 2001).

The requirement for voluntariness does not imply that clinicians should refrain from persuading patients to accept advice. Persuasion involves appealing to the patient's reason in an attempt to help him or her understand and accept the merits of a recommendation (Kuczewski and McCruden, 2001). Although a clinician may attempt to persuade a patient to follow a particular course of action based on medical evidence and clinical judgement, the patient is free to accept or reject this advice.

Why is voluntariness important?

Ethics

Voluntariness is an ethical requirement of valid consent. It is grounded in several related concepts,

An earlier version of this chapter has appeared: Etchells, E., Sharpe, G., Dykeman, M. J., Meslin, E. M., and Singer, P. A. (1996). Voluntariness. *CMAJ* **155**: 1083–6.

including freedom, autonomy, and independence (Faden and Beauchamp, 1986). The goal of the consent process is to maximize the opportunity for decisions to be reached autonomously (Etchells et al., 1999). Clinicians are often faced with an inherent tension between their desire to respect and foster patient autonomy (focusing on the empowerment of the individual) and their a responsibility to act in a patient's best interest (which some might call paternalism). A power imbalance will always exist in the clinician–patient relationship, to the extent that one party has more clinical information and expertise. However, clinicians must be mindful of the fine line between persuasion and coercion: the duty to provide sufficient information and advice to support a patient's autonomous decision making, contrasted against allowing a patient's actions to be substantially controlled by others.

In a presentation on legal and ethical dilemmas delivered to the *Consent and Child Health Workshop* in 1998, New Zealand's Health and Disability Commissioner Ron Paterson stated that "[e]ven for a mature young person, clinicians must be alert to the possibility of coercion or undue influence, for example, by parents on religious matters." (New Zealand Ministry of Health, 1998).

Law

Voluntariness is a legal requirement of valid consent. In *Beausoleil* v. *Sisters of Charity* (1966), a young woman about to undergo spinal surgery repeatedly requested a general anesthetic and refused a spinal anesthetic. After the patient had been sedated, the anesthetist convinced her to have a spinal anesthetic. The patient was subsequently paralyzed as a result of the procedure and successfully sued the anesthetist. In testimony, a witness said that the patient "refused [the spinal anesthetic], but they continued to offer it to her; finally she became tired and said: 'You do as you wish' or something like that" (p. 76). The judge stated that the patient's agreement to the spinal anesthetic was involuntary, because it rested on

"words which denote defeat, exhaustion, and abandonment of the will power." (p. 76).

In *Ferguson* v. *Hamilton Civic Hospitals et al.* (1983), a patient unsuccessfully sued for battery after undergoing an angiogram that resulted in quadriplegia. Although the suit was unsuccessful, the court was critical of the circumstances in which the consent was obtained and suggested "the informing of a patient should occur at an earlier time than when he is on the table immediately before undergoing the procedure" (p. 285). It has been suggested that obtaining consent just before a major procedure is problematic, because "the setting and the immediacy of the medical procedure militate against a patient being able to make a free or voluntary decision" (Picard and Robertson, 1996, p. 55).

The doctrine of undue influence was central to the Court's decision in *Re T* (1992). In that case, a young pregnant woman's refusal of a potentially life-saving blood product was found to be based on the undue influence of her mother, a Jehovah's Witness. The Court differentiated between a patient seeking advice and assistance in reaching a decision about care, versus a decision that is freely given (p. 669).

The real question in each such case is, does the patient really mean what he says or is he merely saying it for a quiet life, to satisfy someone else or because the advice and persuasion to which he has been subjected is such that he can no longer think and decide for himself? In other words, is it a decision expressed in form only, not in reality?

The Court noted that both the strength of the patient's will, and relationship with the persuading party, are central to a finding of undue influence.

In some common law jurisdictions, treatment may be given against an individual's wishes only in rare circumstances, for instance, to protect public safety (as is the case with laws that relate to public health) or to render someone fit to stand trial for a criminal offence. For example, individuals with communicable diseases may be treated against their objection, as in the case of patients with tuberculosis who are non-compliant with treatment [cf. Ontario's Health Protection and Promotion Act (1990)]. Many jurisdictions also permit individuals to be treated without consent in emergency situations where it is impossible to obtain the individual's consent (or that of his or her substitute decision maker).

Most common law jurisdictions allow for the involuntary admission of patients to psychiatric facilities, provided they present a serious, significant, or immediate risk to themselves (the language varies among statutes) or others, or are unable to take care of themselves. However, there is some variation between jurisdictions as to whether consent for treatment related to the mental illness is required for involuntarily admitted patients (although the usual consent rules would continue to apply to other healthcare decisions). Because of the coercive nature of such circumstances, extra care should be taken in obtaining a valid consent to treatment from patients who have been admitted involuntarily.

Finally, voluntariness for certain medical procedures involving minors has more recently been the subject of both legal and ethical debate. Consent to treatment of minors poses additional challenges with respect to voluntariness, given a potentially broader power imbalance between the minor and the clinician, as well as the wish of some parents to make decisions on behalf of their children. This issue was considered in the Canadian case of *Re Dueck* (1999) and in the English case *Re E* (1993) each involving a 15-year-old boy of Jehovah's Witness faith who refused a life-saving blood transfusion.

Policy

Voluntariness is an essential component of valid consent, and obtaining valid consent is generally a policy of professional bodies regulating clinicians. The UK's General Medical Council created a standard for ensuring voluntary decision making (General Medical Council, 1998). For example, discussions with patients about informed consent should provide a balanced view of available options, as well as making clear any potential conflicts of interest. Patients should also understand their right to decline a proposed treatment. The UK's Department of Health (2001) has noted that voluntary consent to treatment (or refusal of that treatment) requires an absence of pressure and undue influence on a patient and that pressure may come from clinicians, as well as from the patient's family members. Clinicians are advised to be alert to this possibility and arrange to meet privately with patients so they are making their own care decisions.

The guidelines for consent to treatment established by the Association of Anaesthetists of Great Britain and Ireland (AAGBI) has been criticized for failing to require that a separate consent be obtained from patients undergoing anesthesia. This criticism rests in part on the fact that, in addition to having adopted a lower standard than some other jurisdictions, the present guidelines make no reference to voluntariness (White and Baldwin, 2003).

Empirical studies

Psychiatric inpatients may be subject to explicit or implicit coercion even when their admission has been voluntary (Reed and Lewis, 1990; Rogers, 1993). However, even patients who require involuntary admission can be given some measure of control over their situation by being allowed to choose the method of restraint (Sheline and Nelson, 1993). An additional dilemma faces those working in forensic mental health, where the individual's consent to be examined or detained may not be necessary and subsequent consent to treatment may not be sought; for example, in the case of court-ordered treatment to render the individual fit to stand trial (Fernie, 2005).

Institutionalization in non-psychiatric hospitals or long-term care facilities can also be coercive. Even simple instructions to patients (e.g., "Don't get out of bed until after your breakfast") can give the patient a sense of diminished control (Hewison, 1995). Interventions that enhance the ability of long-term residents to exert control result in a greater sense of well-being (Langer and Rodin, 1976). Further, many long-term care facilities have developed successful programs to reduce the use of restraints, in some instances as best practice while in others as a result of legislative change (Miles and Meyers, 1994).

Outpatients are less likely than inpatients to be subjected to force and coercion (Connelly and Campbell, 1987) but they may be susceptible to manipulation. Although we are unaware of any data on the incidence of manipulation, studies indicate that decisions can easily by influenced by the manner in which information is presented (Sutherland *et al.*, 1991; Mazur and Hickham, 1994). It is possible for such manipulation to occur in clinical practice. A recent study examined voluntariness in the decisions of adolescents (Schachter *et al.*, 2005).

How should I approach voluntariness in practice?

Internal and external controlling factors can affect patients' decisions about treatment. For example, a patient with metastatic prostate cancer and bone pain is subject to internal controlling factors. A symptom-free life without treatment is not possible, and the patient must make some decisions while suffering severe pain, at least until the pain is treated. These internal factors arise from the patient's medical condition rather than from an external source, such as any action by the clinician. The clinician's role is to minimize the potential controlling effect of these internal factors to the best of their ability. For example, the clinician can reduce the impact of acute pain on decision making by deferring non-urgent decisions until the pain has been treated.

External controlling factors may be related to the clinician, the healthcare setting or to other people such as family and friends. We will focus here on the clinician and the healthcare setting; however, problems can also arise when family, friends, or others exert excessive control.

In the few circumstances in which it is acceptable for clinicians to use force, the least restrictive technique possible should be preferred. For example, if a patient is at immediate risk of harming himself or herself, simple observation in a supervised environment, rather than physical restraint or sedation, may be sufficient. Similarly, an elderly patient with delirium who is falling out of bed can be moved to a mattress on the floor so that the risk of falling is eliminated without physical restraint.

In psychiatric and long-term care institutions, a patient advocate can help the clinician to ensure that consent is not coerced. Clinicians can also take steps to minimize the coercive nature of institutions by enhancing the patient's sense of choice. Useful strategies might include encouraging patients to involve their family or friends in decisions, encouraging them to ask questions, and promoting their awareness of the choices available to them (e.g., "I would like you to have a test tomorrow. Do you want to talk about this with someone you are close to? Is there any reason to delay?").

Clinicians can also take steps to minimize the potential for manipulation. Firstly, because patients can be manipulated when the information they receive is incomplete, clinicians should ensure that adequate information has been disclosed to the patient. Secondly, manipulation can occur when information is presented in a biased fashion. A useful strategy is to ask patients to review information in their own words. Also, if a patient who accepts therapy because of its potential benefits continues to accept it when its potential risks are emphasized, then the clinician can be more confident that this decision has not been manipulated (Redelmeier *et al.*, 1993).

The cases

The endoscopist asks Mr. F to review the reasons for having the test in his own words. Mr. F says that he has "no choice but to have the test" because "my doctor won't let me leave until I do." Mr. F expresses that he is self-employed and cannot afford to be off work any longer. Because the endoscopy is not an emergency, the endoscopist calls the attending physician, who agrees that the test should be delayed. After a further discussion that afternoon, Mr. F consents to the endoscopy, which is performed the next morning before Mr. F's next shift.

In a team meeting that same day, the discussion focuses on Ms. G and her custody battle. The social worker had not previously been aware that Ms. G was divorced, nor that the release of information to the husband could have drastic consequences. In a follow-up meeting with Ms. G, the social worker has an opportunity to discuss her recovery as well as her right to choose how and with whom her information is shared. Ms. G now understands that, in spite of her husband's threats, nobody at the health facility will share information without her consent or other legal authority to disclose as permitted or required by law. Ms. G and her husband ultimately share joint custody of their children.

REFERENCES

Beausoleil v. *Sisters of Charity* (1966) 56 DLR 65 (Que CA).

Connelly, J. E. and Campbell, C. (1987). Patients who refuse treatment in medical offices. *Arch Intern Med* **47**: 1829–33.

Etchells, E., Sharpe, G., Walsh, P. *et al.* (1999). Consent. In *Bioethics at the Bedside: A Clinician's Guide*, ed. P. A. Singer. Ottawa: *CMAJ*, pp. 17–24.

Faden, R. R. and Beauchamp, T. L. (1986). *A History and Theory of Informed Consent*. New York: Oxford University Press.

Ferguson v. *Hamilton Civic Hospitals et al.,* [1983] 23 CCLT 254.

Fernie, G. (2005). Consent and the individual detained in custody. *Med Law* **24**: 515–23.

General Medical Council (1998). *Seeking Patients' Consent: the Ethical Considerations*. London: General Medical Council (http://www.gmc-uk.org/guidance/library/consent.asp#ensuring).

Health Protection and Promotion Act, R.S.O. 1990 c. H.7. Toronto: Ontario Ministry of Health.

Hewison, A. (1995). Nurses' power in interactions with patients, *J Adv Nurs* **21**: 75–82.

Kuczewski, M. and McCruden, P. J. (2001). Informed consent: does it take a village? The problem of culture and truth telling. *Camb Q Health Ethics* **10**: 34–46.

Langer, E. J. and Rodin, J. (1976). The effects of choice and enhanced personal responsibility for the aged: a field experiment in an institutional setting. *J Pers Soc Psychol* **34**: 191–8.

Mazur, D. J. and Hickam, D. H. (1994). The effect of physicians' explanations on patients' treatment preferences. *Med Decis Making* **14**: 255–8.

Miles, S. H. and Meyers, R. (1994). Untying the elderly: 1989 to 1993 update. *Clin Geriatr Med* **10**: 513–25.

New Zealand Ministry of Health (1998). *Consent in Child and Youth Health: Information for Practitioners*. Wellington: Ministry of Health.

Picard, E. and Robertson, G. (1996). *Legal Liability of Doctors and Hospitals in Canada*, 3rd edn. Toronto: Carswell.

Redelmeier, P. A., Rozin, P., and Kahneman, D. (1993). Understanding patients' decisions: cognitive and emotional perspectives. *JAMA* **270**: 72–6.

Re Dueck [1999] 171 D.L.R. (4th) 761 (Sask. Q.B.).

Re E (1993) 1 FLR 386.

Re T [1992] 4 All ER 649.

Reed, S. C. and Lewis, D. A. (1990). The negotiation of involuntary admission in Chicago's state mental hospitals. *J Psychiatr Law* **18**: 137–63.

Rogers, A. (1993). Coercion and "voluntary" admission: an examination of psychiatric patient views. *Behav Sci Law* **11**: 259–67.

Schachter, D., Kleinman, I., and Harvey, W. (2005). Informed Consent and Adolescents. *Can J Psychiatry* **50**: 534–40.

Sheline, Y. and Nelson, T. (1993). Patient choice: deciding between psychotropic medication and physical restraints in an emergency. *Bull Am Acad Psychiatry Law* **21**: 321–9.

Sutherland, H. J., Lockwood, G. A., Tritchler, D. L., *et al.* (1991). Communicating probabilistic information to cancer patients: Is there "noise" on the line? *Soc Sci Med* **32**: 725–31.

UK Department of Health (2001). *Reference Guide to the Consent for Examination or Treatment*. London: The Stationery Office.

White, S. M. and Baldwin, T. J. (2003). Consent for anaesthesia. *Anaesthesia* **58L**: 760–74.

6

Truth telling

Philip C. Hébert, Barry Hoffmaster, and Kathleen C. Glass

Mr. H is 26 years old and has recently joined a general practitioner's list. The patient's past medical history is most notable for an episode several years previously of unilateral arm weakness and visual blurring without headache that resolved within 12 hours. He was referred to a neurologist, who did many tests and told him it was likely a transient viral infection and he should return if the symptoms recurred. Mr. H thought no more about it and has had no similar episodes since then. His medical records contain a letter from the neurologist to the previous family physician stating that Mr. H almost certainly has multiple sclerosis. The neurologist explains that he does not disclose the diagnosis in the early stages because he is concerned about causing excessive worry.

Ms. I is a 56-year-old dishwasher admitted with jaundice and anemia. Investigations have revealed advanced cholangiocarcinoma. Her family insists she not be told, explaining that families in their culture act on behalf of ill relatives. They argue that telling her the diagnosis of cancer would cause her to lose hope and so forbid its disclosure to her by medical staff. "Leave it to us to tell her what she needs to know," they say. A staff member who speaks their language overhears them telling Ms. F that everything will be fine and that she will be able to go home soon.

What is truth telling?

Truth telling in healthcare may be defined as the practice and attitude of being open and forthright with patients; that is, it is about encouraging authenticity and genuineness in the relationship between healthcare professional and patient. Truth telling requires the belief that, in general, truth is better than deception. It also requires an intent and effort to be as accurate and honest as possible with patients and includes the duty to disclose information for consent purposes.

Why is truth telling important?

Ethics

Truthfulness with patients comports well, of course, with democratic policy and practices. Without accurate information, patients are less able to make informed decisions about care. Scientific medicine has provided patients with new treatment opportunities and requires clinicians to be knowledgeable about these and share that knowledge with patients – thus, the harms of non-disclosure have increased as the options for care have expanded over time. Informed patients may also make decisions affecting their lives as a whole that they could not have made had they been unaware of the true nature of their condition.

Regardless of consequences, patients should be told the truth because of the respect owing to them as persons. Interviews with patients support this perspective. For example, in a study carried out

An earlier version of this chapter has appeared: Hébert, P. C., Hoffmaster, B., Glass, K. C., and Singer, P. A. (1997). Truth telling. *CMAJ* **156**: 225–8.

before any treatment for multiple sclerosis existed, many patients with the disease felt they had a right to know what was wrong with them. Some were angry about being asked why they wished to know. One said: "Do I have to explain why? Just so that I know" (Elian and Dean, 1985). Cabot's (1903) view that physicians should strive to create a "true impression" in the mind of the patient about his or her condition fostered the covenant of trust between physician and patient that is central to the practice of medicine (Cassel, 1996). This contrasts with the centuries-old Hippocratic cautioning against veracity with patients (Bok, 1979).

Deception by physicians is sometimes implicitly recommended as a way of preventing the possible harms of truth telling (Nyberg, 1993). Patients, especially when ill, are presumed to have difficulty handling the unvarnished truth and so it is/was the doctor's duty to keep the "whole truth" from them. Some cultures and families believe truth telling is cruel as it may cause avoidable worry in patients. This "protective deception" has some credence, especially at times when, and in those places where, medicine could offer little tangible help to patients. Nonetheless, although very ill patients may want someone to look after and guide them (Ingelfinger, 1980), this does not necessarily entail a preference for ignorance. Allowing others to make decisions for oneself, to be "taken care of" in the full sense of this phrase, can be consistent with wishing to remain informed about one's condition. Physicians should "sound out" patients about their preferences in this regard irrespective of cultural differences.

Law

Truth telling, as conceived in this chapter, includes the broader notion of accurate and honest communication practices. The jurisprudence relevant to this varies among countries and is largely focused on negligent disclosure for consent purposes (see Chapter 2 for more information). Canadian courts have long recognized the physician's obligation to provide information that would be required by a reasonable patient in the plaintiff's position (*Reibl* v. *Hughes*, 1980). Australian (*Rogers* v. *Whitaker*, 1992; *Chappel* v. *Hart*, 1998) and most American jurisdictions (*Canterbury* v. *Spence*, 1972) similarly use this so-called modified-subjective standard while British courts seem largely to adhere to a profession-based standard of disclosure (what a reasonable professional would disclose) (*Bolam* v. *Friern Hospital Management Committee*, 1957).

Recent developments have expanded legally required disclosure to include, as part of a physician's fiduciary duties, telling patients and/or their families about "unexpected outcomes of care," that is, adverse events or errors. For example, failure to tell a patient about the accidental puncture of his spleen during a lung biopsy was held to breach the physician's duty to inform the patient, particularly because the patient had asked what had occurred during the procedure. The judge concluded that litigation arose from a "less than satisfactory physician–patient relationship" caused by the failure of the physician to take the patient "into his confidence" (*Stamos* v. *Davies*, 1985, p. 25).

In another case, a physician was found negligent for failing to tell a patient of his risk of having (possibly) acquired infection with the human immunodeficiency virus from a transfusion. While the doctor argued he had done so to protect the patient from information that would only cause him psychological harm, the court held that *this* patient would have wanted to know this information, even though, at the time, there was little that could be done for HIV (*Pittman Estate* v. *Bain*, 1994).

Courts in the USA (*Arato* v. *Avedon*, 1993), Canada (*Hopp* v. *Lepp*, 1980; *Reibl* v. *Hughes*, 1980), and the UK (*Chester* v. *Afshar*, 2004) have granted that there may be exceptions to truth telling, for example when the patient's emotional condition is such that the disclosure of bad news could itself cause harm. The most relevant test for non-disclosure is "whether the disclosure would in itself cause physical and mental harm to this patient" (Picard 1984, p. 99). Physicians should start with the assumption that all patients are able to cope with the facts, and reserve non-disclosure for the less usual cases in which more harm will result from telling the truth than from not telling it.

Policy

The American College of Physicians (2005, p. 563) recommended that "[h]owever uncomfortable for the clinician, information that is essential to and desired by the patient must be disclosed. How and when to disclose information, and to whom, are important concerns that must be addressed with respect for patient wishes." It adds that the professional duty to be honest with patients requires that the "disclosure and the communication of health information should never be a mechanical or perfunctory process. Upsetting news and information should be presented to the patient in a way that minimizes distress."

The British Medical Association (2004, p. 43) noted that the "relationship of trust depends upon 'reciprocal honesty' between patient and doctor" and also encourages the sensitive delivery of bad news. The Canadian Medical Association's (1996) Code of Ethics recommends that physicians provide patients with whatever information that might, from the patient's perspective, have a bearing on medical care decision making and to communicate that information in a way that is comprehensible to the patient.

Empirical studies

Physicians

In a landmark study in 1961, 90% of a sample of 219 US physicians reported they would not disclose a diagnosis of cancer to a patient (Oken, 1961). Of the 264 physicians surveyed almost 20 years later, 97% stated that they would disclose a diagnosis of cancer (Novack et al., 1979), indicating a complete reversal of professional attitudes toward truth telling, at least in the context of a diagnosis of cancer.

Cultural values appear to influence physicians' attitudes toward truth telling. In one US study,

physicians who reported that they commonly told cancer patients the truth said that they did so in a way intended to preserve "hope" and "the will to live," both valued notions in US society (Good et al., 1990). Compared with their North American counterparts, gastroenterologists from southern and eastern Europe are less likely to be candid with patients about serious disease, believing this to be the best way to preserve "hope" (Thomsen et al., 1993).

Patients

The literature suggests that most North American patients want to be informed about their medical situation. For example, in a study involving 560 patients with cancer and their families, 87% of respondents felt that patients should be told the truth about their illness (Samp and Curreri, 1957). A 1982 survey indicated that 94% of patients wanted to know everything about their condition; 96% wanted to be informed of a diagnosis of cancer, and 85% wanted to be given a realistic estimate of their time to live, even if this were less than one year (President's Commission for the Study of Ethical Problems in Medicine, 1982). Studies of older patients, sometimes thought to be less interested in the truth, have shown that almost 90% want to be told the diagnosis of cancer (e.g., Erde et al., 1988). Studies have found that over 90% of patients want to be told a diagnosis of Alzheimer disease (Ajaj et al., 2001), and that over 80% of patients with amyotrophic lateral sclerosis wanted to be given as much information as possible (Silverstein et al., 1991).

However, lack of effective treatment has generally been taken to justify medicine's traditional avoidance of truth telling and is thought to be one reason, even today, why many patients at risk for Huntington disease do not seek to know their genetic status (Terrenoire, 1992). Other studies suggest cultural influences upon truth telling. For example, one study found a larger percentage of Korean-born patients preferred to be given less information than did US-born patients (Blackhall et al., 1995). In Italy, lack of candor about the diagnosis of Alzheimer disease is common (Pucci *et al.*, 2003). A larger percentage of patients in Japan (65%) than in the USA (22%) would want their families to be told a diagnosis of cancer before being informed themselves, and many more Japanese (80%) than US (6%) doctors agreed with this (Ruhnke *et al.*, 2000). As a result, patients with advanced cancer in Japan are told their prognosis only if the patient's family consents (Akabayashi *et al.*, 1999).

Outcomes

Good physician communication skills, which are part of the art of truth telling generally, improve patient satisfaction and the quality of medical care (Brown *et al.*, 1999). It has been estimated that an extra two to three minutes for consultation improves rapport with the patient (Levinson *et al.*, 1997). Truth telling increases patient compliance (concordance) with prescribed medications (Greenhalgh, 2005), reduces morbidity such as pain (Egbert *et al.*, 1964) and anxiety (Luck *et al.*, 1999) associated with medical interventions, and improves health outcomes (Stewart, 1995). Informed patients are more satisfied with their care and less apt to change physicians than those not well informed (Kaplan *et al.*, 1996). Even very young children, facing major surgery, are able to handle difficult news (Alderson, 1993). Failing to be honest with children can have lasting negative psychological consequences (Wallace, 2001). In one study, parents who were able to be candid about death with their dying child felt such open discussion helped them and their child. Parents who were unable to be so forthright later regretted their reticence (Kreicbergs *et al.*, 2004).

Some studies, however, suggest that truth telling can have negative consequences. Poor disclosure, even if accurate, can have devastating consequences for patients (Anon., 2000) – such disclosure is typically done too hurriedly, in the wrong setting, without appreciation of the patient's circumstances, and without addressing the patient's real needs and fears.

Truth telling can result in "labeling" patients. For example, patients told they had hypertension exhibited decreased emotional well-being and more frequent absence from work (MacDonald *et al.*, 1984). In another study, more information to patients with cancer resulted in higher anxiety levels among patients (Jenkins *et al.*, 2001). Concerns regarding the purportedly very bad outcomes of disclosure – loss of hope, premature death, or suicide – are anecdotal and lack any real empirical foundation.

How should I approach truth telling in practice?

Truth telling can be difficult in practice because of uncertainty – both in medicine and in the patient in terms of what he or she wishes to know – and the concern that the "truth" might harm the patient. It can also be difficult because truth telling is not a simple task and often requires, for its proper exercise, a longitudinal relationship between doctor and patient.

The uncertainty of an early diagnosis of a lethal condition may make the clinician wary of premature disclosure. Nevertheless, this uncertainty can and should be shared with patients (Logan and Scott, 1996). Telling patients about the clinical uncertainties and the range of options available allows them to appreciate the complexities of medicine, to ask questions, to make informed realistic decisions, to assume responsibility for those decisions, and to be better prepared just in case the dire prognosis turns out to be correct.

Predicting what information a patient will find upsetting, or foreseeing how upsetting certain information will be, can be difficult. Patients may indicate, explicitly or implicitly (Pisetsky, 1996), their desire not to know the truth about their situation. When such desires are authentic and realistic they should be respected. It is possible to deliver the truth in a way that softens its impact; many books provide practical suggestions on telling bad news (Buckman, 1992; Tate, 1995). The truth may be brutal, but "the telling of it should not be" (Jonsen *et al.*, 1992). Indeed, the task for physicians is how to combine honesty and respect for patient autonomy with caring and compassion.

For example, some patients with terminal illnesses may indicate that they do not want to know the full truth about their situation (Surbone, 1992). Physicians should explore these preferences sensitively to ascertain whether they are indeed authentic. There should be an attempt to canvas the patient's views on disclosure by "offering the truth" to the patient (Freedman, 1993). When a patient has a serious illness such as cancer, it may be helpful to document his or her preferences regarding the involvement of family members. Families who resist disclosure should be counseled about the importance of truth telling, much as they might be counseled about the appropriate management of any medical problem. Ongoing and respectful communication often, but not always, can overcome family and cultural barriers to disclosure (Chiu *et al.*, 2000).

Physicians are increasingly expected to disclose the occurrence of adverse events resulting from medical care to patients (Hébert, 2001), but they frequently do not do so (Berlin, 2006). The disclosure of such events is not an admission of substandard practice. Telling the truth can defuse resentment on the part of the patient and reduce the risk of legal action (Ritchie and Davies, 1995). Patients sometimes sue physicians out of a "need for explanation – to know how the injury happened and why" (Vincent *et al.*, 1994).

Despite this chapter's emphasis on truth telling, studies suggest that 10–20% of all patients do not want to know the details of their condition. For such patients, truth should be offered but not forced on them. In all cases of disclosure, just how and when to discuss the patient's situation, and how much to say at any one time, will vary from one patient to the next (Shattner, 2002). This is the art of truth telling, which relies on the skills and attitudes of the doctor to "take the patient into his (or her) confidence" and give him (or her) a "true impression" of his (her) illness.

The cases

If the neurologist seriously considered multiple sclerosis as a likely or working diagnosis, he was not justified in withholding this information from Mr. H. A general worry about causing anxiety is not sufficient to exempt a physician from his or her responsibility to tell the patient the truth – which in this case is the possibility (or probability) of serious disease. Physicians need not and should not wait for certainty before they disclose information to patients. Patients may be empowered to watch for symptoms of disease progression or be encouraged to do things that might prevent progression. If Mr. H is not told about his condition and makes a decision he would otherwise not have made had he been better informed, his physicians would bear some moral responsibility and perhaps even legal liability.

Ms. I should be spoken to on her own with a translator who is not a relative to have her views on disclosure assessed. Does she want to be informed of all the details of her illness or would she prefer the physicians to speak first with her family? The patient's authentic wishes ought to be respected. Where they diverge from the family's views, these differences should be acknowledged and help offered to the family in accommodating to them.

REFERENCES

Ajaj, A., Singh, M. P., and Abdulla, A. J. (2001). Should elderly patients be told they have cancer? Questionnaire survey of older people. *BMJ* **323**: 1160.

Akabayashi, A., Kai, I., Takemura, H., and Okazaki, H. (1999). Truth telling in the case of a pessimistic diagnosis in Japan. *Lancet* **354**: 1263.

Alderson, P. (1993). *Children's Consent to Surgery*. Buckingham: Open University Press.

American College of Physicians (2005). Ethics manual, 5th edn. *Ann Intern Med* **142**: 560–82.

Anon. (2000). Delivering bad news. *BMJ* **321**: 1233.

Arato v. *Avedon* [1993] 23 Cal. Rptr. 2d 140.

Berlin, L. (2006). Communicating radiology results. *Lancet* **367**: 373–5.

Blackhall, L. J., Murphy, S. T., Frank, G., Michel, V., and Azen, S. (1995). Ethnicity and attitudes toward patient autonomy. *JAMA* **274**: 820–5.

Bok, S. (1979). *Lying: Moral Choice in Public and Private Life*. New York: Vintage Books.

Bolam v. *Friern Hospital Management Committee* [1957] 1 WLR 582, 586.

British Medical Association (2004). *Medical Ethics Today: The BMA's Handbook of Ethics and Law*, 2nd edn, London: BMJ books.

Brown, J., Boles, M., Mullooly, J., and Levinson, W. (1999). Effect of clinician communication skills training on patient satisfaction: a randomized, controlled trial. *Ann Intern Med* **131**: 822–9.

Buckman, R. (1992). *How to Break Bad News*. Baltimore, MD: Johns Hopkins University Press.

Cabot, R. C. (1903). The use of truth and falsehood in medicine: an experimental study. *Am Med* **5**: 344–9.

Canadian Medical Association (1996). Code of ethics. *CMAJ* **155**: 1176A–B.

Canterbury v. *Spence* [1972] 464 F 2d 772.

Cassel, C. (1996). The patient–physician covenant: an affirmation of Asklepios. *Ann Intern Med* **124**: 604–6.

Chappel v. *Hart* [1998] 195 CLR 232.

Chester v. *Afshar* [2004] UKHL 41 (14 October 2004).

Chiu, T. Y., Hu, W. Y., Cheng, S. Y., and Chen, C. Y. (2000). Ethical dilemmas in palliative care: a study in Taiwan. *J Med Ethics* **26**: 353–7.

Egbert, L., Battit, G., Welch, C., and Bartlett, M. (1964). Reduction of postoperative pain by encouragement and instruction of patients. *N Engl J Med* **270**: 825–7.

Elian, M. and Dean, G. (1985). To tell or not to tell the diagnosis of multiple sclerosis. *Lancet* **ii**: 27–8.

Erde, E., Nadal, E., and Scholl, T. (1988). On truth telling and the diagnosis of Alzheimer's disease. *J Fam Pract* **26**: 401–4.

Freedman, B. (1993). Offering truth: one ethical approach to the uninformed cancer patient. *Arch Intern Med* **153**: 572–6.

Good, M., Good, B., Schaffer, C., and Lind, S. (1990). American oncology and the discourse on hope. *Cult Med Psychiatr* **14**: 59–79.

Greenhalgh, T. (2005). Barriers to concordance with antidiabetic drugs: cultural differences or human nature? *BMJ* **330**: 1250.

Hébert, P. (2001). Disclosure of adverse events and errors in health care: an ethical perspective. *Drug Safety* **15**: 1095–104.

Hopp v. *Lepp* [1980] SCR:192.

Ingelfinger, F. J. (1980). Arrogance. *N Engl J Med* **303**: 1507–11.

Jenkins, V., Fallowfield, L., and Saul, J. (2001). Information needs of patients with cancer: results from a large study in UK cancer centers. *Br J Cancer* **84**: 48–51.

Jonsen, A., Siegler, M., and Winslade, W. (1992). *Clinical Ethics*, 3rd edn, New York: McGraw–Hill.

Kaplan, S., Greenfield, S., Gandek, B., Rogers, W., and Ware, J. (1996). Characteristics of physicians with participatory decision-making styles. *Ann Intern Med* **124**: 497–504.

Kreicbergs, U., Valdimarsdóttir, U., Onelöv, E., Henter, J.-I., and Steineck, G. (2004). Talking about death with children who have severe malignant disease. *N Engl J Med* **351**: 1175–86.

Levinson, W., Roter, D. L., Mullooly, J. P., Dull, V. T., and Frankel, R. M. (1997). Physician–patient communication. The relationship with malpractice claims among primary care physicians and surgeons. *JAMA* **277**: 553–9.

Logan, R. and Scott, P. (1996). Uncertainty in clinical practice: implications for quality and costs of health care. *Lancet* **347**: 595–8.

Luck, A., Pearson, S., Maddern, G., and Hewett, P. (1999). Effects of video information on pre-colonoscopy anxiety and knowledge: a randomized trial. *Lancet* **354**: 2032–5.

MacDonald, L., Sackett, D., Haynes, R., and Taylor, D. (1984). Labelling in hypertension: a review of the behavioral and psychological consequences. *J Chronic Dis* **37**: 933–42.

Novack, D., Plumer, R., Smith, R., *et al.* (1979). Changes in physicians' attitudes toward telling the cancer patient. *JAMA* **241**: 897–900.

Nyberg, D. (1993). *The Varnished Truth: Truth Telling and Deceiving in Ordinary Life*. Chicago, IL: University of Chicago Press.

Oken, D. (1961). What to tell cancer patients: a study of medical attitudes. *JAMA* **175**: 1120–8.

Picard, E. (1984). *Legal Liability of Doctors and Hospitals in Canada*, 2nd edn, Toronto: Carswell Legal Publications.

Pisetsky, D. (1996). The breakthrough. *Ann Intern Med* **124**: 345–7.

Pittman Estate v. *Bain* [1994], 112 DLR (4th) 257 (Ont Gen Div).

President's Commission for the Study of Ethical Problems in Medicine (1982). *Making Health Care Decisions*, Vol. 1. Washington, DC: US Government Printing Office, pp. 69–111.

Pucci, E., Belardinelli, N., Borsetti, G. and Giuliani, G. (2003). Relatives' attitudes towards informing patients about the diagnosis of Alzheimer's disease. *J Med Ethics* **29**: 51–4.

Reibl v. *Hughes* [1980] 2 S.C.R.

Ritchie, J. and Davies, S. (1995). Professional negligence: a duty of candid disclosure? *BMJ* **310**: 888–9.

Rogers v. *Whitaker* [1992] 175 CLR 479, 490.

Ruhnke, G., Wilson, S., Akamatsu, T. *et al.* (2000). Ethical decision-making and patient autonomy: a comparison of physicians and patients in Japan and the United States. *Chest* **118**: 1172–82.

Samp, R. and Curreri, A. (1957). Questionnaire survey on public cancer education obtained from cancer patients and their families. *Cancer* **10**: 382–4.

Shattner, A. (2002). What do patients really want to know? *Q J Med* **95**: 135–6.

Silverstein, M., Stocking, C., Antel, J., Beckwith, J., and Siegler, M. (1991). ALS and life-sustaining therapy: patients' desires for information, participation in decision-making, and life-sustaining therapy. *Mayo Clin Proc* **66**: 906–13.

Stamos v. *Davies* [1985] 52 OR (2d) 11: 25–6.

Stewart, M. A. (1995). Effective physician–patient communication and health outcomes: a review. *CMAJ* **152**: 1423–33.

Surbone, A. (1992). Letter from Italy: truth telling to the patient. *JAMA* **268**: 1661–2.

Tate, P. (1995). *The Doctor's Communication Handbook.* Oxford: Radcliffe Medical Press.

Terrenoire, G. (1992). Huntington's Disease and the ethics of genetic prediction. *J Med Ethics* **18**: 79–85.

Thomsen, O., Wulff, H., Martin, A., and Singer, P. A. (1993). What do gastroenterologists in Europe tell cancer patients? *Lancet* **341**: 473–6.

Vincent, C., Young, M., and Phillips, A. (1994). Why do people sue doctors? A study of patients and relatives taking legal action. *Lancet* **343**: 1609–13.

Wallace, F. (2001). All children deserve to know the truth. *BMJ* **322**: 3665.

7

Confidentiality

Anne Slowther and Irwin Kleinman

Mr. J is 35 years old. He has had unprotected sex with prostitutes on at least two occasions. Although he is asymptomatic he is worried about the possibility that he may have contracted a sexually transmitted disease and consults his physician. After conducting a careful physical examination and providing appropriate counseling, the physician orders a number of investigations. The blood test comes back with a positive result for HIV. The physician offers to meet with Mr. J and his wife to assist with the disclosure of this information, but Mr. J states that he does not want his wife to know about his condition.

Ms. K is 29 years old and has epilepsy. Her driving license was revoked when she was first diagnosed with epilepsy and she has continued to have seizures every three to four months while on treatment. Ms. K mentions in passing to her physician that she sometimes drives short distances to get groceries. When her physician challenges her about this she says her seizures are very infrequent. Finally, the physician tells her he may have to notify the authorities. Ms. K asks what more the authorities can do as they have already revoked her license. Are they going to leave a police car outside her house to make sure she doesn't drive?

What is confidentiality?

If a person gives information to another in confidence there is an obligation on the person receiving the information not to disclose it to someone else. This obligation, or duty, of confidentiality can be invoked explicitly by the provider of information stating that the information must not be shared, or it can be implicit in the nature of the relationship between the provider and receiver of information. Consequently, there is both an individual and a public expectation that information given to a health professional in the context of the clinical relationship will not be disclosed to third parties. The duty of confidentiality provides the foundation for trust in the therapeutic relationship. Professional organizations and regulatory bodies place great importance on the duty of confidentiality, and health professionals who breach confidentiality may be subject to disciplinary proceedings.

However, there is also an understanding that confidentiality cannot be absolute and that sometimes it may be permissible, or even legally required, to breach confidentiality. The increasing capability to generate and disseminate information in healthcare, together with the increasing complexity of healthcare provision, has implications for our understanding of the nature and limits of confidentiality. Development of multidisciplinary healthcare teams raises questions of how much information can be shared within the team, and who is recognized as a team member for this purpose. Access to electronic patient records for research and management purposes provides a "public interest" challenge to individual confidentiality, which expands the boundary of confidentiality beyond the context of individual patient care

An earlier version of this chapter has appeared: Kleinman, I., Baylis, F., Rodgers, S., and Singer, P. A. (1997). Confidentiality, *CMAJ* **156**: 521–4.

(Ingelfinger and Drazen, 2004; Peto *et al.*, 2004; Powell and Buchan, 2005). Advances in genetic testing have prompted debate about whether genetic information creates different responsibilities regarding confidentiality (Hallowell *et al.*, 2003; Plantinga *et al.*, 2003; Parker and Lucassen, 2004).

Breach of confidentiality is generally perceived as a deliberate disclosure of information to a third party. However, inadvertent breaches of confidentiality that are easily preventable may also occur in healthcare: a conversation about an "interesting case" in the hospital elevator, patients' names and/or diagnoses displayed in a manner visible to non-treating individuals. Healthcare workers should be aware of the risks of inadvertent breaches of confidentiality and take steps to avoid them.

Why is confidentiality important?

Ethics

There are a number of moral foundations for the importance of confidentiality in healthcare. The expectation that information disclosed to a health professional will remain confidential encourages patients to be open with their clinician. If patients thought this was not the case, they may withhold important information that is necessary for effective treatment or for protection of others. For example, some patients may not feel secure in confiding their dependence on drugs or alcohol and, therefore, not receive appropriate treatment. The benefit generated by the rule of confidentiality is usually considered to outweigh any harm or disadvantage, for example restrictions on research or management inefficiencies. Of equal, if not greater, importance than this consequentialist justification for confidentiality is the clinician's duty to respect patient autonomy in medical decision making. Competent patients have a right to control the use of information pertaining to themselves. A clinician who shares that information with others, without the patient's consent, does not respect the patient's autonomy and will,

therefore, have behaved in a morally questionable way – even if no harm results, indeed even if the patient is unaware of the breach of confidentiality. A further moral consideration for the importance of confidentiality in the clinician–patient relationship arises from the nature of the relationship and the duties generated by that relationship. There is an implied promise that confidences will be respected in this particular relationship and the clinician has a duty to keep this promise. Breaking such a promise is a betrayal of trust.

Although there are strong moral arguments for taking confidentiality very seriously, there are counter-arguments to support breach of confidentiality in some circumstances. While considerations of utility generally provide a strong argument for maintaining confidentiality, they could also justify breaching confidentiality if there is a risk of serious harm to either the patient or others. This line of reasoning is also used to argue for greater access to patient data for research and public health purposes, for instance, the benefit to the common good outweighs the harm to the individuals' loss of control over their personal data.

Even the principle of autonomy is not absolute. As John Stuart Mill observed in 1859, personal freedom may legitimately be constrained when the exercise of such freedom places others at risk of harm (Mill, 1962). In the context of confidentiality, this suggests that a patient's right to control how personal information is shared with others is constrained by an obligation not to harm others. When harm is threatened, the primacy of autonomy, and hence the duty to preserve confidentiality, no longer takes precedence, and disclosure without the patient's authorization may be permissible or required.

Law

The principle of confidentiality is also underpinned by law. In the UK, the courts have stated that there is a public interest in maintaining medical confidentiality against which any breach of confidentiality in the public interest must be weighed

(*W* v. *Edgell*, 1990). In some countries, there is statutory legislation requiring physicians to respect patient confidentiality. A legislative survey of confidentiality laws in the USA found that 37 US states impose a duty on physicians to maintain confidentiality of medical records, and 42 states protected information received during a clinical consultation from disclosure in court proceedings with some exceptions (Gostin, *et al.*, 1996). Several countries have legislation to protect written and electronic information held as part of a medical record, for example the UK Data Protection Act (1998), State legislation in the USA (Gostin *et al.*, 1996), and the Federal Privacy Act in Australia (1988).

Legal requirements to disclose certain kinds of information are defined in statutory legislation in many countries. These requirements commonly relate to information about specified diseases, suspicion of child abuse, and some criminal proceedings. Some US state legislation permits disclosure of health information for epidemiological and research purposes (Gostin *et al.*, 1996). The UK Data Protection Act (1998) allows disclosure of anonymized information for certain types of research. In addition to statutes, the common law recognizes that breach of confidentiality is lawful in some circumstances, mainly when there is a risk of serious harm to others if confidentiality is maintained. In the case of *W* v. *Edgell* (1990) in the UK, the Court of Appeal held that the breach of confidence in this case regarding a prisoner in a secure hospital was justified in the public interest, in order to protect the public from dangerous criminal acts. However, the Court said the risk must be "real, immediate and serious" to justify such a breach. A key US case was that of *Tarassoff* v. *Regents of the University of California* (1976). This involved a psychologist who had reason to believe that his patient would kill a woman (Ms. Tarassoff). At the psychologist's request, the campus police arrested the patient, but he was later released. Ms. Tarassoff was not informed and was later killed by the patient. The California Supreme Court established a duty to protect that may or may not include a warning to the potential victim or to the police. Both the Tarassoff and Edgell judgments rested on the risk of serious harm to others if confidentiality was not breached. This raises the question of what level of risk and harm are necessary to justify a breach of confidence, or underpin a duty to warn. Recent advances in genetic diagnosis have led to a debate on the nature of the duty of physicians to inform family members of the risk of hereditary disease, and the US courts have already considered cases brought against physicians in this area with conflicting results (Offit *et al.*, 2004).

Policy

The Hippocratic Oath explicitly demands confidentiality in physicians' dealings with patients (Edelstein, 1943): "What I may see or hear in the course of the treatment in regard to the life of men, which on no account one must spread abroad, I will keep to myself, holding such things shameless to be spoken about." The Hippocratic Oath, and subsequent codes of ethics, such as the *International Code of Ethics* of the World Medical Association (1949), admit no exceptions to the duty of confidentiality. However, more recent professional guidance does accept that breaches of confidentiality may be justified, or even required, in some circumstances. Professional codes of ethics (American Medical Association, 1995; Australian Medical Association, 2004; Canadian Medical Association, 2004; General Medical Council, 2004) specify that confidentiality can be breached if required by law, or in circumstances where there is a significant risk of serious harm to others.

Most professional guidance emphasizes the importance of seeking consent from the patient to disclose information if possible, or that the patient is informed that disclosure will occur if the patient refuses to give consent and the risk of harm is thought to justify disclosure. Guidance on informing family members of genetic risk is less clear, unless it falls into the category of representing a significant risk of serious harm. The American

Medical Association (2006) advises that the duty of the physician is to inform the patient of the need to discuss implications of test results with family members, and to offer to facilitate this discussion.

Sharing information within the healthcare team or with others involved in the patient's care is usually seen as acceptable if the information is necessary for effective patient care. Implied consent for this type of disclosure is assumed. However, if information is to be shared with other organizations outside healthcare, for example social services, then patient's consent may be required. In some instances, a professional body may advise that disclosure of information in the public interest is necessary even if not specifically required by legislation.

Empirical studies

An increasing number of empirical studies have looked at the attitudes of patients and healthcare professionals to issues of confidentiality. Sankar *et al.* (2003) conducted a literature review of studies of patients' perceptions of confidentiality and concluded that many patients are unaware of, or misunderstand, the legal and ethical duty of confidentiality, and a significant minority of patients distrust clinicians to protect confidential information to the extent that they will delay or forgo medical care because of this concern. Patients have different views about what information should be kept confidential (Jenkins *et al.*, 2005). Implicit consent to sharing of medical information between healthcare professionals cannot always be assumed. Schers *et al.* (2003) found that patients did not always accept that on-call general practitioners should have full access to their medical records. Carman and Britten (1995) found that patients viewed access by hospital staff to their records as less of a concern than access by staff within their general practice clinic. Young people may be more concerned about their confidentiality being preserved than older adults, and concern over confidentiality in relation to sexual health

services for teenage girls may impede uptake of such services (Reddy *et al.*, 2002; Carlisle *et al.*, 2006). Studies of health professionals also show confusion in this area. Marshall and Solomon (2003) found that 54% of providers of mental health services were confused over what type of information is confidential, and that conservative approaches to confidentiality were thought to be a barrier to collaborative care of patients with mental illness.

Physicians' attitudes to confidentiality vary depending on the country in which they practice. French general practitioners are more likely to be paternalistic in their attitude to patient confidentiality than those in Denmark (Mabeck, 1985). In the Netherlands, 35% of general practitioners would only disclose information to another physician (Lako *et al.*, 1990). A study of family doctors in Spain found that 95% would disclose information to a patient's family, and 35% would do so without seeking the patient's permission (Perez-Carceles *et al.*, 2005). Health professionals may inadvertently breach confidentiality through carelessness or because of physical limitations of privacy in an institutional setting. Several studies have found that hospital lifts are a common setting for breaches of patient confidentiality (Ubel *et al.*, 1995; Vigod *et al.*, 2003) and in one study of privacy in an emergency department, 36% of patients heard conversations from another room or the corridor (Olsen and Sabin, 2003).

How should I approach confidentiality in practice?

Clinicians must respect their patients' confidences. Private information, particularly if identifiable, should only be disclosed to a third party with the consent of the patient. If the patient lacks competence then, depending on jurisdiction, either the consent of the patient's representative is required or disclosure should be discussed with the patient's representatives and only occur if it is in the patient's best interests. Clinicians should be aware of the legal requirements for disclosure of patient information in their own countries, and whenever possible discuss such disclosures with patients beforehand.

When there is a significant risk of serious harm to another person or persons if information is not shared, and there is no statutory requirement to disclose, the duty to protect or warn may override the duty of confidentiality. In considering a breach of confidentiality in such cases it is important to balance the harm likely to arise if the information is not disclosed with the harm resulting from a breach of confidentiality. In determining the proportionality of these harms, the clinician must exercise his or her judgement. If in doubt, it would be prudent to seek advice from a professional organization or medical defense union. Prior to disclosing information, the clinician should seek to persuade the patient to consent to the disclosure, and if disclosure is made without consent, the patient should be informed that this will occur.

When disclosing information, it is necessary to consider to whom the information should be given and how much should be disclosed. Any breach of confidentiality should be limited to that necessary to prevent foreseeable harm. In situations where patient information is shared without explicit consent (e.g. with other health professionals, or use of data for research or disease registers), it is good practice to inform patients that this may occur, for example by explaining this in patient literature or notices in the clinic.

The cases

Mr. J's physician should advise him that his wife needs to be made aware of his condition, and that if necessary his wife will be informed without his consent. It is important to explain the reasons why his confidence may be breached in this situation, and to make every effort to maintain a therapeutic relationship with him, as he will require ongoing treatment and support for his condition. Spending some time discussing his concerns about disclosure and offering support to deal with these

concerns may bring about a change of mind on his part. In jurisdictions where notification of HIV status to a public health authority is legally required, this may provide further persuasion for Mr. J to consent to the sharing of information. The risk of serious harm to Mr. J's wife would be the justification for a breach of confidentiality. Clinicians need to be aware of the local legal and professional standards concerning how they should inform partners in a way that protects them from liability. Therefore, if the conclusion is that Mr. J's wife should be informed without his consent, discussion with a professional or defense organization, or the institutional legal advisor, would be sensible.

Ms. K's physician needs to consider the harm that may occur to her and others if she continues to drive and has a seizure while at the wheel. Apart from Ms. K, there is no clearly identifiable person who is in danger, unlike the case of Mr. J. The risk of her having a seizure while driving is low, given that she drives only for short journeys two or three times a week and has fairly infrequent seizures. However, the potential harm that could occur is very serious, including the possibility of death for several people. Ms. K's physician should counsel her regarding the risks to other people and to herself (including the financial risk as she will not be insured in the event of an accident). This may prove effective in persuading her to face up to her illness and the need to alter her lifestyle as a consequence. If she continues to drive, the physician must decide if the potential harm is sufficiently great to breach her confidence. Professional and legal guidance may vary on this issue in different countries or US States. In the UK, the General Medical Council (2004) provides clear direction that if the physician cannot persuade the patient to stop driving, or is given evidence that a patient is continuing to drive contrary to advice, relevant medical information should be disclosed immediately, in confidence, to the Medical Advisor of the Driver and Vehicle Licensing Authority (General Medical Council, 2004).

REFERENCES

American Medical Association (1995). *AMA Code of Ethics: Policy Statement on Confidentiality*. Washington, DC: American Medical Association.

American Medical Association (2006). *Disclosure of Familial Risk in Genetic Testing, Policy statement E.2.131*. Washington, DC: American Medical Association.

Australian Medical Association (2004). *Code of Ethics*. Barton, ACT: Australian Medical Association (http://www.ama.com.au/web.nsf/doc/WEEN-5WW598).

Canadian Medical Association (2004). *Code of Ethics*. Ottawa: Canadian Medical Association (http://policybase.cma.ca/PolicyPDF/PD04-06.pdf).

Carlisle, J., Shickle, D., Cork, M., and McDonagh, A. (2006). Concerns over confidentiality may deter adolescents from consulting their doctors. A qualitative exploration. *J Med Ethics* **32**: 133–7.

Carman, D. and Britten, N. (1995). Confidentiality of medical records: the patient's perspective. *Br J Gen Pract* **45**: 485–8.

Data Protection Act (1998). London: The Stationary Office (http://www.opsi.gov.uk/ACTS/acts1998/19980029.htm).

Edelstein, L. (1943). *Hippocratic Oath: Text, Translation and Interpretation*. Baltimore, MD: Johns Hopkins University Press.

Federal Privacy Act (1988). Canberra: Government Printing Office (http://www.privacy.gov.au/publications/privacy88_021205.pdf).

General Medical Council (2004). *Confidentiality: Protecting and Providing Information*. London: General Medical Council (http://www.gmc–uk.org/guidance/library/confidentiality.asp).

Gostin, L. O., Lazzarini, Z., and Flaherty, K. M. (1996). Legislative Survey of state confidentiality laws, with specific emphasis on HIV and immunization. *JAMA* **275**: 1921–7.

Hallowell, N., Foster, C., Eeles, R., *et al.* (2003). Balancing autonomy and responsibility: the ethics of generating and disclosing genetic information. *J Med Ethics* **29**: 74–9.

Ingelfinger, J. R. and Drazen, J. M. (2004). Registry research and medical privacy. *N Engl J Med* **350**: 1452–3.

Jenkins, G., Merz, J. F. and Sankar, P. (2005). A qualitative study of women's views on medical confidentiality. *J Med Ethics* **31**: 499–504.

Lako, C. J., Huygen, F. J., Lindenthal, J. J., and Persoon, J. M. (1990). Handling of confidentiality in general practice: a survey among general practitioners in the Netherlands. *Fam Pract* **7**: 34–8.

Mabeck, C. E. (1985). Confidentiality in general practice. *Fam Pract* **2**: 199–204.

Marshall, T. and Solomon, P. (2003). Professionals' responsibilities in releasing information to families of adults with mental illness. *Psychiatr Serv* **54**: 1622–8.

Mill, J. S. (1962). On liberty. In *Utilitarianism: John Stuart Mill*, ed. M. Warnock. Glasgow: HarperCollins, pp. 126–250.

Offit, K., Groeger, E., Turner, S., Wadsworth, E. A., and Weiser, M. A. (2004). The "duty to warn" a patient's family members about hereditary disease risks. *JAMA* **292**: 1469–73.

Olsen, J. C. and Sabin, B. R. (2003). Emergency department patient perceptions of privacy and confidentiality. *J Emerg Med* **25**: 329–33.

Parker, M. and Lucassen, A. M. (2004). Genetic information: a joint account? *BMJ* **329**: 165–7.

Perez-Carceles, M. D., Pereniguez, J. E., Osuna, E., and Luna, A. (2005). Balancing confidentiality and the information provided to families of patients in primary care. *J Med Ethics* **31**: 531–5.

Peto, J., Fletcher, O., and Gilham, C. (2004). Data protection, informed consent, and research. *BMJ* **328**: 1029–30.

Plantinga, L., Natowicz, M. R., Kass, N. E. *et al.* (2003). Disclosure, confidentiality, and families: experiences and attitudes of those with genetic versus nongenetic medical conditions. *Am J Med Genet C Semin Med Genet* **119**: 51–9.

Powell, J. and Buchan, I. (2005). Electronic health records should support clinical research. *J Med Internet Res* **7**: e4.

Reddy, D. M., Fleming, R., and Swain, C. (2002). Effect of mandatory parental notification on adolescent girls' use of sexual health care services. *JAMA* **288**: 710–14.

Sankar, P., Mora, S., Merz, J. F., and Jones, N. L. (2003). Patient perspectives of medical confidentiality: a review of the literature. *J Gen Intern Med* **18**: 659–69.

Schers, H., van den Horst, H., Grol, R., and van den Berg, W. (2003). Continuity of information in general practice. Patient views on confidentiality. *Scand J Prim Health Care* **21**: 21–6.

Tarassoff v. *Regents of the University of California* [1976] 529 P 2d 553 118, Cal Rptr 333.

Ubel, P. A., Zell, M. M., Miller, D. J., *et al.* (1995). Elevator talk: observational study of inappropriate comments in a public space. *Am J Med* **99**: 190–4.

Vigod, S. N., Bell, C. M. and Bohnen, J. M. (2003). Privacy of patients' information in hospital lifts: observational study. *BMJ* **327**: 1024–25.

W v. *Edgell* 1 All ER 835. High Court ([1990]).

World Medical Association (1949). *International Code of Ethics*. Washington, DC: World Medical Association (http://www.wma.net/e/policy/c8.htm).

End of life care

Introduction

James A. Tulsky

Dying patients confront complex and unique challenges that threaten their physical, psychosocial, and spiritual integrity. Many patients die prolonged and painful deaths, receiving unwanted, expensive, and invasive care. Patients' suffering at the end of life can be profound, yet healthcare providers are too frequently ill-equipped to respond to this suffering. Excellent palliative care demands careful attention to diagnostic, prognostic, and therapeutic challenges. The clinician must demonstrate sensitivity to psychosocial and spiritual concerns and provide thoughtful, empathic communication with patients and families. Yet, even when these are done with superb skill, patients and providers will still find that the experience of living with life-limiting illness presents ethical dilemmas. Some are subtle and, perhaps, not recognized. Other dilemmas are easily apparent. This section outlines the key ethical challenges in caring for patients at the end of life.

Chapter 8 is on quality end of life care and presents a conceptual framework with three main elements: (i) control of pain and other symptoms, (ii) decisions on the use of life-sustaining treatments, and (iii) support of dying patients and their families. These elements are key to delivering quality care. They are also the nexus upon which ethical conflicts arise. For example, control of pain, in its extreme, may hasten death. Decisions on the use of life-sustaining treatments depend upon advance care planning and, in its absence, substitute decision making. And support of dying patients and their families recognizes the important role for healthcare providers even when conflicts arise.

Chapters 9 and 10 focus on decision making. The first covers what to do when someone is ill, cannot make decisions for themselves, and has not left clear instructions in the form of an advance directive. This chapter offers detailed suggestions for walking through this process. Chapter 10, on advance care planning, describes the conceptual underpinning of decision making in palliative medicine. The chapter argues that advance care planning is a process with multiple goals, not all of which are directly related to decision making. From the perspective of patients and families, advance care planning also allows them to maintain a sense of control, relieve the burden on loved ones, and strengthen relationships. The process also highlights critical culture differences, always important in bioethics, but which emerge prominently at the end of life. When advance care planning is considered in this total sense, satisfying multiple objectives, clinicians recognize the need to approach patients and families as partners with curiosity and compassion.

We then consider the thorny issues related to euthanasia and assisted suicide (Ch. 11). In many ways, this topic has driven much of the debate about palliative care, even though relatively few people express a true desire to control the time and place of their death in this way. Assisted dying has likely become a flashpoint because such a choice explores most directly questions of what is killing versus letting die at the end of life, and whether such decisions are justified in the face of overwhelming suffering. There is a fair amount of public support for the concept of assisted death, yet it remains illegal in most jurisdictions and these laws are unlikely to change. This probably reflects the high regard for life in all societies, and the strong hesitation to lessen prohibitions against killing, even when some may feel it is the most compassionate option.

Chapter 12 addresses conflict in the healthcare setting at end of life. As much as assisted suicide has dominated news about end of life care in recent years, for the clinician, it is bedside conflicts around treatment decisions that are most prevalent and troubling. Whereas landmark bioethics cases such as Quinlan and Cruzan focused on families wishing to withdraw life-sustaining interventions, most conflicts today arise between clinicians who wish to withhold what they perceive as futile care and families requesting more aggressive treatment. This chapter offers an approach that examines family, healthcare provider, and social/organizational features contributing to these conflicts, and it encourages identifying responsible factors prior to negotiating a solution.

Finally, the last chapter in this section discusses brain death. The diagnosis is described, differentiated from other phenomena such as vegetative state, and criteria given. The authors also discuss the social and legal implications of using a brain death standard and offer an approach to its application in practice.

Caring for patients facing the end of life is difficult for all involved. Frequently, the ethical questions are considerably more challenging than the medical care itself. We hope this section provides the reader with a framework within which to approach these questions.

8

Quality end of life care

Peter A. Singer, Neil MacDonald, and James A. Tulsky

Dr. A is sitting at home enjoying dinner when the phone rings. The caller is Mr. B, an acquaintance. He is distraught. He asks how much air must be injected into an intravenous line to cause a person to die. When asked why he wants to know, he explains that his 72-year-old father, currently a patient in a local hospital, has end-stage metastatic lung cancer and is in excruciating pain. Mr. B cannot bear to see his father in such pain and wants to end his suffering by means of an air embolism.

Mr. C, a 68-year-old man with a 100 pack-per-year history of smoking and known chronic obstructive pulmonary disease, presents to the emergency department with pneumonia and respiratory failure. He has been intubated four times before for respiratory failure. He uses oxygen at home and is dyspneic at rest. He has hypoxemia, hypercapnia, and is delirious. The emergency physician, Dr. D, tries to stabilize his condition with oxygen, bronchodilators, steroids, and non-invasive ventilation, but Mr. C's respiratory status worsens. Dr. D cannot locate Mr. C's family. She calls Mr. C's family physician and respirologist to find out whether they have ever discussed re-intubation, but unfortunately neither has done so. Although she is uncomfortable with this situation because of the uncertainty about the patient's wishes, Dr. D decides to perform the intubation.

What is quality end of life care?

A clinician who receives a call from the emergency department to see a patient with heart failure will have a clear concept of what heart failure is,

as well as a framework within which to approach the condition and its management. Unfortunately, clinicians may not have an analogous conceptual framework for approaching end of life care. Several aspects of end of life care are addressed in other chapters, especially those on truth telling, consent, capacity, substitute decision making, advance care planning, euthanasia and assisted suicide, and conflict in the healthcare setting at end of life. Care of patients at the end of life is best provided by, or in consultation with, clinicians with expert training in palliative care. The World Health Organization (WHO) defines palliative care as "an approach that improves the quality of life of patients and their families facing the problem associated with life-threatening illness, through the prevention and relief of suffering by means of early identification and impeccable assessment and treatment of pain and other problems, physical, psychosocial and spiritual" (http://www.who.int/cancer/palliative/definition/en/). However, in practice, much care for dying patients is provided by other physicians and healthcare workers. By "quality end of life care" we mean a coherent conceptual framework that clinicians can use to approach the care of patients at the end of life. It is a term that pulls together concepts that previously had been fragmented across fields such as bioethics and palliative care. We also want to emphasize that quality of care for patients at the end of life is just as important as at other

An earlier version of this chapter has appeared: Singer, P. A. and MacDonald, N. (1998). Quality end-of-life care. *CMAJ* **159**: 159–62.

times, although historically this has not been mirrored in the care patients receive. A framework for quality end of life care is described in greater detail on p. 55. It has three main elements: control of pain and other symptoms, decisions on the use of life-sustaining treatment, and support of dying patients and their families. These elements are based on empirical research described in the relevant section below.

Why is quality end of life care important?

Ethics and law

From an ethical perspective, beneficence requires that pain and other symptoms be controlled. The legal status of control of pain and other symptoms is not absolutely clear, but clinicians should not risk legal peril if they follow established guidelines distinguishing these practices from euthanasia. (Hawryluck *et al.*, 2002). Advance care planning is used to justify much decision making at the end of life and is ethically supported by respect for autonomy and is legally recognized in most Western countries. Decisions by patients or substitute decision makers to withhold or withdraw life-sustaining treatment proposed by a clinician are also supported by the ethical principle of respect for autonomy and the legal doctrine of informed consent (Etchells *et al.*, 1996a, b; Lazar *et al.*, 1996). In contrast, the ethical and legal issues related to inappropriate use of life-sustaining treatments demanded by patients and substitute decisions makers over the objections of physicians are not as clear (Weijer *et al.*, 1998). Both euthanasia and assisted suicide are illegal in all but a few jurisdictions (see Ch. 11 for more information).

Policy

Advocates have framed end of life care as an issue in healthcare quality: a positive development in that it focuses organizational commitment to quality on the problem of end of life care. But what does quality end of life care entail? The WHO definition of palliative care cited above was the earliest attempt to describe what was needed for patients facing death. The Committee on Care at the End of Life of the US Institute of Medicine, National Academy of Sciences, has proposed the following six categories of quality end of life care: overall quality of life, physical well-being and functioning, psychosocial well-being and functioning, spiritual well-being, patient perception of care, and family well-being and perceptions (Field and Cassel, 1997). The National Consensus Project *Clinical Practice Guidelines for Quality Palliative Care* built upon these categories (National Consensus Project, 2005). This document, endorsed by all major US palliative care organizations, defined the following aspects of care as critical to quality: structure and processes; physical, psychological and psychiatric, social, spiritual, religious and existential, cultural care of the imminently dying patient; and ethical and legal aspects of care.

Empirical studies

Although euthanasia has often consumed the attention of the media, the critical ethical issues vexing clinicians, patients, and families lie elsewhere. Singer *et al.* (1999) published a study identifying the domains of quality end of life care from the patient's perspective: this can be seen as the evidence basis for the approach outlined below. In a survey of 1462 patients, bereaved family members, and healthcare providers, the following factors were considered of greatest importance at the end of life: pain and symptom management, preparation for death, achieving a sense of completion, decisions about treatment preferences, and being treated as a "whole person" (Steinhauser *et al.*, 2000). Respondents ranked freedom from pain and being at peace with God as most important. Unfortunately, pain is often poorly managed (Portenoy *et al.*, 1992; Cleeland *et al.*, 1994; SUPPORT Principal Investigators, 1995). In one study of older patients who were conscious during the last three days of life, 4 in 10 had severe pain most of the time (Lynn *et al.*, 1997). Decision making is also problematic. In a survey of physicians and nurses at five US hospitals, 47% of respondents reported that they had acted against their conscience in providing care to the terminally ill, and 55% reported that they sometimes felt the treatments they offered patients were overly burdensome (Solomon *et al.*, 1993). Consistent with the recent focus of policy efforts, quality-improvement strategies have been applied at the organizational level to the problem of end of life care (Baker *et al.*, 1998; Cleary and Edgman-Levitan, 1997). For example, a randomized, controlled trial examined the effect of a clinical care path containing ethics consultations on the outcomes of seriously ill in intensive care units patients (Schneiderman *et al.*, 2003). The intervention resulted in more rapid withdrawal of life-sustaining treatments, with increased provider and patient surrogate satisfaction. Processes such as these or, for instance, focusing traditional "morbidity and mortality rounds" on quality end of life care, can change the culture within an institution such that quality healthcare includes attending to the needs of dying patients.

How should I approach quality end of life care in practice?

To address this question, we recommend a conceptual framework with three main elements: (i) control of pain and other symptoms, (ii) decisions on the use of life-sustaining treatments, and (iii) support of dying patients and their families. We do not believe that a conceptual framework will magically solve the documented problems in end of life care; we do, however, believe that this is an important step.

Control of pain and other symptoms

No patient should die in pain or with other treatable symptoms. Indeed, before social, psychosocial, and spiritual problems can be properly addressed, good symptom control must first be achieved: it is difficult to contemplate spiritual issues or to reflect on life's accomplishments when in pain or with kidney

basin in hand. The undertreatment of pain and other symptoms is well documented, but aside from inadequate training of health professionals (Von Roenn *et al.*, 1993; MacDonald *et al.*, 1997), the causes are complicated and not well understood. On occasion, clinicians may be concerned about balancing good symptom control with the risk of hastening death. Guidelines have been developed to assist clinicians in distinguishing appropriate analgesia from euthanasia by lethal injection (Hawryluck *et al.*, 2002). Controlling other symptoms, such as nausea, fatigue and breathlessness, may be even more challenging than controlling pain, but effective approaches have been developed (von Gunten, 2005). Clinicians must keep in mind that the problems of dying patients have their genesis at an earlier time in the trajectory of illness. Therefore, palliative care should not be isolated as simply an end of life option; it must be intermeshed with therapies aimed at prolongation of life or cure. As in other areas of medicine, prevention or early control of a symptom is preferable to a rescue attempt on preventable, but now out of control, suffering. All clinicians who care for dying patients should ensure that they have adequate skills in this domain, as well as access to skilled consultative help from palliative care specialists.

Use of life-sustaining treatments

To the extent possible, patients and their families should be able to choose the site and nature of the care that the patient will receive in the last days of life and should be encouraged to discuss in advance their desires regarding life-sustaining treatments and personal care. Clinicians should facilitate this advance care planning (Teno *et al.*, 1994; Emanuel *et al.*, 1995; Singer *et al.*, 1996, 1998; Martin *et al.*, 1999) and guide and support the patient and the family through the process of giving consent to treatment and arranging for substitute decision making (Lazar *et al.*, 1996). A key skill here is empathic communication with patients and families (Tulsky, 2005). In addition, physicians need to develop an approach to the opposite problem when the patient or the family demands treatment that the physician feels is inappropriate (see Ch. 12). Another key skill here is the ability to negotiate a treatment plan that is acceptable to the patient, the family, and the healthcare team (Fisher and Ury, 1991).

Support of patients and their families

The support that each patient and his or her family needs from the clinician is unique. The best way to find out what support will be appropriate in a particular situation is to use reflective listening skills and to be available to help. Attention to psychosocial issues demands involvement of the patients and their families as partners. Although clinicians should be sensitive to the range of psychosocial distress and social disruption common to dying patients and their families, they may not be as available or as skilled as nurses, social workers, and other healthcare professionals in addressing certain issues. An interdisciplinary healthcare team can help in these areas. Spiritual issues often come to the fore as one is dying, and pastoral care teams and other interventions should be available to assist the patient's own clergy in counseling (Chochinov and Cann, 2005). A simple question such as "Are you at Peace?" may identify those patients with spiritual suffering (Steinhauser *et al.*, 2006). Although not all families need or desire follow-up after the death of a loved one, many appreciate a letter or a telephone call from the physician or a member of the palliative care team (Bedell *et al.*, 2001). Some families will need more specific help. Clinicians should be sensitive to risk factors for poor adjustment to bereavement and should be knowledgeable about local bereavement services (El-Jawahri and Prigerson, 2007).

The cases

Both of the cases presented at the beginning of this chapter represent failures in end of life care. In the first, inadequate pain control led to a desire for euthanasia. What was needed was not an air

embolism but better pain control. When this was achieved, Mr. B was relieved and did not pursue the idea of euthanasia. This case also illustrates that physicians should not take requests for euthanasia at face value; rather, they should explore and address the suffering that might have led to such requests. The second case represents a failure of communication about life-sustaining treatments. Mr. C had end-stage lung disease and had been intubated four times previously, so he was ideally situated to know whether he wanted to undergo the procedure again. Indeed, it is very likely that he had considered this possibility. If he did want intubation, knowledge of his wishes would have relieved Dr. D's anxiety. (Although death was looming, it would be difficult to claim that intubation would be futile in this case, given that it had worked before.) If Mr. C did not want to undergo intubation, he missed his opportunity to communicate this desire. Arguably, the family physician and the respirologist should have broached this issue with him and helped him to make his wishes known in such a way that they would be effectively communicated when respiratory failure occurred.

In summary, physicians caring for patients at the end of their lives should ask themselves three questions. Am I managing this patient's pain and other symptoms adequately? Have I addressed the relevant issues with respect to the use of life-sustaining treatment? Am I supporting this person and his or her family?

REFERENCES

Baker, G. R., Gelmon, S., Headrick, L., *et al.* (1998). Collaborating for improvement in health professions education. *Qual Manag Health Care* **6**: 1–11.

Bedell, S. E., Cadenhead, K., and Graboys, T. B. (2001). The doctor's letter of condolence. *N Engl J Med* **344**: 1162–4.

Chochinov, H. M. and Cann, B. J. (2005). Interventions to enhance the spiritual aspects of dying. *J Palliat Med* **8**(Suppl 1): S103–15.

Cleary, P. D. and Edgman-Levitan, S. (1997). Health care quality. Incorporating consumer perspectives. *JAMA* **278**: 1608–12.

Cleeland, C. S., Gonin, R., Hatfield, A. K., *et al.* (1994). Pain and its treatment in outpatients with metastatic cancer. *N Engl J Med* **330**: 592–6.

El-Jawahri, A. R. and Prigerson, H. G. (2007). Bereavement care. In *Principles and Practice of Palliative Care and Supportive Oncology*, 3rd edn, ed. A. M. Berger, J. L. Shuster, and J. H. von Roenn. Philadelphia, PA: Lippincott Williams and Wilkins, pp. 645–53.

Emanuel, L. L., Danis, M., Pearlman, R. A., and Singer, P. A. (1995). Advance care planning as a process: structuring the discussions in practice. *J Am Geriatr Soc* **43**: 440–6.

Etchells, E., Sharpe, G., Elliott, C., and Singer, P. A. (1996a). Bioethics for clinicians: 3. Capacity. *CMAJ* **155**: 657–61.

Etchells, E., Sharpe, G., Walsh, P., Williams, J. R., and Singer, P. A. (1996b). Bioethics for clinicians: 1. Consent. *CMAJ* **155**: 177–80.

Field, M. J. and Cassel, C. K. (1997). *Approaching Death: Improving Care at the End of Life*. Washington, DC: Institute of Medicine.

Fisher, R. and Ury, W. (1991). *Getting to Yes: Negotiating Agreement Without Giving In*. New York: Penguin Books.

Hawryluck, L. A., Harvey, W. R. C., Lemieux-Charles, L., and Singer, P. A. (2002). Consensus guidelines on analgesia and sedation in dying intensive care patients. *BMC Med Ethics* **3**: 3.

Lazar, N. M., Greiner, G. G., Robertson, G., and Singer, P. A. (1996). Bioethics for clinicians: 5. Substitute decision-making. *CMAJ* **155**: 1435–7.

Lynn, J., Teno, J. M., Phillips, R. S., *et al.* (1997). Perceptions by family members of the dying experience of older and seriously ill patients. *Ann Intern Med* **126**: 97–106.

MacDonald, N., Findlay, H. P., Bruera, E., Dudgeon, D., and Kramer, J. (1997). A Canadian survey of issues in cancer pain management. *J Pain Symptom Manage* **14**: 332–42.

Martin, D. K., Thiel, E. C., and Singer, P. A. (1999). A new model of advance care planning: observations from people with HIV. *Arch Intern Med* **159**: 86–92.

National Consensus Project (2005). *Clinical Practice Guidelines for Quality Palliative Care*. Pittsberg, PA: American Academy of Hospice and Palliative Care (www.nationalconsensusproject.org).

Portenoy, R. K., Miransky, J., Thaler, H. T., *et al.* (1992). Pain in ambulatory patients with lung or colon cancer.

Prevalence, characteristics, and effect. *Cancer* **70**: 1616–24.

Schneiderman, L. J., Gilmer, T., Teetzel, H. D., *et al.* (2003). Effect of ethics consultations on nonbeneficial life-sustaining treatments in the intensive care setting: a randomized controlled trial. *JAMA* **290**: 1166–72.

Singer, P. A., Robertson, G., and Roy, D. J. (1996). Bioethics for clinicians: 6. Advance care planning. *CMAJ* **155**: 1689–92.

Singer, P. A., Martin, D. K., Lavery, J. V., *et al.* (1998). Reconceptualizing advance care planning from the patient's perspective. *Arch Intern Med* **158**: 879–84.

Singer P. A., Martin D. K., and Kelner M. (1999). Quality end of life care: patients' perspectives. *JAMA* **281**: 163–8.

Solomon, M. Z., O'Donnell, L., Jennings, B., *et al.* (1993). Decisions near the end of life: professional views on life-sustaining treatments. *Am J Public Health* **83**: 14–23.

Steinhauser, K. E., Christakis, N. A., Clipp, E. C., *et al.* (2000). Factors considered important at the end of life by patients, family, physicians, and other care providers. *JAMA* **284**: 2476–82.

Steinhauser, K. E., Voils, C. I., Clipp, E. C., *et al.* (2006). "Are you at peace?": one item to probe spiritual concerns at the end of life. *Arch Intern Med* **166**: 101–5.

SUPPORT Principal Investigators (1995). A controlled trial to improve care for seriously ill hospitalized patients: The study to understand prognosis and preferences for outcomes and risks of treatments (SUPPORT). *JAMA* **274**: 1591–8.

Teno, J. M., Nelson, H. L., and Lynn, J. (1994). Advance care planning. Priorities for ethical and empirical research. *Hastings Cent Rep* **24**: S32–6.

Tulsky, J. A. (2005). Beyond advance directives: importance of communication skills at the end of life. *JAMA* **294**: 359–65.

Von Gunten, C. F. (2005). Interventions to manage symptoms at the end of life. *J Palliat Med* **8**: (Suppl. 1): S88–94.

Von Roenn, J. H., Cleeland, C. S., Gonin, R., Hatfield, A. K., and Pandya, K. J. (1993). Physician attitudes and practice in cancer pain management. A survey from the Eastern Cooperative Oncology Group. *Ann Intern Med* **119**: 121–6.

Weijer, C., Singer, P. A., Dickens, B. M., and Workman, S., (1998). Bioethics for clinicians: 16. Dealing with demands for inappropriate treatment. *CMAJ* **159**: 817–21.

9

Substitute decision making

Robert A. Pearlman

Mr. E is a 35-year-old man with advanced AIDS who has recently been diagnosed with AIDS-related dementia. When he still had decision-making capacity he told his partner, but not his close family members, that if he ever "lost his mind" because of his HIV infection, he would want to receive only comfort measures for any new medical problem. During the past two weeks Mr. E's caregivers have noticed that he is having increasing difficulty breathing. In view of his medical history they think he probably has a recurrence of Pneumocystis carinii *pneumonia (PCP). Mr. E is brought to the hospital for a chest X-ray to confirm these impressions. This shows probable PCP. The physician knows that Mr. E has had a lot of difficulty with adverse drug reactions in the past and wonders whether or not the patient should be admitted to the hospital for further investigations and treatment.*

Mrs. F is an 83-year-old widow with advanced chronic obstructive pulmonary disease (COPD) and osteoporosis. Approximately six months ago Mrs. F was hospitalized for six days because of an acute exacerbation of her COPD. Since discharge, her breathing has not improved to her prehospitalization status. Three months ago, she moved into a nursing home because of her deteriorating health and difficulty in caring for herself. In the nursing home, she has shortness of breath at rest, which is made worse with eating. Her closest family members are her three married children. One daughter lives in the same city, and the other two children live more than an hour away by car. Earlier today, Mrs. F's breathing deteriorated suddenly and she was transferred to the hospital for assessment and treatment. When she is seen in the emergency department she is confused because of either

respiratory failure or the toxic effects of an infection. Blood analysis reveals hypoxemia and respiratory acidosis. The attending physician wonders whether or not Mrs. F should be intubated, especially if her situation does not improve with additional bronchodilators and steroids. She has never required intubation before, and her hospital records give no instructions with regard to resuscitation. Mrs. F's daughter has just arrived and is waiting to talk to the physician.

What is substitute decision making?

Patients with decision-making capacity may accept or refuse medical recommendations and this often occurs after they weigh the trade offs between likely benefits and risks of a proposed test or treatment. Healthcare providers assess the medical situation and offer recommendations, but patients' preferences and values reframe the information into patient-centered decisions. When a patient loses the capacity to participate meaningfully in the decision at hand, a mechanism must exist to make decisions that represent the patient's goals, preferences, and interests. This mechanism is substitute decision making, and it usually occurs when a spouse, partner, close family member, or friend assumes this responsibility on behalf of the incapacitated patient.

This model of decision making is based on two principal assumptions: the individual is the primary

An earlier version of this chapter has appeared: Lazar, N.M., Greiner, G.G., Robertson, G., and Singer, P.A. (1996). Substitute decision-making. *CMAJ* **155**: 1435–37.

decision maker and decisions are the result of a rational weighing of benefits and risks. Both of these assumptions can be challenged. It is important that healthcare providers know whether their patients and substitute decision makers share these values. For example, in some cultural groups, the family unit or the oldest male is the appropriate decision maker. Therefore, although the remainder of this chapter proceeds assuming the dominant model of the rational, individual decision maker, healthcare providers need to be sensitive and responsive to cultural differences.

Why is substitute decision making important?

Ethics

The approach to medical decision making described above is rooted in the Western tradition of respect for patient autonomy and the right to self-determination (Buchanan and Brock, 1989). It is expressed most clearly in the practice of informed consent. Substitute decision making is an attempt, albeit an imperfect one, to extend patients control over their own healthcare after they can no longer exert direct control.

Healthcare providers often believe that they know what is best for the patient. Historically, healthcare providers frequently made decisions for patients without discussing it with them or their family members. However, the power to make medical decisions has been tempered over the last several decades, with greater appreciation for sharing information with patients and an appreciation for the patient's moral authority to decide what is done to his or her body. Moreover, healthcare providers often have values that are distinct from those of their patients and have difficulty predicting accurately their patients' preferences for life-sustaining treatments (Uhlmann *et al.*, 1988; Seckler *et al.*, 1991; Tsevat *et al.*, 1995). This lack of understanding of patients' preferences has even been demonstrated with physicians who report having talked to their long-term patients about their preferences and values (Uhlmann *et al.*, 1988).

Under certain conditions, healthcare providers may experience moral distress when caring for patients who have lost decision-making capacity. For example, when hospital-based healthcare providers confront major decisions for patients without decision-making capacity and without a substitute decision maker, there may be uncertainty about how to proceed. Uncertainty, by itself, and the decision to continue all active therapies without clear guidance anchored to goals of care are challenging situations for clinicians. The decision to keep treating without guidance also occurs when family members disagree about the right course of action. These situations have been associated with moral distress, especially for nurses, and moral distress is associated with burn-out and turnover (Jameton, 1984).

Law

In the USA and Canada, for instance, the legal approach to substitute decision making has primarily been two-pronged. In association with passage of the Patient Self-Determination Act (1990) and growing interest in advance directives, laws have been passed that enable individuals to designate the person they wish to make healthcare decisions for them once they lose decision-making capacity. In addition, laws pertaining to informed consent have given family members the right to make decisions on behalf of incapacitated patients. In some statutes, a hierarchy of substitute decision makers is provided. For example, in the state of Washington, the order of surrogacy is the court-appointed guardian, healthcare agent (through a durable power of attorney for healthcare), spouse, adult children, parents, and adult siblings (Washington State Legislature, 2006). An alternative to family-based substitute decision making is using the courts, such as assigning a court-appointed guardian. This mechanism exists in both the USA and Canada.

Policy

Substitute decision making is an important part of policies of healthcare facilities and professional organizations. For instance, the Canadian Medical Association policy on resuscitative interventions includes provisions related to substitute decision making (Canadian Medical Association, 1995). Similarly, the American Geriatric Society endorses the value of substitute decision making for patients who have lost decision-making capacity (American Geriatrics Society Ethics Committee, 1996). In the Veterans Health Administration (VHA), the largest healthcare system in the USA, the informed consent policy refers to substitute decision makers as surrogates. The policy states that, when a patient lacks decision-making capacity, the practitioner must make a reasonable inquiry as to the availability and authority of an advance directive naming a healthcare agent. If no healthcare agent is authorized and available, the practitioner must make a reasonable inquiry as to the availability of other possible surrogates according to the order of priority (legal guardian, spouse, adult child, parent, sibling, grandparent, grandchild, close friend) (Veterans Health Administration, 2003). This policy also outlines procedures for managing disagreements between healthcare providers and substitute decision makers.

Empirical studies

Empirical studies pertaining to substitute decision making have primarily focused on the role and experience of the substitute decision maker, and the level of concordance between patients' preferences and those of substitute decision makers. When patients are asked who they would want to represent them, the majority opt for their own family members (High, 1994). Although the primary role of substitute decision makers is to make healthcare decisions, their role is more complicated. Substitute decision makers usually try to do the right thing for their loved one while realistically taking into consideration their own interests. They also try to present to the healthcare providers a

more holistic picture of their loved one than that of a patient. In addition, they often serve a role in safeguarding the loved one's dignity (Chambers-Evans and Carnevale, 2005).

Research has demonstrated that family members have difficulty predicting accurately their loved one's preferences for life-sustaining treatments (Uhlmann et al., 1988; Pearlman et al., 2005). This has been shown even among family members involved in a study of advance care planning (Pearlman et al., 2005). Yet, if a conflict were to arise between a patient's prior wishes and what the substitute decision maker believes to be the best decision, patients prefer that the substitute decision maker's decision take priority over their previously stated wishes (Terry et al., 1999).

How should I approach substitute decision making in practice?

Any individual can become so sick that they cannot speak for themselves. Consequently, asking who is the preferred substitute decision maker should occur early in the development of a patient–provider relationship. In the outpatient setting, this can be raised in the context of getting to know the patient and his or her preferences better. Some patients lose decision-making capacity when they are hospitalized for an acute illness. Therefore, hospitalization is another opportunity for raising the question of substitute decision making.

Healthcare providers are able to identify patients at increased risk for losing decision-making capacity. They also understand that patients with families in conflict or without family pose a high risk for future problems should the patient lose decision-making capacity. Therefore, healthcare providers should target these patients for discussion about substitute decision makers if the need arises. These high risk situations include:

- early dementia
- history of a stroke
- health conditions that predispose to a future stroke (e.g., uncontrolled hypertension)

- health conditions that predispose to delirium (e.g., frailty, advanced age)
- terminal illness
- engaging in risky behaviors that are associated with brain injuries (e.g., riding convertible cars without using seat belts)
- recurrent severe psychiatric illnesses (e.g., severe dementia, mania, psychosis)
- families with conflicts
- social isolation (e.g., no family members or close friends).

Who should make the decision for the person who has lost decision-making capacity?

The substitute decision maker should be the person or persons with the best knowledge of the patient's specific wishes, or of the patient's values and beliefs, as they pertain to the present situation. In general, close relatives are preferred as substitute decision makers in the belief that they will know the patient well enough to replicate the decision that the patient would make if he or she were capable. However, the patient may be estranged from his or her spouse, parents, children, or siblings, and in some instances a friend will know the patient's wishes best.

In order to help patients to decide on the ideal candidates to be their substitute decision makers, healthcare providers may review with patients the following attributes:

- meets local legal requirements, if they exist, such as being a competent adult or at least 18 years of age (this is important if the person wishes to empower a healthcare agent through a durable power of attorney for healthcare)
- knows the patient well and is willing to speak on behalf of him or her
- is willing to talk with the patient now about sensitive issues
- would be able to act on/advocate for the patient's wishes and separate their own feelings
- would be able to solicit input from other intimates if the surrogate is unclear regarding what patient's wishes would have been

- ability to handle the responsibility, physically and emotionally
- available to meet with healthcare providers if needed
- ability to speak to healthcare providers as equal partners in decision making
- ability to handle conflicting opinions between family members, friends, and/or healthcare providers.

Sometimes a substitute decision maker is not available or appears to be making decisions that conflict with the patient's previously expressed preferences or best interests. In these circumstances a substitute decision maker may need to be appointed by a court of law. In many jurisdictions this takes significant amounts of time and adds to the costs of care (Teno *et al.*, 1995).

How should decisions be made for persons who have lost decision-making capacity?

The task of substitute decision makers is not to decide how they would want to be treated were they in the patient's situation but, rather, to decide how the patient would want to be treated. This is critically important, and healthcare providers must help to ensure that substitute decision makers understand this role. The criteria on which the decision should be based are: (i) the specific wishes previously expressed by the patient; (ii) if specific wishes are not known, the patient's known values and beliefs; and (iii) if neither specific wishes or values and beliefs are known, the patient's best interests. Patients' wishes are those preferences expressed while they had capacity that seem to apply to the decision that needs to be currently made. Values and beliefs are less specific than wishes but allow substitute decision makers to infer, in light of other choices the patient has made and their general approach to life, what patients would decide in the present situation. Despite the best intentions and most sincere efforts of those involved, it sometimes remains unknown or unclear what the patient would have chosen. When good information about patients' wishes, or values and beliefs, is lacking, or when the available information is contradictory, decision makers may be forced to make a judgement as to patients' best interests in particular circumstances. The calculation of a patient's best interests is based on objective estimates of the benefits and burdens of treatment to the patient.

When relatives disagree, they should be encouraged to focus their attention on the question of what the patient would want to be done given the current goal of treatment or what is in the patient's best interests. Both of these questions need to be answered with an understanding of the current goals of care. For example, a patient's preference for a treatment, especially a life-sustaining one, usually varies depending on whether the goal of care is palliative comfort care or curative treatment. Often, disagreements between family members abate over time because a shared understanding of the clinical situation and prognosis develops. Chaplains may be of assistance, especially if one or more family members are invoking religious interpretations or perceiving religious implications of the decision. On occasion, a court-appointed guardian becomes involved to help to decide which of the family members should be the official decision maker.

How can substitute decision making be improved?

Often substitute decision makers never anticipated that they would be in this role. The role was not previously discussed with the patient, and so they often feel unprepared. Healthcare providers can initiate the discussion with patients and their loved ones about substitute decision making.

Of course, helping them engage in a meaningful and useful conversation becomes the more challenging step. It is important for patients and their family members to know how decision making would likely occur without explicit planning. If a friend or unmarried partner is the desired substitute decision maker, then in some areas these individuals might be excluded from the decision-making

process unless they were formally appointed as a healthcare agent. For example, in the USA the appointment of a healthcare agent is the mechanism to empower a non-family member, and this occurs through a durable power of attorney for healthcare.

The next task for healthcare providers is to guide patients and their surrogates through a discussion. Often, these discussions immediately focus on cardiopulmonary resuscitation (e.g., do-not-resuscitate orders) or what should be done if the person ended up in a permanent coma (Tulsky et al., 1998). More nuanced discussion is required. One increasingly popular approach is to identify whether there are any particular situations in which the patient would not want to receive life-sustaining treatment. This might be prolonged coma, severe dementia, or dying anyway from a terminal illness. Studies have shown that a "state worse than death" usually leads people to want to forgo life-sustaining treatments (Patrick et al., 1997). Thus, the identification of these conditions can serve as a proxy for preferences about treatments. Three questions can help to focus this conversation

1. "Are there any situations that you've read about in the newspaper, or heard about on the radio, or seen on TV where you've said to yourself, I would never want to live like that."

2. "What makes each of these situations so unacceptable?" Asking this helps the patient to identify core values that should help guide decision making if a situation arises that requires a substitute decision maker for something different from what was specifically talked about.

3. As a check on these preferences and values, the healthcare provider should ask if the following interpretation is correct: "Does this mean that if you end up like [X], you would not want treatment for a life-threatening event that would serve to prolong this existence?" If the answer is yes, then the construct is supported. If the answer is no, then asking why should identify other core values that need to be understood and factored into future decision making.

If patients decide to formalize preferences through an advance directive (Ch. 10), then healthcare providers should reinforce the importance of ensuring that substitute decision makers have access to the document (and any future updates). Moreover, the healthcare provider should ensure that the information is readily available in the medical record to ensure that other providers, if needed, have access to this information.

Healthcare providers need to understand and be trained in their important role of facilitating the process of substitute decision making by providing information that will enable the substitute to make an informed choice on the patient's behalf. Healthcare professionals should guide substitute decision makers to consider the patients' previously expressed wishes, values and beliefs, or best interests (in this order). When it is apparent that the substitute decision maker is making a choice that is significantly different from what the patient might have chosen, healthcare providers find themselves in a difficult situation and should seek advice from colleagues, ethics consultants, or legal counsel.

The cases

Mr. E is incapable of participating in the decision making because of AIDS-related dementia. The physician speaks to Mr. E's partner, who agrees that he would not want to be admitted to hospital to undergo any invasive procedures. The partner believes he would want to go home, perhaps with supplemental oxygen therapy to relieve some of his distress. He tells the physician that after his last episode of PCP, Mr. E instructed him that he would never wish to go through the necessary treatment again. Before palliative home oxygen therapy is arranged, Mr. E's family members arrive at the hospital and express the desire that he receive "everything," including aggressive life-sustaining treatment if indicated. Mr. E's partner talks to the family and shows them a durable power of attorney for healthcare form that Mr. E completed that empowers him to make medical decisions on his behalf. After a series of discussions, the family members appreciate the importance of respecting Mr. E's preferences and values, including having his partner function as the primary decision maker on his behalf. Jointly, the healthcare agent (i.e., the partner and formal substitute decision maker) and the family agree to palliative home oxygen. The patient is sent home with hospice follow-up and dies comfortably several days later.

Mrs. F is judged to be temporarily incapacitated during this COPD exacerbation. After discussing the patient's incapacity, the physician asks the daughter whether she knows what her mother would want if the situation deteriorates further. The daughter says that Mrs. F's quality of life has been declining since her dad died two years ago, but seems to have taken a marked fall recently since the latest hospitalization. Although she has never discussed this sort of situation directly with her mother, she does not think that her mother would want resuscitation (CPR) or mechanical ventilation. However, she is uncomfortable making this decision on her own. The physician suggests that she consult with her siblings. The physician says that in the meantime everything possible will be done to avoid intubation; however, intubation will proceed if it becomes medically necessary. Two hours later the daughter reports to the physician that all of the children feel that Mrs. F would refuse CPR and intubation if she had the capacity to communicate her wishes. Although the physician makes it clear that Mrs. F might be able to make this decision herself if she recovers from the current episode, the daughter requests that "do not intubate" and "do-not-attempt-resuscitation" orders be placed on the patient's chart. The rationale is that the family members believe (and the physician concurs) that their mother's recovery, at best, would be short lived, and that she would not want to spend her remaining days suffering with shortness of breath. The physician agrees to write the order and plans to discuss it with the patient if her capacity improves.

REFERENCES

American Geriatrics Society Ethics Committee (1996). Making treatment decisions for incapacitated elderly patients without advance directives. *J Am Geriatr Soc* **44**: 986–7.

Buchanan, A. E. and Brock, D. W. (1989). *Deciding for Others: The Ethics of Surrogate Decision-Making.* Cambridge, UK: Cambridge University Press.

Canadian Medical Association (1995). Joint statement on resuscitative interventions. *CMAJ* **153**: 1652A–C.

Chambers-Evans, J. and Carnevale, F. A. (2005). Dawning of awareness: the experience of surrogate decision making at the end of life. *J Clin Ethics* **16**: 28–45.

High, D. M. (1994). Families roles in advance directives. *Hastings Cent Rep* **24**: 516–18.

Jameton, A. (1984). *Nursing Practice: The Ethical Issues.* Englewood Cliffs, NJ: Prentice Hall.

Patrick, D. L., Pearlman, R, A., Starks, H. E., *et al.* (1997). Validation of life-sustaining treatment preferences: implications for advance care planning. *Ann Intern Med* **127**: 509–17.

Pearlman, R. A., Starks, H., Cain, K. C., and Cole, W. G. (2005). Improvements in advance care planning in the VA: results of a multifaceted intervention. *Arch Intern Med* **165**: 667–74.

Seckler, A. B., Meier, D. E., Mulvihill, M., and Paris, B. E. (1991). Substituted judgment: how accurate are proxy predictions? *Ann Intern Med* **115**: 92–8.

Teno, J. M., Hakim, R. B., Knaus, W. A., *et al.* (1995). Preferences for cardiopulmonary resuscitation: physician–patient agreement and hospital resource use. *J Gen Intern Med* **10**: 179–86.

Terry, P. B., Vettese, M., Song, J., *et al.* (1999). End of life decision making: when patients and surrogates disagree. *J Clin Ethics* **10**: 286–93.

Tsevat, J., Cook, E. F., Green, M. L., *et al.* (1995). Health values of the seriously ill. *Ann Intern Med* **122**: 514–20.

Tulsky, J. A., Fischer, G. S., Rose, M. R., and Arnold, R. M. (1998). Opening the black box: how do physicians communicate about advance directives? *Ann Intern Med* **129**: 441–9.

Uhlmann, R. F., Pearlman, R. A., and Cain, K. C.. (1988). Physicians' and spouses' predictions of elderly patients' resuscitation preferences. *J Gerontol* **43**: M115–21.

Veterans Health Administration (2003). *VHA Handbook 1004.1: VHA Informed Consent for Clinical Treatments and Procedures.* Washington, DC: Department of Veterans Affairs.

Washington State Legislature (2006). RCW: Informed consent – persons authorized to provide for patients who are not competent – priority. Olympia, WA: Statute Law Committee.

10

Advance care planning

James A. Tulsky, Linda L. Emanuel, Douglas K. Martin and Peter A. Singer

Mrs. G is 63 years old and has no significant history of illness. She presents for a routine visit to her family physician. She has read newspaper articles about living wills and thought that this was something she ought to address, but had never taken it further. In the physician's waiting room, she sees a leaflet on advance directives and decides that today would be a good day to learn more about this.

Mr. H is a 40-year-old man who was diagnosed 6 months ago with advanced glioblastoma multiforme, an incurable brain tumor. He presents to his oncologist with symptoms of early cognitive dysfunction. The physician considers what Mr. H should be told about advance directives.

What is advance care planning?

Advance care planning is a process whereby a patient, in consultation with healthcare providers, family members, and important others, makes decisions about his or her future healthcare (Teno *et al.*, 1994). This planning may involve the preparation of a written advance directive (Emanuel *et al.*, 1991). Completed by patients when they are capable, advance directives are invoked in the event that the patient loses decision making capacity. Advance directives may indicate what interventions patients would or would not want in

various situations, and whom they would want to name as healthcare surrogates to make treatment decisions on their behalf.

Why is advance care planning important?

Ethics, law, and policy

Advance care planning helps to ensure that the norm of consent is respected when sick people are no longer able to discuss their treatment options with physicians and thereby exercise control over the course of their care. This norm is grounded in the principle of self-determination and respect for autonomy, a classic expression of which is Justice Benjamin Cardozo's statement in 1914 that "Every human being of adult years and sound mind has the right to determine what shall be done with his own body" (Faden *et al.*, 1986).

Advance care planning also rests on the principle of respect for persons, and this respect must extend to those whose cultural values emphasize the interdependence of human beings and the well-being of the family or community as a whole. Advance care planning recognizes that sick people suffer a loss of dignity when they cannot command respect for their considered and cherished intentions and that such

An earlier version of this chapter has appeared: Singer, P. A., Robertson, G., and Roy, D. J. (1996). Advance care planning. *CMAJ* **155**: 1689–92. Portions from the following sources were also used: Martin, D. K., Emanuel, L. L., and Singer, P. A. (2000). Planning for the end of life. *Lancet* **356**: 1672–6; Fischer, G. S., Tulsky, J. A., and Arnold, R. M. (2004). Advance Directives. In *Encyclopedia of Bioethics*, 3rd edn, ed. S. G. Post. New York: Macmillan Reference USA.

intentions may be shaped by cultural values (Kagawa-Singer and Blackhall, 2001).

In the USA, state laws allow individuals to complete advance directive documents and to name surrogate healthcare decision makers, and a federal law requires all patients admitted to hospital to be notified of this right (US Congress, 1990). Most European countries have followed suit with provisions for advance care planning (Fassier *et al.*, 2005).

Empirical studies

Despite considerable interest and widespread legislation in favor of advance directives, advance care planning has not been as successful as proponents would wish. In multiple surveys, patients and providers expressed positive attitudes towards advance directives (Lo *et al.*, 1986; Shmerling *et al.*, 1988; Frankl *et al.*, 1989; Stolman *et al.*, 1990; Emanuel *et al.*, 1991; Gamble *et al.*, 1991; Joos *et al.*, 1993), yet they seldom complete such forms (Emanuel *et al.*, 1991). With considerable effort, a variety of interventions can increase the use of advance directives (Cohen-Mansfield *et al.*, 1991; Hare and Nelson, 1991; Sachs *et al.*, 1992; High, 1993; Markson *et al.*, 1994; Rubin *et al.*, 1994) but only to modest levels and with minimal effect on care (Hanson *et al.*, 1997a; Landry *et al.*, 1997). One large study to assess the effectiveness of advance care planning in the care of dying patients (SUPPORT) found that it had no impact on physician–patient communication, incidence, or timing of written do-not-resuscitate (DNR) orders, physicians' knowledge of patients' preferences, the number of days spent in the intensive care unit receiving mechanical ventilation, the level of reported pain, or the use of hospital resources (SUPPORT Principal Investigators, 1995).

This lack of effect may result from several issues. The communication between clinicians and patients that guides the creation of advance directives may be flawed (Tulsky *et al.*, 1998). Some patients change their views as time passes (Emanuel *et al.*, 1994; Danis *et al.*, 1994) and others

request life-prolonging interventions that subsequently prove to be unrealistic. Substitute decision makers are not always sure that a patient's situation is equivalent to that described in an advance directive (Tulsky, 2005). Furthermore, cultural values play an important role in advance care planning, and advance directives may not be acceptable to some groups of people or may be variably interpreted (Caralis *et al.*, 1993; Blackhall *et al.*, 1995; Carrese and Rhodes, 1995). In a review of more than 100 research articles, advance care planning, and advanced directive forms, Miles and colleagues (1996) concluded, "Advance treatment preferences have been shown to be difficult to form, communicate, and implement." The key question is why?

One answer may be that the traditional conceptual framework underlying advance care planning and use of advance directive forms is not rooted in the needs and experiences of patients. Traditionally, advance care planning was thought to help people to prepare for treatment decisions in times of incapacity, to be based on the ethical principle of autonomy, and to focus on completing written advance directive forms within the context of the physician–patient relationship. However, from the perspective of patients, advance care planning also helps patients to prepare for death, is influenced by personal relationships, is a social process, and occurs within the context of family and loved ones (Singer *et al.*, 1998). Thus, the process of advance care planning and outcome measures used in previous research may not have focused on the issues of greatest importance to patients and their loved ones.

How should I approach advance care planning in practice?

The original goal of the movement for advance care planning – from the perspective of ethicists and legal scholars – was to assist patients to make treatment decisions for the event of incapacity. However, from the patient's perspective, the primary goal of advance care planning is more commonly preparing for death and dying (Martin *et al.*, 1999). People struggle to find ways to cope with death (Field and Cassel, 1997). Once a central ritual of social and religious life, death has been privatized, desacralized, hidden behind institutional walls, and implicitly made taboo. Advance care planning can help people to prepare for death, which, from the patient's perspective, tends to mean helping them to achieve a sense of control, relieving burdens on loved ones, and strengthening or reaching closure in relationships with loved ones (Martin *et al.*, 1999). Given this reconceptualization, clinicians approaching patients to discuss advance care planning ought to keep in mind the following goals for the process (Martin *et al.*, 2000).

Maintaining a sense of control

Autonomy is central to advance care planning, but not primarily in the sense of controlling each treatment decision, as has generally been assumed. Bereaved family members feel that improved communication would improve end of life care, but that focusing on specific treatment decisions avoids considerations of death and ''may not satisfy the real needs of dying patients and their families'' (Hanson *et al.*, 1997b). Achieving an overall sense of control in the dying experience is an important psychosocial outcome. Advance care planning can help people to achieve a sense of control by thinking beyond an itemized list of concrete objectives to a situation that maps a personal approach to dying by considering the values and goals that should guide their dying (Singer *et al.*, 1998; Martin *et al.*, 1999).

Relieving the burden

People who are dying want to attend to the needs of their loved ones, and patients fear that loved ones may bear the burdens of a protracted terminal illness. Advance care planning allows people to determine settings for care and limits for life-sustaining treatments that may inappropri-
ately lengthen dying, and it facilitates reflective discussion of values, goals, and preferences with loved ones in a non-crisis environment. This may help loved ones who bear the burdens of anxiety and physical care through a protracted dying process. Advance care planning may also help to prepare those who serve as substitute decision makers in a crisis, and mitigate the guilt felt by loved ones who must make difficult substitute decisions with respect to life-sustaining treatment. Advance care planning can also help the healthcare team to be prepared for the patient's death.

Strengthening relationships

People live in a web of social ties and generally fear dying in isolation. Advance care planning facilitates communication about death and thus provides an opportunity to strengthen relationships with loved ones. Advance care planning may help people to settle their differences with loved ones, including giving or seeking forgiveness for past disagreements. Reflecting on life and the meaning of death, and sharing those reflections with loved ones may also help to strengthen personal relationships.

Respecting culture

Decision making about end of life is influenced by culturally shaped values. The principle of autonomy is the dominant ethic of healthcare in North America and Western Europe. Yet for many other people, autonomy may not be the dominant value. For example, a study of attitudes toward end of life decision making among people of Chinese origin found that they were indifferent or negatively disposed to advance care planning. These people reflected a world view that values interdependence, compassion, and protection, by contrast with independence and autonomy. Consequently, to be consistent with a patient-centered approach, healthcare professionals should discuss patient's goals about end of life decision making.

A practical approach

Advance care planning discussions vary depending on a patient's state of health. Patients who are in good health may benefit from selecting a healthcare proxy and thinking about whether there are any situations so intolerable that they would not want their lives prolonged. When patients are older or have more serious chronic illnesses, physicians may wish to begin a discussion that is broader in scope.

Although many view advance care planning as an opportunity for patients to make known their "preferences" for treatment, many patients do not have well-formed treatment preferences. By careful exploration of patients' values, healthcare providers can help patients to discover these preferences. Patients can be asked to talk about their goals for life, their fears about disability, their hopes for what the end of their life will look like, and their ideas about states worse than death (Pearlman *et al.*, 1993). This expanded view of advance care planning allows people to think about their mortality and legacy. From such discussions, healthcare providers can help patients to consider specifically whether there are certain treatments that they might wish to forgo, and to think about the circumstances under which they might forgo them.

When the patient's illness has progressed to its final stages, healthcare providers can use the groundwork from these earlier discussions to make specific plans about what is to be done when the inevitable worsening occurs. Among other things, the patient and the healthcare providers can decide the following. Should an ambulance be called? Should the patient come to the hospital? Which life-prolonging treatments should be employed and which should be forgone? Are there particular treatments aimed at symptomatic relief that should be employed?

Even with this emphasis on the discussion and process, advance directive forms remain useful as they provide a legal, written record of the patient's values and preferences that may be useful in some end of life scenarios. Numerous advance directive forms have been developed by organizations, governments, and academics. Instruction directives (also called living wills) describe what type of care a person would or would not want in various situations. Proxy directives (sometimes called durable powers of attorney for healthcare) indicate who a person would want to make treatment decisions on his or her behalf. These two types of directive are designed to accomplish different, important, and complementary objectives.

For most situations, we recommend that advance directive forms contain both instruction and proxy directives. Furthermore, we recommend detailed instruction directives that systematically lead people through a process that helps them to think about the form and to articulate values, goals, and preferences relevant to healthcare decisions. Most function as a worksheet and then a form for documentation. Non-detailed instruction directives instead provide limited space, usually a few lines, in which people may write instructions. General instructions noted on a non-detailed directive are generally inconsistent with specific treatment preferences (Schneiderman *et al.*, 1992). Moreover, compared with a detailed advance directive, a non-detailed advance directive results in less-uniform interpretation by physicians (Mower and Baraff, 1993).

When detailed, scenario-based instruction directives with intervention choices are used, it is possible to derive a patient's personal thresholds for intervention (Emanuel, 2007). These can be particularly helpful when inferring from scenarios in a prior statement to real situations. For instance, in some documents, scenarios are arrayed in a sequence that approximates a gradient of prognosis severity (Emanuel *et al.*, 1991). For each scenario, potential interventions are arranged approximately by level of burdensomeness. Individuals tend to have thresholds regarding burdensomeness and prognosis that can be seen when all the options are filled in. This approach is supported by the finding that most patients are concerned about prognosis and treatment burden when they engage in advance care planning (Weeks *et al.*, 1998; Fried *et al.*, 2002; Fried and Bradley, 2003).

Yet, as carefully as such documents may be completed, rarely do advance directives clearly dictate the care that should be given to a patient who lacks decision-making capacity (Fischer *et al.*, 2004). Generally, some interpretation of the document is required, a responsibility left to the named surrogate decision maker, other family members, and the healthcare team.

When a patient who has an advance directive lacks decision-making capacity and is seriously ill, the clinicians should discuss the situation with the named proxy and other appropriate loved ones. Reviewing the advance directive, those involved should decide what they think the patient would have wanted under the current circumstances. It is easiest when the situation under consideration matches well the scenarios described in the advance directive. However, frequently the advance directive form may not be sufficiently detailed to guide treatment, in which case it may be necessary to proceed almost as if there were no advance directive. In such situations, prior discussions involving the patient, his or her loved ones, and clinicians about the patient's values regarding medical treatments would be extremely useful.

Even when there seems to be an applicable advance directive, there may be disagreement among family members or between family members and the healthcare team regarding the patient's care (Fischer *et al.*, 2004). Loved ones may disagree with the content of the advance directive, believe that the patient changed his or her mind, or believe that the patient made an error. Disagreements may occur because of differing interpretations of the document, such as the meaning of a "reasonable chance of recovery." In these situations, it helps to focus the decision makers on what the patient would have wanted and why the advance directive was written in the first place.

Although it is best to gain a consensus of all the interested parties, especially about forgoing life-sustaining treatment, ultimately a named proxy has the final decision. Healthcare providers who wish to override proxies based on a patient's written advance directive should be wary. It is not clear that all patients would want their proxy's or loved one's wishes overruled. One study showed that over half of a group of patients on dialysis thought their doctors or proxies should have at least some leeway to interpret their advance directive (Sehgal *et al.*, 1992). In such situations, clinicians may be best off consulting with the hospital ethics committee.

Advance care planning enables clinicians to respect patients' wishes for medical care in the event of future incompetence. The goals of advance care planning will be different for patients at different stages of life and health, but the aim in all cases is to help patients to articulate health-related values in a manner that can assist decision makers, allow patients to maintain control, relieve burdens on others, and strengthen important personal relationships.

The cases

Mrs. G is requesting information about advance care planning. Her physician should refer her to one of the available information sources or provide her a form and encourage her to begin the process of advance care planning with her preferred proxy decision maker. After a period of time, Mrs. G and her substitute might together meet with the physician. At this meeting, the physician can review Mrs. G's treatment preferences to ensure that she has understood the information in the advance directive form and is capable of completing it. If her health situation changes, the physician should recommend that Mrs. G update her advance directive.

Mr. H, unfortunately, may soon be incapable of making healthcare decisions. The physician should raise the subject of advance care planning with him in a sensitive manner and follow the same steps as described for Mrs. G. However, in the case of Mr. H, the physician will have to pay particular attention to the issue of capacity. This situation also represents an opportunity for the physician to tailor the information considered by Mr. H in advance care planning to the likely future of progressive cognitive deterioration. It is also an opportunity for the patient, his family, and the physician to begin to prepare for his impending death.

REFERENCES

Blackhall, L. J., Murphy, S. T., Frank, G., Michel, V., and Azen, S. (1995). Ethnicity and attitudes toward patient autonomy. *JAMA* **274**: 820–5.

Caralis, P. V., Davis, B., Wright, K., and Marcial, E. (1993). The influence of ethnicity and race on attitudes toward advance directives, life-prolonging treatments, and euthanasia. *J Clin Ethics* **4**: 155–65.

Carrese, J. A. and Rhodes, L. A. (1995). Western bioethics on the Navajo reservation. Benefit or harm? *JAMA* **274**: 826–9.

Cohen-Mansfield, J., Rabinovich, B. A., Lipson, S., *et al.* (1991). The decision to execute a durable power of attorney for healthcare and preferences regarding the utilization of life-sustaining treatments in nursing home residents. *Arch Intern Med* **151**: 289–94.

Danis, M., Garrett, J., Harris, R., and Patrick, D. L. (1994). Stability of choices about life-sustaining treatments. *Ann Intern Med* **120**: 567–73.

Emanuel, L. L. (2007). Advance directives and assessment of decision-making capacity. In *Principles and Practice of Palliative Care and Supportive Oncology*, 3rd edn, ed. A. M. Berger, J. L. Shuster, and J. H. Von Roenn. Philadelphia, PA: Lippincott, Williams and Wilkins, pp. 687–95.

Emanuel, L. L., Barry, M. J., Stoeckle, J. D., Ettelson, L. M., and Emanuel, E. J. (1991). Advance directives for medical care: a case for greater use. *N Engl J Med* **324**: 889–95.

Emanuel, L. L., Emanuel, E. J., Stoeckle, J. D., Hummel, L. R., and Barry, M. J. (1994). Advance directives. Stability of patients' treatment choices. *Arch Intern Med* **154**: 209–17.

Faden, R., Beauchamp, T. L., and King, N. M. P. (1986). *A History and Theory of Informed Consent.* New York: Oxford University Press.

Fassier, T., Lautrette, A., Ciroldi, M., and Azoulay, E. (2005). Care at the end of life in critically ill patients: the European perspective. *Curr Opin Crit Care* **11**: 616–23.

Field, M. J. and Cassel, C. K. (1997). *Approaching Death: Improving Care at the End of Life.* Washington, DC: Institute of Medicine.

Fischer, G. S., Tulsky, J. A., and Arnold, R. M. (2004). Advance Directives. In *Encyclopedia of Bioethics*, 3rd edn, ed. S. G. Post. New York: Macmillan Reference USA.

Frankl, D., Oye, R. K., and Bellamy, P. E. (1989). Attitudes of hospitalized patients toward life support: a survey of 200 medical inpatients. *Am J Med* **86**: 645–8.

Fried, T. R. and Bradley, E. H. (2003). What matters to seriously ill older persons making end of life treatment decisions? A qualitative study. *J Palliat Med* **6**: 237–44.

Fried, T. R., Bradley, E. H., Towle, V. R., and Allore, H. (2002). Understanding the treatment preferences of seriously ill patients. *N Engl J Med* **346**: 1061–6.

Gamble, E. R., McDonald, P. J., and Lichstein, P. R. (1991). Knowledge, attitudes, and behavior of elderly persons regarding living wills. *Arch Intern Med* **151**: 277–80.

Hanson, L. C., Tulsky, J. A., and Danis, M. (1997a). Can clinical interventions change care at the end of life? *Ann Intern Med* **126**: 381–8.

Hanson, L. C., Danis, M., and Garrett, J. (1997b). What is wrong with end of life care? Opinions of bereaved family members. *J Am Geriatr Soc* **45**: 1339–44.

Hare, J. and Nelson, C. (1991). Will outpatients complete living wills? A comparison of two interventions. *J Gen Intern Med* **6**: 41–6.

High, D. M. (1993). Advance directives and the elderly: a study of intervention strategies to increase use. *Gerontologist* **33**: 342–9.

Joos, S. K., Reuler, J. B., Powell, J. L., and Hickam, D. H. (1993). Outpatients' attitudes and understanding regarding living wills. *J Gen Intern Med* **8**: 259–63.

Kagawa-Singer, M. and Blackhall, L. J. (2001). Negotiating cross-cultural issues at the end of life: "You got to go where he lives." *JAMA* **286**: 2993–3001.

Landry, F. J., Kroenke, K., Lucas, C., and Reeder, J. (1997). Increasing the use of advance directives in medical outpatients. *J Gen Intern Med* **12**: 412–5.

Lo, B., Mcleod, G. A., and Saika, G. (1986). Patient attitudes to discussing life-sustaining treatment. *Arch Intern Med* **146**: 1613–5.

Markson, L. J., Fanale, J., Steel, K., Kern, D., and Annas, G. (1994). Implementing advance directives in the primary care setting. *Arch Intern Med* **154**: 2321–7.

Martin, D. K., Thiel, E. C., and Singer, P. A. (1999). A new model of advance care planning: observations from people with HIV. *Arch Intern Med* **159**: 86–92.

Martin, D. K., Emanuel, L. L., and Singer, P. A. (2000). Planning for the end of life. *Lancet* **356**: 1672–6.

Miles, S. H., Koepp, R., and Weber, E. P. (1996). Advance end of life treatment planning. A research review. *Arch Intern Med* **156**: 1062–8.

Mower, W. R. and Baraff, L. J. (1993). Advance directives. Effect of type of directive on physicians' therapeutic decisions. *Arch Intern Med* **153**: 375–81.

Pearlman, R. A., Cain, K. C., Patrick, D. L., *et al.* (1993). Insights pertaining to patient assessments of states worse than death. *J Clin Ethics* **4**: 33–41.

Rubin, S. M., Strull, W. M., Fialkow, M. F., Weiss, S. J., and Lo, B. (1994). Increasing the completion of the durable power of attorney for healthcare. A randomized, controlled trial. *JAMA* **271**: 209–12.

Sachs, G. A., Stocking, C. B., and Miles, S. H. (1992). Empowerment of the older patient? A randomized, controlled trial to increase discussion and use of advance directives. *J Am Geriatr Soc* **40**: 269–73.

Schneiderman, L. J., Pearlman, R. A., Kaplan, R. M., Anderson, J. P., and Rosenberg, E. M. (1992). Relationship of general advance directive instructions to specific life-sustaining treatment preferences in patients with serious illness. *Arch Intern Med* **152**: 2114–22.

Sehgal, A., Galbraith, A., Chesney, M., *et al.* (1992). How strictly do dialysis patients want their advance directives followed? *JAMA* **267**: 59–63.

Shmerling, R. H., Bedell, S. E., Lilienfeld, A., and Delbanco, T. L. (1988). Discussing cardiopulmonary resuscitation: a study of elderly outpatients. *J Gen Intern Med* **3**: 317–21.

Singer, P. A., Martin, D. K., Lavery, J. V., *et al.* (1998). Reconceptualizing advance care planning from the patient's perspective. *Arch Intern Med* **158**: 879–84.

Stolman, C. J., Gregory, J. J., Dunn, D., and Levine, J. L. (1990). Evaluation of patient, physician, nurse, and family attitudes toward do not resuscitate orders. *Arch Intern Med* **150**: 653–8.

SUPPORT Principal Investigators (1995). A controlled trial to improve care for seriously ill hospitalized patients: the study to understand prognosis and preferences for outcomes and risks of treatments (SUPPORT). *JAMA* **274**: 1591–98.

Teno, J. M., Nelson, H. L., and Lynn, J. (1994). Advance care planning. Priorities for ethical and empirical research. *Hastings Cent Rep* **24**: S32–6.

Tulsky, J. A. (2005). Beyond advance directives: importance of communication skills at the end of life. *JAMA* **294**: 359–65.

Tulsky, J. A., Fischer, G. S., Rose, M. R., and Arnold, R. M. (1998). Opening the black box: how do physicians communicate about advance directives? *Ann Intern Med* **129**: 441–9.

US Congress (1990). Patient Self-Determination Act, Omnibus Budget Reconciliation Act (OBRA) (PL 101–508). Washington, DC: Government Printing Office.

Weeks, J. C., Cook, E. F., O'Day, S. J., *et al* (1998). Relationship between cancer patients' predictions of prognosis and their treatment preferences. *JAMA* **279**: 1709–14.

11

Euthanasia and assisted suicide

Bernard M. Dickens, Joseph M. Boyle Jr., and Linda Ganzini

Ms. I is 32 years old and has advanced gastric cancer that has resulted in constant severe pain and poorly controlled vomiting. Despite steady increases in her opioid dose, her pain has worsened greatly over the last two days. Death is imminent, but the patient pleads incessantly with the hospital staff to "put her out of her misery."

Mr. J is a 39-year-old injection drug user with a history of alcoholism and depression. He presents at an emergency department, insisting that he no longer wishes to live. He repeatedly requests euthanasia on the grounds that he is no longer able to bear his suffering (although he is not in any physical pain). A psychiatrist rules out clinical depression.

What are euthanasia and assisted suicide?

Euthanasia has been defined as a deliberate act undertaken by one person with the intention of ending the life of another person to relieve that person's suffering. Euthanasia may be "voluntary," "involuntary," or "non-voluntary," depending on (i) the competence of the recipient, (ii) whether or not the act is consistent with the recipient's wishes (if these are known), and (iii) whether or not the recipient is aware that euthanasia is to be performed. Assisted suicide has been defined as "the act of intentionally killing oneself with the assistance of another who deliberately provides the knowledge, means, or both" (Special Senate Committee on Euthanasia and Assisted Suicide, 1995). In "physician-assisted suicide," a physician provides the assistance.

Why are euthanasia and assisted suicide important?

States all over the world have debated recently the question of whether physicians and other health-care professionals should in certain circumstances participate in intentionally bringing about the death of a patient, and whether these practices should be accepted by society as a whole. The ethical, legal, and public-policy implications of these questions merit careful consideration.

Ethics

There is considerable disagreement about whether euthanasia and assisted suicide are ethically distinct from decisions to forgo life-sustaining treatments (Gillion, 1988; Roy, 1990; Brock, 1992; Dickens, 1993; Annas, 1996) and the issue has formed the basis of a number of legal actions (*Sue Rodriguez* v. *British Columbia (Attorney General)*, 1993; *Quill* v. *Vacco*, 1996; *Compassion in Dying* v. *Washington*, 1996). At the heart of the debate is the ethical significance given to the intentions of those performing

An earlier version of this chapter has appeared: Lavery, J. V., Dickens, B. M., Boyle, J. M., and Singer, P. A. (1997). Euthanasia and assisted suicide. *CMAJ* **156**: 1405–8.

these acts (Brody, 1993; Quill, 1993). Supporters of euthanasia and assisted suicide reject the argument that there is an ethical distinction between these acts and acts of forgoing life-sustaining treatment. They claim, instead, that euthanasia and assisted suicide are consistent with the right of patients to make autonomous choices about the time and manner of their own death (Brock, 1992; Angell, 1997). Opponents of euthanasia and assisted suicide claim that death is a predictable consequence of the morally justified withdrawal of life-sustaining treatments only in cases where there is a fatal underlying condition, and that it is the condition, not the action of withdrawing treatment, that causes death (Foley, 1997). A physician who performs euthanasia or assists in a suicide, by comparison, has the death of the patient as his or her primary objective. Although opponents of euthanasia and assisted suicide recognize the importance of self-determination, they argue that individual autonomy has limits and that the right to self-determination should not be given ultimate standing in social policy regarding euthanasia and assisted suicide (Callaghan, 1992). Supporters of euthanasia and assisted suicide believe that these acts benefit terminally ill patients by relieving their suffering (Brody, 1992), while opponents argue that the compassionate grounds for endorsing these acts cannot ensure that euthanasia will be limited to people who request it voluntarily (Kamisar, 1995). Opponents of euthanasia are also concerned that the acceptance of euthanasia may contribute to an increasingly casual attitude toward private killing in society (Kamisar, 1958). Most commentators make no formal ethical distinction between euthanasia and assisted suicide, since in both cases the person performing the euthanasia or assisting the suicide deliberately facilitates the patient's death. Concerns have been expressed, however, about the risk of error, coercion, or abuse that could arise if physicians become the final agents in voluntary euthanasia (Quill *et al.*, 1992). There is also disagreement about whether euthanasia and assisted suicide should rightly be considered ''medical'' procedures (Kinsella, 1991; Drickamer *et al.*, 1997).

Law

Most legal systems recognize a distinction between positive acts intended to cause death and passively allowing natural death to occur. The former is usually considered homicide, including murder and infanticide. Withholding and withdrawing life support can also be homicide, usually manslaughter, when there is a legal duty of maintenance. However, although physicians must render care necessary for their patients' survival, they are usually not bound to provide treatment that in good faith they consider futile or ineffective to sustain their patients' well-being or capacity to function at a conscious, aware level. For instance, patients who remain in a permanent or persistent vegetative state may have means of nutrition and hydration withdrawn when death is predicted to result (*Airedale NHS Trust* v. *Bland*, 1993).

A small but potentially growing number of jurisdictions allow physicians to comply with competent patients' persistent requests that their unbearable pain be relieved by terminal means. The Netherlands pioneered medically induced death, not limited to terminal patients, by a series of judicial rulings in the 1960s and legislation enacted in 2000, and the US state of Oregon and Belgium have amended their legislation to provide conditions under which physicians may (not must) comply with competent patients' requests by undertaking interventions intended to cause death. In the absence of such law, however, a competent patient's consent to such an intervention is not a defense to a criminal charge of homicide or criminal negligence laid against a physician.

Assisted suicide was decriminalized in Switzerland in 1942 (Guillod and Schmidt, 2005), not necessarily limited to physicians' assistance, but this is the exception that proves the general rule that decriminalization of individuals' attempted suicide does not open a way to assistance, by physicians or others. Withdrawal of prohibition of attempted suicide does not create a right to an attempt (*Sue Rodriguez* v. *Attorney-General of British Columbia*, 1993), nor to assistance. Counseling and assisting suicide remain offences in most jurisdictions. However, several jurisdictions such as the Netherlands and Belgium are coming to recognize individuals' capacity for rational choice of suicide, and the right of physicians to give assistance.

A concern regarding approaching euthanasia and medically assisted suicide through criminal law is that enforcement may be ineffective. Physicians may be justified in increasing medications for pain control, as patients' relief from pain at given dosage levels decreases, until a toxic level is predictably reached and is the precipitating cause of death. Patients' deaths result, however, not from their treatment but from their pathologies, which justified and even compelled the pain relief treatment (*R* v. *Adams*, 1957; Williams, 2001). Physicians who withhold indicated measures of pain relief for fear of personal accountability for their patients' deaths are in a conflict of interest. However, prosecutors may find it impossible to show beyond reasonable doubt that physicians' primary intentions are not pain relief but "mercy killing."

Similarly, medications may properly be prescribed for patients' periodic self-administration, which they may hoard and then consume at the same time in order to commit suicide. Physicians may recognize this as a risk, but it may be impossible to show beyond reasonable doubt that they intended this consequence or were negligent. Warning patients of dangers to their lives of over medication may send an ambiguous message.

Empirical studies

A study in 1995 in Canada (Singer *et al.*, 1995) showed that more than 75% of the general public supported voluntary euthanasia and assisted suicide in the case of patients who were unlikely to recover from their illness. Roughly equal numbers, however, opposed these practices for patients with reversible conditions (78% opposed), elderly disabled people who feel they are a burden to others (75% opposed), and elderly people with minor physical ailments (83% opposed) (Genuis *et al.*, 1994). Results of one survey indicated that 24% of

Canadian physicians would be willing to practice euthanasia and 23% would be willing to assist in a suicide if these acts were legal (Wysong, 1996). These findings are similar to the results of surveys conducted in the UK (Ward and Tate, 1994) and in Australia's Northern Territory (Anon., 1996). Surveys of physicians in the Australian state of Victoria (Kuhse and Singer, 1988), as well as surveys in Oregon (Lee *et al.*, 1996), Washington (Shapiro *et al.*, 1994), and Michigan (Bachman *et al.*, 1996) indicated that a majority of physicians in these jurisdictions supported euthanasia and assisted suicide in principle and favored their decriminalization. Physicians in certain specialties, such as palliative care, appear to be less willing to participate in euthanasia and assisted suicide than physicians in other specialties.

Approximately 3% of all deaths in the Netherlands result from euthanasia or assisted suicide (van der Maas *et al.*, 1996). Most of these patients have cancer, though one in five patients with amyotrophic lateral sclerosis die of euthanasia or assisted suicide (Veldink *et al.*, 2002). Physicians report that Dutch patients pursue euthanasia because of loss of dignity, "unworthy dying," and dependence on others. Pain was mentioned as a reason for pursuing hastened death by almost half of patients, but in only 5% was it the sole reason (van der Maas *et al.*, 1996).

In a national US sample of almost 2000 physicians, one in six reported having received a request from a patient for assistance with suicide; 11% had received a request for a lethal injection; 3% reported that they had written at least one prescription to be used to hasten death; and 4.7% said that they had administered at least one lethal injection. The most common reasons for the request were discomfort other than pain, loss of dignity, fear of uncontrollable symptoms, pain, and loss of meaning in life (Meier *et al.*, 1998). Physicians were more likely to honor the requests of patients with severe pain or discomfort who had a life expectancy of less than one month and were not assessed as depressed at the time of the request (Meier *et al.*, 2003).

Assisted suicide became lawful in Oregon in 1997, and each year approximately 0.1% of deaths in that state are by lethal prescription. One in six explicit requests for physician aid in dying are honored. Individuals who access lethal prescriptions under the law are well educated and socio-economically secure compared with other Oregon decedents. Most patients are enrolled in home hospice when they receive the lethal prescription, suggesting that assisted suicide is not a substitute for palliative care. Physicians and hospice workers report that terminally ill individuals request assisted suicide to control the timing and manner of death and to avoid dependence on others. Maintaining independence appears to be a lifelong value for these patients. Uncontrolled pain is rarely a reason for requesting assisted suicide, though fears of worsening symptoms in the future are prominent. Depressive disorders underlie desire for hastened death in a variety of studies, but the prevalence of depression among Oregon residents who die by assisted suicide appears paradoxically low, and may represent underrecognition by clinicians (Ganzini et al., 2000, 2002; Ganzini and Dobscha, 2003). Physicians from Oregon who have received requests reported that the experience is emotionally intense, but those who agreed to participate rarely had regrets (Dobscha et al., 2004).

How should I approach euthanasia and assisted suicide in practice?

Although legal in a handful of countries and states, euthanasia and assisted suicide remain illegal and punishable by imprisonment in most jurisdictions. Physicians who believe that euthanasia and assisted suicide should be legally accepted may pursue these convictions through various legal and democratic means at their disposal: the courts and the legislature. In approaching these issues in a clinical setting, it is important to (i) thoroughly explore the reasons for the request; (ii) respect competent decisions to forgo treatment, such as discontinuing mechanical ventilation at the request

of a patient who is unable to breathe independently, which is legal; (iii) support the patient's autonomy and attempts to maintain control in other areas of life; and (iv) provide appropriate palliative measures.

The cases

The case of Ms. I involves a competent, terminally ill patient who is imminently dying and in intractable pain. The case of Mr. J involves an apparently competent patient who is not dying but is experiencing extreme mental suffering. In both cases, the physician is confronted with a possible request to participate in euthanasia or assisted suicide. Ms. I is suffering and close to death. In consultation with her and her family, the medical team should aggressively control pain and symptoms, calling on the assistance of palliative care specialists if available. Some physicians may be concerned that this type of assertive sedation and pain management may hasten death and thus constitutes euthanasia. This approach, however, is ethically permissible as long as the goal of care is to decrease suffering, euthanasia is not the physician's intention, and death is not the means for alleviating suffering (Williams, 2001).

In the case of Mr. J, the clinical team should explore the source of his despair and respond with psychosocial support and efforts to decrease suffering that do not end the patient's life. Despite the absence of clinical depression, assistance from mental health experts may be beneficial.

REFERENCES

Airedale NHS Trust v. Bland [1993] 1 All ER 821 (House of Lords, England).
Angell, M. (1997). The Supreme Court and physician-assisted suicide: the ultimate right. N Engl J Med **336**: 50–3.
Annas, G. J. (1996). The promised end: constitutional aspects of physician-assisted suicide. N Engl J Med **335**: 683–7.

Anon. (1996). Managing a comfortable death. *Lancet* **347**: 1777.

Bachman, J. G., Alcser, K. H., Doukas, D. J., *et al.* (1996). Attitudes of Michigan physicians and the public toward legalizing physician-assisted suicide and voluntary euthanasia. *N Engl J Med* **334**: 303–9.

Brock, D. W. (1992). Voluntary active euthanasia. *Hastings Cent Rep* **22**: 10–22.

Brody, H. (1992). Assisted death: a compassionate response to a medical failure. *N Engl J Med* **327**: 1384–8.

Brody, H. (1993). Causing, intending, and assisting death. *J Clin Ethics* **4**: 112–17.

Callaghan, D. (1992). When self-determination runs amok. *Hastings Cent Rep* **22**: 52–5.

Compassion in Dying v. *Washington* [1996] 79 F 3d 790 (9th Cir).

Dickens, B. M. (1993). Medically assisted death: *Nancy B.* v. *Hotel–Dieu de Quebec. McGill Law J* **38**: 1053–70.

Dobscha, S. K., Heintz, R. T., Press, N., and Ganzini, L. (2004). Oregon physicians' responses to requests for assisted suicide: a qualitative study. *J Palliat Med* **7**: 450–61.

Drickamer, M. A., Lee, M. A., and Ganzini, L. (1997). Practical issues in physician-assisted suicide. *Ann Intern Med* **126**: 146–51.

Foley, K. M. (1997). Competent care for the dying instead of physician-assisted suicide. *N Engl J Med* **336**: 54–8.

Ganzini, L. and Dobscha, S. K. (2003). If it isn't depression. *J Palliat Med* **6**: 927–30.

Ganzini, L., Nelson, H. D., Schmidt, T. A., *et al.* (2000). Physicians' experiences with the Oregon Death with Dignity Act. *N Engl J Med* **342**: 557–63.

Ganzini, L., Harvath, T. A., Jackson, A., *et al.* (2002). Experiences of Oregon nurses and social workers with hospice patients who requested assistance with suicide. *N Engl J Med* **347**: 582–8.

Genuis, S. J., Genuis, S. K., and Chang, W. C. (1994). Public attitudes toward the right to die. *CMAJ* **150**: 701–8.

Gillon, R. (1988). Euthanasia, withholding life-prolonging treatment, and moral differences between killing and letting die. *J Med Ethics* **14**: 115–7.

Guillod, O. and Schmidt, A. (2005). Assisted suicide under Swiss law. *Eur J Health Law* **12**: 25–38.

Kamisar, Y. (1958). Some non-religious views against proposed ''mercy killing'' legislation. *Minnesota Law Rev* **42**: 969–1042.

Kamisar, Y. (1995). Against assisted suicide: even a very limited form. *Univ Detroit Mercy Law Rev* **72**: 735–69.

Kinsella, D. T. (1991). Will euthanasia kill medicine? *Ann R Coll Physic Surg Canada* **24**: 489–92.

Kuhse, H. and Singer, P. (1988). Doctors' practices and attitudes regarding voluntary euthanasia. *Med J Aust* **148**: 623–7.

Lee, M. A., Nelson, H. D., Tilden, V. P., *et al.* (1996). Legalizing assisted suicide: views of physicians in Oregon. *N Engl J Med* **334**: 310–15.

Meier, D. E., Emmons, C. A., Wallenstein, S., *et al.* (1998). A national survey of physician-assisted suicide and euthanasia in the United States. *N Engl J Med* **338**: 1193–201.

Meier, D. E., Emmons, C. A., Litke, A., Wallenstein, S., and Morrison, R. S. (2003). Characteristics of patients requesting and receiving physician-assisted suicide. *Arch Intern Med* **163**: 1537–42.

Quill, T. E. (1993). The ambiguity of clinical intentions. *N Engl J Med* **329**: 1039–40.

Quill, T. E., Cassel, C. K., and Meier, D. E. (1992). Care of the hopelessly ill. Proposed clinical criteria for physician-assisted suicide. *N Engl J Med* **327**: 1380–4.

Quill v. *Vacco* [1996] 80 F 3d 716 (2nd Cir).

R v. *Adams* (1957). *Crim LR* 365.

Rachels, J. (1975). Active and passive euthanasia. *N Engl J Med* **292**: 78–80.

Rodriguez v. *Attorney-General of British Columbia* (1993) 107 DLR (4d) 342 (Supreme Court of Canada).

Roy, D. J. (1990). Euthanasia: where to go after taking a stand? *J Palliat Care* **6**: 3–5.

Shapiro, R. S., Derse, A. R., Gottlieb, M., Schiedermayer, D., and Olson, M. (1994). Willingness to perform euthanasia. A survey of physician attitudes. *Arch Intern Med* **154**: 575–84.

Singer, P. A., Choudhry, S., Armstrong, J., Meslin, E. M., and Lowy, F. H. (1995). Public opinion regarding end of life decisions: influence of prognosis, practice and process. *Soc Sci Med* **41**: 1517–21.

Special Senate Committee on Euthanasia and Assisted Suicide (1995). *Of Life or Death*. Ottawa: Supply and Services Canada.

Sue Rodriguez v. *British Columbia (Attorney General)* (1993) 3 SCR 519 [See Justice Cory's dissent].

van der Maas, P. J., van der Wal, G., Haverkate, I., *et al.* (1996). Euthanasia, physician-assisted suicide, and other medical practices involving the end of life in the Netherlands, 1990–1995. *N Engl J Med* **335**: 1699–705.

Veldink, J. H., Wokke, J. H., van der Wal, G., Vianney de Jong, J. M., and van den Berg, L. H. (2002). Euthanasia and physician-assisted suicide among patients with amyotrophic lateral sclerosis in the Netherlands. *N Engl J Med* **346**: 1638–44.

Ward, B. J. and Tate, P. A. (1994). Attitudes among NHS doctors to requests for euthanasia. *BMJ* **308**: 1332–4.

Williams, G. (2001). The principle of double effect and terminal sedation. *Med Law Rev* **9**: 41–53.

Wysong, P. (1996). Doctors divided on euthanasia acceptance: preference is to refer euthanasia to another doctor. *Med Post* **32**: **1**: 90.

12

Conflict in the healthcare setting at the end of life

Susan Dorr Goold, Brent C. Williams, and Robert Arnold

Mrs. K, an 82-year-old woman with moderate to severe Alzheimer's dementia, advanced heart failure, emphysema, and diabetes mellitus with neuropathy and nephropathy has just been readmitted with difficulty breathing, two days after being discharged to the care of her daughter. In the previous admission for the same problem, she was treated in the intensive care unit, narrowly avoiding intubation by the use of aggressive pulmonary toilet, antibiotics, and diuretics for possible pneumonia and congestive heart failure. Just after her second admission, the attending physician approached Mrs. K's daughter to discuss forgoing life-sustaining treatment. "In my opinion, if your mother should have a cardiac arrest, resuscitating her would be futile," said Mrs. K's physician. The daughter reacted angrily and insisted that "everything be done," because her mom is strong and can get better (as she has previously).

What is conflict in the healthcare setting at the end of life?

Conflict may be defined as disagreement between people when a decision must be made or an action taken. Healthcare providers encounter conflict in everyday practice, and one of the most difficult and distressing situations physicians face is conflict with family members over forgoing life-sustaining treatment. What should be a cooperative effort to achieve treatment goals turns into an exercise in frustration and distress.

Why is conflict in the healthcare setting at the end of life important?

In the hospital, death is routine to the caregivers, but not to patients and families. Given the emotional impact of decisions surrounding death and dying, conflicts are not surprising but are still disturbing to all parties involved and can diminish trust between doctor and patient or family. This impaired trust profoundly influences the ability of families to believe or understand the prognosis and accept physicians' recommendations based on the patient's goals. Physicians, meanwhile, may be angry and frustrated, distrust the family's motives, worry about litigation, or believe that they are asked to violate their professional ethos by providing care that "does not work." Although physicians and patients (or families) may disagree about the proper course of action in other settings, conflicts in the context of severe illness involve high stakes, great vulnerability, deep fears, and strongly held beliefs. The focus here is on clinician–family conflicts, and not conflicts between clinicians and patients, because when decisions about withholding or withdrawing life-sustaining treatment are contemplated, patients are often incapacitated. Furthermore, a competent patient's wishes are justifiably given much more respect than the judgements of surrogates.

An earlier version of this chapter has appeared: Goold, S. D., Williams, B., and Arnold, R.M. Conflicts around decisions to limit treatment: a differential diagnosis. *Journal of the American Medical Association* Feb. 16, 2000; **283**(7): 909–14. Copyright (2000), American Medical Association. All Rights Reserved.

Decisions about withholding or withdrawing life-sustaining treatment can receive a great deal of publicity. While some cases, such as Terri Schiavo in the USA, reach the courts and media, most conflicts about end of life decisions do not. Even without legal or media attention, these conflicts can have serious consequences. They negatively affect the quality of care and decision making, as well as the satisfaction of both family members and healthcare providers.

Ethics

Decisions about withdrawing, withholding, or continuing life-sustaining treatment require consideration of moral as well as medical concerns. Clinicians may feel that they are violating professional norms to "do no harm" when they are asked to continue burdensome interventions that they consider to be of little or no benefit. Recognizing moral dimensions is an important first step, including professional obligations of compassion, respect for patients' and families' values and beliefs (which may differ substantially from those of the physician), competence (e.g., in prognosticating and communicating), honesty, and humility. Humility, and its antithesis arrogance, bear particular weight when families face the need to trust physicians' prognoses and recommendations.

Law

Statutes and legal precedents from a number of jurisdictions frequently apply to end of life decision making. Many courts have addressed "right to die" cases permitting the withdrawing or withholding of life-sustaining treatment, although the standard of evidence required regarding what the patient would have wanted may vary. For example, the US Supreme Court decision in *Cruzan* v. *Director, Missouri Dep't. of Health* (1990) clarified the circumstances under which a patient may refuse medical treatment or authorize another to speak for him or her, and permitted states to develop their own right to die laws. Statutes may legitimize advance directives (living wills and/or durable powers of attorney for healthcare), address the circumstances under which

a patient can refuse medical treatment, provide guidance for surrogate decision making, address physician-assisted suicide, or require healthcare organizations or doctors to inquire about advance directives. Professionals should be familiar with laws in their own country and locality, and know how to access legal advice when necessary.

Policy

Besides policies set by governments, institutions (hospitals, nursing homes, health systems) frequently include end of life issues in their policies. Some healthcare institutions have "futility" policies; most will have policies about withdrawing and withholding life-sustaining treatment (e.g., do not resuscitate orders) and surrogate decision making. Other relevant policies may not be formal or obvious, for instance intensive care units and emergency rooms may restrict family access to patients during certain hours or certain events (e.g., resuscitation) (Kopelman *et al.*, 2005).

Empirical studies

End of life decision making and care have attracted an enormous amount of research, ranging from comparisons of patients' and surrogates' preferences to interventional studies aiming to increase advance directive use or discussions about limiting treatment (Lynn *et al.*, 2000; Prendergast, 2001). Most of these studies portray an unfortunate reality: the wishes of patients are rarely known, poorly predicted by surrogates, unreliably followed when they *are* known, and patients' symptoms remain inadequately treated (Fagerlin and Schneider, 2004; Silveira *et al.*, 2005). The approach below integrates, when available, evidence about end of life decision making.

How should I approach conflict in the healthcare setting at the end of life in practice?

As for other problems in medicine, developing a differential diagnosis for end of life conflicts can help clinicians to consider carefully all of the possible explanations for the disagreement. Rather than reacting to the manifest problem (e.g., establishing code status), the first crucial step is to actively inquire what are some possible root causes of the conflict. After reflecting on root causes, addressing conflicts in end of life care should begin with a few open-ended questions. Asking the family about the patient's past history, what other clinicians have told them about their loved one's condition, and their choices (e.g., "Can you tell me why you are leaning toward resuscitation in the event she stops breathing?") allows one to identify the reasons behind decisions, as well as assess understanding. With that information, clinicians can explicitly create a differential diagnosis of the sources of conflict, which fall into three general categories: family features, healthcare provider features, and contextual (organizational and social) features. These are often present in combination and may interact.

Family features that contribute to conflicts

"Family" refers here to a patient's collection of intimates, who may or may not be related by blood ties. Two types of circumstance can explain the family's role in conflict. In the first, families do not understand the medical issues. In the second, they understand the clinical situation but reach a different conclusion from healthcare providers.

Inadequate understanding of the medical situation by the family could include a completely different understanding of the prognosis. An optimistic belief that cardiopulmonary resuscitation will succeed, for instance, could reflect its 77% success rate on television (Diem *et al.*, 1996). Consultants or nurses may inadvertently convey a different prognosis to the family than the primary physicians, so it is often useful to choose one healthcare professional to serve as the primary communicator, while other clinicians convey information *through* this spokesperson. Families often poorly process and imperfectly remember "bad news," even when it is clearly and consistently provided. Repeating key concepts, giving written as well as verbal information, encouraging questions ("I expect you will have questions about what we discussed today. Write them down for our talk tomorrow") and periodically assessing understanding of the situation may improve information transfer and decrease frustration.

Denial – the inability to explicitly recognize a set of facts because of its unacceptable psychological consequences – commonly affects the ability to understand medical situations. Symptoms of denial include displacement – a focus of concern on trivial, but controllable, matters – and an inability to discuss "bad news" (Weissman, 2004). Mrs. K's daughter, in the case described, asked about her mother's oxygen level and laboratory results; conversations about the "big picture" were quickly turned into discussions about relatively unimportant medical processes. Effective techniques for managing denial include open-ended listening; non-defensive, neutral responses; silence; and frequent, regular opportunities for the patient or family member to communicate with a consistent healthcare provider. Reflecting and validating family members' emotions can be especially valuable. Saying "It must be very hard for you to see your mother so ill," and "You've been a wonderful caregiver for her for many years" may prompt an exchange that begins to deal with the grief, guilt, or anger that can cause denial.

Finally, healthcare language can adversely affect understanding. Problems associated with interpretation of language can be avoided by using language appropriate to the family's educational level, by frequently assessing understanding, and by avoiding shorthand terms. Phrases like "usually," "most of the time," or "we cannot rule out," used by physicians to convey uncertainty, may be interpreted variably (Knapp *et al.*, 2004). Families are more likely to understand "out of 100 patients like your mother, about half will survive six months or longer" (Morrison, 2000) than "your mother has a 50% six month survival rate." Some caution is in order, however, given the impossibility of precise prognoses for individual patients (Fox *et al.*, 1999). Providing a range of possible outcomes can usefully convey uncertainty, for example "Almost all patients like this will not survive to be discharged from the hospital; some die within hours or days, others might stay alive for weeks or even months with in-hospital treatments. A rare few beat all the odds." Other language commonly used in discussions with families ("death with dignity," "everything done") contribute to misunderstandings. In Mrs. K's case, her daughter may have interpreted use of the term "futile" to mean that the physician did not think her mother was worth treating.

Grief can contribute to an inability to make *any* decisions, especially decisions that may result in a loved one's death. When Mrs. K's daughter said "I will not be able to live without her," it reflected her inability to cope with her mother's death. Supportive, open-ended dialogue allows the family to recognize, express, and begin to work through grief. Family members' guilt, often manifest during times of crisis, may also contribute to an unwillingness to make decisions. Guilt is recognizable when family members say, "I cannot do this," or "I will not be able to live with myself." Physicians may unwittingly increase feelings of guilt when they ask the family to take responsibility for medical decisions (e.g., "Do you want us to resuscitate her?" rather than, "What do you think *your mother* would want us to do?") (Tomlinson *et al.*, 1990). Even if surrogates do not always make decisions that patients would make (Fagerlin and Schneider, 2004), inaccuracy in no way undermines the family's role in decision making. Another way to treat the family's guilt is to take responsibility for medical decisions (e.g., "You tell me about what was important to your mother, and I will recommend what we should do for her"). The family can set positive goals and objectives of treatment (e.g., maximizing comfort) and clinicians recommend actions to achieve those goals. Clinicians should also praise family members, when appropriate, for respecting their loved one's values and wishes at the end of life.

Occasionally, secondary gain ("conflict of interest") may lead a family to make a decision with which the healthcare team disagrees. Secondary gain, often suspected when conflict arises, is always present to some degree when intimates make decisions for and about each other (Goold, 2000). Identifying potential sources of secondary gain – avoiding unbearable grief, avoiding overwhelming caregiving responsibilities, or avoiding financial ruin – is nonetheless illuminating. Addressing wishes to postpone the death of a spouse because of grief and loneliness requires a very different approach, for instance, than addressing wishes to keep a spouse or parent alive to collect a pension.

Even if they understand and accept the situation, family members may make decisions with which the healthcare team disagrees. Clinicians' values and those of patients or families differ. Individuals may have vastly different ideas about what constitutes a reasonable chance worth pursuing, a good quality of life, or a "good death." If Mrs. K's daughter, deciding according to her best understanding of her mother's wishes, chooses resuscitation because it might prolong her mother's life for a few days, weeks, or months even though the chance of survival to discharge is very small, this decision probably reflects a difference in values and should be respected. Empirical data suggest that these conflicts occur infrequently; with good communication, doctors and families usually come to mutually agreeable moral decisions.

Healthcare provider features

Clinicians, like patients, may be uncomfortable with prognostic uncertainty (Spikes and Holland, 1975; Kahneman *et al.*, 1982; Novack *et al.*, 1997; Christakis and Lamont, 2000; Meier *et al.*, 2001), which may lead them to approach limiting treatment decisions in overly hesitant or overly confident ways. Statements like "She won't leave the hospital alive" or "She has less than six months to live" fail to take into account the near-universal uncertainty in prognosis (Christakis and Lamont, 2000), and can make families suspicious they are not being told the whole story. Likewise, communicating information or recommendations too vaguely can lead to confusion or false hope. Clinicians who have known the patient for a long time might provide overly optimistic prognoses.

Like patients and families, healthcare providers are often uncomfortable discussing death; anxiety about one's own mortality may lead clinicians to avoid frank discussions about death or to provide false reassurance that "everything is OK." Clinicians also face the troubling thought of a medical "failure" (Spikes and Holland, 1975). Healthcare providers tend to underestimate the quality of life of chronically ill patients, especially for demented patients, and are more likely than patients or families to think that such patients would choose to forgo life-sustaining treatment. Other clinician attitudes that influence conflict include beliefs about the sanctity of life, the proper role of family members, difficulty with radically different values, or insecurity about one's competence or skill. Insight into one's own limitations and beliefs helps clinicians to understand feelings of anger and frustration with certain families and then to discuss with the family areas of disagreement (Novack et al., 1997; Meier et al., 2001).

Similarly, knowledge or skill deficits can catalyze clinician–family conflicts. Clinicians may be unaware of the prognosis or treatment options and misinform the family, although now numerous resources provide information on prognostic indicators for patients with a variety of clinical conditions (Gage et al., 2000). They may not understand ethical, legal, or hospital policies surrounding end of life care. Mistaken beliefs regarding the legality of withdrawing ventilators or artificial nutrition, for example, may lead a provider to refuse to accede to the family's desire. A lack of training in palliative care and symptom management can make interventions more burdensome for the patient, and hence lead clinicians to perceive they are inflicting suffering. Finally, healthcare providers may be ill-trained in interpersonal communication regarding end of life decisions, leading to misunderstandings, confusion, and frustrations (Tulsky et al., 1995, 1998). Fortunately, skills training is now more widely available.

Healthcare professionals, like patients and families, can be overworked, fatigued, frustrated, stressed, and otherwise beset by competing concerns. Physicians in training have heavy workloads and may be poorly motivated to spend additional time with patients or care for more of them and hence especially intent on making decisions quickly. The intern caring for Mrs. K may feel that her scarcest resource, time, is "wasted" on a demented, terminally ill woman. The culture of the hospital, with its prioritization of emergency, life and death decisions, high technology, and speedy discharges, as well as (in some systems) poor reimbursement for conversations with families, contributes to an emphasis on "high-tech" interventions and the avoidance of time-consuming family conferences. Insight into one's emotional status may help, although larger cultural changes in medicine will probably be needed (Scott et al., 1995; Field and Cassel, 1997; Mildred and Solomon, 2000).

Social and organizational features

Both the immediate and the general context in which clinician–family communication occurs can influence conflict. Conversations about end of life decisions that are unexpected (to the family), unannounced, or unplanned are more likely to result in conflict than those preceded by preliminary communication between clinicians and family, that occur at a preplanned time and location, and that have agreed-upon participants. As no competent surgeon would begin an operation without a plan for the procedure, clinicians should enter family discussions prepared with information about prognoses and with prepared methods to communicate information and ask and answer questions. The actual participants are important. Trust, which often accompanies long-standing doctor–patient relationships, can be invaluable for effective, solution-oriented communication. With the increasing use of hospitalists, seeking the input and participation of continuity clinicians may help in communication.

System-wide social and organizational factors also contribute to conflicts. Hospitals and health systems are worried about finances; doctors are under pressure to constrain the use of limited resources, and there is a pervasive social feeling that too much money is spent on medical care. Consequently, when a patient's prognosis seems to be hopeless, clinicians may feel, on the one hand, that life-prolonging treatment should be stopped quickly. On the other hand, some incentives such as reporting mortality rates for surgeons may encourage physician over treatment.

Patients and families face economic pressures of their own from serious illness; in the USA, medical expenses are the most common cause of personal bankruptcy. Families may prolong inpatient treatment because it costs them less than caring for a patient at home, or end things quickly if they bear substantial financial costs of care. Sadly, economic circumstances predict greater suffering at the end of life, and the availability of hospice care can depend on where a patient lives, their particular diagnosis, and whether or not they are insured (Silveira *et al.*, 2003, 2005).

Hospital policies may also promote conflicts in end of life decisions. When intensive care and other units restrict visiting hours, this minimizes contact between families and patients and may impair communication between them, and keeps families from seeing what their loved one is going through (Rosenczweig, 1998; Kopelman *et al.*, 2005). Similarly, requiring physicians to sign orders limiting life-support treatments may lead to unwanted resuscitation, particularly in settings (e.g., nursing facilities) staffed primarily by other clinicians. Organizations as well as doctors have legal fears regarding end of life decisions. In most of the major court cases in the USA since the mid 1980s, organizations refused to accede to family wishes, leading to legal action.

By considering this list of potential sources of conflict, clinicians can more readily and accurately identify the causes of difficult interactions with families of desperately ill patients around decisions to limit treatment. Improving the quality of end of life care requires development and research in interventions designed to identify and decrease these sources of conflicts. Training may help to improve physicians' capacity to elicit and identify psychological and social factors at play in conflicts at the end of life (Smith *et al.*, 1998) and improve their ability to give bad news, deal with emotions, and negotiate treatment goals. Hospitals and healthcare organizations should also experiment with structural changes, such as changing visiting time or increasing support for family meetings, to minimize conflicts and facilitate acceptable and relatively efficient solutions. It is hoped that by more accurately identifying the "diagnosis," the effective "treatment" (empathic end of life care) and "prevention" (early clinician–patient discussions and institutional change) will follow.

The case

Mrs. K was intubated and transferred to the intensive care unit when she experienced respiratory distress. Her daughter received counseling from clergy. She consistently expressed a request that her mother's treatment not exclude the goal of extending life. Several days after transfer to the intensive care unit, Mrs. K died.

REFERENCES

Christakis, N. A. and Lamont, E. B. (2000). Extent and determinants of error in doctors' prognoses in terminally ill patients: prospective cohort study. *BMJ* **320**: 469–73.

Cruzan v. *Director, Missouri Dep't. of Health* [1990] 110 S. Ct. 2841.

Diem, S. J., Lantos, J. D., and Tulsky, J. A. (1996). Cardiopulmonary resuscitation on television. Miracles and misinformation. *N Engl J Med* **334**: 1578–82.

Fagerlin, A. and Schneider, C. E. (2004). Enough: the failure of the living will. *Hastings Cent Rep* **34**: 30–42.

Field, M. J. and Cassel, C. K., for the Committee on Care at the End of Life of the Institute of Medicine (1997). *Approaching Death: Improving Care at the End of Life.* Washington, DC: Institute of Medicine.

Fox, E., Landrum-McNiff, K., Zhon, Z., *et al.*, for the SUPPORT Investigators (1999). Evaluation of prognostic criteria for determining hospice eligibility in patients with advanced lung, heart, or liver disease. Study to Understand Prognoses and Preferences for Outcomes and Risks of Treatments. *JAMA* **282**: 1638–45.

Gage, B., Miller, S. C., Coppola, K., *et al.*, for the MEDSTAT Group (2000). *Important Questions for Hospice in the Next Century.* Washington, DC: Government Printing Office (http://aspe.hhs.gov/daltcp/Reports/impquesa.htm). Accessed 5 July 2006.

Goold, S. D. (2000). Conflicts of interest and obligation. In *Ethics in Primary Care*, ed. J. Sugarman. New York: McGraw-Hill, pp. 93–101.

Kahneman, D., Slovic, P., and Tversky, A. (ed.) (1982). *Judgement under Uncertainty: Heuristics and Biases.* New York: Cambridge University Press.

Knapp, P., Raynor, D. K., and Berry, D. C. (2004). Comparison of two methods of presenting risk information to patients about the side effects of medicines. *Qual Safety Healthcare* **13**: 176–80.

Kopelman, M. B., Ubel, P. A., and Engel, K. G. (2005). Changing times, changing opinions: history informing the family presence debate. *Acad Emerg Med* **12**: 999–1002.

Lynn, J., De Vries, K. O., Arkes, H. R., *et al.* (2000). Ineffectiveness of the SUPPORT intervention: review of explanations. *J Am Geriatr Soc* **48**(Suppl. 5): S206–13.

Meier, D. E., Back, A. L., and Morrison, R. S. (2001). The inner life of physicians and care of the seriously ill. *JAMA* **286**: 3007–14.

Mildred, Z. and Solomon, M. Z. (2000). Institutional accountability in end of life care: organizational leadership, measurement, and consumer demand. *J Palliat Med* **3**: 225–8.

Morrison, R. S. and Siu, A. L. (2000). Survival in end–stage dementia following acute illness. *JAMA* **284**: 47–52.

Novack, D. H., Suchman, A. L., Clark, W., *et al.* (1997). Calibrating the physician. Personal awareness and effective patient care. Working Group on Promoting Physician Personal Awareness, American Academy on Physician and Patient. *JAMA* **278**: 502–9.

Prendergast, T. J. (2001). Advance care planning: pitfalls, progress, promise. *Critical Care Medicine* **29**(Suppl. 2): N34–9.

Rosenczweig, C. (1998). Should relatives witness resuscitation: ethical issues and practical considerations. *CMAJ* **158**: 617–20.

Scott, R. A., Aiken, L. H., Mechanic, D., and Moravcsik, J. (1995). Organizational aspects of caring. *Milbank Quart* **73**: 77–95.

Silveira, M. J., Goold, S. D., and McMahon, L. F., Jr. (2003). Access to hospice under Medicare; some for all, or all for some? *J Gen Intern Med* **18**: 217.

Silveira, M. J., Kabeto, M., and Langa, K. M. (2005). Net worth predicts symptom burden for at the end of life. *J Palliat Med* **8**: 827–37.

Smith, R. C., Lyles, J. S., Mettler, J., *et al.* (1998). The effectiveness of intensive training for residents in interviewing. A randomized, controlled study. *Ann Intern Med* **128**: 139–41.

Spikes, J. and Holland, J. (1975). The physician's response to the dying patient. In *Psychological Care of the Medically Ill: A Primer in Liaison Psychiatry* ed. J. J. Strain and S. Grossman. New York: Appleton-Century-Crofts, pp. 138–48.

Tomlinson, T., Howe, K., Notman, M., and Rossmiller, D. (1990). An empirical study of proxy consent for elderly persons. *Gerontologist* **30**: 54–64.

Tulsky, J. A., Chesney, M. A., and Lo, (1995). How do medical residents discuss resuscitation with patients? *J Gen Intern Med* **10**: 436–42.

Tulsky, J. A., Fischer, G. S., Rose, M. R., and Arnold, R. M. (1998). Opening the black box: how do physicians communicate about advance directives? *Ann Intern Med* **129**: 441–9.

Weissman, D. E. (2004). Decision making at a time of crisis near the end of life. *JAMA* **292**: 1738–43.

13

Brain death

Sam D. Shemie, Neil Lazar, and Bernard M. Dickens

Mr. L is a 35-year-old man who has a sudden, excruciating headache and collapses in his chair at dinner. At the emergency department, a CT scan reveals a subarachnoid hemorrhage. Mr. L is admitted to the intensive care unit for monitoring and supportive measures aimed at controlling the intracranial pressure. The next morning he is noted to be unresponsive, with non-reactive, mid-position pupils.

A $3\frac{1}{2}$-year-old boy, M, is playing near the backyard pool under supervision of his babysitter. The caretaker goes into the house to answer the telephone. Upon returning, she discovers the child face down in the pool. The paramedic team arrives and finds the child's vital signs are absent. Basic life support is started, and the boy is taken to the hospital. He is resuscitated with intubation, ventilation, and intravenous epinephrine injection. The minimum documented duration of absent vital signs is 30 minutes. He is comatose and unresponsive, with spontaneous breathing, reactive pupils and intermittent generalized seizures.

What is brain death?

Medicine and society continue to struggle thoughtfully with the definition of death, particularly with the progression of sophisticated life-support systems that challenge traditional concepts. The questions of when a disease is irreversible, when further treatment is ineffective, or when death has occurred are of great consequence.

These questions are independent of, and galvanized by, the practice of organ donation.

Brain death is defined as the absence of all brain function demonstrated by profound coma with the irreversible loss of capacity for consciousness, loss of the ability to breathe and absence of all brain stem reflexes. Analogous to a cardiac arrest, it is better understood as brain arrest – the loss of all clinical brain function. If a proximate cause is known and there are no reversible conditions present, death is determined by documenting the absence of brain function by clinical examination. In most cases, brain death can be diagnosed at the bedside. Common causes include trauma, intracranial hemorrhage, cerebrovascular accidents, hypoxia owing to resuscitation after cardiac arrest, drug overdose or near drowning, primary brain tumor, meningitis, homicide, and suicide.

The clinical entity was first described in the medical literature by the French and termed ''coma dépassé'' (Mollaret and Goulon, 1959; Wertheimer *et al.*, 1959), a state beyond coma. It was placed into practice in the next decade with the use of specific clinical criteria, arising from the landmark work by the Ad Hoc Committee of the Harvard Medial School to Examine the Definition of Brain Death (1968). The concept of brain death was influenced by two major health care advances in the 1960s: the development of intensive care units, with artificial airways and mechanical ventilators

An earlier version of this chapter has appeared: Lazar, N. M., Shemie, S., Webster, G. C., and Dickens, B. M. (2001). Brain death. *CMAJ* **164**: 833–6.

to treat irreversible apnea, thus interrupting the natural evolution from brain failure to cardiac arrest, and the emergence of organ donation arising from the new discipline of transplant surgery. An ethical consensus existed that the donation itself must not cause the death of the donor, commonly referred to as the "dead donor" rule (Truog and Robinson, 2003).

Advanced technologies also revealed the existing limitations in the lexicon of death. The word "death" may be inadequate to describe the event or process in the various domains in which it can be defined, including medical–biological, legal, social, bioethical, philosophical, religious, spiritual, and existential. Brain death as a criterion for determining the death of a person is a medicolegal and social formulation. It implies a notion of irreversible loss of personhood and integrative functions of the brain. The diagnosis uncovers cultural and religious diversity in a pluralistic society.

Why is brain death important?

Ethics

Social formulation

For centuries, determining the death of another person was seen to be a rather straightforward matter. The cessation of cardiac and respiratory functions was thought to be sufficient to conclude that a person had died. The advent of neurological or brain-based criteria to establish the death of a person was a significant departure from the traditional way of defining death. Regardless of which criteria are used, agreement about when death occurs is not simply an agreement about medical or biological criteria for death but is also a "social formulation" (Capron, 1995). On this point, Karen Gervais (1995) noted "that even in pre-technological culture, use of the traditional cardiopulmonary criteria was a choice, an imposition of values on biological data. It was a choice based on a decision

concerning significant function, that is, a decision concerning what is so essentially significant to the nature of the human being that its irreversible cessation constitutes human death."

Medical–biological formulation

Death in medicine may be fulfilled by the complete and irreversible absence of (i) circulation, as a consequence of cardiac arrest; or (ii) brain function, as a consequence of brain arrest.

The concept of brain death has been criticized as a social construct created for utilitarian purposes to permit transplantation (Taylor, 1997). Scientific advances have diminished the legitimacy of these historical arguments. Traditional cardiopulmonary definitions of death (asystolic cardiocirculatory arrest) are no longer sufficient in the face of advancing technology that may support and/or replace complete and irreversible loss of heart and/or lung function. Every solid organ can be supported by technology in the intensive care unit or replaced by transplantation, except the brain. If the heart is completely and irreversibly arrested, death has not occurred if the circulation is being supported by a machine such as the extracorporeal membrane oxygenator or other forms of artificial heart technology, as long as the prospect for recovery of neurological function is maintained. The concept of irreversibility in cardiac death is itself being questioned, in favor of definitions based on permanence (Bernat, 2006).

Cardiorespiratory function can be sustained in any form or severity of brain failure. It was once considered that brain death invariably leads to hemodynamic instability and cardiac arrest (Lagiewska *et al.*, 1996). However, it is now clear that aggressive cardiorespiratory support, hormonal therapy, and nursing care can maintain somatic functions indefinitely, as demonstrated in individuals who become brain dead during pregnancy (Powner and Bernstein, 2003). These continued advances in technology and transplantation have made brain-based determination of death more relevant today than in their original conception.

Personhood

Conceptually, complete loss of brain function is seen to be a significant threshold separating one who is living from one who is dead. Recognizing and accepting this threshold allows clinicians and patients' families to consent to organ donation without fear of violating the dead donor rule. It also permits clinicians to proceed with discontinuation of cardiorespiratory support without fear or belief that they are causing the death of their patient. Those who accept brain-based definitions of death argue that those brain functions necessary for the integrated functioning of the person are irreversibly lost, and without artificial support, the person would not be able to spontaneously sustain those necessary functions.

Some have even argued that the whole-brain definition of death should be amended to incorporate people in a persistent vegetative state, that is, those who have experienced the irreversible loss of so-called higher-brain functions (Truog and Robinson, 2003). Proponents of this higher-brain definition of death argue that consciousness and the capacity to relate to other people and the wider world is a defining characteristic of human beings. In this view, the death of that part of the brain responsible for consciousness and interaction with the world is equivalent to the death of the person. Although the whole-brain definition of death has gained wide acceptance, the higher-brain definition has not. Concern about the implications of this higher-brain definition of death can be found in the early work of the US President's Commission for the Study of Ethical Problems in Medicine and Biomedical and Behavioral Research (1981a). The implication of the personhood and personal identity arguments is that a patient like Karen Quinlan, who retains brainstem function and breathes spontaneously, is just as dead as a corpse in the traditional sense. The Commission rejected this conclusion and the further implication that such patients could be buried or otherwise treated as dead persons.

Cultural and religious diversity

Understanding, defining, and determining brain death continue to be ethically challenging and complex undertakings in many cultures. Various cultural and religious groups (e.g., some Canadian First Nations and Asian cultures, and ultra-orthodox Judaism) have been reluctant to accept that death has occurred until all vital functions have ceased. Furthermore, in the clinical setting, some families simply may not accept that a relative is dead. Many experience a certain discomfort when they view a person who is brain dead but who appears to be alive because vital bodily functions are being sustained by technological support. Some jurisdictions have even made legal exemptions based on religious perspectives (Olick, 1991).

Trust

Surveys of public attitudes towards organ donation show remarkable levels of support, exceeding 95% in Canada for example (Canadian Council for Donation and Transplantation, 2005). The public's perceptions of brain death, and the distinction between cardiac and brain death, however, remain poorly understood. Any residual public ambivalence toward organ donation and retrieval may be rooted in the experience of witnessing a person declared brain dead who is sustained on technological support. This concern may not only be about accurately determining death but may also reflect fears that death will be declared prematurely for the sake of organ and tissue retrieval. This should not be underestimated by clinicians caring for the critically ill or by those involved in the procurement of tissue and organs. Without an enduring trust between doctors and their patients, brain death will remain an enigma to most of the general public.

Law

The law approaches death as an event rather than a process, and as a matter of status rather than as a medical condition. Death marks the time from which certain legal consequences follow, including termination of obligations to provide resuscitative measures, termination of individual legal rights, execution of a will or other distribution of an estate, eligibility for autopsy and organ or tissue donation, lawful disposal of bodily remains, and, for instance, beneficiaries' claims under life insurance policies and other entitlements.

The law sets the criteria by which death is determined. Legislation or judge-declared law may specify that death occurs on irreversible cessation of heart function and/or respiration but may provide, in addition or instead, that death occurs on irreversible cessation of total brain function. Physicians usually determine whether the legal criteria of death are satisfied. When death may be determined by neurological criteria, the assessment is legally decisive even if other criteria relating to cessation of heart beat and respiration are being artificially resisted, such as for preservation of transplantable organs. Laws may alternatively not set criteria of death but only a process of determination. For instance in Canada, legislation in Ontario provides that "for the purposes of a post-mortem transplant, the fact of death shall be determined by at least two physicians in accordance with accepted medical practice" (Shemie *et al.*, 2006).

In many of the world's jurisdictions, there are laws to prevent conflicts of interest in a physician determining death and caring for a potential recipient of the deceased person's organ. Provisions commonly preclude a physician who has any association with the likely recipient of a deceased person's organ from participation in or influence over determination of that person's death. A physician is similarly precluded from participation in transplantation into a recipient of an organ or tissues from the body of a person whose death the physician participated in determining, including deciding on allocation of such person's organs and/or tissues.

Policy

Many national critical care, neurological, and neurosurgical societies have drafted policies and practice guidelines for the declaration of brain death (Medical Consultants on the Diagnosis of Death to the President's Commission, 1981; Task Force for the Determination of Brain Death in Children, 1987; American Academy of Neurology, 1995; Royal College of Physicians Working Party, 1995; Shemie *et al.*, 2006). While variability in brain-death practices have been well described (Wijdicks, 2002; Powner *et al.*, 2004; Hornby *et al.*, 2006), the clinical criteria for the determination are remarkably consistent across jurisdictions (Wijdicks, 2002; Powner *et al.*, 2004). Brain death is fundamentally a clinical evaluation, where the clinical criteria have primacy and routine ancillary laboratory testing has fallen into disfavor. Ancillary testing is recommended only when the usual clinical criteria cannot be completed at the bedside, when confounding conditions exist, or specific to infants (Wijdicks, 2002). While many countries still utilize electroencephalography because of its widespread availability and historical use, it has well-known shortcomings that limit its applicability (Young *et al.*, 2006). Demonstrating the absence of brain blood flow is increasingly recommended as the preferred ancillary test in both children and adults (Shemie *et al.*, 2006; Young *et al.*, 2006).

How should I approach brain death in practice?

Physicians who participate in the declaration of brain death should be experienced in the care of critically ill brain-injured patients, relevant clinical criteria, and diagnostic procedures. National or institutional checklists for testing and documentation are useful assets (Shemie *et al.*, 2006). In cases of potential organ donation, it has been seen that physicians declaring death must not have any association with the identified transplant recipient and must not participate in any way in the transplant procedures.

Brain death is a detailed clinical examination that documents the complete and irreversible loss of consciousness and absence of brainstem function, including the capacity to breathe. The following criteria apply (Shemie *et al.*, 2006).

1. Established etiology capable of causing brain death in the absence of reversible conditions capable of mimicking brain death
2. Deep unresponsive coma
3. Absent brainstem reflexes as defined by absent gag and cough reflexes, corneal responses, pupillary responses to light with pupils at mid size or greater and vestibulo-ocular responses
4. Bilateral absence of motor responses, excluding spinal reflexes
5. Absent respiratory effort based on the apnea test
6. Absent confounding factors.

An absolute prerequisite is the absence of clinical neurological function with a known, proximate cause that is irreversible. There must be definite clinical and/or neuroimaging evidence of an acute central nervous system event that is consistent with the irreversible loss of neurological function. Coma of unclear mechanism precludes the diagnosis. Deep unresponsive coma implies an absence of centrally mediated response to pain. Any motor response in the cranial nerve distribution, central nervous system-mediated motor response to pain in any distribution, seizures, and decorticate and/or decerebrate responses are not compatible with the diagnosis.

Spinal reflexes, or motor responses confined to spinal distribution, may persist. A proportion of patients may continue to display some reflex spinal activity, which can confuse the bedside staff or the inexperienced clinician and can be disturbing to family members. They should be anticipated and explanations should be provided to families. Observed spinal reflex activity may range from subtle twitches to the more complex "Lazarus sign" and may be seen in 13–39% of cases (Saposnik *et al.*, 2000; Dosemeci *et al.*, 2004). Reversible conditions such as hypothermia and the influence of central nervous system depressants and muscle relaxants need to be excluded. Independent confirmation

and/or determining the irreversibility of coma may require a period of observation, with recommendations varying from 0 to 24 hours, depending on the individual's age and the cause of the coma (Wijdicks, 2002; Hornby *et al.*, 2006). In clinical practice, distinguishing between brain death and persistent vegetative state is not difficult. In a persistent vegetative state, spontaneous respiration and other rudimentary brainstem reflexes are present and persistent.

In the USA, a whole-brain definition (cerebral hemispheres and the brainstem) for brain death is codified based on the irreversible cessation of all functions of the brain, including the brainstem (President's Commission for the Study of Ethical Problems in Medicine and Biomedical and Behavioral Research, 1981b). This is distinct from the UK, where a brainstem-based definition of death is in place (Pallis and Harley, 1996). It must be understood that the basic clinical evaluation for loss of neurological function in brain death examinations only detects the absence of *brainstem* function. The clinical examination cannot distinguish between the complete loss of whole-brain function versus brainstem function. The distinction between whole-brain versus brainstem death can be made based on etiology of brain injury and neuroimaging. It can only be confirmed by the use of an ancillary test that shows absence of electroencephalographic activity, or the absence of brain blood flow. For this reason, ancillary testing is commonly used in the USA but only rarely in the UK.

Once brain death has been diagnosed according to the clinical criteria outlined above, physicians and families must realize that brain death equals the death of the patient. Families should be told in no uncertain terms that the patient has died. Issues for the family to consider at this time include organ or tissue donation, autopsy examination and funeral arrangements. Organ-support technologies should be removed unless organ donation is being considered. If there is conflict regarding the diagnosis of brain death that cannot be resolved by the clinicians and the family at the bedside, the coroner may be called in to evaluate the case and possibly complete the medical certificate of death.

Two possible exceptions to this approach have been discussed in the literature. The first is the unusual circumstance of an apparently brain-dead patient who is pregnant at the time of diagnosis. A small number of such cases have been described in the literature, some with attempts made to maintain the pregnancy until viability of the fetus (Powner and Bernstein, 2003). No consensus has been reached as to whether this should be attempted (Sperling, 2006). Another exception might be based on religious objections to the acceptance of brain death as a criterion for declaring death. New York State adopted a religious exception to brain death in 1987 and New Jersey in 1991 (Olick, 1991). Limitation of support interventions, rather than withdrawal, would normally be accepted and would typically lead to cardiovascular instability and death over a period of days.

The cases

Mr. L probably has progressed to clinical brain death. His doctors will have to perform a formal evaluation at the bedside to determine this status. A careful review of the medication record fails to reveal any sedative or neuromuscular-blocking drugs administered. The patient is not hypothermic. No stimulation evokes a response except for spinal reflexes of the lower extremities. All brain stem reflexes are absent when tested with adequate stimuli. His family is informed of the results of these tests and is asked whether Mr. L was in favor of organ donation. The family agrees to consider organ donation. Mr. L is formally declared brain dead by two qualified physicians. Nine other patients benefit from transplants of his organs.

The condition of the boy, M, deteriorates over the ensuing 48 hours, with signs of brainstem herniation, including fixed and dilated pupils, diabetes insipidus, and impaired thermoregulation. A computed tomography (CT) scan of the head shows severe cerebral edema consistent with hypoxic–ischemic injury. Examination by two independent specialists on two separate occasions confirms the clinical diagnosis of brain death. The family is counseled on multiple occasions regarding the diagnosis of brain death and consents to organ donation. Seven patients benefit from transplants of the child's organs.

REFERENCES

Ad Hoc Committee of the Harvard Medical School to Examine the Definition of Brain Death (1968). A definition of irreversible coma. *JAMA* **205**: 337–40.

American Academy of Neurology (1995). Practice parameters for determining brain death in adults: report of the Quality Standards Subcommittee of the American Academy of Neurology. *Neurology* **45**: 1012–14.

Bernat, J. L. (2006). Are organ donors after cardiac death really dead? *J Clin Ethics* **17**: 122–32.

Canadian Council for Donation and Transplantation (2005). *Public Survey*. Ottawa: Canadian Council for Donation and Transplantation (www.ccdt.ca).

Capron, A. (1995). Legal issues in pronouncing death. In *Encyclopedia of Bioethics*, revised edn, ed. W. T. Reich. New York: Simon and Schuster Macmillan, pp. 534–9.

Dosemeci, L., Cengiz, M., Yilmaz, M., and Ramazanoglu, A. (2004). Frequency of spinal reflex movements in brain-dead patients. *Transplant Proc* **36**: 17.

Gervais, K. G. (1995). Death, definition and determination: philosophical and theological perspectives. In *Encyclopedia of bioethics*, revised edn, ed. W. T. Reich. New York: Simon and Schuster Macmillan, pp. 540–8.

Hornby, K., Shemie, S. D., Teitelbaum, J., and Doig, C. (2006). Variability of hospital based brain death guidelines in Canada. *Can J Anes* **53**: 613–19.

Lagiewska, B., Pacholczyk, M., Szostek, M., Walaszewski, J., and Rowinski, W. (1996). Hemodynamic and metabolic disturbances observed in brain dead organ donors. *Transplant Proc* **28**: 165–6.

Medical Consultants on the Diagnosis of Death to the President's Commission (1981). Guidelines for the determination of death. *JAMA* **246**: 2184–5.

Mollaret, P. and Goulon, M. (1959). Le coma dépassé. *Rev Neurol (Paris)* **101**: 3–15.

Olick, R. S. (1991). Brain death, religious freedom, and public policy: New Jersey's landmark legislative initiative. *Kennedy Inst Ethics J* **1**: 275–92.

Pallis, C. and Harley, D. H. (1996). *ABC of Brainstem Death*, 2nd edn. London: BMJ Publishing, pp. 8–12.

Powner, D. J. and Bernstein, I. M. (2003). Extended somatic support for pregnant women after brain death. *Crit Care Med* **31**: 1241–9.

Powner, D. J., Hernandez, M., and Rives, T. E. (2004). Variability among hospital policies for determining brain death in adults. *Crit Care Med* **31**: 1284–88.

President's Commission for the Study of Ethical Problems in Medicine and Biomedical and Behavioral Research (1981a). *Defining Death: A Report on the Medical, Legal and Ethical Issues in the Determination of Death.* Washington, DC: The President's Commission.

President's Commission for the Study of Ethical Problems in Medicine and Biomedical and Behavioral Research (1981b). Defining death. *JAMA* **246**: 2184–6.

Royal College of Physicians Working Party (1995). Criteria for the diagnosis of brain stem death. *J R Coll Physicians Lond* **29**: 381–2.

Saposnik, G., Bueri, J. A., Maurino, J., Saizar, R., and Garretto, N. S. (2000). Spontaneous and reflex movements in brain death. *Neurology* **54**: 221–3.

Shemie, S. D., Doig, C., Dickens, B., *et al.* (2006). Severe brain injury to neurological determination of death: Canadian forum recommendations. *CMAJ* **174**: S1–12.

Sperling, D. (2006). *Management of Post-mortem Pregnancy: Legal and Philosophical Aspects.* Aldershot: Ashgate.

Task Force for the Determination of Brain Death in Children (1987). Guidelines for the determination of brain death in children. *Arch Neurol* **44**: 587–8.

Taylor, R. M. (1997). Reexamining the definition and criteria of death. *Semin Neurol* **17**: 265–70.

Truog, R. D. and Robinson, W. M. (2003). Role of brain death and the dead-donor rule in the ethics of organ transplantation. *Crit Care Med* **31**: 2391–6.

Wertheimer, P., Jouvet, M., and Descotes, J. (1959). A propos du diagnostic de la mort du système nerveux dans les comas avec arrêt respiratoire traités par respiration artificielle. *Presse Med* **67**: 87–8.

Wijdicks, E. F. M. (2002). Brain death worldwide: accepted fact but no global consensus in diagnostic criteria. *Neurology* **58**: 20–5.

Young, B., Shemie, S. D., Doig, C., and Teitelbaum, J. (2006). Brief review: the role of ancillary tests in the neurological determination of death. *Can J Anes* **53**: 620–7.

Pregnant women and children

Introduction

John Lantos

The clinical care of pregnant women and children raises unique and complex ethical issues for three reasons. Firstly, unlike in other areas of medicine where the primary ethical principle is respect for patient autonomy, the care of pregnant women and children requires a balancing act. During pregnancy, the balancing act may involve the weighing of actual physical risks to the pregnant woman against potential benefits for her fetus. After the birth of the child, the balancing requires us to weigh the child's medical interests against the psychological, spiritual, or economic interests of his or her parents and family. This balancing requires that decisions reflect considerations other than the values, desires, or stated wishes of the patient. Parents, doctors, ethics committees, judges, or other adults must decide what is or is not permissible for a given child or a group of children.

Obstetrics and pediatrics are also especially complicated because the goal of clinical medicine in these areas is fundamentally different from that in other areas of medicine. In other areas, medicine works against the inevitable. Everybody will get sick. Everybody will die. In obstetrics and pediatrics, however, the hope and the goal is that everyone will be healthy. In fact, most pregnancies turn out well, most children do not get seriously ill, and very few die during childbirth or childhood. The goal in obstetrics and pediatrics is to preserve and protect good health, rather than to diagnose and cure disease. Both are, fundamentally, preventive. However, the means by which disease is prevented are themselves becoming more and more invasive. Prenatal testing, newborn screening, and immunizations all require sophisticated medical interventions. These interventions are beneficial, but not always risk free.

A unique aspect of pediatrics that distinguishes it from both obstetrics and adult medicine is the way in which it must take into account the progressive and evolving capacity of children to participate in medical decisions. This evolving capacity takes children from absolute inability to participate – during fetal life or infancy – toward the full capacity to participate that they generally acquire by late adolescence.

One must read the following chapters with these three factors in mind. Each confronts these differences and avoids the easy procedural trap of trying to transform the ethics dilemmas of obstetrics and pediatrics into dilemmas of surrogate decision making. That trap tempts us to attempt an end run around the difficult dilemmas of this clinical domain by simply assigning decision-making authority to one or another adult. Thus, we may say, "Let the parents decide. After all, they are the ones who must live with the consequences of the decision." Or "Let the parents decide. After all, they must know their child best." Or, "Let the doctors decide. They have special insight into the medical facts that ought to be considered in this decision." Each of these procedural shortcuts tries to substitute an efficient simplicity for a messy confrontation with the fundamental complexities of understanding the moral claims that our children make upon us, and deciding what our best response ought to be.

The section is divided into two halves. The first half deals with the ethical dilemmas of caring for pregnant women in high-risk obstetrical situations, with the dilemmas of our expanding capabilities to screen fetuses and newborns for diseases that we cannot yet treat, and with the complexities of infertility treatment. The second half focuses more on dilemmas that arise in pediatric practice: questions about when and whether to report child abuse, about when a non-therapeutic intervention might be appropriate, and the dilemmas raised by the evolving competencies of children as they move through adolescence. The authors of the various chapters in this section take on a range of such difficult issues in pediatrics. They highlight the conceptual issues as well as the practical ones, offering not just concrete recommendations for clinicians but theoretical ethical justifications for their actions as well.

The ethics of providing clinical care for pregnant women and children is primarily about obligations, rather than rights. The authors of chapters in this section attempt to clarify the nature and scope of those obligations in different contexts. The focus upon obligations, rather than rights, sometimes leads them as writers and us as readers into uncomfortable territory, but it is necessary to follow the path. It does not make sense to talk about whether an unconceived child has a right to be conceived. Instead, we must talk about the sorts of safeguards that must be put into place to help doctors and parents who confront infertility to do so in a way that serves the needs of all. It does not make sense to talk about the rights of a newborn to be screened for certain diseases. Instead, we must focus on our duties and obligations to provide or not provide screening in particular situations. To the extent that we, collectively, have an obligation to children, that obligation falls equally upon parents, doctors, policy makers, and the community that collectively subsidizes obstetrical and pediatric therapies.

14

Ethical dilemmas in the care of pregnant women: rethinking "maternal–fetal conflicts"

Françoise Baylis, Sanda Rodgers, and David Young

Ms. A is 19 years old and 25 weeks pregnant. Although her pregnancy was unplanned, at no time has she considered pregnancy termination. During a prenatal office visit, Ms. A reveals that she has a daily drug habit that includes crack cocaine and intravenous narcotics. She refuses to consider a change in her behavior, despite a thorough review of the potential effects of her substance abuse on her pregnancy outcome. Specifically, she refuses to participate in a methadone or other substance-abuse program.

Ms. B is 24 years old and has been in labor for 18 hours. The cervical dilatation has not progressed past 3 cm. The fetal heart rate tracing has been worrisome but is now seriously abnormal, showing a profound bradycardia of 65 beats per minute. This bradycardia does not resolve with conservative measures. Repeat pelvic examination reveals no prolapsed cord and confirms a vertex presentation at 3 cm dilatation. The obstetrician explains to Ms. B that a cesarean section will be necessary because of suspected fetal distress. Ms. B absolutely refuses, saying "No surgery."

What are ethical dilemmas in the care of pregnant women?

When a pregnant woman engages in behavior(s) that may be harmful to her fetus, or refuses a recommended diagnostic or therapeutic intervention aimed at enhancing fetal health and well-being, her physician may experience an ethical dilemma. An ethical dilemma arises when a person has an ethical obligation to pursue two (or more) conflicting courses of action (Beauchamp and Childress, 1994), as when a physician believes that he or she has an obligation both to respect a patient's decision and to protect the fetus from harm.

Ethical dilemmas in the care of pregnant women can arise because of women's personal healthcare choices, lifestyle and behaviors, and occupational situation. These dilemmas are often described as maternal–fetal conflicts (Hornstra, 1998; Oduncu *et al.*, 2003; Wallace *et al.*, 1997). Use of this term is problematic, however, for several reasons. Firstly, the term maternal–fetal conflict situates the conflict between the pregnant woman and the fetus. In so doing, it misdirects attention away from the conflict that needs to be addressed: namely the conflict between the pregnant woman and others (such as child welfare agencies, physicians, and other healthcare providers) who believe they know best how to protect the fetus. Secondly, the term perpetuates the underlying, but unfounded, assumption that the problem involves the opposition of maternal rights and fetal rights when, at most, there is a conflict between the woman's autonomy and the best interest of the fetus. Finally, the term maternal–fetal conflict is factually incorrect. The term maternal suggests the existence of parental obligations toward the fetus, whereas the woman is *yet to become* a mother to the fetus she is carrying. Although maternal–fetal conflict has

An earlier version of this chapter has appeared: Flagler, E., Baylis, F., and Rodgers, S. (1997). Ethical dilemmas that arise in the care of pregnant women: rethinking "maternal–fetal conflicts." *CMAJ* **156**: 1729–32.

some currency, we advocate the use of the more accurate, descriptive phrase, "ethical dilemmas in the care of pregnant women."

Why are ethical dilemmas in the care of pregnant women important?

Ethics

The principle of reproductive freedom stipulates that people have the right to make their own reproductive choices and that the state has an obligation to foster conditions under which this can occur (Sherwin, 1992). For some, this principle is morally objectionable because it grants women the right to make decisions concerning the termination of unwanted pregnancies. In their view, whatever rights pregnant women may or may not have, they do not override the fetus' right to life (Kluge, 1988) or prenatal care (Keyserlingk, 1984; Fasouliotis and Schenker, 2000). The problem with this view is that it rests on the highly contested belief that the fetus has a right to life and a "right to be born of sound mind and body."

Others endorse the principle of reproductive freedom but advocate for what they believe to be legitimate restrictions on this principle as it applies to pregnant women. They maintain that a woman has a limited right to terminate her pregnancy but that once she has chosen to continue her pregnancy, she incurs obligations to protect and promote the health and well-being of her fetus and the state incurs obligations to limit or preclude actions that would irreversibly harm the future person. These obligations to the fetus are grounded in the belief that the fetus has a right not to be damaged and a right not to be deliberately or negligently harmed. (For a brief description of the difference between the right to be born of sound mind and body, the right not to be damaged and the right not to be deliberately or negligently harmed, see Bewley [2002]). The problem with this alternative view in support of state intervention is that it erroneously assumes that continuing a pregnancy

involves a deliberate active choice on the part of the woman, and that behaviors that ultimately may harm a fetus can properly be described as choices – consider, for example, addictive behaviors (Baylis, 1998; Harris, 2000). Further, this view egregiously suggests an opposition between the interests of the woman and those of the fetus, when in fact these interests are inextricably linked.

A third perspective on state intervention in the lives of pregnant women insists that forced screening, forced incarceration to prevent continued substance abuse, and forced obstetrical interventions are always indefensible. Such coercion is an unacceptable infringement of the woman's rights to personal autonomy, inviolability, and bodily integrity (Annas, 1987; Mahowald, 1993; Hornstra, 1998; Harris and Paltrow, 2003).

State coercion is also deeply problematic when considered in its broader social and political context. One of the justifications for state intervention in pregnancy is the belief that such intervention benefits the fetus. In fact, however, the harm to women that results from state coercion often occurs without any countervailing benefit to the fetus. Consider, for example, reports of healthy infants delivered after women have refused consent for cesarean section (Kolder et al., 1987; American College of Obstetricians and Gynecologists, 2006). Also, at times, no benefit accrues to the fetus from state intervention because by the time the health need is identified and state intervention is contemplated, irreversible fetal harm has already occurred.

State intervention is also counter-productive relative to the goal of promoting fetal health and well-being as it undermines the trust between pregnant women and physicians that is necessary to foster the education which would promote the birth of healthier babies. When trust is diminished or absent, women whose fetuses may be most at risk may be discouraged from seeking appropriate care from physicians whom they perceive as merely "agents of the state."

It is also important to note that state intervention in pregnancy to save fetal lives is far in excess of any non-voluntary action that would be tolerated to save non-fetal lives. For example, parents are not coerced to become organ donors, even if failure to do so would likely result in the death of their child. We may consider a parent's refusal to make such a donation morally reprehensible, but not within the realm of state authority.

Finally, state intervention to promote fetal well-being is hypocritical given the inconsistency between aggressive efforts to rescue a few fetuses from a few women in unfortunate situations, when there is widespread tolerance for unacceptable and sometimes dangerous living conditions for many children whose moral status (unlike that of the developing fetus) is not contested. Here, it is also important to emphasize that the attention paid to pregnant women's behaviors and choices overlooks the fact that "malnutrition, violence, chaotic lives, serious maternal health problems and lack of medical care" (Pollitt, 1990, p. 411) have a significant impact on the health and well-being of the fetus.

Law

In general, both domestic laws and international covenants address issues relevant to this discussion, confirming both the absence of fetal rights and the competent woman's right to make her own treatment decisions: For example, see cases such as *Re MB* (1997), *St George's NHS Trust* v. *S* (1999), *Regina* v. *Collins* (1999) in the UK; *Harrild* v. *Director of Proceedings* (2003) in New Zealand; *R* v. *Phillip Nathan King* (2003) in Australia; *Paton* v. *UK* (1980), *RH* v. *Norway* (1992), *Boso* v. *Italy* (2002), and *Vo* v. *France* (2004), all at the European Court of Human Rights.

In many countries, the courts have recognized that the fetus does not have legal rights until it is born alive and with complete delivery from the body of the pregnant woman (*R* v. Sullivan, 1991; Rodgers, 1993; Martin and Coleman, 1995). Because the fetus has no legal rights until born, child protection legislation (which, under certain circumstances, authorizes state intervention on behalf of a child at risk) does not apply to the fetus.

Additionally, a number of international instruments affirm that legal rights attach only at birth, making clear that the fetus has no legal rights that could override the pregnant woman's right to determine her own healthcare (Council of Europe, 1989; United Nations, 1989, 1966, 1994; Cook *et al.*, 2003; Copelon *et al.*, 2005). The *Universal Declaration of Human Rights* (United Nations, 1994) states that "All human beings are *born* free and equal in dignity and rights." The *Convention on the Elimination of All Forms of Discrimination Against Women* (United Nations, 1979) provides that all women have "The same rights to decide freely and responsibly on the number and spacing of their children and to have access to the information, education and means to enable them to exercise these rights."

As regards the right of pregnant women to make their own healthcare choices – physicians who treat competent patients (including competent pregnant patients) without their consent put themselves at risk of both criminal and civil liability (cf. *Malette* v. *Shulman*, 1990). Courts considering cases from various jurisdictions, including England, France, Italy, New South Wales, New Zealand, and the USA, all have confirmed the right of pregnant women to make decisions concerning their own healthcare. In *Paton* v. *UK* (1980), for example, the European Commission held that "The life of the fetus is intimately connected with, and it cannot be regarded in isolation of, the life of the pregnant woman ..." They held that to preclude abortion would mean that "... the 'unborn life' of the fetus would be regarded as being of a higher value than the life of the pregnant woman."

Also, in many jurisdictions, decisions refer to and rely on a decision of the Supreme Court of Canada in *Winnipeg Child and Family Services (Northwest Area)* v. *G. (D.F.)* (1997). At issue was whether there was legal authority to order a pregnant woman to undergo counseling and hospital admission to manage a drug addiction in the absence of her consent. The Supreme Court held that forced detention and treatment would violate the woman's constitutional rights and that there was no legal basis on which to do so. This decision also confirmed that the fetus is not protected before birth and that courts have no legal grounds on which to order a competent pregnant woman to undergo a medical intervention that she does not want. The Court held (paragraph 43) that imposing legal liability on pregnant women for injury to their fetus during pregnancy was not likely to result in improved pregnancy outcome:

It is far from clear that the proposed [legal duty of the mother] will decrease the incidence of substance-injured children. Indeed, the evidence suggests that such a duty might have negative effects on the health of infants. No clear consensus emerges from the debate on the question of whether ordering women into "places of safety" and mandating medical treatment provide the best solution or, on the contrary, create additional problems.

The Court added (paragraph 44) that imposing liability might:

... tend to drive the problems underground. Pregnant women suffering from alcohol or substance abuse addictions may not seek prenatal care for fear that their problems would be detected and they would be confined involuntarily and/or ordered to undergo mandatory treatment. As a result, there is a real possibility that those women most in need of proper prenatal care may be the ones who will go without and a judicial intervention designed to improve the health of the fetus and the mother may actually put both at serious health risk. ... In the end, orders made to protect a fetus' health could ultimately result in its destruction.

Policy

The legal position is supported by the policies of a number of important professional organizations. For example, the Society of Obstetricians and Gynecologists of Canada (1997), the American College of Obstetricians and Gynecologists (2004, 2006) and the International Federation of Gynecology and Obstetrics (FIGO) (2003a,b) all have policies that recognize the authority of the pregnant woman to make healthcare decisions and underline that this is in the best interests of both the woman and the fetus. The FIGO (2003a) policy

on *Professional and Ethical Responsibilities Concerning Sexual and Reproductive Rights* enjoins its member societies to:

Support a decision-making process, free from bias or coercion, which allows women to make informed choices regarding their sexual and reproductive health. This includes the need to act only on the basis of a fully informed consent or dissent, based on adequate provision of information and education to the patient regarding the nature, management implications, options and outcomes of choices. In this way, healthcare professionals provide women with the opportunity to consider and evaluate treatment options in the context of their own life circumstances and culture.

When a physician's view of the best interest of the fetus conflicts with the view of the pregnant woman, the role of the physician is to provide counseling and persuasion, but not coercion. Codes of ethics that apply to medical practice in many countries support the same. For example, the Royal College of Obstetricians and Gynaecologists (1996) in the UK stipulates that: "Obstetricians must respect the woman's legal liberty to ignore or reject professional advice, even to her own detriment and that of her fetus."

Empirical studies

Unfortunately, there is no standardized system for documenting and assessing cases where pregnant women refuse medical advice and physicians seek judicial intervention to overcome refusals of treatment.

A recent survey of physician (obstetrician–gynecologist, pediatrician, and family physician) attitudes towards mandatory screening and legal coercion of pregnant women with problems of alcohol and illicit drug abuse found that half (or more) supported such measures (Abel and Kruger, 2002). This finding indicates that physician attitudes are at variance with recent court cases and the policy statements of professional organizations. As regards physician attitudes to court-ordered treatment (particularly surgery), a recent survey of directors of maternal–fetal medicine programs revealed strong opposition to such efforts and a continuing decline in the number of requests for this type of judicial intervention (Adams *et al.*, 2003).

Of note, a review of relevant data shows unequivocally that state intervention is disproportionately oppressive of poor women, aboriginal women, and women who are members of other racial and ethnic minorities (Chasnoff *et al.*, 1990; Royal Commission on New Reproductive Technologies, 1993). This finding is cause for concern. Of equal concern is the almost exclusive focus on the impact of pregnant women's behaviors and choices on the health and well-being of the fetus when there is ample evidence to show that paternal drug and alcohol abuse, excessive caffeine and nicotine use, spousal abuse, and certain paternal occupations are also potentially hazardous to the fetus (Olshan *et al.*, 1991; Zhang and Ratcliffe, 1993; Losco and Shublack, 1994; Schroedel and Peretz, 1994; Chavkin, 2001; Frank *et al.*, 2001; Uncu *et al.*, 2005).

How should I approach ethical dilemmas that arise in the care of pregnant women in practice?

Although many jurisdictions do not recognize fetal rights, fetal interests are taken into consideration by physicians and their pregnant patients. In fact, with the development of detailed ultrasound imaging, excellent perinatal technology, and the ability to improve outcomes for very small infants, it is hard for many physicians not to envision the fetus as a patient. Thus, some physicians see themselves as having responsibility for two "patients" in one body. It is extraordinarily difficult for a physician to stand by while a fetus dies or becomes irreparably harmed, when an intervention might prevent this result. Nonetheless, it is inappropriate to coerce a patient to undergo an intervention or to abandon her.

Difficult as it may be, the physician must respect the competent woman's right to make decisions for herself and her fetus. Moreover, care must be taken not to question the competence of the woman merely because she does not concur with the physician's recommendation(s). There are many reasons why competent women reject medical advice, and to counsel these women effectively it is important to understand their particular reason(s) for rejecting medical advice.

As one of us has argued elsewhere (Baylis and Sherwin, 2002, pp. 295–6), sometimes women do not accept medical advice because of value conflicts, epistemological conflicts, or lack of trust in the medical profession:

> . . . [W]omen sometimes make a deliberate decision to reject their physician's advice because it runs contrary to their values . . . In other cases, women may agree with the values that inform the physician's recommendation (e.g., promotion of their own health and that of their fetuses), but question the medical knowledge on which that advice is based . . . [In still other cases] women who intentionally reject medical advice do so not because of conflicting values, or problematic knowledge claims, but rather because of a deep-seated mistrust of physicians and the medical profession as a whole.

In addition to the above, sometimes medical advice may not be followed because of ignorance, failure to understand, fear or apprehension, denial, and bias toward the present and near future.

Communication, understanding, and respect for women are essential in the management of these difficult situations. However, no matter how skilled a communicator the physician may be, a woman may not alter her decision or behavior. The physician's communication skills may be significantly tested in such cases (especially when a decision is needed urgently), and it may be difficult to develop the trust that is integral to the physician–patient relationship. As in other challenging medical situations, consultation with a colleague may be extremely helpful.

The cases

As Ms. A's pregnancy progresses, she develops a rapport with her physicians and the perinatal staff. An ultrasound shows a modestly growth-restricted fetus, with increased resistance noted in umbilical artery Doppler flow studies. With the help and support of her care providers, Ms. A decides to enter a methadone support program. Had she not voluntarily decided to do this, her care providers would have continued to follow her pregnancy (as much as she would allow) and sought to provide advice on timing of the birth and on subsequent treatment options for her newborn.

In the second case, further discussion clarifies that Ms. B is terrified of general anesthesia because her mother died from anesthesia complications. Moreover, Ms. B has a strong distrust of physicians and believes that too many cesarean sections are done. When it is explained that the cesarean can be done with spinal anesthesia, and in view of the risks of the ongoing bradycardia, Ms. B agrees to the surgery. However, if the patient had continued to refuse the surgery, the physician would have been obliged to respect her decision despite the serious risks to the fetus.

REFERENCES

Abel, E. L. and Kruger, M. (2002). Physician attitudes concerning legal coercion of pregnant alcohol and drug abusers. *Am J Obstet Gynecol* **186**: 768–72.

Adams, S. F., Mahowald, M. B., and Gallagher, J. (2003). Refusal of treatment during pregnancy. *Clin Perinatol* **30**: 127–40.

American College of Obstetricians and Gynecologists (2004). Patient choice in the maternal–fetal relationship. In *Ethics in Obstetrics and Gynecology*, 2nd edn. Washington, DC: American College of Obstetricians and Gynecologists, pp. 34–6.

American College of Obstetricians and Gynecologists (2006). Maternal decision making, ethics, and the law. In *Compendium of Selected Publications*. Washington, DC: American College of Obstetricians and Gynecologists, pp. 111–20.

Annas, G. J. (1987). Protecting the liberty of pregnant patients. *N Engl J Med* **316**: 1213–14.

Baylis, F. (1998). Dissenting with the dissent: *Winnipeg Child and Family Services* (*Northwest Area*) v. *G.* (D.F.). *Alberta Law Rev* **36**: 785–98.

Baylis, F. and Sherwin, S. (2002). Judgements of non-compliance in pregnancy. In *Ethical Issues in Maternal–Fetal Medicine*, ed. D. Dickenson. Cambridge: Cambridge University Press, pp. 285–301.

Beauchamp, T. L. and Childress, J. F. (1994). *Principles of Biomedical Ethics*, 4th edn, New York: Oxford University Press.

Bewley, S. (2002). Restricting the freedom of pregnant women. In *Ethical Issues in Maternal–Fetal Medicine*, ed. D. Dickenson, Cambridge University Press, Cambridge, pp. 131–46.

Boso v. *Italy* (2002). App. No. 50490/99, European Commission on Human Rights (September 2002). American Declaration, OAS Off. Rec. OEA/Ser.L/V/II.82, Doc. 6, Rev.1.

Chasnoff, I. J., Landress, H. J., and Barrett, M. E. (1990). The prevalence of illicit-drug or alcohol use during pregnancy and discrepancies in mandatory reporting in Pinellas County, Florida. *N Engl J Med* **322**: 1202–6.

Chavkin, W. (2001). Cocaine and pregnancy: time to look at the evidence. *JAMA* **285**: 1626–8.

Cook, R. J., Dickens, B. M., and Fathalla, M. F. (2003). *Reproductive Health and Human Rights*. Oxford: Oxford University Press.

Copelon, R., Zampas, C., Brusie, E., and de Vore, J. (2005). Human rights begin at birth: international law and the claim of fetal rights. *Reprod Health Matt* **13**: 120–9.

Council of Europe (1989). *The European Convention for the Protection of Human Rights and Fundamental Freedoms*, 312 UNTS 221 (entered into force on 3 September 1953), as amended by protocols 4, 6, 7, 12, and 13. Strasbourg: Council of Europe.

Fasouliotis, S. J. and Schenker, J. G. (2000). Maternal–fetal conflict. *Eur J Obstet Gynecol Reprod Biol* **89**: 101–7.

Frank, D. A., Augustyn, M., Knight, W. G., Pell, T., and Zuckerman, B. (2001). Growth, development, and behavior in early childhood following prenatal cocaine exposure: a systematic review. *JAMA* **285**: 1613–25.

Harrild v. *Director of Proceedings* [2003] 3 NZLR 289.

Harris, L. H. (2000). Rethinking maternal–fetal conflict: gender and equality in perinatal ethics. *Obstet Gynecol* **96**: 786–91.

Harris, L. H. and Paltrow, L. (2003). The status of pregnant women and fetuses in US criminal law. *JAMA* **289**: 1697–9.

Hornstra, D. (1998). A realistic approach to maternal–fetal conflict. *Hastings Cent Rep* **28**: 7–12.

International Federation of Gynecology and Obstetrics (FIGO) (2003a). *Professional and Ethical Responsibilities Concerning Sexual and Reproductive Rights*. London:

FIGO (http://www.sogc.org/iwhp/pdf/FIGOCODEOFH
UMANRIGHTSBASEDETHICS.pdf) accessed 2 May 2006.

International Federation of Gynecology and Obstetrics
(FIGO) (2003b). *Recommendations on Ethical Issues in
Obstetrics and Gynecology by the FIGO Committee for the
Ethical Aspects of Human Reproduction and Women's
Health*. London: FIGO (http://www.figo.org/content/PDF/
ethics–guidelines–text_2003.pdf) accessed 2 May 2006.

Keyserlingk, E. W. (1984). *McGill Legal Studies The Unborn
Child's Right to Prenatal Care: A Comparative Law
Perspective*, No. 5: Montreal: Quebec Research Centre of
Private and Comparative Law.

Kluge, E. H. (1988). When caesarian section operations
imposed by a court are justified. *J Med Ethics* **14**: 206–11.

Kolder, V. E. B., Gallagher, J., and Parsons, M. T. (1987).
Court-ordered obstetrical interventions. *N Engl J Med*
316: 1192–6.

Losco, J. and Shublack, M. (1994). Paternal–fetal conflict:
an examination of paternal responsibilities to the fetus.
Politics Life Sci **13**: 63–75.

Mahowald, M. B. (1993). *Women and Children in Health Care:
An Unequal Majority*. New York: Oxford University Press.

Malette v. *Shulman* [1990] 67 DLR (4th) (Ont CA) 338.

Martin, S. and Coleman, M. (1995). Judicial intervention
in pregnancy. *McGill Law J* **41**: 973–80.

Oduncu, F. S., Kimmig, R., Hepp, H., and Emmerich, B.
(2003). Cancer in pregnancy: maternal–fetal conflict.
J Cancer Res Clin Oncol **129**: 133–46.

Olshan, A. F., Teschke, K., and Baird, P. A. (1991). Paternal
occupation and congenital anomalies in offspring. *Am J
Indust Med* **20**: 447–75.

Paton v. *UK* (1981) App. No. 8317/78, European Commission on Human Rights, 13 May 1980, 3 European
Human Rights Rep. 408 (1981) (Commission report).

Pollitt, K. (1990). Fetal rights: a new assault on feminism.
The Nation, 26 March: 409–18.

R v. *Phillip Nathan King* [2003] NSWCCA 399.

R v. *Sullivan* [1991] 1 SCR 489.

Re C [2003] 1 HKC 248.

Re MB [1997] 2 FLR 426.

Regina v. *Collins* [1999] Fam 26.

RH v. *Norway* (1992). Decision on Admissibility, App. No.
17004/90,73 European Commission on Human Rights
Et Rep. 155 (19 May 1992).

Rodgers, S. (1993). Judicial interference with gestation and
birth. In *Legal and Ethical Issues in New Reproductive
Technologies: Pregnancy and Parenthood*, Vol. 4, ed.
Royal Commission on New Reproductive Technologies.
Ottawa: Minister of Supply and Services Canada.

Royal College of Obstetricians and Gynaecologists Royal
College of Obstetricians and Gynaecologists (1996). *A
Consideration of the Law and Ethics in Relation to
Court-Authorised Obstetric Intervention*, revised edn,
London: Royal College of Obstetricians and Gynaecol-
ogists (http://www.rcog.org.uk) accessed 2 May 2006.

Royal Commission on New Reproductive Technologies
(1993). *Proceed with Care: Final report of the Royal
Commission on New Reproductive Technologies*, Vol. 2.
Ottawa: Minister of Government Services.

St George's NHS Trust v. *S* [1999] Fam 26.

Schroedel, J. R. and Peretz, P. (1994). A gender analysis of
policy formation: the case of fetal abuse. *J Health Polit
Policy Law* **19**: 335–60.

Sherwin, S. (1992). *No Longer Patient: Feminist Ethics and
Health Care*. Philadelphia, PA: Temple University Press.

Society of Obstetricians and Gynaecologists of Canada
Ethics Committee (1997). *Policy Statement* No. 67:
*Involuntary Intervention in the Lives of Pregnant
Women*. Ottawa: Society of Obstetricians and Gynae-
cologists of Canada (http://www.sogc.org/guidelines/
pdf/ps67.pdf) accessed 2 May 2006.

United Nations (1979). *The Convention on the Elimination
of All Forms of Discrimination Against Women*, GA Res.
34/180 (18 December). New York: United Nations.

United Nations (1989). *The Convention on the Rights of the
Child*, GA Res. 44/25, Annex, UN GAOR 44th Session,
Suppl. No. 49 at 166, UN Doc. A/44/49 (entered into
force 2 September 1990). New York: United Nations.

United Nations (1966). *The International Covenant on
Civil and Political Rights*, 16 December 1966, 993 UNTS
171, entered into force 23 March 1976. New York:
United Nations.

United Nations (1994). *The Universal Declaration of
Human Rights*, UN Doc. A/CONF.171/13. New York:
United Nations.

Uncu, Y., Ozcakir, A., Ercan, I., Bilgel, N., and Uncu, G.
(2005). Pregnant women quit smoking; what about
fathers? Survey study in Bursa Region, Turkey. *Croat
Med J* **46**: 832–7.

Vo v. *France* [2004] 2 FCR 577, European Court of Human
Rights.

Wallace, R., Wiegand, F., and Warren, C. (1997). Beneficence toward whom? Ethical decision-making in a
maternal–fetal conflict. *AACN Clin Issues* **8**: 586–94.

Winnipeg Child and Family Services (*Northwest Area*) v. *G.*
(*D.F.*) [1997] 3 SCR 925.

Zhang, J. and Ratcliffe, J. M. (1993). Paternal smoking and
birthweight in Shanghai. *Am J Public Health* **83**: 207–10.

15

Prenatal testing and newborn screening

Lainie Friedman Ross

Ms. C is 34 and she is getting married for the first-time. She tells her obstetrician/gynecologist that she and Mr. D are hoping to conceive quickly. Both Ms. C and Mr. D are of Ashkenazi Jewish descent. Ms. C's physician recommends that she undergo prenatal testing for a number of diseases more common in people of Jewish ancestry. Currently, the Ashkenazi Jewish panel includes up to 10 conditions depending on the laboratory (Leib et al., 2005). The conditions include severe conditions such as Tay Sachs disease and more mild conditions such as Gaucher disease type 1. Ms. C has never heard of any of the conditions, but she agrees to follow her physician's advice.

E is a healthy full-term infant male, who was born 24 hours ago. The nurses inform you that E's mother refused routine vitamin K supplementation given intramuscularly and the hepatitis B immunization because she does not want to put her son through any more discomfort than the birth process. You come to draw the newborn screen for phenylketonuria and other metabolic conditions before discharge, but she refuses.

What is prenatal testing and newborn screening?

Prenatal testing includes a number of clinical tools to provide reproductive information to individuals or couples either preconception or during pregnancy about their risks of having a child with a health disorder or condition. Prenatal testing involves a number of different types of test including genetic carrier testing, ultrasound, amniocentesis or chorionic villus sampling (CVS), or preimplantation

genetic diagnosis. An individual or couple may be referred for prenatal testing because of genetic risk factors, maternal illnesses that are associated with various birth defects (e.g., maternal diabetes is associated with spina bifida and congenital heart disease), or advanced maternal age (which is a risk factor for certain chromosomal anomalies).

Genetic carrier testing is offered to women and couples to provide risk information about having a child with one or more genetic conditions. Tay Sachs Disease was one of the first conditions for which prenatal carrier testing was developed (Kaback and O'Brien, 1973). It is an autosomal recessive condition, which means that if both parents have one abnormal allele they are asymptomatic carriers who have a 25% chance of having a child affected with the disease. Today, many additional genetic conditions can be tested for depending on prospective parental interest, family history, or ethnicity, with various modes of inheritance. Ideally, carrier testing is performed preconception because this allows for greater decision-making latitude.

Ultrasound is one of the most common screening tests used during pregnancy. In the first trimester, ultrasound is often used to determine that the pregnancy is intrauterine and to determine the number of fetuses. In the first trimester, nuchal translucency can be examined as a screening tool for Down syndrome. In the second trimester, level-2 ultrasound is used to look for congenital anomalies of various organs (e.g., four-chamber examination of the heart).

More invasive techniques are usually reserved for "high-risk" women and "at-risk" couples and fetuses. Both CVS and amniocentesis are techniques that allow for chromosomal analysis of the fetus. While CVS can be done earlier than amniocentesis, it has a slightly higher risk of miscarriage from the procedure itself. Alternatively, some couples will seek preimplantation genetic diagnosis: genetic analysis of embryos during assisted reproduction prior to implantation.

Newborn screening (NBS), by comparison, is a population-based program that seeks to screen newborns for early-onset treatable conditions. Unlike prenatal testing, which targets individuals or couples who are at risk, NBS is designed as a universal public health program. It began in the early 1960s with the development by Robert Guthrie of both an assay to test for elevated levels of phenylalanine, which is diagnostic of phenylketonuria (PKU), and a stable way to collect and store the blood samples using filter paper (the Guthrie card) (Guthrie and Susi, 1963). The Guthrie card allows for the efficient and economical testing of large numbers of samples.

Guthrie piloted the PKU test and the cards in Massachusetts in 1961. The pilot was a success, but the initial medical response was to promote further testing and piloting before widespread implementation (Reilly, 1977). Guthrie and the National Association for Retarded Children (NARC) were impatient and advocated for legislative mandate to ensure universal screening of all infants. By 1976, over 40 states had legislative statutes (Reilly, 1977).

Today, PKU screening is performed universally in all US states, Canadian provinces, and many other countries around the world (National Newborn Screening Status Report, 2006). Many states and countries also test for other conditions, but there is wide variability regarding which conditions are included (Saxena, 2003). In the USA, the most common tests are for PKU, hypothyroidism, hemoglobinopathies (including sickle-cell disease), congenital adrenal hyperplasia, and galactosemia (National Newborn Screening Status Report, 2006). Each of these conditions meets the criteria for

universal screening as enumerated by Wilson and Jungner (1968). These criteria include (i) that the condition represents an important health problem; (ii) that the natural history of the condition is well understood; (iii) that there is an accepted cost-effective treatment which, if begun early, can prevent many if not all of the negative sequelae of the condition; (iv) that the screening test is simple and cheap and acceptable to the population; and (v) that the follow-up diagnostic testing is highly accurate (Wilson and Jungner, 1968).

Since the mid 1990s, newborn screening programs have expanded rapidly because of the development of tandem mass spectrometry, which allows for testing for numerous conditions at one time (McCandless, 2004). While some of these conditions clearly meet the Wilson and Jungner criteria for population screening, others are not as well understood and may not have available therapies (Pandor et al., 2004). In addition, other screening programs have been developed that do not depend upon the Guthrie card. The most widespread program is hearing screening using otoacoustic emissions or brain stem audio-evoked responses (Davis et al., 1997; Kerschner, 2004).

Why is prenatal testing and newborn screening important?

Ethics

Prenatal testing is important because it promotes informed reproductive decision making, particularly when provided with pre- and post-test genetic counseling. Prenatal testing and genetic counseling help individuals and couples to understand their personal risk for having a child with an inherited condition. The risk may be as high as 100% (e.g., the risk that a couple who both have sickle-cell anemia will pass the disease on to their child) or lower than 1% (e.g., the risk that a woman under 40 years old will give birth to a child with a chromosome abnormality such as Down syndrome). But knowing the probability of inheriting a gene mutation does not necessarily tell one how severe the condition will be ("variable expression"), or whether it will present at all ("variable penetrance").

Yet not everyone embraces the expansion of prenatal testing. Disability rights advocates question the assumptions that underlie prenatal testing, because positive results often lead to pregnancy termination (Parens and Asch, 2000). Even disability rights advocates who are pro-choice are disturbed by this sequence because they believe that the parents are making a misguided choice, electing to abort a wanted pregnancy based on one trait of the child rather than seeing the fetus as a future child with many traits. They also fear that increased use of prenatal testing will lead to greater discrimination against those who are already living with a particular disability and to greater intolerance for those parents who elect to continue a pregnancy of a child with a known disability (Parens and Asch, 2000).

Newborn screening is important because it allows for the early detection of treatable conditions and thereby prevents serious morbidity and mortality. However, there has been rapid expansion to include conditions that do not meet the traditional public health screening criteria (Botkin *et al.*, 2006). This raises questions about the goals of screening. Historically, the goal was to promote the medical well-being of the child, but now there are those who advocate for NBS to inform parents of future reproductive risks and to promote broader family benefits even if the testing does not offer any direct benefit to the child (Bailey *et al.*, 2005).

Law and policy

Alpha-fetoprotein (AFP) is a marker for fetal neural tube defects and Down syndrome. In 1985, the Department of Professional Liability of the American College of Obstetricians and Gynecologists issued an "Alert" entitled *Professional Liability Implications of AFP Tests*. The Alert declared that it was "*imperative* that every prenatal patient be advised of the availability of this test" (American

College of Obstetricians and Gynecologists, 1985). As a result of these liability concerns, maternal serum screening for AFP became the standard of care. This was reinforced in California in 1986 when legislation mandated that all healthcare providers offer such testing to every pregnant patient who begins prenatal care prior to the 20th week of pregnancy (California Code of Regulations, 2002). Today, even greater sensitivity and specificity are achieved by the use of triple screens (AFP, maternal serum human chorionic gondatropin and unconjugated estriol) and quadruple screens (which add dimeric inhibin-A). Serum markers are often used in conjunction with ultrasound for ever greater sensitivity (Reddy and Mennuti, 2006).

The main liability concern for failing to screen women using serum markers is a wrongful birth lawsuit. Wrongful birth cases are becoming more widely recognized in a wide variety of situations in which physicians failed to warn prospective parents that they are at risk of conceiving or giving birth to a child with a serious genetic disorder (Bernstein, 2001; Howlett *et al.*, 2002; Strasser, 2003). In addition, parents can also bring wrongful life suits on behalf of the children. These are more controversial because they must allege that the child would have been better off not being born.

Currently, NBS is a mandatory public health program in most US states. Wyoming and Maryland are the only two states that require informed consent for newborn screening, although 13 other states require that parents be informed about newborn screening before testing (Nelson *et al.*, 2001). All states except South Dakota and Nebraska permit parental refusal of newborn screening for religious or personal reasons (Nelson *et al.*, 2001; *Douglas County, Nebraska* v. *Josue Anaya and Mary Anaya*, 2005).

Empirical studies

One of the most controversial questions in prenatal testing is "what counts as success?" (Chadwick, 1993; Clarke, 1993). Is it a success only if parents choose to terminate a pregnancy because a fetal disorder is discovered, or is it a success if informed parents decide to continue the pregnancy? Depending on what one views as success might influence how one counsels prospective parents. The data show that non-geneticist healthcare practitioners (e.g., primary care physicians and obstetricians) are generally more directive than genetic counselors regarding an abnormal prenatal test (Geller *et al.*, 1993; Marteau *et al.*, 1994). That said, there are data that even genetic counselors show bias (Michie *et al.*, 1997) or that patients read between the lines (Anderson, 1999). There are also empirical data that show wide variation with respect to how individuals and couples use the prenatal testing information both within and between countries (Drake *et al.*, 1996; Mansfield *et al.*, 1999).

Although disability rights advocates are concerned that increased prenatal testing will lead to decreased support and increased stigmatization of persons with disabilities, the empirical data do not support this concern. Rather, the period since the mid 1980s has been quite progressive in the legislation and policies designed to promote opportunities for individual with disabilities. In the USA, the passage of the Americans with Disabilities Act (ADA) of 1990 has been heralded as an important advance in promoting opportunities for persons with disabilities (Blanck and Marti, 1996; Befort, 2004; McCleary-Jones, 2005). There are also global initiatives aimed at improving the lives of individuals with disabilities (Walsh, 2004; International Disability Alliance, 2006) as well as specific legislation and policies in many countries (Canadian Human Rights Commission, 2005; Directgov (UK), 2006).

Empirical studies in NBS are scant. Clearly more studies are needed to determine if early diagnosis improves outcome. This is particularly important as we move away from newborn screening for conditions that represent a medical emergency in the newborn period to conditions with natural histories that are less well known or that are currently untreatable (Grosse *et al.*, 2006). National and international collaborative studies are needed

to understand genotypic–phenotypic correlations and to rigorously test various treatments in rare metabolic conditions (Guttler *et al.*, 1999; Emery and Rutgers, 2001; Goss *et al.*, 2002). They are also needed to determine short-term and long-term impact of false-positive results (Sorenson *et al.*, 1984; Tluczek *et al.*, 1992; Gurain *et al.*, 2006). Because of the rarity of many conditions, Botkin (2005) has argued that expanded NBS should only be done with parental permission under a research protocol.

The evaluation of NBS must include all aspects of the screening program, which begins with blood spot acquisition and includes confirmatory testing and long-term management (American Academy of Pediatrics, Newborn Screening Task Force, 2000). Empirical data show that there are many loopholes in the process (Stoddard and Farrell, 1997; Desposito *et al.*, 2001; Farrell *et al.*, 2001; Mandl *et al.*, 2002; Hoff and Hoyt, 2006; Therrell *et al.*, 2006). A study of pediatricians found that many did not have a system in place to ensure that testing had occurred but assumed that no news was good news (Desposito *et al.*, 2001). In addition, each US state has a different process by which to add or subtract new conditions (Hiller *et al.*, 1997; Therrell *et al.*, 2006). There is also wide variation in standards between the different US state laboratories and how states track long-term results (Hoff and Hoyt, 2006; Therrell *et al.*, 2006).

How should I approach prenatal testing and newborn screening in practice?

Individuals and couples may not be aware that they carry certain gene mutations which may affect the health or well-being of their fetus. Taking a detailed family health history as well as reviewing the woman's health and health management (e.g., what medications she is taking) can provide great insight into the risks of having a child with a disorder or condition. The number of conditions that can be tested for prenatally is growing rapidly. Prenatal counseling should always precede prenatal testing in order to allow women and couples to think about what type of testing they wish to undergo. It should not be presumed that anything that can be screened for should be screened for, nor should it be presumed that all individuals and couples share similar attitudes about specific disabilities or disorders. Rather, the decision to undergo different types of prenatal test is a personal issue that will reflect how a woman or couple balances risks and benefits of testing. Healthcare providers should discuss with women and couples about how they want to proceed with a pregnancy, what they understand about their own health risks and the potential risks to the fetus, and determine other risk factors.

Clearly, women and couples have a moral and legal right to know what is available, and what are their risks based on clinical and social factors (e.g., whether or not they smoke or drink), their demography, and their family health histories. Preconception testing offers individuals and couples greater options in terms of using donor gametes or other forms of assisted reproduction, pre-implantation diagnosis, or adoption. For a couple where a pregnancy already exists at the time they learn of genetic risk factors, this new awareness can be anxiety provoking, require rapid decision making, and put a substantial amount of stress on the couple (Ormond and Ross, 2006). When deciding whether or not to have prenatal diagnosis, prospective parents need to think about the perceived burden associated with having an affected child, what level of risk (e.g., miscarriage of a healthy fetus) they are willing to take in order to obtain information regarding specific genetic diseases, and the degree of certainty that testing will provide (Ormond and Ross, 2006). For example, a couple might weigh the potentially beneficial and highly accurate information that invasive prenatal diagnosis can provide against the increased risk of miscarriage that is associated with these procedures.

Pediatricians and other healthcare providers who take care of newborns need to be aware of the NBS laws that exist in their jurisdiction. They ought to be aware of what conditions are tested for, what is available for those parents who want expanded screening, and whether parents can refuse state screening. Healthcare providers should encourage parents to screen their children, particularly for those conditions that meet the Wilson and Jungner (1968) criteria because clinical diagnoses may not occur until after irreversible morbidity has developed. Parents need to understand that the blood spot is a screening test and that definitive testing may be necessary to confirm or refute a positive screen. Parents also need to understand that even if a child is not found to have a disease, some of the screening tests uncover carrier information and that this may have implications about their own future reproductive risks as well as for their families (Laird *et al.*, 1996; Parsons *et al.*, 2003).

The cases

Ms. C was tested and found to be a carrier of cystic fibrosis and Tay Sachs disease. Her husband underwent the full panel as well and he was found not to be a carrier of any of the conditions. The couple was informed that they were not at risk for Tay Sachs Disease and that their risk for having a child with cystic fibrosis was low (<0.05%), but not zero because there are over 1100 mutations, and the prenatal panel only includes the more common mutations (Palomaki *et al.*, 2004; American College of Obstetricians and Gynecologists Committee on Genetics, 2005). They could get greater certainty but not 100% by doing a full gene analysis at a cost of $1500, which they elected not to do. Ms. C and her husband gave birth 1 year later to a healthy baby boy. He has no signs or symptoms consistent with cystic fibrosis.

Despite repeated attempts to convince E's mother to have her child undergo the newborn screen, she refused. Prior to discharge, the physician emphasized the importance of discussing her refusal with her child's pediatrician, and encouraged E's mother to bring the Guthrie card to her child's first pediatric appointment. E's mother did bring the Guthrie card to her pediatrician and discussed the "pros and cons" of testing, the meaning of a screening test, and the probability of a false positive, a true positive, and a true negative. The pediatrician explained to E's mother and father that the mode of inheritance for most of these conditions made it unlikely that one could determine risk by family history; and that clinical diagnoses could be too little too late. The pediatrician explained that she was very supportive of the screening program, and in fact, that she often recommended that her patients purchase an expanded screen that included conditions not currently screened for in their state. She provided brochures for the private laboratories that perform expanded newborn screening. The physician also stated that she was willing to respect their refusal, in part because the likelihood of a positive result was small, but that a delayed diagnosis could lead to a worse outcome for the infant. After further conversation, the parents elected to have the child screened by the state but did not want to send an additional sample to a private laboratory. The state screen was negative.

REFERENCES

American Academy of Pediatrics Newborn Screening Task Force (2000). Serving the family from birth to the medical home: newborn screening a blueprint for the future. *Pediatrics* **106**: 389–427.

American College of Obstetricians and Gynecologists (1985). *Professional Liability: Implications of AFP Testing* (Liability Alert). Washington, DC: American College of Obstetricians and Gynecologists.

American College of Obstetricians and Gynecologists, Committee on Genetics (2005). Committee Opinion Number 325, December 2005. Update on carrier screening for cystic fibrosis. *Obstet Gynecol* **106**: 1465–8.

Anderson, G. (1999). Nondirectiveness in prenatal genetics: patients read between the lines. *Nurs Ethics* **6**: 126–36.

Bailey, D. B., Jr., Skinner, D., and Warren, S. F. (2005). Newborn screening for developmental disabilities: reframing presumptive benefit. *Am J Public Health* **95**: 1889–93.

Befort, S. F. (2004). Accommodation at work: lessons from the Americans with Disabilities Act and possibilities for alleviating the American worker time crunch. *Cornell J Law Public Policy* **13**: 615–36.

Bernstein, P. (2001). Comment: fitting a square peg in a round hole: why traditional tort principles do not apply to wrongful birth actions. *J Contemp Health Law Policy* **18**: 297–322.

Blanck, P. D. and Marti, M. W. (1996). Genetic discrimination and the employment provisions of the Americans with Disabilities Act: emerging legal, empirical, and policy implications. *Behav Sci Law* **14**: 411–32.

Botkin, J. R. (2005). Research for newborn screening: developing a national framework. *Pediatrics* **116**: 862–71.

Botkin, J. R., Clayton, E. W., Fost, N. C., *et al.* (2006). Newborn screening technology: proceed with caution. *Pediatrics* **117**: 1793–9.

California Code of Regulations (2002). Tit 17 §. 6527.

Canadian Human Rights Commission (2005). *Practical Guide for Employment Accommodation for People with Disabilities*. Ottawa: Canadian Human Rights Commission (http://www.chrc-ccdp.ca/discrimination/barrier_free–en.asp) accessed 31 August 2006.

Chadwick, R. F. (1993). What counts as success in genetic counselling? *J Med Ethics* **19**: 43–6.

Clarke, A. (1993). Response to: "What counts as success in genetic counselling?" *J Med Ethics* **19**: 47–9.

Davis, A., Bamford, J., Wilson, I., *et al.* (1997). A critical review of the role of neonatal hearing screening in the detection of congenital hearing impairment. *Health Technol Assess* **1**: 1–176.

Desposito, F., Lloyd-Puryear, M. A., Tonniges, T. F., Rhein, F., and Mann, M. (2001). Survey of pediatrician practices in retrieving statewide authorized newborn screening results. *Pediatrics* **108**: E22.

Directgov (UK) (2006). *Disabled People*. London: Directgov (http://www.direct.gov.uk/DisabledPeople/fs/en) accessed 31 August 2006.

Douglas County, Nebraska, appellee, v. Josue Anaya and Mary Anaya, husband and wife, as parents of Rosa Ariel Anaya, a minor child, appellants (2005) No. S-03-1446. Supreme Court of Nebraska 269 Neb. 552; 694 N. W.2d 601.

Drake, H., Reid, M., and Marteau, T. (1996). Attitudes towards termination for fetal abnormality: comparisons in three European countries. *Clin Genet* **49**: 134–40.

Emery, A. and Rutgers, M. (2001). European collaboration in research into rare diseases: experience of the European Neuromuscular Centre. *Clin Med* **1**: 200–2.

Farrell, M., Certain, L., and Farrell, P. (2001). Genetic counseling and risk communication services of newborn screening programs. *Arch Pediatr Adolesc Med* **155**: 120–6.

Geller, G., Tambor, E. S., Chase, G. A., *et al.* (1993). Incorporation of genetics in primary care practice: will physicians do the counseling and will they be directive? *Arch Fam Med* **2**: 1119–25.

Goss, C. H., Mayer-Hamblett, N., Kronmal, R. A., and Ramsey, B. W. (2002). The cystic fibrosis therapeutics development network (CF TDN): a paradigm of a clinical trials network for genetic and orphan diseases. *Adv Drug Deliv Rev* **54**: 1505–28.

Grosse, S. D., Boyle, C. A., Kenneson, A., Khoury, M. J., and Wilfond, B. S. (2006). From public health emergency to public health service: the implications of evolving criteria for newborn screening panels. *Pediatrics* **117**: 923–9.

Gurain, E. A., Kinnamon, D. D., Henry, J. J., and Waisbren, S. E. (2006). Expanded newborn screening for biochemical disorders: the effect of a false-positive result. *Pediatrics* **117**: 1915–22.

Guthrie, R. and Susi, A. (1963). A simple phenylalanine method for detecting phenylketonuria in large populations of newborn infants. *Pediatrics* **32**: 338–43.

Guttler, F., Azen, C., Guldberg, P., *et al.* (1999). Relationship among genotype, biochemical phenotype, and cognitive performance in females with phenylalanine hydroxylase deficiency: report from the Maternal Phenylketonuria Collaborative Study. *Pediatrics* **104**: 258–62.

Hiller, E. H., Landenburger, G., and Natowicz, M. R. (1997). Public participation in medical policy-making and the status of consumer autonomy: the example of newborn-screening programs in the United States. *Am J Public Health* **87**: 1280–8.

Hoff, T. and Hoyt, A. (2006). Practices and perception of long-term follow-up among state newborn screening programs. *Pediatrics* **117**: 1922–30.

Howlett, M. J., Avard, D., and Knoppers, B. M. (2002). Physicians and genetic malpractice. *Med Law* **21**: 661–80.

International Disability Alliance (2006). http://www. internationaldisabilityalliance.org/ (last accessed 31 August 2006).

Kaback, M. M. and O'Brien, J. S. (1973). Tay Sachs: prototype for prevention of genetic disease. *Hosp Pract* **8**: 107–116.

Kerschner, J. E. (2004). Neonatal hearing screening: to do or not to do. *Pediatr Clin North Am* **51**: 725–36.

Laird, L., Dezateux, C., and Anionwu, E. N. (1996). Neonatal screening for sickle cell disorders: what about the carrier infants? *BMJ* **313**: 407–11.

Leib, J. R., Gollust, S. E., Hull, S. C., and Wilfond, B. S. (2005). Carrier screening panels for Ashkenazi Jews: is more better? *Genet Med* **7**: 185–90.

Mandl, K. D., Feit, S., Larson, C., and Kohane, I. S. (2002). Newborn screening program practices in the United States: notification, research, and consent. *Pediatrics* **109**: 269–73.

Mansfield, C., Hopfer, S., Marteau, T. M. on behalf of a European Concerted Action: DADA (1999). Termination rates after prenatal diagnosis of Down syndrome, spina bifida, anencephaly, and Turner and Klinefelter syndromes: a systematic literature review. *Prenat Diagn* **19**: 808–12.

Marteau, T., Drake, H., and Bobrow, M. (1994). Counselling following diagnosis of a fetal abnormality: the differing approaches of obstetricians, clinical geneticists, and genetic nurses. *J Med Genet* **31**: 864–7.

McCandless, S. E. (2004). A primer on expanded newborn screening by tandem mass spectrometry. *Primary Care Clin Office Pract* **31**: 583–604.

McCleary-Jones, V. (2005). The Americans with Disabilities Act of 1990 and its impact on higher education and nursing education. *ABNF [Association of Black Nursing Faculty] J* **16**: 24–7.

Michie, S., Bron, F., Bobrow, M., and Marteau, T. M. (1997). Nondirectiveness in genetic counseling: an empirical study. *Am J Hum Gen* **60**: 40–7.

National Newborn Screening Status Report (2006). http://genes–r–us.uthscsa.edu/nbsdisorders.pdf (updated monthly; accessed 31 August 2006).

Nelson, R. M., Botkin, J. R., Kodish, E. D., *et al.*, for the American Academy of Pediatrics, Committee on Bioethics (2001). Ethical issues with genetic testing in pediatrics. *Pediatrics* **107**: 1451–5.

Ormond, K. and Ross, L. F. (2006). Ethical issues in reproductive genetics. In *Individuals, Families, and the New Era of Genetics*, ed. S. M. Miller, S. H. McDaniel, J. S. Rolland, and S. L. Feetham. New York: WW Norton, pp. 465–85.

Palomaki, G. E., FitzSimmons, S. C., and Haddow, J. E. (2004). Clinical sensitivity of prenatal screening for cystic fibrosis via CFTR carrier testing in a United States panethnic population. *Genet Med* **6**: 405–14.

Pandor, A., Eastham, J., Beverley, C., Chilcott, J., and Paisley, S. (2004). Clinical effectiveness and cost-effectiveness of neonatal screening for inborn errors of metabolism using tandem mass spectrometry: a systematic review. *Health Technol Assess* **8**: 1–121.

Parens, E. and Asch, A. (2000). The disability rights critique of prenatal genetic testing: reflections and recommendations. In *Prenatal Testing and Disability Rights*, ed. E. Parens, and A. Asch. Washington, DC: Georgetown University Press, pp. 3–43.

Parsons, E. P., Clarke, A. J., and Bradley, D. M. (2003). Implications of carrier identification in newborn screening for cystic fibrosis. *Arch Dis Childh Fet Neonat Edn* **88**: F467–71.

Reddy, U. M. and Mennuti, M. T. (2006). Incorporating first-trimester Down syndrome studies into prenatal screening: executive summary of the National Institute of Child Health and Human Development Workshop. *Obstet Gynecol* **107**: 167–73.

Reilly, P. (1977). *Genetics, Law and Social Policy*. Cambridge, MA: Harvard University Press.

Saxena, A. (2003). Issues in newborn screening. *Genet Test* **7**: 131–4.

Sorenson, J. R., Levy, H. L., Mangione, T. W., and Sepe, S. J. (1984). Parental response to repeat testing of infants with "false-positive" results in a newborn screening program. *Pediatrics* **73**: 183–7.

Stoddard, J. J. and Farrell, P. M. (1997). State-to-state variations in newborn screening policies. *Arch Pediatr Adolesc Med* **151**: 561–4.

Strasser, M. (2003). Yes, Virginia, there can be wrongful life: on consistency, public policy, and the birth-related torts. *Georgetown J Gender Law* **4**: 821–60.

Therrell, B. L., Johnson, A., and Williams, D. (2006). Status of newborn screening programs in the United States. *Pediatrics* **117**: S212–52.

Tluczek, A., Mischler, E. H., Farrell, P. M., *et al.* (1992). Parents' knowledge of neonatal screening and response to false positive cystic fibrosis testing. *Devel Behav Pediatr* **13**: 181–6.

Walsh, N. E. (2004). The Walter J. Zeiter Lecture: global initiatives in rehabilitation medicine. *Arch Phys Med Rehabil* **85**: 1395–402.

Wilson, J. M. G. and Jungner, F. (1968). *Public Health Papers, No. 34: Principles and Practice of Screening for Disease*. Geneva: World Health Organization.

16

Assisted reproduction

Roxanne Mykitiuk and Jeff Nisker

Ms. F and Mr. G are trying to have a child. They have been having sexual intercourse approximately three times a week for the past year, and daily around the time when Ms. F thinks she is ovulating. They are both 38 years old. Ms. F has had regular menstrual cycles up to the last three months, in which she has had only two. They are worried they have delayed starting a family too long and will not be able to afford the expensive fertility treatment they may require at Ms. F's age. They have questions regarding the success of in vitro fertilization and the possibility of having twins or triplets.

What is assisted reproduction?

Assisted reproduction enables the deliberate manipulation of the processes and materials of human reproduction outside of sexual intercourse. In describing the practices that constitute assisted reproduction, it must be understood that all such practices are embedded with ethical issues, whether standard therapies such as ovulation induction (Messinis, 2005), insemination with donor sperm (Daniels *et al.*, 2006), and in vitro fertilization (IVF) (Steptoe and Edwards, 1978); emerging practices such as pre-implantation genetic diagnosis (PGD) (Handyside, 1990; Nisker and Gore-Langton, 1995); or practices prohibited under law in many countries, such as the purchase or bartering of oocytes (Gurmankin, 2001; Nisker, 1996, 1997, 2001).

Ovulation induction through clomiphene citrate has been practiced for over 30 years (Messinis, 2005). This oral therapeutic strategy can assist 50–80% of women with ovulatory dysfunction become pregnant, depending on the etiology of their disorder (with the exception of premature ovarian failure) (Messinis, 2005). Aromatase inhibitors are new oral ovulation induction agents (Casper and Mitwally, 2006; Holzer *et al.*, 2006). When these are unsuccessful in inducing ovulation, menotropins (also referred to as gonadotropins) may be used (Messinis, 2005). This is a much riskier strategy, with side effects including ovarian hyperstimulation syndrome (Budev *et al.*, 2005) and the creation of high-order multiple pregnancies (Barrett and Bocking, 2000a, b).

Provision of sperm, by other than the woman's partner, was one of the earliest forms of assisted reproduction and has been encompassed in medical practice for 50 years (Daniels *et al.*, 2006). Sperm donation is a common practice when a woman's partner has sperm of low count or quality or carries a communicable disease, when she is in a lesbian relationship, or if she is single. Oocytes may be provided to women who no longer have an "ovarian reserve," because of their advanced age (Pastor *et al.*, 2005) or having undergone cancer treatment (Byrne *et al.*, 1999; Nisker *et al.*, 2006).

Menotropin ovarian stimulation create multiple oocytes for IVF (Abramov *et al.*, 1999). When the

An earlier version of this chapter has appeared: Shanner, L. and Nisker, J. (2001). Assisted reproductive technologies. *CMAJ* **164**: 1589–1594.

oocytes reach approximately 2 cm in diameter, they are matured with human chorionic gonadotropin and approximately 36 hours later are removed through transvaginal ultrasonographic-guided needles (Yuzpe *et al.*, 1989). The oocytes are placed in Petri dishes under strict sterile conditions, sperm is added, and if fertilization occurs, the embryos are microscopically observed for two days (up to four days if the plan is to transfer blastocysts) (Blake *et al.*, 2002). Embryos are then transferred to the uterus (Min *et al.*, 2006) (one or two embryos preferred, but often more in older women), and the remaining embryos are cryopreserved for transfer in non-treatment cycles (Trounson and Mohr, 1983). Cryopreserved embryos no longer required for reproductive purposes are usually donated to research (Nisker and White, 2005) or discarded. They may, however, be donated to another couple, although this rarely occurs for a number of reasons, including parental fear of allowing a child for another couple that is genetically related to their own (Newton *et al.*, 2003; Nachtigall *et al.*, 2005). Pregnancy rates for IVF exceed 25% per cycle for women/couples whose infertility etiology may be blocked Fallopian tubes, endometriosis, sperm problems (with intracytoplasmic sperm injection) (Van Steirteghem *et al.*, 1994) or unexplained. They become higher following the transfer of cryopreserved embryos (Alsalili *et al.*, 1995; Mishell, 2001). The risks of IVF are in both the menotropin stimulation (Abramov *et al.*, 1999; Buckett *et al.*, 2005) and the surgery (Alsalili *et al.*, 1995). There are also risks to the child and family unit, such as those owing to multiple births (Barrett and Bocking, 2000a, b).

Gestational agreements (Rodgers *et al.*, 1997; Ber, 2000) are often used in conjunction with assisted reproduction practices (Mykitiuk and Wallrap, 2002; Rivard and Hunter, 2005). Although the more common type of gestational agreement occurs when the gestational carrier is impregnated with the sperm of the partner of a woman who, because of medical problems, cannot gestate her own embryo/fetus, gestational agreements may also include those in which the embryo's genetic make-up has resulted from an oocyte other than that of the gestational carrier, sperm other than that of the man for whom the embryo/fetus is being gestated, or both (Rodgers *et al.*, 1997).

A relatively new area relates to the genetic scrutiny of embryos by PGD (Handyside *et al.*, 1990; Nisker and Gore-Langton, 1995), or most recently, preimplantation genetic haplotyping (PGH) (Renwick *et al.*, 2006). The embryos or polar bodies (Verlinsky *et al.*, 1990) are assessed genetically through polymerase chain reaction (Mullis and Faloona, 1987) or fluorescent in situ hybridization (Delhanty *et al.*, 1993). Genetic determinations of an embryo through PGD may be used not only to implant embryos to avoid a specific genetic characteristic but also to implant embryos with particular characteristics, for example embryos of a specific histocompatibility in a savior sibling scenario (Pennings *et al.*, 2002), embryos that will result in a child who is deaf (Levy, 2002) or who has Duchene's dwarfism (Nunes, 2006).

Why is assisted reproduction important?

Assisted reproduction enables subfertile heterosexual couples, single women, and women in lesbian relationships to have children. In addition, individuals and couples who carry genetic conditions may wish to use assisted reproduction in order to avoid passing (or to deliberately pass) these conditions on to their children. Thus, assisted reproduction is important for both medical and social indications.

Assisted reproduction is increasingly important as many women delay having a child until they have employment and financial security. Delay in becoming pregnant predisposes a woman not only to deplete her ovarian reserve but also to develop other etiologies of infertility, such as endometriosis or tubal occlusion, as well as lengthening her exposure to environmental toxins (Younglai *et al.*, 2002), an under-researched area (Royal Commission on New Reproductive Technologies, 1993).

Assisted reproduction is also increasingly important as more women are surviving cancer treatment, including leukemias in girls and adolescents, lymphomas, and breast cancer (Nisker *et al.*, 2006). Women who have received chemotherapy, for example, may have a dramatic decrease in the number of ovarian Follicles that remain, and thus the normal attrition rate frequently causes these women to develop ovarian failure in their thirties (Sklar *et al.*, 2006).

Ethics

Commercialization

Commercialization and commodification of gametes, and commercial gestational agreements, offend a number of ethical precepts including respect for human integrity and dignity through the non-commodification and non-commercialization of the person, her or his bodily parts, tissues, substances and processes; protection of vulnerable persons from coercion or inducement; and respect for the patient–physician relationship by avoiding a conflict of interest between the two parties (Royal Commission on New Reproductive Technologies, 1993; Nisker and White, 2005).

"Donation" is an ethically charged term in that, until the 1990s, in most countries, "donors" of sperm and oocytes have been paid in the range of $100 for sperm and between $1500 and $5000 for oocyte donation (Nisker, 1996, 1997, 2001; Gurmankin, 2001). In addition, oocyte "donors" are almost always economically disadvantaged women who either sell their eggs to support their family or pay tuition, or who barter half of their oocytes in order to undergo an IVF cycle (Royal Commission on New Reproductive Technologies, 1993; Nisker, 1996, 1997, 2001; Mykitiuk and Wallrap, 2002). The ethical problems of these practices is reflected in their prohibition by law in most Western European countries such as France, the UK, and Germany, as well as Australia, New Zealand, and Canada, amongst other countries (see the list of relevant legislation at the end of the chapter). In some of these countries, sperm donors may be offered reimbursement of expenses, and occasionally compensation for their time (Daniels *et al.*, 2006).

Informed choice

Free and informed choice requires that the patient must be informed about the benefits and risks of treatment, alternative courses of action, and the consequences of not having the treatment (Mykitiuk and Wallrap, 2002). This includes the provision of sufficient information for the patient to be able to both understand and appreciate the chances of having a child for that particular patient in that particular infertility clinic, including clarification of the meaning of success rates (as to biochemical pregnancy or live birth), and the specific risks of treatment inherent for that patient (in general and in that particular clinic). Patients should also be informed about the potential for multiple births to have physical and cognitive consequences for children, as well as social consequences for them and their families and financial costs (Barrett and Bocking, 2000a,b; Elster, 2000; Mykitiuk and Wallrap, 2002; Adamson and Baker, 2004).

A free choice process is difficult to ensure for sisters and close friends of infertile women who have been asked to become oocyte "donors" or gestational carriers for them (Rodgers *et al.*, 1997; Ber, 2000). These women have indicated that they would feel that they were a bad sister or a bad friend if they did not comply with the request. Further, even in the best-case scenarios for altruistic oocyte donation or gestational agreements, ethical problems remain.

Informed choice is particularly difficult for those who are soon to undergo cancer treatment (Nisker *et al.*, 2006). In the case of girls and adolescent women, a substitute decision maker, usually a parent or guardian, may base their decision on the belief that the child will want to be a mother. As with adult women, decision making is also complicated by the fact that delaying cancer treatment in order to retrieve and cryopreserve oocytes (or for adult women to possibly undergo IVF to freeze embryos) may be problematic to the success of the cancer treatment. Finally, although encouraging, the success of new techniques such as oocyte vitrification (Lucena *et al.*, 2006) and in vitro maturation (Rao and Tan, 2005) requires further study.

Free and informed choice for research purposes may also be complex in that it is difficult for a woman undergoing fertility treatment not to agree to a request by her physician to participate in research, as she may perceive that the research must be important to the physician or it would not have been offered, and that a negative decision may compromise her clinical care (Sherwin, 1992, 1998; Kenny, 1994; Nisker and White, 2005). Particularly regarding stem cell research, women who "volunteered" to undergo IVF to provide eggs may be coerced (Cyranoski, 2004; Nisker and White, 2005; Chang, 2006).

Access

Access to assisted reproduction is constrained in some jurisdictions by financial considerations and other eligibility criteria. Without public funding, access to IVF is generally limited to economically advantaged women/couples. In most countries where a publicly funded healthcare system exists, access to infertility treatment, including IVF and intracytoplasmic sperm injection, is provided. In some countries, such as Australia, IVF is publicly funded for the number of cycles it takes for the woman to complete her family, while in most Western European countries and Israel, some restrictions are placed on the maximum number of cycles or the maximum number of children for which publicly funded IVF is available (Birenbaum-Carmeli, 2004). Canada is an exception among countries with publicly funded healthcare systems in that no public funding is provided for IVF and corollary therapies, with the exception of the province of Ontario, where IVF is provided for blocked Fallopian tubes only (Mykitiuk and Wallrap, 2002; Nisker, 2004).

Access may also be restricted by the eligibility criteria used by physicians and clinics. Although the access criteria typically center on the potential benefits and risks to the health and safety of participants based on medical factors, including the condition of infertility and the participant's age, some physicians and clinics use non-medical criteria.

These may include a woman's or couple's ability to parent, which may be perceived to be limited by physical or cognitive disability (Gurmankin et al., 2005), low income (Gurmankin et al., 2005), marital status (Vandervort, 2006), and sexual orientation (Mykitiuk and Wallrap, 2002; Peterson, 2005). Individuals and couples may also face barriers to access based on race and ethnicity (Mykitiuk and Wallrap, 2002; Gurmankin et al., 2005). These non-medical barriers to access are ethically suspect, often relying on discriminatory personal or social prejudices and may be subject to human rights challenges (Mykitiuk and Wallrap, 2002).

Genetic determination

Assisted reproduction is now used to determine the potential characteristics of children (Mykitiuk et al., 2006) through PGD (Handyside et al., 1990; Nisker and Gore-Langton, 1995) and PGH (Renwick et al., 2006). Focus on genetic characteristics of an embryo has been used not only to avoid a specific genetic characteristic but also to enhance the chance a child will have a particular characteristic (Pennings et al., 2002). To a limited degree, couples have for more than 10 years purchased sperm from genius sperm banks and oocytes from "Ron's Angels" to enhance the chances of an "intelligent" or conventionally "beautiful" child (Nisker and Gore-Langton, 1995; Nisker, 2002). The use of these strategies, as well as PGD and PGH for such purposes, raises ethical issues about the proper use of medical technology and the physician's role in providing enhancement rather than therapeutic benefits (Nisker, 2002). The use of PGD to avoid specific genetic conditions and diseases is also considered by some to be ethically problematic, resting on discriminatory ideas of disability and difference (Parens and Asch, 1999; Shakespeare, 1999; Taylor and Mykitiuk, 2001; Mykitiuk, 2002a). Also morally complex is the use of PGD to detect embryos of a specific histocompatibility in order to produce a savior sibling for an existing child (Pennings et al., 2002). The potential use of PGD to ascertain embryos that will result in a child who is deaf (Levy, 2002) or who has Duchene's dwarfism (Nunes, 2006) is also ethically problematic.

Social factors

Assisted reproduction also makes possible the creation of novel social arrangements: postmortem insemination, virgin births, postmenopausal pregnancy, multiple parents, anonymous genetic parents, and embryos conceived at one time being born at different times or to different people (Mykitiuk, 2002b). The use of assisted reproduction, therefore, has implications for kinship and also the understanding of the legal, social, and emotional bonds created by heredity and the consequences presumed to ensue from processes of conception and birth (Mykitiuk, 2002b). Social factors include the inappropriate continuation of a male-dominant work ethic that sees women as less valuable employees if they want to become pregnant. This coerces women to delay pregnancy and risk infertility rather than create an obstacle to career advancement or employment.

Law and policy

Western European countries, such as France, Sweden, the UK, and Germany, as well as Australia, New Zealand, Canada, and Israel, have enacted legislation governing assisted reproduction (see the legislation listed at the end of this chapter). However, in many jurisdictions, including the USA and eastern Europe, these practices remain largely unregulated by law. ''Reproductive tourism'' can result when patients and clinicians are prohibited by law from accessing certain practices in their own jurisdiction (Storrow, 2005).

The law generally sets out prohibited practices, usually enforceable through criminal sanctions (e.g., payment for gestational arrangements and oocytes in most jurisdictions) and provides a regulatory framework within which permissible practices must be carried out (e.g., the storage, handling, and use of reproductive materials, and a registry of gamete donors). In addition, national legislation may establish a regulatory or oversight body whose responsibility it is to license, inspect, and monitor all human reproduction clinics. Further, domestic human rights legislation may prohibit discrimination: for example, a single or disabled woman, or lesbian couple being denied access to IVF or donor conception for non-medical reasons.

In most countries where legislation regarding assisted reproduction exists, it is illegal to create an embryo for research purposes (e.g., Canada, France, Germany, and Sweden; see legislation at the end of this chapter). By contrast, in the UK, it is legal to create an embryo for research if legal consent has been given, provided one is licensed to do so (Human Fertilization and Embryology Act, 1990). However, in some countries, such as Canada, France, and Australia, research can be performed on embryos that were created for reproductive purposes but are no longer required for this purpose, pursuant to a license and with consent of the embryo donor. In most countries with legislation, there are also prohibitions on reproductive cloning, ectogenesis, and germ-line modification. For more on issues related to stem cell research and therapeutic cloning, see Chs. 21 and 31.

Professional practice policies are developed in order to set the standard of care by which clinicians should practice in order to provide optimal therapeutic outcome and minimum risk to their patients. As policies impact not only patients, clinicians, and researchers but also social relationships and institutions, good policy making must involve voices and perspectives of all parties who are affected by that policy, as well as those of the general public. In the development of such policies, it should be appreciated that women more than men are affected by assisted reproductive practices (Royal Commission on New Reproductive Technologies, 1993).

How should I approach assisted reproduction in practice?

Understanding that assisted reproduction is an ethically complex area of medicine, whether the clinician is a family physician, general gynecologist, fertility specialist, nurse, social worker, or psychologist, is essential in its practice. Family physicians and general gynecologists may become skilled in many aspects of infertility investigation, including history taking, physical examination, assessment of semen and ovulation characteristics, tubal patency, as well as parameters of general health. As referring physicians, these individuals should be aware of the infertility clinics that provide optimal care. Infertility specialists have the obligation to be educated in all currently clinically proven investigations and treatments. These specialists have an obligation to keep accurate records and report their findings in a manner in which the pregnancy and treatment-complication rates are clearly apparent to patients and referring physicians. All clinicians have the obligation to provide a free and comprehensive informed choice process.

Clinicians need to be mindful of the fact that that there may be both national and state/territorial/provincial legislation governing assisted human reproductive practices. Access to appropriate infertility treatment is problematic in countries such as Canada and the USA where, unlike Western European countries, Australia, and Israel, IVF is not covered under a publicly funded healthcare system, and advocacy for socioeconomically disadvantaged patients is required. Professional practice guidelines should be developed in order to have uniform reporting of data and to advise both fertility specialists and referring physicians as to the standards of care.

The case

The ethical issues embedded in the case include the inability of some women/couples, because of their financial or social situation, to access assisted reproduction and the informed choice process, particularly considering clinical factors (e.g., age of the woman) that may allow for more risky treatment strategies and require different information in the informed choice process. The fact that Ms. F is 38 years of age may allow ethical practice to commence infertility investigation if after one year pregnancy does not occur (or slightly before because of irregular ovulation, as with Ms. F), as well as permitting the transfer of more than one or two embryos during the treatment cycle. This couple should be made aware in the informed choice process that their chance of having a child, biologically related to them, through assisted reproduction or otherwise is much lower than the overall statistics reported by infertility clinics. Further, the additional risk of multiple pregnancy, and the physical and cognitive risks to the child inherent in multiple births, need to be addressed, as the option of more than two embryos being transferred will likely be offered. Ms. F and Mr. G, as all women/couples in their age group (and indeed all women/couples), should be counseled about the possibility of adoption, and about the fact that in most "developed" countries, access to an infant through adoption is very limited, and access to international adoption is restricted to the financially well off.

REFERENCES

Abramov, Y., Elchalal, U., and Schenker, J.G. (1999). Severe OHSS: an "epidemic" of severe OHSS: a price we have to pay? *Hum Reprod* **14**: 2181–3.

Adamson, D. and Baker, V. (2004). Multiple births from assisted reproductive technologies: a challenge that must be met. *Fertil Steril* **81**: 517–22.

Alsalili, M., Yuzpe, A., Tummon, I., *et al.* (1995). Cumulative pregnancy rates and pregnancy outcome after in-vitro fertilization: 5000 cycles at one centre. *Hum Reprod* **10**: 470–4.

Barrett, J. and Bocking, A. (2000a). The SOGC Consensus Statement: Management of Twin Pregnancies Part 1. *Soc Obstet Gynaecol Canada* **22**: 619–29.

Barrett, J. and Bocking, A. (2000b). The SOGC Consensus Statement: Management of Twin Pregnancies Part 2. *Soc Obstet Gynaecol Canada* **22**: 607–10.

Ber, R. (2000). Ethical issues in gestational surrogacy. *Theor Med Bioethics* **21**: 153–69.

Birenbaum-Carmeli, D. (2004). ''Cheaper than a new-comer'': on the social production of IVF policy in Israel. *Soc Health Illness* **26**: 897–92.

Blake, D., Proctor, M., Johnson, N., and Olive, D. (2002). Cleavage stage versus blastocyst stage embryo transfer in assisted conception. *Cochrane Database Syst Rev* **2**: CD002118.

Buckett, W., Chian, R. C., and Tan, S. L. (2005). Can we eliminate severe ovarian hyperstimulation syndrome? Not completely. *Hum Reprod* **20**: 2367 (author reply 2367–8).

Budev, M. M., Arroliga, A. C., and Falcone, T. (2005). Ovarian hyperstimulation syndrome. *Crit Care Med* **33** (Suppl. 10): S301–6.

Byrne, J. (1999). Infertility and premature menopause in childhood cancer survivors. *Med Pediatr Oncol* **33**: 24–8.

Casper, R. F. and Mitwally, M. F. (2006). Review: aromatase inhibitors for ovulation induction. *J Clin Endocrinol Metab* **91**: 760–71.

Chang, S. (2006). Investigations document still more problems for stem cell research. *Science* **311**: 754–5.

Cyranoski, D. (2004). Korea's stem-cell stars dogged by suspicion of ethical breach. *Nature* **429**: 3.

Daniels, K., Feyles, V., Nisker, J., *et al.* (2006). Semen donation: Implications of Canada's Assisted Human Reproduction Act, 2004 on recipients, donors, health professionals, and institutions. *J Obstet Gynaecol Canada* **28**: 608–15.

Delhanty, J. D. E., Griffen, D. K., Handyside, A. H., *et al.* (1993). Detection of aneuploidy and chromosomal mosaicism in human embryos during preimplantation se determination by fluorescent in situ hybridization (FISH). *Hum Mol Genet* **2**: 1183–5.

Elster, N. (2000). Less is more: the risks of multiple births. *Fertil Steril* **74**: 17–23.

Gurmankin, A. D. (2001). Risk information provided to prospective oocyte donors in a preliminary phone call. *Am J Bioethics* **1**: 3–13.

Gurmankin, A. D., Caplan, A. L., and Braverman, A. M. (2005). Screening practices and beliefs of assisted reproductive technology programs. *Fert Steril* **88**: 61–7.

Handyside, A. H., Kontogianni, E. H., Hardy, K., and Winston, R. M. (1990). Pregnancies from biopsied human preimplantation embryos sexed by Y-specific DNA amplification. *Nature* **344**: 768–70.

Holzer, H., Casper, R., and Tulandi, T. (2006). A new era in ovulation induction. *Fert Steril* **85**: 277–84.

Horsey, K. (2005). European Parliament calls for egg trade ban. IVF.net (http://www.ivf.net/content/page-o1326.html) accessed 10 August 2006.

Human Fertilization and Embryology Act 1990. (London: The Stationary Office).

Kenny, N. P. (1994). The ethics of care and the patient–physician relationship. *Ann R Coll Phys Surg Canada* **27**: 356–8.

Levy, N. (2002). Deafness, culture, and choice. *J Med Ethics* **28**: 284–5.

Lucena, E., Bernal, D. P., Lucena, C., *et al.* (2006). Successful ongoing pregnancies after vitrification of oocytes. *Fert Steril* **85**: 108–11.

Messinis, I. E. (2005). Ovulation induction: a mini review. *Hum Reprod* **20**: 2688–97.

Min, J. K., Claman, P., and Hughes, E. (2006). Guidelines for the number of embryos to transfer following in vitro fertilization. *J Obstet Gynaecol Can* **28**: 799–813.

Mishell, D. R., Jr. (2001). Infertility. In *Comprehensive Gynecology*, 4th edn, ed. M. A. Stenchever, W. Droegemueller, A. L. Herbst *et al.*, St. Louis: Mosby, pp. 1169–215.

Mullis, K. B. and Faloona, F. A. (1987). Specific synthesis of DNA in vitro via a polymerase-catalyzed chain reaction. *Meth Enzymol* **155**: 335–50.

Mykitiuk, R. (2002a). Public bodies, private parts: genetics in a post-Keynesian era. In *Privatization, Law and the Challenge to Feminism*, ed. B. Cossman and F. Fudge. Toronto: University of Toronto Press, pp. 311–54.

Mykitiuk, R. (2002b). Beyond conception: legal determinations of filiation in the context of assisted reproductive technologies. *Osgoode Hall Law J* **39**: 771–815.

Mykitiuk R. and Wallrap, A. (2002). Regulating reproductive technologies in Canada. In *Canadian Health Law and Policy*, 2nd edn, ed. J. G. Downie, T. A. Caulfield, and C. Flood. Markham: Butterworth, pp. 367–431.

Mykitiuk, R., Turnham, S., and Lacroix, M. (2006). Prenatal diagnosis and pre-implantation genetic diagnosis: legal and ethical issues. In: *Genetic Testing: Care, Consent and Liability*, ed. N. Sharpe and R. Carter. Hoboken, NJ: John Wiley, pp. 189–218.

Nachtigall, R. D., Becker, G., Friese, C., and Butler, A. (2005). Parents' conceptualization of their frozen embryos complicates the disposition decision. *Fert Steril* **84**: 431–4.

Newton, C., McDermid, A., Tekpetey, F., and Tummon, I. (2003). Embryo donation: attitudes toward donation procedures and factors predicting willingness to donate. *Hum Reprod* **14**: 878–84.

Nisker, J. (1996). J's ladders or how societal situation determines reproductive therapy. *Hum Reprod* **11**: 1162–7.

Nisker, J. (1997). In quest of the perfect analogy for using in vitro fertilization patients as oocyte donors. *Women's Health Issues* **7**: 241–7.

Nisker, J. (2001). Physician obligation in oocyte procurement. *Am J Bioethics* **1**: 22–3.

Nisker, J. (2002). There is no gene for the human spirit. *J Obstet Gynaecol Canada* **24**: 209–10.

Nisker, J. (2004). Anniversary of injustice: April Fool's Day, 1994. *J Obstet Gynaecol Canada* **26**: 321–2.

Nisker, J. and Gore-Langton, R. E. (1995). Pre-implantation genetic diagnosis: a model of progress and concern. *J Obstet Gynaecol Canada* **5**: 247–62.

Nisker, J. and White, A. (2005). The CMA Code of Ethics and the donation of fresh embryos for stem cell research. *CMAJ* **173**: 621–2.

Nisker, J., Baylis, F., and McLeod, C. (2006). Preserving the reproductive capacity of girls and young adolescent women with cancer: informed choice. *Cancer* **107** (suppl 7): 1686–9.

Nunes, R. (2006). Deafness, genetics and dysgenics. *Med Health Care Philos* **9**: 25–31.

Parens, E. and Asch, A. (1999). The disability rights critique of prenatal genetic testing: reflections and recommendations. *Hastings Cent Rep* **29** (Special suppl. 5).

Pastor, C. L., Vanderhoof, V. H., Lim, L.-C., *et al.* (2005). Pilot study investigating the age-related decline in ovarian function of regularly menstruating normal women. *Fertil Steril* **84**: 1462–9.

Pennings, G., Schots, R., and Liebaers, I. (2002). Ethical considerations on preimplantation genetic diagnosis for HLA typing to match a future child as a donor of haematopoietic stem cells to a sibling. *Hum Reprod* **17**: 534–8.

Peterson, M. M. (2005). Assisted reproductive technology and equity of access issues. *J Med Ethics* **31**: 280–5.

Rao, G. D. and Tan, S. L. (2005). In vitro maturation of oocytes. *Semin Reprod Med* **23**: 242–7.

Renwick, P. J., Trussler, J., Ostad-Saffari, E., *et al.* (2006). Proof of principle and first cases using preimplantation genetic haplotyping: a paradigm shift for embryo diagnosis. *Reprod Biomed Online* **13**: 110–19.

Rivard, G. and Hunter, J. (2005). *The Law of Assisted Human Reproduction*. Markham, ON: Lexis Nexis.

Rodgers, S., Baylis, F., Lippman, A., *et al.* (1997). *Practice Guidelines* No. 5: *Preconception Arrangements*. Ottawa: Society of Obstetricians and Gynaecologists of Canada (http://sogc.medical.org/SOGCnet/sogc_docs/common/guide/pdfs/ps59.pdf).

Royal Commission on New Reproductive Technologies [Patricia Baird, Chair] (1993). *Proceed With Care: Final Report. of the Royal Commission on New Reproductive Technologies*. Ottawa: Supply and Services Canada.

Shakespeare, T. (1999). Losing the plot? Medical and activist discourses of contemporary genetics and disability. *Sociol Health Illness* **21**: 669–88.

Sherwin, S. (1992). *No Longer Patient: Feminist Ethics and Health Care*. Philadelphia, PA: Temple University Press.

Sherwin, S. (1998). A relational approach to autonomy in healthcare. In *The Politics of Women's Health: Exploring Agency and Autonomy*, coordinator S. Sherwin. Philadelphia, PA: Temple University Press, pp. 19–47.

Sklar, C. A., Mertens, A. C., Mitby, P. *et al.* (2006). Premature menopause in survivors of childhood cancer: a report from the childhood cancer survivor study. *J Natl Cancer Inst* **98**: 890–6.

Steptoe, P. C. and Edwards, R. G. (1978). Birth after the reimplantation of a human embryo. *Lancet* **ii**: 366.

Storrow, R. (2005). Quests for conception: fertility tourists, globalization and feminist legal theory. *Hastings Law J* **57**: 295–330.

Taylor, K. and Mykitiuk, R. (2001). Genetics, normalcy and disability 2(3). *ISUMA* [*Can J Policy Res*] **2**: 65–71.

Trounson, A. and Mohr, L. (1983). Human pregnancy following cryopreservation, thawing and transfer of an eight-cell embryo. *Nature* **305**: 707–9.

Vandervort, L. (2006). Reproductive choices: screening policy and access to the means of reproduction 28. *Hum Rights Quart* **28**: 438–64.

Van Steirteghem, A., Nagy, Z., Liu, J., *et al.* (1994). Intracytoplasmic sperm injection. *Baillières Clin Obstet and Gynaecol* **8**: 85–93.

Verlinsky, Y., Ginsberg, N., Lifchez, A., *et al.* (1990). Analysis of the first polar body: preconception genetic diagnosis. *Hum Reprod* **5**: 826–9.

Younglai, E. V., Foster, W. G., Hughes, E. G., Trim, K., and Jarrell, J. F. (2002). Levels of environmental contaminants in human follicular fluid, serum, and seminal plasma of couples undergoing in vitro fertilization. *Arch Environ Contam Toxicol* **43**: 121–6.

Yuzpe, A. A., Brown, S. E., Casper, R. F., *et al.* (1989). Transvaginal, ultrasound-guided oocyte retrieval for in vitro fertilization. *J Reprod Med* **34**: 937–42.

LEGISLATION

Australia

Artificial Conception Act 1985 (W.A.).
Reproductive Technology (Clinical Practices) Act 1988 (S.A.).
Human Reproductive Technology Act 1991 (W.A.).
Infertility Treatment Act 1995 (Vic.).
Infertility Regulations Act 1997 (Vic.).
Research Involving Human Embryos Act 2002 (Cth.).
Australian Government, Department of Health and Aging. http://www.health.gov.au/internet/ministers/publishing.nsf/content/health-mediarel-yr2005-ta-abb048.htm?OpenDocument&yr=2005&mth=5 (accessed 10 August 2006).

Canada

Assisted Human Reproduction Act, S.C. 2004, c.2.

France

Art. L152–1 to L152–10, L673–5 C. santé publ.
Art. 16–7 C. civ.

Art. 311–19, 311–20 C. civ.
Art. 511–18, 511–119 C. pén.

Germany

Embryo Protection Act (*Embryonenschutzgestz* – ESchG) (1990). Federal Law Gazette I, 13 December 1990, p. 2746.

Israel

Public Health (Extra-Corporeal Fertilization) Regulations 1987 (Official Gazette, Regulations, 5035 p. 978, 11 June 1987).
Ova Donation for Extra–Corporeal Fertilization Act 2001 (Official Gazette, Statutory Bills, no. 2985 p. 537, 5 March 2001).

New Zealand

Human Assisted Reproductive Technology Act (N.Z.), 2004/9.

Sweden

In Vitro Fertilisation Act SFS 1988: 711.
The Act Concerning Measures for Research or Treatment Involving Fertilised Human Ova, SFS 1991: 115.

17

Respectful involvement of children in medical decision making

Nuala Kenny, Jocelyn Downie, and Christine Harrison

H is a bright, loving, 11-year-old child who has been treated for osteosarcoma. Her left arm has been amputated and she was given a course of chemotherapy. She has been cancer free for 18 months and is doing well in school. She is self-conscious about her prosthesis and sad because she had to give away her cat, Snowy, to decrease her risk of infection. Recent tests indicate that the cancer has recurred and metastasized to her lungs. Her family is devastated by this news but do not want to give up hope. However, even with aggressive treatment, H's chances for remission are less than 20%. H adamantly refuses further treatment. In the first round of treatment, she had initially acquiesced to the treatment but ultimately struggled violently when it was administered. She distrusts her healthcare providers and is angry with them and her parents. She protests, "You already made me give up Snowy and my arm. What more do you want?" Her parents insist that treatment must continue. At the request of her physician, a psychologist and psychiatrist conduct a capacity assessment. They agree that H is incapable of making treatment decisions; her understanding of death is immature and her anxiety level very high. Nursing staff are reluctant to impose treatment. In the past, H's struggling and the need to restrain her caused them serious concern.

What is respectful involvement of children in medical decisions?

Respectful involvement of children in medical decisions requires respect for parental authority and family context as well as careful attention to the communicative and developing decisional needs and abilities of the child.

Why is it important to respectfully involve children in medical decision making?

Ethics

Children have traditionally been excluded from medical decision making. Inclusion was seen to be dependent upon autonomy (the capacity for self-determination) and children were considered non-autonomous. Children were seen as needing substitute decision makers, and parents were generally turned to as substitutes with the right and responsibility to make medical decisions for their children.

However, ethical analysis of the involvement of children in medical decision making has evolved and at least two significant changes must be noted. Firstly, it was recognized that children from infants to teens have dramatically differing levels of capacity for decision making. Three general categories of children were described: those lacking decisional capacity, those with developing decisional capacity, and those with developed decisional capacity (American Academy of Pediatrics, 1995). The focus of respectful involvement of children in medical

An earlier version of this chapter has appeared: Harrison, C., Kenny, N. P., Sidarous, M., and Rowell, M. (1997). Involving children in medical decisions. *CMAJ* **156**: 825–8.

decisions became fixed on decisional maturity. Differing levels of inclusion in decision making, relating to these different categories of decisional capacity, came to be seen as necessary.

The North American standard for clinical decision making, for instance, evolved into parental consent/permission for the first category, the child's consent for the third category, and parental consent/permission *and* child assent for the second category (Canadian Paediatric Society and Bioethics Committee, 2004). It was claimed that assent recognizes the developing capacity of children in this second category. Assent refers to an agreement with a decision or course of action as distinct from consent, which refers to an informed and voluntary choice with respect to a decision or course of action. The capacity to assent assumes a lower standard for each of the elements of informed choice (freedom, information, and decision-making capacity) than the capacity to consent. Assent was said to demonstrate respect for the child's developing autonomy, and parental consent/permission was said to protect the child from assuming unreasonable risks (Rossi *et al.*, 2003).

However, a second change in thinking occurred as assent has presented both practical and theoretical difficulties. Bulford (1997) has identified the lack of standards by which to judge competency and the ad hoc nature of assessment of the child's capacity for participation in the decision. Kenny and Skinner (2003) have noted that identifying the appropriate role for the child is complex. Among other things, it requires an understanding of the neurodevelopmental capacities of children that are necessary for decision making. On a substantive level, the role of assent has become contested, as demonstrated in a special issue of the *American Journal of Bioethics* in 2003. Serious questions have been raised. Is assent required from the child? Is dissent morally binding? If so, in what way is dissent different from competent refusal? Is respectful and meaningful involvement of the child about more than decisional autonomy?

If children are to be treated with respect in medical decisions, it is imperative to have clarity

regarding children's roles and to be more attentive to the developing capacities of child participants. Simpson (2003) and Baylis *et al.* (1999) have suggested that at least four categories of children can be described based on an understanding of the various developing capacities of the child: (i) children with no communication (neonates and young children); (ii) children with some communication but no decisional maturity (younger school-aged children); (iii) children with some communication and developing decisional authority (older school-aged children); and (iv) children with decisional maturity (i.e., equivalent to adult capacity for decisional maturity and mature and emancipated minors).

Building on this, it is argued that the appropriate involvement of the child depends upon an assessment of the child's decision-making capacity, what the child can understand, what the child can benefit from being told (even if not capable of making a decision), what the child wants to know, and what the child needs to know in order to participate appropriately (Baylis *et al.* 1999; Kenny and Skinner 2003).

For example, there is no role in decision making or communication (other than comforting) for an infant. A mature minor, at the other extreme, must be told everything that a competent adult would be told and has the moral authority to make the decision. A child with no decisional capacity, but good language comprehension, should be told what is going to happen to him or her. For instance, it can be morally necessary to share information even where the child has no decisional authority and it can be morally required to ask a child's opinion about various options even if the child may not yet have developed decisional authority. In other words, information sharing should be distinguished from ascribing decisional authority, and the objectives of sharing information and seeking opinions from the child can vary according to the capacities of the child.

Respectful involvement of the child, therefore, involves attention to the communicative as well as decisional needs and abilities of the child. Further, it requires careful and respectful attention to the family context of the child. It has been argued that a family-centered ethic is the best model for understanding the interdependent relationships that are at play in the clinical context. A family-centered approach considers the effects of a decision on all family members, their responsibilities toward one another, and the burdens and benefits of a decision for each member, while acknowledging the special vulnerability of the paediatric patient (Nelson and Nelson 1995; Committee on Pediatric Emergency Medicine, AAP Policy, and American Academy of Pediatrics, 2003). This approach presents special challenges for the healthcare team when there is disagreement between parent(s) and a child. Such a situation raises profound questions about the nature of the physician–patient relationship in pediatric practice. In the care of competent adults, the physician's primary relationship is with the patient. The patient's family may be involved in decision making (i.e., may participate in discussions of diagnosis, prognosis, and treatment options), but it is the patient who defines the bounds of such involvement and it is the patient who has the authority to make any and all decisions. The care of children, by comparison, involves a family-centered relationship in which the child, the parents, and the physician all have a necessary involvement. When there is disagreement between parent and child, the physician may experience some moral discomfort, feeling caught somewhat between the child and parent. The goal, however, must be to ensure the pursuit of the child's best interests and the respectful involvement of the child in the decision-making process (in a fashion appropriate to his or her capacities).

The family-centered approach can also present special challenges for the healthcare team when there is disagreement between the parent(s) and the team with respect to what is in the child's best interests. The assumption that parents best understand what is in the best interest of their child is usually sound. However, situations can arise in which the parents' distress prevents them from understanding or appropriately weighting their child's concerns and wishes. Simply complying with the parents' wishes in such cases is inadequate. Furthermore, the family-centered approach must not be taken to allow family members' interests to trump the child's interests. Rather, it must be seen as recognizing the fact that children are embedded in their families and the interests of the child can be seen as bound up with the interests of other family members. The child's interests must always be the basis for a decision to be followed by the healthcare team. This approach does not discount the parents' concerns and authority but it does recognize the child (albeit as a member of a family) as the particular patient to whom the healthcare team has a primary duty of care.

Law

Apart from exceptional circumstances (e.g., emergency), medical treatment must only be provided or withheld on the basis of a legally valid consent or refusal. To be legally valid, a consent or refusal of medical treatment must be free and informed. It must also be made by a person with appropriate authority who is deemed capable of making the treatment decision, that is, capable of understanding the nature and consequences of the recommended treatment, alternative treatments, and no treatment. If the patient is capable, then the patient has decisional authority. If the patient is a child, parents or legal guardians generally have the legal authority to act as substitute decision makers.

A child's substitute decision maker is obliged to make treatment decisions in the best interests of the child. Healthcare providers who believe that a substitute's decisions are not in the child's best interests should turn to child welfare authorities. Through child welfare legislation, the courts can ensure the appointment of a different substitute decision maker if they believe the current substitute to be acting not in accordance with the child's best interests (legislation usually provides guidance on the content of "best interests"). Courts also have the power to authorize or refuse to authorize treatment if they believe such action to be in the child's best interests. For example, courts have deemed children to be in need of protection and placed them under the care and control of child and family services and courts have themselves ordered blood transfusions in cases in which parents who are Jehovah's Witnesses refuse life-saving transfusions for their children.

Policy

Professional bodies with obligations and duties to children have formally recognized this new and emerging attention to the respectful involvement of children and youth in medical decisions. For example, the Canadian Paediatric Society policy on treatment decisions regarding infants, children, and adolescents states that "to ensure that the best decisions are made for children and adolescents, these decisions should be made jointly by members of the healthcare team, the parents of the child or adolescent, and sometimes the child or adolescent. Children and adolescents should be involved in decision-making to an increasing degree as they develop, until they are capable of making their own decisions about treatment" (Canadian Paediatric Society and Bioethics Committee, 2004, p. 99). The American Academy of Pediatrics (1995, p. 314) statement identifies the joint responsibility of physicians and parents to make decisions for very young patients in their best interest and states that "[p]arents and physicians should not exclude children and adolescents from decision-making without persuasive reasons."

Empirical studies

There is a body of empirical research providing some information on the competence of children for assent and consent (Abramovitch et al., 1995). Miller et al. (2004) have reviewed the empirical literature focusing on the voluntariness and competence of children for medical decisions. This review identified several fundamental dilemmas underlying current approaches to children's consent, demonstrating the differences between a legal (all-or-none) and a psychological (developmental, context dependent, and interactional) perspective; differences between the clinical and research settings; and differences in studies focusing on who makes the decision in contrast to those focusing on which decision is in the child's best interest. They conclude that more research is needed in this area, with particular attention to be paid to the differences between the respectful involvement of the child in clinical and research decisions, examination of the non-cognitive aspects of children's competence, and the importance of context in the development of decisional capacity.

How should healthcare professionals respectfully involve a child in medical decision making in practice?

Healthcare professionals working with children should be sensitive to the particular capacities of each child. Children are constantly developing with respect to their physical, intellectual, emotional, and personal maturity. Although developmental milestones give us a general sense of capacities, there is no bright-line of a particular age that will indicate ability to participate in independent decision making.

Where it is determined that it would not harm the child to be involved in the parental decision making and where there is sufficient language capacity to engage the child, healthcare professionals should discuss the treatment options with the child. Healthcare professionals should seek the child's opinion about the potential benefits and harms of the various options. Then, when assessing what action is in the best interests of the child, they should include a consideration of:

- the potential harm of having something done to you that you do not want done (e.g., frustration, loss of trust in healthcare providers, loss of trust in family)
- the potential harms and benefits to the child of the various options from the child's perspective

as well as the perspectives of the healthcare providers and family members

- the potential harms and benefits to the child's family members and any others that the child's interests are bound up with.

Once the substitute decision maker has made the decision (likely the parents), the healthcare professionals should carefully explain to the child, at an appropriate level and with the family's assistance, what is going to happen to him or her.

The case

For H, resuming aggressive treatment will have a serious negative effect on her quality of life. The chances of remission are small, yet a decision to discontinue treatment will likely result in her death. Because death is irreversible, and decisions with serious consequences require a high level of competence in decision making, the capacity required for this treatment decision is very high. It has been determined that H does not have this decisional capacity and that her parents are her substitute decision makers.

Nevertheless, H is included in discussions about the treatment options and her reasons for not wanting treatment are explored. Members of the team work hard to re-establish trust. Discussions address the hopes and fears of H and her parents, the parents' understanding of the possibility of cure, the meaning for them of the statistics provided by the physicians, as well as H's role in the decision-making process and her access to information. Members of the team include physicians, nurses, a child psychologist, a psychiatrist, a member of the clergy, a bioethicist, a social worker, and a palliative care specialist.

Discussions focus on reaching a common understanding about the goals of treatment for H. Her physician helps her to express her feelings and concerns about the likely effects of continued treatment. Consideration is given to the effects on her physical well-being, quality of life, self-esteem, and dignity of imposing treatment against her

wishes. Spiritual and psychological support for H and her family is acknowledged to be an essential component of the treatment plan. Opportunities are provided for H and her family to speak to others who have had similar experiences, and staff are given the opportunity to voice their concerns.

Ultimately, a decision is made by H's parents to refuse chemotherapy and the goal of treatment shifts from "cure" to "care." H's caregivers assure her and her family that they are not "giving up" but are directing their efforts toward H's physical comfort and her spiritual and psychological needs. H returns home, supported by a community palliative care program, and is allowed to have a new kitten. She dies peacefully.

The healthcare team met after H's death to review her care. They acknowledged that some parents might have made a different decision and discussed what their plan would be should this arise in future. This would include discussions among team members and with the parents to seek consensus about the potential for benefit to the patient, ongoing communication with the parents to ensure mutual understanding of the realistic goals of treatment, and psychosocial and emotional support of the patient during his or her course of treatment. It was acknowledged that in a situation such as H's, her parents' wishes for treatment would take precedence over her dissent. The team did not agree what their approach would be in situations where treatment would not be predicted to have a chance of remission of less than 20%. Some argued that they should refuse to provide treatment in such circumstances. Others argued that, even then, the parents' decision should be respected. It was agreed that should the situation arise they would invite the hospital ethics team to assist with decision making and conflict resolution.

REFERENCES

Abramovitch, R., Freedman, J. L., Henry, K., and Van Brunschot, M. (1995). Children's capacity to agree to psychological research: knowledge of risks and benefits and voluntariness. *Ethics and Behaviour* **5**: 25–48.

American Academy of Pediatrics (1995). Informed consent, parental permission and assent in pediatric practice. *Pediatrics* **95**: 314–17.

Baylis, F., Downie, J., and Kenny, N. P. (1999). Children and decisionmaking in health research. *IRB: Rev Hum Subject Res* **21**: 5–10.

Bulford, R. (1997). Children have rights too. *BMJ* **314**: 1421–2.

Canadian Paediatric Society and Bioethics Committee (2004). Treatment decisions regarding infants, children and adolescents. *Paediatr Child Health* **9**: 99–103.

Committee on Pediatric Emergency Medicine, AAP Policy, and American Academy of Pediatrics (2003). Consent for emergency medical services for children and adolescents. *Pediatrics* **111**: 703–6.

Kenny, N. P. and Skinner, L. E. (2003). Skills for assessing the appropriate role for children in health decisions. In *Pediatric Clinical Skills*, 3rd edn, ed. R. Goldbloom. New York: Saunders, pp. 349–59.

Miller, V. A., Drotor, D., and Kodish, E. (2004). Children's competence for assent and consent: a review of empirical findings. *Ethics Behav* **14**: 255–95.

Nelson, H. L. and Nelson, J. L. (1995). *The Patient in the Family: An Ethics of Medicine and Families*. New York: Routledge.

Rossi, W. C., Reynolds, W., and Nelson, R. M. (2003). Child assent and parental permission in pediatric research. *Theor Med Bioethics* **24**: 131–48.

Simpson, C. (2003). Children and research participation: who makes what decisions. *Health Law Rev* **11**: 20–9.

Various authors (2003). *Am J Bioethics* **3**: issue 4.

18

Non-therapeutic pediatric interventions

David Benatar

A five-year-old boy who has acute lymphoblastic leukemia was originally treated with combination chemotherapy and achieved remission. Within several months his disease relapsed. His doctors have determined that allogenic bone marrow transplantation offers the greatest chance of a sustained remission. His one-year-old sister is the best match. Their mother has agreed to the sister being a donor, but their father has reservations about putting her through the procedure and suggests that his wife, although not quite as good a match, should be the donor.

What are non-therapeutic pediatric interventions?

Non-therapeutic pediatric interventions, such as harvesting a child's bone marrow, are medical interventions that are not intended to benefit medically the child upon whom they are performed. Therefore, where such interventions are proposed or undertaken, they have some other purpose. In the case opening this chapter, the purpose of harvesting J's bone marrow is to save the life of I.

The word "therapeutic" can be understood in broader and narrower ways. In the narrower sense, it excludes prophylactic interventions – namely those that are not intended to cure some condition the child currently has but to prevent an adverse medical condition later. Because prophylactic interventions are morally similar (even if not identical) to narrowly therapeutic ones, I shall group these together and thus use "therapeutic" in the broader sense that includes prophylactic

measures. Non-therapeutic interventions are then those that neither cure nor prevent disease or impairment in those on whom they are performed.

The distinction between therapeutic and non-therapeutic interventions, although clear in theory, is far from clear in practice. This is because it is often a matter of dispute whether an intervention has therapeutic value. In other words, it is often unclear whether an intervention constitutes a net medical benefit to a child. For example, consider male circumcision that is not therapeutic in the narrow sense of curing an existing condition (such as true phimosis). There is considerable disagreement about whether such circumcision is an effective prophylactic measure. Some maintain that circumcision has considerable protective value against urinary tract infection, sexually transmitted diseases, and penile cancer. Others deny that it has any such value. Similar disagreements arise in connection with more radical interventions. For instance, some maintain that surgically assigning some intersex children to one sex or separating some conjoined twins is in those children's interests. Others deny that these children are benefited by such procedures. I shall refer to all these types of intervention as interventions of disputed therapeutic value.

The word "pediatric," like the word "therapeutic," can be understood in narrower and broader ways. It can be used more restrictively to refer only to (prepubescent) children or more expansively to include adolescents. I shall use the term in a broader (but not the broadest) sense. This is because what is important, from an ethical perspective, is to refer to those young people who are insufficiently developed to be competent to make judgements for themselves about whether the intervention should be performed. These include children and younger adolescents, but probably not the oldest adolescents. Competence is a matter of degree and so there is no sharp divide between children and early adolescence. Moreover, there are important distinctions to be drawn within childhood. For example, very young children – infants – have no ability whatsoever to decide for themselves whereas older pre-teens have some capacity to do so. Decision making on their behalf needs to take these developmental stages into account.

Why are non-therapeutic pediatric interventions important?

Non-therapeutic pediatric interventions pose a moral problem because they fall beyond the bounds of the only widely uncontested condition for medical intervention in the lives of those who are unable to consent to medical interventions – namely the therapeutic condition. Generally, in the case of competent people, their consent is a necessary moral condition for medical intervention. Children are not competent to decide which medical interventions may be performed on them and are, consequently, unable to provide valid consent. The absence of this consent, however, does not render all pediatric interventions problematic. It is widely agreed that some form of paternalism towards those who are not competent to make decisions for themselves is at least permissible and usually required. Following this principle of paternalism, pediatric interventions may or must be performed if they are to the child's benefit. Therapeutic interventions clearly fall into this category. However, the paternalistic justification for intervention does not seem to apply to those pediatric interventions that are not (clearly) therapeutic. May such interventions ever be undertaken and, if so, when?

Consider first interventions that are of disputed therapeutic value. What is one to do in such circumstances of uncertainty? To intervene may impose a needless risk or harm if there happens to be no net benefit. However, acting on the principle of "primum non nocere" ("first do no harm") would oversimplify matters, because to fail to intervene may be to withhold an important benefit if the intervention happens to be positively efficacious.

A vital question to ask in such circumstances is whether the uncertainty is a result of one's own ignorance about the best available evidence or whether the best available evidence requires uncertainty. Doctors are often ignorant (or insufficiently critical) of the evidence for or against the purported therapeutic effect of some intervention. They operate on the basis of impression, anecdotal evidence, or received wisdom rather than carefully tracking down the primary data or even reliable reviews. However, sometimes a full inquiry into these matters reveals that the evidence is inconclusive and that agnosticism is the appropriate response. In such cases, there is no clear side of caution on which to err, and reasonable people might disagree about whether to undertake the intervention even if it is believed that therapeutic interventions are the only permissible ones in the pediatric context.

Disagreement about the therapeutic value of an intervention is not always attributable to uncertainty about the medical evidence. Sometimes, the disagreement is at least partly a disagreement about values. For example, some might judge a very small chance of death following circumcision in infancy to be less bad than an equally small chance of death from penile cancer at an older age, while others may hold the opposite view. Some might believe that a life spent joined to one's twin is worse than death, while others might deny that it is bad at all. The presence of such disagreements does not mean that all competing views are always equally good. Sometimes, there may be better arguments for one evaluation than for the other. For this reason, the arguments for the competing views should be explored. However, such exploration may reveal that the arguments for one view are not clearly stronger than the arguments for a competing view. In such cases, reasonable people can disagree: some taking a given intervention to be therapeutic while others deny that it is so.

The fitting response to *reasonable* disagreement about the therapeutic value of an intervention is to judge both the intervention and its avoidance permissible. If this is so, then even those who believe that the only pediatric interventions that are permissible are therapeutic ones must acknowledge that interventions they personally do not judge to be therapeutic should be permissible if others can reasonably regard them to be so.

More controversial than interventions of disputed therapeutic value are those that are performed in order to benefit somebody other than the child on whom they are performed. Consider, for example, research on children. Although children upon whom research is performed may sometimes stand to benefit from the intervention being tested, they may also be harmed by it. The main beneficiaries of the research are future children, who will either benefit from a proven effective intervention or be spared an intervention that at best is useless and at worst harmful. Other interventions, such as bone marrow transplantation from a child to a close family member, provide more certain benefits to others. Such interventions expose the (donor) child to some risk and harm without aiming to benefit that child medically.

Some people maintain that *no* such non-therapeutic pediatric intervention is permissible. In making this claim, they might appeal to the difference between a competent person agreeing to incur a risk or be harmed in order to benefit another and a second party authorizing such risk or harm for a being, such as a child, who has never been competent. However, we can acknowledge this difference without thinking that the latter authorizations are *never* permissible. One might think that authorizations for children may be made only below a lower threshold of risk or harm. It would surely be implausible to judge as

impermissible parents' authorizing one of their children to be a blood donor for another of their children. The costs to the child of blood donation are clearly very minor and the benefits to the recipient clearly sufficiently great to justify such an intervention. Thus we see that an intervention cannot be ruled out simply because it is not therapeutic (for that child). We have to consider how big a risk or cost the intervention involves and how much good it can be expected to do others.

A second consideration that may be adduced in favor of at least some non-therapeutic interventions is that, although they may not benefit the child medically, some of them may benefit the child in other ways. If a child's parent, for example, will likely die without a bone marrow transplant for which the child is the most suitable donor, it may be quite plausible to say that the child would be benefited, all things considered, by donating the bone marrow. The child may be harmed more by the loss of the parent than, for example, by the pain attendant upon harvesting of bone marrow.

How should I approach non-therapeutic pediatric interventions in practice?

Although doctors often recommend pediatric interventions, they are rarely ethically or legally entitled to make the decision that the intervention will be performed on a given child. Authority to make that decision is usually borne by the parents, who are the presumptive surrogate decision makers. However, the presumption that the parents have this authority may sometimes be defeated. In such cases, doctors and others, including sometimes the courts, may or must assume decision-making responsibility. Doctors usually have more power to refuse an intervention than they have power to authorize an intervention. If a parent authorizes an intervention that the doctor believes is clearly unreasonable, the doctor may usually refuse to perform it.

However, whether doctors are working in concert with or in opposition to parents, the underlying practical question that doctors, parents, and others should be asking is how one decides whether an intervention of disputed therapeutic value or of medical benefit only to others should be performed? One helpful decision procedure would be to ask the following series of questions. (i) Is the benefit to self or others greater than the risk or harm? (ii) Is the harm or risk excessive? (iii) Does the child support the intervention?

Is the benefit to self or others greater than the risk or harm?

All the relevant factors must be considered in assessing whether benefit to self or others is greater than the risk or harm. These include not only the medical benefits and harms, but also all other benefits and harms. The evidence for these benefits and harms must be carefully considered. If having considered all this, the question is answered in the negative then the intervention may not be performed. If the answer is positive or it is unclear whether it is negative or positive, then one should proceed to the second question.

Is the harm or risk excessive?

Even if the harms or risks of harm are outweighed by the benefits, they may nonetheless be excessive. That is to say, they may be greater than can reasonably be authorized under the circumstances by a second party on behalf on an incompetent being. What constitutes excessive harm or risk varies depending on whether the expected beneficiary is the child on whom the intervention is performed or others. It is reasonable to run greater risks and inflict greater harms if the beneficiary is the same child than if it is somebody else. What constitutes excessive harm or risk also varies depending on whether the answer to the first question is positive or is uncertain. The less certain the intended benefits, the less the risk or harm that can be sanctioned.

Of course, what constitutes "excessive" in either case is open to some interpretation, but only within a certain range. Some risks or harms will be clearly

excessive and others will clearly not be so. A positive answer to the second question renders the intervention impermissible. If the answer is negative and the child is an infant, then the intervention may be performed. If the answer is negative and the child is partially competent, one should proceed to the third question.

Does the child support the intervention?

There are two relevant variables to consider here. The first is the extent of the child's competence. The more competent the child, the more weight should be put on his or her judgement about whether the intervention should be performed. The second variable is the reasonableness of the child's preference. The smaller the margin whereby the benefits outweigh the harms and the closer the harms are to the excessive threshold the more weight should be attributed to a child's preference *not* to have the intervention performed. The more the benefits outweigh the harms, and the further the harms are from the excessive threshold, the more weight should be given to a child's preference *to* have the intervention performed. The two variables interact in the following way. The more competent the child the less reasonable his or her judgement need be to carry the same weight.

The case

Ordinarily, harvesting bone marrow from a young child in order to save the life of his or her sibling is a justifiable intervention. The risks of serious harm to the donor are negligible. To be sure, the process of harvesting the marrow is quite painful, but this cost is outweighed by the considerable benefit to the child's sibling. The donor also benefits indirectly by not losing a sibling. In addition to the short-term loss of a sibling, there may be a considerable psychological burden later in life, if the would-have-been donor learns, once she grows up, that her deceased sibling could well have survived had she been used as a donor. The sister is too young to understand the situation and thus her (absent) views cannot be taken into account.

There are two complicating factors in our case. Firstly, we need to know how much more suitable a donor the child is than her mother. If the difference is only minor, then the slightly decreased chances of success may be warranted by the preferability of using a consenting adult rather than a non-consenting child as the donor. Second, although the mother is willing to authorize the harvesting of her daughter's bone marrow, the father has reservations. His concerns need to be addressed. If he cannot make a good case for refusing to allow his daughter to be a donor, then he should be persuaded of the justification for permitting the harvesting of her bone marrow. The life of his son is not all that lies in the balance. Unless the mother and father can reach agreement, a deep rift between them is likely to develop, particularly if the daughter is not used as a donor and the son subsequently dies.

RECOMMENDED READING

Benatar, D. (ed.) (2006). *Cutting to the Core: Exploring the Ethics of Contested Surgeries*. Lanham MD: Rowman and Littlefield.

Benatar, M. and Benatar, D. (2003). Between prophylaxis and child abuse: the ethics of neonatal circumcision. *Am J Bioethics* **3**: 35–48.

Carr, C. (1978). Children, medical research and informed consent. *J Soc Philos* **9**: 14–18.

Dawson, A. (2005). The determination of "best interests" in relation to childhood vaccinations. *Bioethics* **19**: 188–205.

Fleck, L. M. (2004). Children and organ donation: some cautionary remarks. *Camb Q Healthc Ethics* **13**: 161–6.

Jansen, L. A. (2004). Child organ donation, family autonomy, and intimate attachments. *Camb Q Healthc Ethics* **13**: 133–42.

Ladd, R. E. (2004). The child as living donor: parental consent and child assent. *Camb Q Healthc Ethics* **13**: 143–8.

Redmon, R. B. (1986). How children can be respected as "ends" yet still be used as subjects in non-therapeutic research. *J Med Ethics* **12**: 77–82.

Sommerville, M. (2000). Altering baby boys' bodies: the ethics of infant male circumcision. In *The Ethical Canary: Science, Society, and the Human Spirit*. Toronto: Viking, pp. 202–19.

Viens, A. M. (2004). Value judgment, harm and religious liberty. *J Med Ethics* **30**: 241–7.

Zinner, S. (2004). Cognitive development and pediatric consent to organ donation. *Camb Q Healthc Ethics* **13**: 125–32.

19

Child abuse and neglect

Benjamin H. Levi

A six-year-old girl and her older sister are brought by their father to be evaluated for a history of cough, runny nose, and low-grade fever. In addition to signs of a cold, the physician notes that the girl's nasal bridge is quite swollen and bruised. When asked what happened, she innocently shrugs her shoulders, and her father's only conjecture is that since she sleepwalks she might have bumped into something. The father sits impatiently, but as questioning progresses becomes increasingly defensive, at one point angrily declaring "we don't beat our kids, if that's what you're asking." Further complicating the situation is information from several nurses that this family is "on the brink" both socially and financially, and that additional stress is likely "to blow this family apart."

What is child abuse and neglect?

The term *child abuse* encompasses physical abuse, sexual abuse, psychological abuse, and neglect – though the phrase "child abuse and neglect" is also common parlance. In its typical usage, child abuse refers to actions (or failures to act) by a parent or caregiver that result in serious physical or emotional harm, sexual abuse or exploitation, or imminent risk of serious harm.

Why are ethical issues regarding child abuse and neglect important?

What could be more simple than the ethics of child abuse? For those who commit it, don't. For everyone else, do what you can to protect children from it. As one looks more deeply, though, definitions, interpretations, conflicting responsibilities, and, most prominently, uncertainty (on a range of issues) raise difficult questions. What exactly counts as abuse? How should we understand *reasonable suspicion* (which serves as the trigger for mandated reporting)? How sure must we be that abuse has occurred before initiating a child abuse investigation? Knowing that biases are inevitable in our assessments of risk and probability, how can we treat families fairly in our efforts to protect children from abuse? Finally, what should we as mandated reporters do when we do not think that reporting abuse is in a given child's best interest?

In addressing these questions, there are several important things to understand about child abuse. Firstly, it is prevalent. In one Canadian study of over 10 000 households, 21% of women and 31% of men reported having been physically abused as children (MacMillan *et al.*, 1997). In the USA in 2004 there were over 3.4 million investigations for suspected child abuse, with 872 088 confirmed cases, and at least 1490 deaths (Gaudiosi, 2006). Moreover, there is reason to believe that these numbers significantly underestimate the true incidence of abuse (Finkelhor, 1990; Herman-Giddens *et al.*, 1999; Crume *et al.*, 2002). Secondly, it is ubiquitous. One finds child abuse occurring in every community and at all levels of society (Finkelhor, 1994; Wyatt *et al.*, 1999; Lampe, 2002; Lalor, 2004; Daro, 2006; Gaudiosi, 2006), though a variety of risk factors do make abuse more likely. Those at increased risk include children who are younger, acutely ill, have chronic medical conditions and/or behavioral disorders, or have low intelligence (Warner and Hansen, 1994; Levitzky and Cooper, 2000; Gaudiosi, 2006). Family characteristics that predispose to abuse include increased stress, marital conflict, a young and/or single parent, unwanted pregnancy, and poverty (Warner and Hansen, 1994; Kotch *et al.*, 1995; Brown *et al.*, 1998; Drake and Zuravin, 1998; Overpeck *et al.*, 1998). Thirdly, it has significant sequelae: bruises, lacerations, sexually transmitted diseases, pregnancy, post-traumatic stress disorder, chronic somatic disorders, serious brain injury, plus acute and chronic medical care (Irazuzta *et al.*, 1997; Emery and Laumann-Billings, 1998; Widom, 1999; Discala *et al.*, 2000; MacMillan *et al.*, 2001; Diaz *et al.*, 2002; Fein *et al.*, 2002; Lansford *et al.*, 2002; Scheid, 2003). Recent estimates for the USA alone put the total direct costs related to child abuse at more than $24 billion annually, with indirect costs exceeding $64 billion (Fromm, 2001).

There are significant interpersonal and cultural variations in terms of what counts as child abuse (Hansen, 1997; Dubowitz *et al.*, 1998; FitzSimmons *et al.*, 1998; Daro, 2006). An illustration of this is recounted by Dr. Catherine DeAngelis, editor of the *Journal of the American Medical Association*, from her years teaching police officers about child abuse: "I started each new class by asking how many had ever spanked a child; almost all hands were raised. I then asked how many had ever beaten a child; no hand was ever raised. I then asked them to explain the difference, and the fun began" (Fargason *et al.*, 1996).

At root, DeAngelis' question is about harm and proportionality. In meting out punishment, how much harm is acceptable before the threshold into abuse has been crossed? Research tells us that our answers are heavily influenced by individual attitudes regarding discipline, as well as our personal experiences with corporal punishment (Howe *et al.*, 1988; Hansen, 1997; Bonardi, 2000; Jankowski and Martin, 2003; Tirosh *et al.*, 2003). So, too, significant cultural norms come into play (Daro, 2006). Some communities hold that beating children is a sign of love and commitment (Visser and Miller, 2002; Rakundo, 2006) whereas others (e.g., almost half of European countries) have outlawed even routine spanking (Daro, 2006). At times, it will be difficult to identify precise cutoffs, and inevitably reasonable people will disagree whether a given practice qualifies as legitimate discipline or abuse. But no reasonable person would dispute the notion that an adult who non-accidentally inflicts serious harm on a child commits an act of abuse (Chen, 2004; Maiter and Alaggia, 2004; Daro, 2006).

Though less central than harm, *intention* also figures into what we consider abuse. A parent can bruise their child by accident, or out of anger, or by pulling them out of harm's way, or even by administering non-traditional medical therapy. In each case, the parent's intention influences not only the nature of our response but also our judgement whether their action qualifies as abuse. Again, there are cultural components to this. Certain practices (e.g., coining, circumcision, scarification, and other body manipulations) are accepted because, within their cultural context, they are not intended to harm. But good intentions do not render *any* practice immune from being judged abuse. Children have the right to an open future (Feinberg, 1980) as well as the right to protection from serious harm (Archard, 2002). "Well-intended" culturally bound practices that violate these rights, and in so doing cause significant harm, do constitute abuse. Examples include severe shaking of an infant to raise a sunken fontanelle (i.e., *caida de Mollera*) or cutting off a girl's clitoris and labia, then sewing her vagina shut (i.e., clitoridectomy and infibulation). The *intention* of these acts may mitigate our reactions to the adults who carry them out. But the lasting injuries and impairment and psychological damage that befall children who are subjected to such acts are testament to the abusive nature of these practices (Barstow, 1999; Chalmers and Hashi, 2000; el-Defrawi *et al.*, 2001; Refaat *et al.*, 2001; Whitehorn *et al.*, 2002; Nour, 2003; K. M. Yount and D. L. Balk, unpublished data). The growing criticism from within cultures that engage in these practices simply reinforces the judgement that they are indeed abusive (Adinma, 1999; Eke and Nkanginieme, 1999; Nkwo and Onah, 2001; Msuya *et al.*, 2002; Nour, 2003).

Separate from concerns about intention or even thresholds for harm are questions about what should count as cause to suspect child abuse and when is it appropriate to actually report suspected abuse to child protective services (CPS) agencies. According to a recent report, 82% of countries sanction voluntary reporting of suspected child abuse, while 65% require reporting from at least certain individuals (Daro, 2006). In the USA, CPS agencies screen approximately 60 000 reports of alleged abuse per week, investigating two-thirds of them (Gaudiosi, 2006). Most reports are initiated by individuals who qualify as mandated reporters in that their professional work brings them into routine contact with children. At a minimum, this includes teachers, law-enforcement personnel, firefighters, healthcare professionals, social services providers, and child care workers – though in 18 US states *any competent adult* qualifies as a mandated reporter (National Clearinghouse on Child Abuse and Neglect Information, 2001, 2003). Of note, countries that have mandatory reporting have a significantly lower mortality rate for children under five years of age (−0.46; $p < 0.0001$; Daro, 2006).

As mentioned above, there are known risk factors for abuse. So, too, there is an extensive medical and social science literature that documents clinical indicators of abuse (Kempe *et al.*, 1962; Warner and Hansen, 1994; Reece and Ludwig, 2001; Giardino and Giardino, 2002; Vasquez and Pitts, 2006). At times, these resources combined with good interviewing skills and clinical acumen will cause mandated reporters to be certain in their judgement that abuse has occurred. Still, we will be less than certain in most instances. Hence our judgement and eventual decision to report will of necessity be grounded in a calculus, whose cofactors will include physical findings, observed behavior, risk factors, and so on. Though such a calculus is itself unavoidable, several ethical issues arise in how it is utilized.

The first has to do with bias, in terms of whom we suspect and report, and why. We know from research that mandated reporters are more likely to suspect and report children whose ethnic and socioeconomic profiles do not resemble their own (Hampton and Newberger, 1985; Brosig and Kalichman, 1992; Bonardi, 2000). Perhaps we presume that people like ourselves are not likely to have abused a child. But it is interesting that ethnic and socioeconomic resemblance seem to make us more prone to identify with a child's caregiver, exonerating them from suspicions of abuse, rather than make us more protective of the child who has been harmed (Adler, 1995). However this bias is to be explained, it is a problem of justice that minorities are several times more likely to be reported and investigated for suspected abuse (Sinal *et al.*, 1997; Lane *et al.*, 2002).

Were there little downside to being reported and investigated, this might be of minor concern. However, reports and investigations of child abuse are events that can destroy families and careers (Renke 1999). The ideal, of course, is that CPS agencies will carefully and sensitively investigate reports of child abuse, coordinate with social services and law enforcement to rehabilitate or remove offenders, and work with at-risk families to stabilize the home environment. But the reality is that families are stressed and disrupted – and sometimes blown apart – by the very process of state intervention into their lives (Thompson-Cooper *et al.*, 1993; Beck and Coloff, 1995; Richman, 2000). Moreover, because the CPS system is fundamentally underfunded and overburdened, support services frequently do not materialize, leaving families no better off than before (Murphy-Berman, 1994; Melton *et al.*, 1995; Melton, 2005; Gaudiosi, 2006). For these reasons, significant numbers of mandated reporters who have had experience with CPS agencies are wary of reporting further cases of suspected abuse (Applebaum, 1999; Flaherty *et al.*, 2002; Melton, 2002; Flaherty *et al.*, 2004).

None of this is to say that reporting suspected child abuse is, on balance, wrong to do. Rather it is to acknowledge that as currently configured the system is not without risks – which must be entered into our calculus of whether to report.

A second and related ethical issue has to do with the threshold that has been set to trigger mandated reporting, which varies from country to country, and even region to region. Across the USA, for example, there are 11 distinct thresholds; five use some variant of *belief*, while six use some variant of *suspicion* (National Clearinghouse on Child Abuse and Neglect Information, 2003). From a conceptual standpoint, there are important differences between believing and suspecting (White, 1993; Levi and Loeben, 2004), and various statutes have been changed in recognition of this (National Clearinghouse on Child Abuse and Neglect Information, 2001). In an nutshell, the problem with "belief" is that it involves holding an idea to be true, whereas in the context of mandated reporting one is seldom *sure* that abuse occurred but instead concerned that it *might* have occurred.

Collectively, the various statutory thresholds are referred to by the legal penumbra of *reasonable suspicion*. As such, mandated reporters typically are instructed that reporting is required any time they have reasonable suspicion that a child has been abused (Myers, 2001). The problem, however, is that there is no consensus what reasonable suspicion means (Deisz *et al.*, 1996; Kalichman, 1999; Levi and Loeben, 2004; Levi and Brown, 2005; Levi *et al.*, 2006). For some, it means whenever the thought of *child abuse* goes through your head, even if it goes right out (Deisz *et al.*, 1996). For others, it requires a substantial likelihood that abuse actually occurred. For example, one survey of over 2000 pediatricians found that 15% of respondents indicated that abuse would need to be over 75% likely to qualify as *reasonable suspicion*; while a quarter of respondents set the threshold at a 60–70% likelihood; another quarter set it at 40–50%, and 35% of respondents set the threshold as low as 10–35% probability (Levi and Brown, 2005).

Surprisingly, the professional literature on child abuse provides no substantive clarification on this (Deisz *et al.*, 1996; Kalichman, 1999; Levi and Loeben, 2004), nor does the law (Myers, 2001; Levi and Loeben, 2004). Mandated reporters are "left to define their own personal standards for what constitutes a reasonable suspicion of child abuse" (Kalichman, 1999): the result being an ad hoc system that ensures neither equal protection for children nor justice for those who are reported. In addition, this absence of a standard can create significant burdens for conscientious mandated reporters trying to determine the right thing to do (Flaherty *et al.*, 2004). So, too, it can foster conceptual confusion, as was shown in one study where physicians interpreted *reasonable suspicion* differently for severe versus minor injuries (Levi *et al.*, 2006). Though perhaps clinically understandable, this is conceptually problematic because the question is not whether physicians should have a heightened level of suspicion when the stakes are higher, it is whether they are clear on the concept itself. By way of analogy, it may be more important to look for fever in an obtunded patient than in someone with an itchy rash; but what constitutes "fever" (i.e., the properties that make up one's conceptual understanding of *fever*) should not vary with the clinical situation. Moreover, because the vast majority of child abuse cases do not involve severe injury (and prior severity of injury is not predictive of subsequent severity; Levy *et al.*, 1995), to safeguard children it is important that mandated reporters regard *all* instances of harm with the same level of careful consideration.

From a systems standpoint, the absence of a standard is equally troubling. Imagine that police were directed to write speeding tickets for motorists driving "too fast" but given no clear guidelines for judging what should count as "too fast." In the case of mandated reporting, the result is a system of indiscriminate reporting (Blacker, 1998) that not only disrupts families in which no abuse has occurred, and misses cases that warrant investigation, but also diminishes the effectiveness of CPS by dispersing already scarce resources and by eroding confidence in the legitimacy of child abuse investigations (Applebaum, 1999; Flaherty *et al.*, 2000; Richman, 2000; Melton, 2005).

Preliminary evidence suggests that statutory wording can significantly influence how individuals interpret and apply the threshold for mandated reporting. Two studies in particular have shown that mandated reporters express significantly greater willingness to report abuse when the threshold is defined as there being a 25% chance or greater that abuse occurred (Blacker, 1998; Flieger, 1998). This is not to say that "25% probability" is the appropriate threshold to endorse. But it does demonstrate that specifying the threshold in more concrete terms makes a significant difference.

A third ethical issue in our calculus of when to report abuse is where society should set the threshold for mandated reporting. Setting the threshold too low – say, 10% estimated probability – not only would bring about considerable disruption to families where no abuse has occurred but also would greatly stretch already limited CPS resources. Moreover, it would potentially overload the legal system, strain relationships between parents and mandated reporters, and (if reporting requirements are seen as unreasonable) increase disrespect for the law (Applebaum, 1999; Melton, 2005). These implications are further compounded when mandated reporters have immunity from criminal and civil prosecution, as occurs in the USA (*State of Minnesota* v. *Curtis Lowell Grover*, 1989). In point of fact, mandated reporting systems often provide little check or balance of mandated reporters' power, little recourse for non-malicious reporting injustices, and no ready mechanism for constructive feedback to educate mandated reporters (Thompson-Cooper *et al.*, 1993; Kalichman, 1999). So, setting an extremely low threshold risks indiscriminate reporting with little prospect for amelioration.

By contrast, setting the threshold for mandated reporting too high – say, 75% estimated probability – risks overlooking children who have been abused, since the signs of child abuse are often ambiguous (Giardino and Giardino, 2002). Consequently, some balancing is in order to identify an appropriate threshold. This, in turn, will require deciding how much we are willing to invest to protect children from abuse, as well as how much harm and what kinds of harm we are willing to tolerate. For this, we will need public dialogue and debate, as well as a

much better understanding of the costs and benefits of various cutoff points: 25% estimated probability versus 35%, 50%, and so on.

A temptation to be resisted is the construction of different thresholds for different kinds of abuse, depending on the severity of risks in play. The reason is that there is simply too great a variability in education and expertise among the millions of mandated reporters to expect individuals to discern accurately which threshold ought to apply for one kind of abuse versus another.

Even if there was a well-defined threshold, however, there is a fourth ethical issue in our calculus of when to report abuse. What should we do when we *have* reasonable suspicion that a child has been abused, but do not think that their interests are best served by reporting the abuse? From a legal standpoint, the answer is clear: mandated reporters are required to report whenever they have reasonable suspicion of abuse and the suspected abuser is either a parent or a person responsible for the child's welfare. In many jurisdictions (e.g., throughout the USA), failure to report makes one guilty of a misdemeanor (punishable by a fine and up to several months in jail) and civilly liable for damages if the abused child (or another child) is further victimized because of the failure to report.

Despite this, large numbers of mandated reporters regularly do not report suspected abuse (Singley 1998; Kalichman 1999; Delaronde *et al.*, 2000; Flaherty and Sege, 2005), though prosecutions for this are rare (Singley 1998; *State of Missouri* v. *Leslie A. Brown*, 2004). Reasons that mandated reporters do not report suspected abuse include the many ambiguities and uncertainties discussed above, as well as competing interests that mandated reporters often experience – such as worries about their relationship with a family, costs (financial, social, professional), and so on. In addition, the decision whether to report suspected abuse weighs heavily on many mandated reporters precisely because reporting does not always benefit the child (Johnson, 1999; Flaherty *et al.*, 2000, 2004). Relatedly, some competing interests can be intricately intertwined with the interests of a given child. For example, we know that child abuse is present in 50–80% of families in which domestic violence occurs (Garbarino *et al.*, 1991; Appel and Holden, 1998; Edleson, 1999), but it is not at all clear that it is in the interests of all (or even most) children exposed to domestic violence to be reported for suspected child abuse just because of the known association between the two. Another, and perhaps more problematic, example of intertwined interests involves instances where a parent who has committed child abuse is in therapy. Here, the concern is that reporting parents' abusive behavior could impede not only their own rehabilitation, but also (if such reporting were standard practice) prevent other child abusers from coming forward for help (Berlin *et al.*, 1991; Budai, 1996).

How should I approach child abuse and neglect in practice?

Putting such twists aside, the question remains whether a mandated reporter should follow the law and report suspected abuse when doing so does not appear to be in a child's interest. At root, it is a matter of conflicting obligations: obligation to follow the law versus obligation to protect children from harm. What makes the matter particularly difficult is that, unlike many laws or countervailing ethical principles such as patient confidentiality (see Ch. 7), mandated reporting laws were constructed with the protection and well-being of children specifically in mind. Hence, the tension is between following a rule specifically designed to protect children from abuse and following one's own judgement about how best to ensure a child's safety and well-being.

I think it is possible ethically to justify such acts of conscientious refusal (Rawls, 1971) that are grounded in one's professional principles and responsibilities. But to do so certain conditions must be met: (i) you genuinely believe that reporting the suspected abuse will result in a net harm for this child; (ii) you are confident that the child is not at risk for subsequent injury, and you are willing to

take responsibility for their safety; (iii) all other law-abiding alternatives would (in your estimation) also conduce to significant harm; and (iv) you are prepared to defend your decision publicly, and if need be accept the legal penalties for not carrying out your responsibilities as a mandated reporter.

What these conditions reflect is the strength of conviction necessary for true conscientious refusal of mandated reporting. In weighing one's resolve, however, one must be careful of overconfidence in predicting either a child's safety or one's ability to intervene on their behalf (Adler, 1995). However imperfect, CPS agencies provide the only systematic approach for investigating and safeguarding a child's well-being.

The case

In the case presented at the outset, a careful physical examination revealed no other injuries, and a thorough review disclosed no evidence of prior suspicious injuries, frequent visits to the emergency room, or bleeding abnormalities. While the evidence does not point to abuse as the most likely explanation for the injury, it is not ruled out. In this case, the default decision must be to report suspected abuse, unless the physician has a strong relationship with the family and can meet the four criteria for conscientious refusal mentioned above.

REFERENCES

Adinma, J. I. B. (1999). Practice and perceptions of female genital mutilation among Nigerian Igbo women. *J Obstet Gynaec* **19**: 44–8.

Adler, R. (1995). To tell or not to tell: the psychiatrist and child abuse. *Aust N Z J Psychiatry* **29**: 190–8.

Appel, A. E. and Holden, G. W. (1998). The co-occurrence of spouse and physical child abuse: a review and appraisal. *J Fam Psychol* **12**: 578–99.

Applebaum, P. S. (1999). Law and psychiatry: child abuse reporting laws: time for reform? *Law Psychiatry* **50**: 27–9.

Archard, D. W. (2002). Children's rights. *The Stanford Encyclopedia of Philosophy*, ed. E. N. Zalta. Palo Alto, CA: Stanford University Press (plato.stanford.edu/).

Barstow, D. G. (1999). Female genital mutilation: the penultimate gender abuse. *Child Abuse Negl* **23**: 501–10.

Beck, K. A. and Coloff, J. R. (1995). Child abuse reporting in British Columbia. *Res Pract* **26**: 245–51.

Berlin, F. S., Malin, H. M. and Dean, S. (1991). Effects of statutes requiring psychiatrists to report suspected sexual abuse of children. *Am J Psychiatry* **148**: 449–53.

Blacker, D. M. (1998). Reporting of child sexual abuse: the effects of varying definitions of reasonable suspicion on psychologists' reporting behavior. Ph.D. Thesis, California School of Professional Psychology, Berkeley/Alameda.

Bonardi D. J. (2000). Teachers' decisions to report child abuse: the effects of ethnicity, attitudes, and experiences. Ph.D. Thesis, Pacific Graduate School of Psychology, Palo Alto, CA.

Brosig, C. L. and Kalichman, S. C. (1992). Clinicians' reporting of suspected child abuse: a review of the empirical literature. *Clin Psychol* **12**: 155–68.

Brown, J., Cohen, P., Johnson, J. G. and Salzinger, S. (1998). A longitudinal analysis of risk factors for child maltreatment: findings of a 17-year prospective study of officially recorded and self-reported child abuse and neglect. *Child Abuse Negl* **22**: 1065–78.

Budai, P. (1996). Mandatory reporting of child abuse: is it in the best interest of the child? *Aust N Z J Psychiatry* **30**: 794–804.

Chalmers, B. and Hashi, K. O. (2000). 432 Somali women's birth experiences in Canada after earlier female genital mutilation. *Birth* **27**: 227–34.

Chen, J., Dunne, M. P., and Han, P. (2004). Child sexual abuse in China: a study of adolescents in four provinces. *Child Abuse Negl* **28**: 1171–86.

Crume, T. L., DiGuiseppi, C., Byers, T., Sirotnak, A. P., Garrett, C. J. (2002). Underascertainment of child maltreatment fatalities by death certificates, 1990–1998. *Pediatrics* **110**: e18.

Daro, D. (2006). *World Perspectives On Child Abuse*. New Haven, CT: International Society for Prevention of Child Abuse and Neglect.

Deisz, R., Doueck, H., and George, N. (1996). Reasonable cause: a qualitative study of mandated reporting. *Child Abuse Negl* **20**: 275–87.

Delaronde, S., King, G., Bendel, R., and Reece, R. (2000). Opinions among mandated reporters toward child maltreatment reporting policies. *Child Abuse Negl* **24**: 901–10.

Diaz, A., Simantov, E., and Rickert, V. I. (2002). Effect of abuse on health. *Arch Pediatr Adolesc Med* **156**: 811–17.

Discala, C., Sege, R., Li, G., and Reece, R. M. (2000). Child abuse and unintentional injuries. *Arch Pediatr Adolesc Med* **154**: 16–22.

Drake, B. and Zuravin, S. (1998). Bias in child maltreatment reporting: revisiting the myth of classlessness. *Am J Orthopsychiatry* **68**: 295–304.

Dubowitz, H., Klockner, A., Starr, R. H., Jr., and Black, M. M. (1998). Community and professional definitions of child neglect. *Child Maltreat* **3**: 235–43.

Edleson, J. L. (1999). The overlap between child maltreatment and woman battering. *Violence Against Women* **5**: 134–54.

Eke, N. and Nkanginieme, K. E. (1999). Female genital mutilation: a global bug that should not cross the millennium bridge. *World J Surg* **23**: 1082–6.

el-Defrawi, M. H., Lotfy, G., Dandash, K. F., Refaat, A. H., and Eyada, M. (2001). Female genital mutilation and its psychosexual impact. *J Sex Marital Ther* **27**: 465–73.

Emery, R. E. and Laumann-Billings, L. (1998). An overview of the nature, causes, and consequences of abusive family relationships: toward differentiating maltreatment and violence. *Am Psychol* **53**: 121–35.

Fargason, C. A., Chernoff, R. G., and Socolar, R. R. S. (1996). Attitudes of academic pediatricians with a specific interest in child abuse toward the spanking of children. *Arch Pediatr Adolesc Med* **150**: 1049–153.

Fein, J. A., Kassam-Adams, N., Gavin, M., *et al.* (2002). Persistence of posttraumatic stress in violently injured youth seen in the emergency department. *Arch Pediatr Adolesc Med* **156**: 836–40.

Feinberg, J. (1980). A Child's right to an open future. In *Whose Child? Parental Rights, Parental Authority and State Power*, ed. W. Aiken, H. LaFollette. Totowa, NJ: Littlefield, Adams, pp. 124–53.

Finkelhor, D. (1990). Is child abuse over-reported? The data rebut arguments for less intervention. *Public Welf* **48**: 22–9.

Finkelhor, D. (1994). The international epidemiology of child sexual abuse. *Child Abuse Negl* **18**: 409–17.

FitzSimmons, E., Prost, J. H., and Peniston, S. (1998). Infant head molding: a cultural practice. *Arch Fam Med* **7**: 88–90.

Flaherty, E. G. and Sege, R. (2005). Barriers to physician identification and reporting of child abuse. *Pediatr Ann* **34**: 349–56.

Flaherty, E. G., Sege, R., Binns, H. J., Mattson, C. L., and Christoffel, K. K. (2000). Health care providers' experience reporting child abuse in the primary care setting. *Arch Pediatr Adolesc Med* **154**: 489–93.

Flaherty, E. G., Sege, R., Mattson, C. L., and Binns, H. J. (2002). Assessment of suspicion of abuse in the primary care setting. *Ambul Pediatr* **2**: 120–6.

Flaherty, E. G., Jones, R., and Sege, R. (2004). Telling their stories: primary care practitioners' experience evaluating and reporting injuries caused by child abuse. *Child Abuse Negl* **28**: 939–45.

Flieger, C. L. (1998). Reporting child physical abuse: the effects of varying legal definitions of reasonable suspicion on psychologists' child abuse reporting. Ph.D. Thesis, California School of Professional Psychology, Berkeley/Alameda.

Fromm, S. (2001). *Total Estimated Cost of Child Abuse and Neglect in the United States*. New York: Prevent Child Abuse America, Edna McConnell Clark Foundation.

Garbarino, J., Kostelny, and Dubrow, N. (1991). What children can tell us about living in danger. *Am Psychol* **46**: 376–83.

Gaudiosi J. A. (2006). *Child Maltreatment 2004*, Chs. 3 and 4. Washington, DC: US Department of Health and Human Services, Administration for Children and Families.

Giardino, A. P. and Giardino, E. R. (2002). *Recognition of Child Abuse for the Mandated Reporter*. St. Louis, MO: G.W. Medical Publishing.

Hampton, R. L. and Newberger, E. (1985). Child abuse incidence and reporting by hospitals: significance of severity, class, and race. *Am J Public Health* **75**: 56–68.

Hansen, K. K. (1997). Folk remedies and child abuse: a review with emphasis on caida de mollera and its relationship to shaken baby syndrome. *Child Abuse Negl* **22**: 117–27.

Herman-Giddens, M., Brown, G., Verbiest, S., *et al.* (1999). Underascertainment of child abuse mortality in the United States. *JAMA* **282**: 463–7.

Howe, A. C., Herzberger, S., and Tennen, H. (1988). The influence of personal history of abuse and gender on clinicians' judgments of child abuse. *J Fam Viol* **3**: 105–19.

Irazuzta, J. E., McJunkin, J. E., Danadian, K., Arnold, F., and Zhang, J. (1997). Outcome and cost of child abuse. *Child Abuse Negl* **21**: 751–7.

Jankowski, P. J. and Martin, M. J. (2003). Reporting cases of child maltreatment: decision-making processes of family therapists in Illinois. *Contemp Fam Ther* **25**: 311–32.

Johnson, C. F. (1999). Child abuse as a stressor of pediatricians. *Pediatr Emerg Care* **15**: 84–9.

Kalichman, S. C. (1999). *Mandated Reporting of Suspected Child Abuse: Ethics, Law, and Policy*. Washington, DC: American Psychological Association.

Kempe, C. H., Silverman, F. N., Steele, B. F., Droegemueller, W., and Silver, H. K. (1962). The battered child syndrome. *JAMA* **181**: 17–24.

Kotch, J. B., Browne, D. C., Ringwalt, C. L., *et al.* (1995). Risk of child abuse or neglect in a cohort of low-income children. *Child Abuse Negl* **19**: 1115–30.

Lalor, K. (2004). Child sexual abuse in sub-Saharan Africa: a literature review. *Child Abuse Negl* **28**: 439–60.

Lampe, A. (2002). [The prevalence of childhood sexual abuse, physical abuse and emotional neglect in Europe.] *Z Psychosom Med Psychother* **48**: 370–80.

Lane, W. G., Rubin, D. M., Monteith, R., and Christian, C. W. (2002). Racial differences in the evaluation of pediatric fractures for physical abuse. *JAMA* **288**: 1603–9.

Lansford, J. E., Dodge, K. A., Pettit, G. S., *et al.* (2002). A 12-year prospective study of the long-term effects of early child physical maltreatment on psychological, behavioral, and academic problems in adolescence. *Arch Pediatr and Adolesc Med* **156**: 824–30.

Levi, B. H. and Brown, G. (2005). Reasonable suspicion: a study of Pennsylvania pediatricians regarding child abuse. *Pediatrics* **116**: e5–12.

Levi, B. H. and Loeben, G. (2004). Index of suspicion: feeling not believing. *Theor Med Bioethics* **25**: 1–34.

Levi, B. H., Brown, G., and Erb, C. (2006). Reasonable suspicion: a pilot study of pediatric residents. *Child Abuse Negl* **30**: 345–56.

Levitzky, S. and Cooper, R. (2000). Infant colic syndrome: maternal fantasies of aggression and infanticide. *Clin Pediatr* **39**: 395–400.

Levy, H. B., Markovic, J., Chaudhry, U., Ahart, S., and Torres, H. (1995). Reabuse rates in a sample of children followed for 5 years after discharge from a child abuse inpatient assessment program. *Child Abuse Negl* **19**: 1363–77.

MacMillan, H. I.., Fleming, J. E., Streiner, D. L., *et al.* (1997). Prevalence of child physical and sexual abuse in the community: results from the Ontario Health Supplement. *JAMA* **278**: 131–5.

MacMillan, H. L., Fleming, J. E., Trocme, N., *et al.* (2001). Childhood abuse and lifetime psychopathology in a community sample. *Am J Psychiatry* **158**: 1878–83.

Maiter, S. and Alaggia, R. (2004). Perceptions of child maltreatment by parents from the Indian subcontinent:

challenging myths about culturally based abusive parenting practices. *Child Maltreat* **9**: 309–24.

Melton, G. B. (2002). Chronic neglect of family violence: more than a decade of reports to guide US policy. *Child Abuse Negl* **26**: 569–86.

Melton, G. B. (2005). Mandated reporting: a policy without reason. *Child Abuse Negl* **29**: 9–18.

Melton, G. B., Goodman, G. S., Kalichman, S. C., *et al.* (1995). Empirical research on child maltreatment and the law. *J Clin Child Psychol* **24**(Suppl.): 47–77.

Msuya, S. E., Mbizvo, E., Hussain, A., *et al.* (2002). Female genital cutting in Kilimanjaro, Tanzania: changing attitudes? *Trop Med Int Health* **7**: 159–65.

Murphy-Berman, V. (1994). A conceptual framework for thinking about risk assessment and case management in child protective service. *Child Abuse Negl* **18**: 193–201.

Myers, J. E. B. (2001). Medicolegal aspects of suspected child abuse. In *Child Abuse: Medical Diagnosis and Treatment*, ed. R. M. Reece and S. Ludwig. Philadelphia, PA: Lippincott, Williams and Wilkins, pp. 545–63.

National Clearinghouse on Child Abuse and Neglect Information (2001). *Child Abuse and Neglect State Statute Elements*, No. 2: *Mandatory Reporters of Child Abuse and Neglect*. Washington, DC: US Department of Health and Human Resources, p. 50.

National Clearinghouse on Child Abuse and Neglect Information (2003). *Statutes at a Glance: Mandatory Reporters of Child Abuse and Neglect*. Washington, DC: US Department of Health and Human Services, p. 9.

Nkwo, P. O. and Onah, H. E. (2001). Decrease in female genital mutilation among Nigerian Ibo girls. *Int J Gynaecol Obstet* **75**: 321–2.

Nour, N. M. (2003). Female genital cutting: a need for reform. *Obstet Gynecol* **101**: 1051–2.

Overpeck, M. D., R. A. Brenner, *et al.* (1998). Risk factors for infant homicide in the United States. *N Engl J Med* **339**: 1211–16.

Rakundo, L. (2006). Spare the rod and spoil the child. *New Times*, Kigali, Rwanda, 11 July.

Rawls, J. (1971). *A Theory of Justice*. Cambridge, MA: Harvard University Press.

Reece, R. M. and Ludwig, S. (eds.) (2001). *Child Abuse: Medical Diagnosis and Treatment*. Philadelphia, PA: Lippincott, Williams and Wilkins.

Refaat, A., Dandash, K. F., el Defrawi, M. H., and Eyada, M. (2001). Female genital mutilation and domestic violence among Egyptian women. *J Sex Marit Ther* **27**: 593–8.

Renke, W. N. (1999). The mandatory reporting of child abuse under the Child Welfare Act. *Health Law J* **7**: 91–140.

Richman, H. A. (2000). Neuhauser Lecture. From a radiologist's judgment to public policy on child abuse and neglect: what have we wrought? *Pediatr Radiol* **30**: 219–28.

Scheid, J. M. (2003). Recognizing and managing long-term sequelae of childhood maltreatment. *Pediatr Ann* **32**: 391–401.

Sinal, S. H., Lawless, M. R., Rainey, D. Y., *et al.* (1997). Clinician agreement on physical findings in child sexual abuse cases. *Arch Pediatr Adolesc Med* **151**: 497–501.

Singley, S. J. (1998). Failure to report suspect child abuse: civil liability of mandated reporters. *J Juven Law* **19**: 236–71.

State of Minnesota v. *Curtis Lowell Grover* [1989] N.W.2d, Minnesota Supreme Court 437: 60.

State of Missouri v. *Leslie A. Brown* [2004] Missouri Supreme Court.

Thompson-Cooper, I., Fugere, R., and Cormier, B. M. (1993). The child abuse reporting laws: an ethical dilemma for professionals. *Can J Psychiatry* **38**: 557–62.

Tirosh, E., Offer S., Cohen, A., and Jaffe, M. (2003). Attitudes towards corporal punishment and reporting of abuse. *Child Abuse Negl* **27**: 929–37.

Vasquez, E. and Pitts, K. (2006). Red flags during home visitation: infants and toddlers. *J Commun Health Nurs* **23**: 123–31.

Visser, S. and Miller, J. Y. (2002). Child discipline at root of church trial. *Atlanta J Constit* 9 October.

Warner, J. E. and Hansen, D. J. (1994). The identification and reporting of physical abuse by physicians: a review and implications for research. *Child Abuse Negl* **18**: 11–25.

White, A. R. (1993). Suspicion. In *Wittgenstein's Intentions* ed. J. V. Canfield. Hamden: Garland, pp. 81–5.

Whitehorn, J., Ayonrinde, O., and Maingay, S. (2002). Female genital mutilation: cultural and psychological implications. *Sex Relat Ther* **17**: 161–70.

Widom, C. S. (1999). Posttraumatic stress disorder in abused and neglected children grown up. *Am J Psychiatry* **156**: 1223–9.

Wyatt, G. A., Burns Loeb, T., Solis, B., and Vargas Carmona, J. (1999). The prevalence and circumstances of child sexual abuse: changes across a decade. *Child Abuse Negl* **23**: 45–60.

Genetics and biotechnology

Introduction

Abdallah S. Daar

This section deals with complex technological issues that we often read about in the media because they are either very new or are controversial. The ethical issues are broad, falling under the umbrella of ELSI (ethical, legal, and social issues) or, for example in Canada, under GE3LS (genetic ethics, environmental, economic, and legal issues).

Chapter 20, deals with traditional organ transplantation, which has been one of the notable biomedical successes of the second half of the twentieth century. It has raised a host of difficult bioethical issues, many of which revolve around organ donation. In the 1980s, it was considered unseemly to consider donation other than from the dead or from genetically related living donors. Today, the range of ethically acceptable potential donors, both cadaveric and living, has expanded substantially in response to the rising need and demand – a measure of transplantation's success. Living donations from spouses and friends are common, and those from acquaintances and even strangers (Good Samaritans) are increasing. Donations from the recently deceased now include the controversial non-heart-beating donors of various types (actually harking back to the early days of cadaveric donation). The two cases discussed in Ch. 20 illustrate a number of important transplant-related issues such as consent, altruism, systems of just allocation of public resources, transplant tourism as well as and other substantive issues.

The life sciences are developing so rapidly that it is perfectly possible to think of regenerative medicine as the next stage in the evolution of organ transplantation, and indeed of organ function-replacement therapies. The tools of regenerative medicine include the controversial, highly charged, and politicized technology of stem cells. The two cases used in Ch. 21 illustrate the challenges encountered by primary physicians faced with patients seeking information about, and access to, cutting edge experimental therapies that they have read about in the media or on the Internet. Regenerative medicine is new even to specialists in other fields, and so Ch. 21 begins by defining the field and then goes on to highlight issues and approaches in experimental, innovative therapies. It talks of the distinction between therapy and enhancement, of media hype, the regulation of embryo and stem cell research internationally, and the obligation of clinicians to keep abreast of scientific and technological developments. It just touches upon neuroregenerative therapy and hints at the whole emerging and important domain of scholarly inquiry, dealt with in Ch. 63.

Much has been written about genetic testing, but it takes a world expert of the caliber of Ruth Chadwick to lucidly tease out the many complex, confusing, and evolving issues surrounding this subject. She asks the perennial question ''Is there something special about genetic information?'' and goes on to discuss confidentiality, sharing of information, the right not to know, stigmatization, testing of children, etc. Her discussion of secondary use of data derived from DNA analysis in Ch. 22 sets the scene very well for the next chapter, on bio-banking.

Another world expert, Bartha Maria Knoppers, who has enormous international experience in the field of bio-banking, joins with Madelaine Saginur to discuss the many issues surrounding a subject that is not of trivial scope or significance. Chapter 23 addresses stored tissue samples, handling of data, and consent and authorization models for legal and ethical secondary use of genetic data, especially for unknown future research projects. These are all crucial issues in the planning, establishment, and management of bio-banks in a responsible, transparent, and socially just fashion.

Finally, the section moves to a very controversial subject that spans a number of difficult territories, including genetics, eugenics, racism, and neuroethics, namely behavioral genetics. Jason Scott Robert masterfully negotiates his way through these subjects in Ch. 24. The two cases he has chosen to base this chapter on are superb, yet eminently realistic. The very question "Is there a genetic basis for 'normal' and 'abnormal' behavior" sends a shudder down the informed spine, evoking as it does visions of floodgates opening onto courtrooms all the way to supreme courts that will guide human society on how to interpret what scientists find in their laboratories and clinics. Robert notes that "advances in behavioral genetics may threaten or reinforce long-cherished personal and social values and stereotypes, perception of group differences, and even perception of ourselves and our human nature." Not trivial or insignificant at all. Maybe one day the science will be adequate to give us comfort, but at present this is more a minefield than a scientific field because of the paucity of scientifically reliable and generalizable evidence, other than in a few circumscribed instances. There are also definitional and methodological difficulties. Perhaps the most worrying fear is the likelihood of political agendas being used in the skewed social interpretation of incomplete, emerging data. Yet this is a valid and promising field of research. In years to come, we will undoubtedly read of "criminal genes," the interplay of genetics and early childhood experience (e.g., abuse), discrimination, and stigmatization. The field will inform not only the nature versus nurture debate but also the more philosophically exciting discourse on free will and determinism. What an exciting minefield. Time to get the sappers trained!

20

Organ transplantation

Linda Wright, Kelley Ross, and Abdallah S. Daar

A 53-year-old single mother offers to donate a kidney to a work colleague whom she knows distantly. Although the recovery time needed away from work after donation will strain her modest income, the woman tells the transplant team that she understands this and is willing to go ahead. She explains that her motivation to donate is purely to help another human being.

A man involved in a serious road traffic accident has suffered severe injuries and has been placed on life support while investigations are completed. The results indicate he will not survive. His relatives are not present at the hospital. The junior physician treating the patient considers withdrawing supportive treatment. He wonders whether the patient would be a candidate for non-heart-beating donation after cardiac death is pronounced.

What is organ transplantation?

Organ transplantation is both a life-extending and a life-saving medical procedure in which a whole or partial organ (or cells in cell therapy) from a deceased or living person is transplanted into another individual, replacing the recipient's non-functioning organ with the donor's functioning organ. Advances in the science of organ transplantation since the 1980s have significantly broadened the range of transplantable organs and improved transplant outcomes. Transplant centers in different parts of the world successfully transplant kidneys, livers, lungs, hearts, pancreases, and intestinal organs, and the procedure is considered the preferred treatment for several indications. Since the first kidney transplant in 1954, the increasing success

of, and innovations in, transplantation have created a demand for organs that greatly exceeds the supply in most countries.

The scarcity of organs is a major impetus behind the continuing search for, and development of, alternative ways to expand the pool of organs and tissues available for transplantation (O'Connor and Delmonico, 2005). A major development is the procurement of organs from family members, and most recently from friends and even from strangers (Matas *et al.*, 2000; Gohh *et al.*, 2001; Hilhorst *et al.*, 2005). We are also witnessing desperate patients soliciting organs on the Internet (Wright and Campbell, 2006), the compensation of living donors for related expenses or even the bestowing of financial rewards for donation (Larijani *et al.*, 2004), and the experimental use of organs from animals (i.e., xenotransplantation; Daar and Chapman, 2004). These recent trends are at the forefront of current ethical debate on transplantation, and they are gaining varying levels of acceptance in different countries by both the public and the transplant community. The sale of organs is another highly complex subject that has received much attention (Radcliffe-Richards *et al.*, 1998; Phadke and Anandh, 2002; Taylor, 2002; Daar, 2003, 2004a).

Why is organ transplantation important?

Ethics

Organ transplantation presents several ethical challenges. Amongst these are issues related to the determination of death, organ procurement, and organ allocation (Veatch, 2000). Definitions of death attempt to establish the point at which a person's loss of critical bodily functions alters his or her status from living to dead (Lazar *et al.*, 2001) and therefore when, in the context of transplantation, it is morally acceptable to procure organs from the deceased. There is now widespread acceptance, especially among intensivists and the transplant community, but with much public support in many countries, of brain death criteria for diagnosing death (US President's Commission, 1981; Dossetor and Daar, 2001). Some cultures do not accept this, preferring instead the traditional definition of death as the irreversible cessation of cardiorespiratory functions. These different perspectives obviously influence the formulation of legal and medical criteria for the posthumous procurement of organs.

One of the questions being debated is whether, after death, an individual's organs are a societal resource to be automatically recovered or an individual's personal property, requiring his or her approval to organ recovery (Truog, 2005). The vast majority maintain that organs belong to the potential donor and thus the most prevalent deceased donation model requires a person's consent to donate through signing a donor card while alive, or more commonly, through the agency and consent of next-of-kin, after death. This model is based on respect for individual autonomy (Veatch, 2000). The practice of obtaining consent to donation of deceased organs from a substitute decision maker raises, for some people, ethical concerns about presuming another's wishes if the subject of donation had not been discussed with the deceased while he or she was alive (Veatch, 2004).

A variation of this model is what is known as presumed consent (Kennedy *et al.*, 1998), which permits the removal of organs unless the person has formally opposed it while living. This model emphasizes the greatest net benefit for society (Veatch, 2000), but apart from a few European countries, it has not been successfully adopted and implemented internationally.

Organ procurement from the living is more accepted in some parts of the world than others. Donation is assessed by weighing the benefit to the recipient against the physical harm and psychological benefit to the donor (Matas *et al.*, 2000). Many agree that a donation between relatives is ethical because the familial relationship appears to justify the risks involved. Some, however, have expressed reservations about the propriety of living donation from non-family members, and especially from strangers. They argue that, in the absence of a genetic or emotional link between the donor and recipient, the donor's motives are more questionable or that the psychological benefit of donation does not justify the physical risks. However, altruism is an acceptable basis for living donation, and some argue that altruism is foremost expressed through donation to non-relatives and strangers than to relatives (Evans, 1989; Daar, 2002). Some further contend that, because a stranger's offer to donate is altruistically motivated, there is a greater chance that he or she is acting autonomously and in the absence of undue external pressure to donate (Gohh *et al.*, 2001). The debate continues as to whether strangers should be allowed to assume the same level of risk as other living donors when being considered for donation (Abecassis *et al.*, 2000; Spital, 2002; Daar, 2002; Ross *et al.*, 2002).

The scarcity of organs for transplantation necessitates the establishment of criteria on which to base allocation decisions, particularly for organs from deceased donors. The distribution formula commonly used draws mainly on two general ethical principles: utility and justice (Veatch, 2000). Utility is calculated according to medical benefit and justice is assessed on the equity of distribution, requiring (on some accounts) that the sickest or worst off be given some priority to ensure that all are afforded an equal chance to be healthy (Veatch, 2000). Many allocation decisions require trade offs in favor of either utility or justice, and thus attempt an acceptable compromise.

Law

The laws enacted to regulate organ transplantation vary with jurisdictions around the world. They generally cater to definitions of death, donor consent, and, often, the prohibition of the commercial trade in organs. The laws in most North American, Asian, and European countries permit organ removal when the patient is pronounced dead. These laws most commonly define death as the irreversible cessation of the entire brain function, although Japanese law allows the individual while living to choose between the cardiac- and brain-based definitions of death according to his or her beliefs (Morioka, 2001; Bagheri, 2005).

The laws in most countries require donor consent to posthumous organ donation. The Uniform Anatomical Gift Act (USA) and the Human Tissue Gift Act (Canada) each require an individual's express consent to the removal of his or her organs after death. "Opt-in" donor consent is common internationally. In contrast, the laws in some European countries (Kennedy et al., 1998; Abadie and Gay, 2006), and with rare exception elsewhere, as in Singapore (Schmidt and Lim, 2004), allow the procurement of organs based on presumed consent, but permit individuals to "opt-out" of donation. Japanese law does not allow for a substitute decision maker but requires both a signed donor card and family approval of organ removal (Bagheri, 2005). Internationally, transplantation laws generally permit the removal of organs from a living individual with his or her consent.

Many countries have enacted legislation against commerce in organs. Partly as a result of these legal prohibitions, the phenomenon of transplant tourism has emerged (Daar, 2004a). In India, for example, the sale of organs is illegal but the legislation established to prevent it has proven ineffective (Daar, 2004a; Young, 2005), and the practice apparently continues to flourish, with some foreigners traveling to India to buy kidneys for transplantation. China has recently pledged to outlaw the sale of organs from executed prisoners in an attempt to eliminate a widely criticized market in human organs (BBC News, 2006).

Unlike payment for organs, the compensation for expenses incurred by donation is considered completely justified. Genuine compensation is allowed in most countries, although there has been little work done to define acceptable limits of reimbursement and, more importantly, to develop schemes to reduce disincentives to donation. The US law grants a 30-day paid leave of absence to federal employees for organ transplantation (Delmonico et al., 2002). Iran is the only country so far that has openly institutionalized the formal payment of donors. The Iranian model, which gives money to kidney donors as a social reward, is still evolving. Although it has been criticized, the model has resulted in Iran completely eliminating its kidney transplant waiting list (Gohds and Nasrollahzadeh, 2005).

Policy

Government agencies, transplant regulatory bodies, and healthcare institutions recommend and set policies that, in addition to legislation, guide transplant practice with respect to definitions of death, allocation decisions, and organ procurement. Despite the widely adopted legal definition of brain death, individual hospitals have varying practices used by physicians to certify death. It would be advisable to have uniformity (Powner et al., 2004).

Organs from the deceased are commonly allocated according to policies established by regional, national, or international transplant organizations. In Canada, the Trillium Gift of Life Network and the British Columbia Transplant Society are among the largest regional organizations handling the collaborative development and implementation of policies governing organ distribution. Policy management is undertaken in the USA by a national organization, the United Network for Organ Sharing, and in several European countries by an international organization, the Eurotransplant International Foundation. Generally, these transplant organizations use computer programs to allocate organs to recipients on a waiting list, and position recipients on the list based on acceptable criteria such as organ compatibility, medical need, wait time, and geographical distance between the organ and the recipient (British Columbia Transplant Society, Eurotransplant International Foundation, Trillium Gift of Life Network, and the United Network for Organ Sharing).

Policies on living donation at most transplant centers support donations from relatives. Donations from friends and altruistic strangers are increasingly being accepted. Although policies allow donors to direct their organ to a known recipient, transplant centers that permit donations from altruistic strangers, in which the recipient is unknown, are reluctant to allow such donors to direct organs to a recipient of a specific social group (Matas *et al.*, 2000). Instead the recipient is selected according to the same waiting list criteria as for deceased donor organs (Hilhorst *et al.*, 2005).

At a conference in Munich in 2002 (Warren, 2003), the following resolution was passed on the complex issue of payments related to transplantation:

The well-established position of transplantation societies against commerce in organs has not been effective in stopping the rapid growth of such transplants around the world. Individual countries will need to study alternative, locally relevant models, considered ethical in their societies, which would increase the number of transplants, protect and respect the donor, and reduce the likelihood of rampant, unregulated commerce.

Empirical studies

A 2001 study indicated that a significant percentage of Americans surveyed found kidney donations from close friends (90%) and strangers (80%) acceptable (Spital, 2001). Related national and international social research data spanning the period from the late 1970s show that a sizeable proportion of individuals (studies vary from 11% to 45%) would be willing to donate a kidney to a stranger while living (Henderson *et al.*, 2003). Despite general public approval of altruistic stranger donation, a noteworthy 2003 Canadian study (Landolt *et al.*, 2003) sought to measure the relationship between people's willingness to donate to a stranger, while living, and their actual behavior. Results indicated that of the 52 respondents who were

hypothetically prepared to donate and underwent a psychosocial assessment parallel to living donors, 31% qualified as committed to donate. The study concluded that, because the respondents generally had no prior knowledge of altruistic stranger donation, some people would be candidates for this form of donation if informed about the need and given accurate information about the procedure (Landolt *et al.*, 2003).

Several related studies have measured public opinion on the recent debate over altruistic stranger-directed donation. Results from a recent study (Spital, 2003) indicated that the majority of American respondents would not permit altruistic strangers to direct their organs to recipients on the basis of their membership in a particular racial or religious group (two-thirds), although 74% would allow directed donation to children. The study conclude that current local and national policies against altruistic stranger-directed donation are rightly aligned with public views, although some raise concerns about using the general public's attitudes to determine policy (Hilhorst, 2005).

Public acceptance of xenotransplantation, or the transplantation of organs, cells, or tissues from animals into humans, has been empirically evaluated. A 2004 study (Rios *et al.*, 2004) indicated that, if animal organs had similar results to human organs, 74% of American respondents would accept the use of animal organs and, when compared with all organ donation options, it was the favored option. In Canada, an exemplary government-sponsored public consultation on xenotransplantation (Canadian Public Health Association, 2001) found that of the most informed participants, 34% did not want xenotransplantation to proceed under any conditions; 19% indicated that it was too soon; and 46% were in favor of proceeding if safe and effective. The study resulted in the government recommending that Canada "not proceed with xenotransplantation involving humans at this time as there are critical issues that first need to be resolved" (Canadian Public Health Association, 2001). Despite this verdict, some argue that a different rendering of the study's data reveals more favorable attitudes toward proceeding with xenotransplantation (Wright, 2004).

How should I approach organ transplantation in practice?

Practice guidelines for deceased donation, in instances in which a person's death is expected but has not yet occurred, urge that declarations of death or the decision to withdraw life support be made by a physician who is not a member of the transplant team and before approaching the family about donation. Usually, the family is given information about the option to donate and the possible outcomes, is asked about the patient's intention to donate, if known, and is asked to give consent to such donation. These tasks are often handled by regional organ procurement agencies, which upon being notified of a potential donor by the transplant center, find a suitable recipient and coordinate the recovery and transportation of organs (United Network for Organ Sharing).

Consensus statements and recommended ethical practice guidelines on living donation identify several practical elements as essential to ensuring the well-being of living donors. With respect to informed consent, a donor must be fully and accurately informed about, and demonstrate an understanding of, the risks and benefits of donation as it affects themselves and the recipient (Abecassis et al., 2000; Ethics Committee of the Transplantation Society, 2004; Wright et al., 2004; Zink, 2005), as well as the different treatment options available to the recipient. A period of time between consent and the operation is recommended, during which the donor has an opportunity to reconsider his or her decision. The transplant center must ensure that the donor's decision to donate is voluntary and is not influenced unduly by material gain, coercion, or other factors that may reduce individual autonomy. It is recommended that, if possible, the donor and the recipient be assigned separate care teams or advocates to protect their individual interests (Abecassis et al., 2000; Ethics Committee of the Transplantation Society, 2004; Wright et al., 2004), as well as to enhance confidentiality and avoid conflicts of interest.

Assessments of medical suitability will depend on which organ is being donated and will be carried out by the transplant team physicians. The donor's psychosocial suitability must be evaluated to rule out psychological risk factors such as severe mental disorder. It is also advisable to evaluate other factors such as economic constraints or domestic issues. These evaluations help to determine whether the donor is mentally competent to give informed consent, and if his or her decision is voluntary (Abecassis et al., 2000; Wright et al., 2004).

Altruistic stranger donation should follow the same guidelines as those established for donations from relatives, with an emphasis on the psychosocial assessment. In addition, the relationship between the donor and recipient, whether strangers or familial, should not affect the degree of acceptable risk to the donor (Abecassis et al., 2000).

The cases

It would be useful to have transplant unit policies on living donations from non-relatives, especially as they are becoming increasingly common. In the first case, the transplant unit must balance the need to explore ulterior motives such as covert payments with the need to respond to a genuinely altruistically motivated donor. A psychosocial evaluation, preferably by an independent expert in living organ donation, is usually administered, but it is difficult to establish ulterior motives. In addition, transplant units cannot control the exchange of material rewards or other events that may transpire after a transplant is completed. These are also matters of concerns in donations from relatives.

The transplant center planned ahead to ensure that the donor had sufficient support, including legitimate financial support, during her recovery from the operation. The recipient was a distant work colleague, which made this, in the absence of any coercion, a truly altruistic donation. The donor was fully informed about, and understood, the risks and benefits of her donation, and the donation process. The transplant team concluded that the woman was a willing, informed, altruistically motivated individual, wishing to donate for rational reasons that were important to her, and she was, therefore, a suitable donor.

If there is consensus that non-heart-beating donation should be undertaken in the second case described, it should be done exclusively at institutions with clearly established protocols. The Maastricht classification divides the five donation types into uncontrolled and controlled groups depending on whether cardiac death was anticipated (Ridley *et al.*, 2005). Several decisions must be made under emergency conditions when a patient is brought in either dead according to cardiopulmonary criteria (uncontrolled) or is in extremis with no hope for survival (controlled). In the controlled group (as in this patient), if the patient's relatives are not present, should preparation for organ retrieval proceed while they are sought? This usually takes the form of cooling the organs and may involve administering drugs to protect the organs, neither of which will benefit the injured and dying patient. If the relatives cannot be contacted, should organ retrieval proceed? These pressing issues are currently being explored with much interest at many centers.

If the relatives are present, there are minor differences in the consent procedures used currently in standard practice in which the potential donor is pronounced dead according to neurological criteria (i.e., brain death). In fact, deceased organ transplantation originally started with donation after cardiac death, not by applying brain death criteria, which entered transplant practice later. Brain death criteria continue, in some places, to be controversial.

If the heart is still beating, another question arises, based on the tension between a desire to confirm death absolutely and the desire to obtain organs that have not been damaged by ischemia: how long should the surgeon wait after the heart has stopped, following withdrawal of life support, before removing the organs (Daar, 2004b)? In this case, the relatives were found quickly and they consented first to withdrawal of life support and later to donation only of the kidneys. The physicians proceeded to cool the

kidneys via an abdominal catheter but chose not to administer any drugs to help to preserve them. The patient was taken to the operating theatre, life support was withdrawn (Maastricht type 3), and the surgeon waited a full 10 minutes before removing the kidneys, which were offered to two recipients with their full knowledge that the kidneys came from a non-heart-beating donor. One kidney functioned straight away, while the other had mild ischemic damage but began functioning well three days later. Both recipients are alive with functioning kidneys four years later.

REFERENCES

Abadie, A., and Gay, S. (2006). The impact of presumed consent legislation on cadaveric organ donation: A cross-country study. *J Health Econ* **25**: 599–620.

Abecassis, M., Adams, M., Adams, P., *et al.*, for the Live Organ Donor Consensus Group (2000). Consensus statement on the live organ donor. *JAMA* **284**: 2919–26.

Bagheri, A. (2005). Organ transplantation laws in Asian countries: a comparative study. *Transplant Proc* **37**: 4159–62.

BBC News (2006). China ''selling prisoners'' organs. http://news.bbc.co.uk/2/hi/asia-pacific/4921116.stm

Canadian Public Health Association (2001). *Animal-to-Human Transplantation: Should Canada Proceed? A Public Consultation on Xenotransplantation*. Ottawa: Supply and Services Canada (http://www.xeno.cpha.ca/english/bigissue/animal.htm).

Daar, A. S. (2002). Strangers, intimates, and altruism in organ donation. *Transplantation* **74**: 424–6.

Daar, A. S. (2003). Paid organ donation and organ commerce: continuing the ethical discourse. *Transplant Proc* **35**: 1207–9.

Daar, A. S. (2004a). Money and organ procurement: narratives from the real world. In *Ethical, Legal and Social Issues in Organ Transplantation*, ed. T. Gutmann, A. S. Daar, R. A. Sells, and W. Land. Lengerich: Pabst Science, pp. 298–317.

Daar, A. S. (2004b). Non-heart-beating donation: ten evidence-based ethical recommendations. *Transplant Proc* **36**: 1885–7.

Daar, A. S. and Chapman, L. E. (2004). Xenotransplantation. In *Encyclopedia of Bioethics*, 3rd edn, Vol. 5, ed. S. G. Post. New York: Macmillan Reference USA, pp. 2601–12.

Delmonico, F., Arnold, R., Scheper-Hughes, N., *et al.* (2002). Ethical incentives – not payment – for organ donation. *N Engl J Med* **346**: 2002–5.

Dossetor, J. B. and Daar, A. S. (2001). Ethics in transplantation: allotransplantation and xenotransplantation. In *Kidney Transplantation: Principles and Practice*, 5th edn, ed. P. J. Morris. Philadelphia, PA: Saunders, pp. 732–44.

Ethics Committee of the Transplantation Society (2004). The consensus statement of the Amsterdam Forum on the Care of the Live Kidney Donor. *Transplantation* **78**: 491–2.

Evans M. (1989). Organ donations should not be restricted to relatives. *J Med Ethics* **15**: 17–20.

Ghods, A. J. and Nasrollahzadeh, D. (2005). Transplant tourism and the Iranian model of renal transplantation program: ethical considerations. *Exp Clin Transplant* **3**: 351–4.

Gohh, R. Y., Morrissey, P. E., Madras, P. N., and Monaco, A. P. (2001). Controversies in organ donation: the altruistic living donor. *Nephrol Dial Transplant* **16**: 619–21.

Henderson, A. J., Landolt, M. A., McDonald, M. F., *et al.* (2003). The living anonymous kidney donor: lunatic or saint? *Am J Transplant* **3**: 203–13.

Hilhorst, M. T., Kranenburg, L. W., Zuidema, W., *et al.* (2005). Altruistic living kidney donation challenges psychosocial research and policy: a response to previous articles. *Transplantation* **79**: 1470–4.

Kennedy, I., Sells, R. A., Daar, A. S., *et al.* (1998). The case for "presumed consent" in organ donation. International Forum for Transplant Ethics. *Lancet* **351**: 1650–2.

Landolt, M. A., Henderson, A. J., Gourlay, W., *et al.* (2003). They talk the talk: surveying attitudes and judging behavior about living anonymous kidney donation. *Transplantation* **76**: 1437–44.

Larijani, B., Zahedi, F., and Ghafouri-Fard, S. (2004). Rewarded gift for living renal donors. *Transplant Proc* **36**: 2539–42.

Lazar, N. M., Shemie, S., Webster, G. C., and Dickens, B. M. (2001). Bioethics for clinicians: 24. Brain death. *CMAJ* **164**: 833–6.

Matas, A. J., Garvey, C. A., Jacobs, C. L., and Kahn, J. P. (2000). Nondirected donation of kidneys from living donors. *N Engl J Med* **343**: 433–6.

Morioka, M. (2001). Reconsidering brain death: a lesson from Japan's fifteen years of experience. *Hasting Cent Rep* **31**: 41–6.

O'Connor, K. J. and Delmonico, F. L. (2005). Increasing the supply of kidneys for transplantation. *Semin Dial* **18**: 460–2.

Phadke, K. D. and Anandh, U. (2002). Ethics of paid organ donation. *Pediatr Nephrol* **17**: 309–11.

Powner, D. J., Hernandez, M., and Rives, T. E. (2004). Variability among hospital policies for determining brain death in adults. *Crit Care Med* **32**: 1284–8.

Radcliffe-Richards, J., Daar, A. S., Guttmann, R. D., *et al.* (1998). The case for allowing kidney sales. International Forum for Transplant Ethics. *Lancet* **27**: 1950–2.

Ridley, S., Bonner, S., Bray, K., *et al.*, for the Intensive Care Society's Working Group on Organ and Tissue Donation (2005). UK guidance for non-heart-beating donation. *Br J Anaesth* **95**: 592–5.

Rios, A. R., Conesa, C. C., Ramirez, P., Rodriguez, M. M., and Parrilla, P. (2004). Public attitude toward xenotransplantation: opinion survey. *Transplant Proc* **36**: 2901–5.

Ross, L. F., Glannon, W., Josephson, M. A., and Thistlethwaite J. R. (2002). Should all living donors be treated equally? *Transplantation* **74**: 418–21.

Schmidt, V. H. and Lim, C. H. (2004). Organ transplantation in Singapore: history, problems, and policies. *Soc Sci Med* **59**: 2173–82.

Spital, A. (2001). Public attitudes toward kidney donation by friends and altruistic strangers in the United States. *Transplantation* **71**: 1061–4.

Spital, A. (2002). Justification of living-organ donation requires benefit for the donor that balances the risk: commentary on Ross *et al. Transplantation* **74**: 423–4.

Spital, A. (2003). Should people who donate a kidney to a stranger be permitted to choose their recipients? Views of the United States public. *Transplantation* **76**: 1252–6.

Taylor J. S. (2002). Autonomy, constraining options, and organ sales. *J Appl Philos* **19**: 273–85.

Truog, R. D. (2005). Are organs personal property or a societal resource? *Am J Bioethics* **5**: 14–16.

United Network for Organ Sharing. Richmond, VA: United Network for Organ Sharing. www.unos.org/.

US President's Commission for the Study of Ethical Problems in Medicine and Biomedical and Behavioural Research (1981). *Defining Death*. Washington, DC: Government Printing Office.

Veatch, R. M. (2000). *Transplantation Ethics*. Washington, DC: Georgetown University Press.

Warren, J. (2003). Commerce in organs acceptable in some cultures, guidelines needed, ethics congress recommends. *Transplant News* **13**: 1–3.

Wright, J. R., Jr. (2004). Public consultation on xenotransplantation. *Transplantation* **78**: 1112–13.

Wright, L. and Campbell, M. (2006). Soliciting kidneys on web sites: is it fair? *Semin Dial* **19**: 5–7.

Wright, L., Faith, K, Richardson, R., *et al.*, for the Joint Centre for Bioethics of the University of Toronto (2004). Ethical guidelines for the evaluation of living organ donors. *Can J Surg* **47**: 408–13.

Young, E. (2005). Laws fail to stop India's organ trade. *New Sci* **188**: 20.

Zink, S., Weinreib, R., Sparling, T., and Caplan, A. L. (2005). Living donation: focus on public concerns. *Clin Transplant* **19**: 581–5.

Transplantation organizations

British Columbia Transplant Society. Vancouver, BC: British Columbia Transplant Society (www.transplant.bc.ca/.

Eurotransplant International Foundation. Leiden, Germany: Eurotransplant International Foundation. www.transplant.org/.

Trillium Gift of Life Network. www.unos.org/.

21

Regenerative medicine

Heather L. Greenwood and Abdallah S. Daar

A 56-year-old man with severe angina pectoris visits a cardiac specialist for a consultation. During the course of the examination, the patient excitedly describes a story from the news about an experimental gene therapy that aims to stimulate new blood vessel growth in patients with coronary artery disease. He feels that such therapy could dramatically improve his condition and expresses a strong desire to enroll in the clinical trial. The clinician has some familiarity with the details of the trial and wonders how she should counsel her patient.

A 24-year-old woman with abnormal bladder development and function resulting from spina bifida visits her physician for a routine check-up. The patient would also like to discuss a new therapy she has heard about that involves the growth of a replacement bladder for transplantation using the patient's own cells. This therapy has been successfully applied in a number of other patients with spina bifida. Her physician wonders how to approach the discussion with his patient.

What is regenerative medicine?

Regenerative medicine has been the focus of substantial funding and research efforts worldwide (Attorney General of California, 2004; Greenwood *et al.*, 2006). Additionally, it has engaged public attention through highly publicized political debates (Press, 2006; Wagner, 2006), media accounts of "miracle" cures (Kuntzman, 2004), and strong lobbying from voluntary health organizations (Perry, 2000). As a newly emerging and evolving field, there is to date no consensus definition of regenerative medicine (Mironov *et al.*, 2004). For the purposes of

this discussion, we define regenerative medicine as follows:

Regenerative medicine is an emerging interdisciplinary field of research and clinical applications focused on the repair, replacement, or regeneration of cells, tissues, or organs to restore impaired function resulting from any cause, including congenital defects, disease, trauma, and aging. It uses a combination of several technological approaches that moves it beyond traditional transplantation and replacement therapies. These approaches may include, but are not limited to, the use of soluble molecules, gene therapy, stem cell transplantation, tissue engineering, and the reprogramming of cell and tissue types.

Regenerative medicine can be thought of as the next phase in the evolution of organ transplantation and replacement therapies (Haseltine, 2003; Daar, 2005). Instead of simply replacing cells, tissues, and organs, however, regenerative medicine aims to provide the elements required for in vivo repair, to design replacements that seamlessly interact with the living body, and to stimulate the body's intrinsic capacities to regenerate (Greenwood *et al.*, 2006). Disciplines contributing to this field include genetics and molecular biology, materials science, stem cell biology, transplantation, developmental biology, and tissue engineering (Haseltine, 2001; Greenwood *et al.*, 2006). In the realm of tissue engineering, for example, researchers aim to design and grow new tissues and organs using cells, scaffold material, and soluble molecules to guide growth. Such developments could help to overcome challenges facing traditional transplantation, such as immune rejection and shortages of donor material (Cortesini, 2005).

It has been estimated that stem cell-based therapies, one aspect of regenerative medicine, could potentially benefit over a hundred million patients in the USA alone for conditions such as diabetes mellitus, autoimmune diseases, cardiovascular disease, cancer, and neurodegenerative diseases (Commission on Life Sciences, 2002). Though still in the early stages of development, regenerative medicine has produced several therapies currently available on the market. These include the tissue-engineered skin substitute Apligraf (Petit-Zeman, 2001) and the adult stem-cell-containing bone regenerating therapy Osteocel (http://www.osiristx.com/products_osteocel.php).

Given the new therapies that regenerative medicine is likely to produce, the high level of media and public attention the field is receiving, and the experimental nature of many of the regenerative medicine therapies currently available, how should clinicians respond to patients' inquiries and what ethical issues does this field raise?

Why is regenerative medicine important?

Ethics

Regenerative medicine raises a number of ethical issues, some of which, such as the moral status of the embryo, are relevant at the broad societal and policy levels. This section focuses specifically on ethical issues that are likely to be encountered in everyday clinical practice: informed consent, decision-making capacity, therapy versus enhancement, and transplantation ethics. Each of these four issues will be discussed in turn.

Firstly, regenerative medicine presents new challenges to the process of informed consent. This is partly the case because many regenerative medicine therapies are currently available only through clinical trials, and clinicians will, therefore, face the question of whether or not their patients should enroll in such trials. In these cases, extra weight is placed on the importance of proper informed consent because the potential risks associated with

such experimental therapies are largely unknown (McKneally and Daar, 2003; Kimmelman, 2005). Certain regenerative medicine therapies, such as gene therapy, are associated with a higher degree of uncertainty than traditional therapeutics because they are not backed by a long history of pharmacological data that can provide a degree of predictability (Kimmelman, 2005). It is also the case that patients, particularly severely ill patients, can inaccurately perceive the purpose of a trial as one designed to provide direct therapeutic benefit rather than to produce generalizable knowledge (Lo *et al.*, 2005). Clinicians, therefore, must be particularly alert to their obligation to fully disclose and explain potential risks, benefits, and areas of uncertainty in order to allow their patients to give true and full informed consent to treatment.

Regenerative medicine also presents challenges to the informed consent process because of its innovative nature. As an innovative technology, regenerative medicine raises questions regarding a patient's ability to consent fully to treatment given that the therapies are often complex and unfamiliar (Lo *et al.*, 2005). Simplifying complex material so that patients can appropriately comprehend potential therapies can be challenging. Clinicians, however, have an ethical obligation to provide clear and reliable information to patients and to verify that the patient has fully understood this discussion (Lo *et al.*, 2005). The duty to inform patients accurately and thoroughly is of particular relevance in the face of media attention and hype, which may lead to unrealistic expectations of potential therapeutic outcomes.

Secondly, regenerative medicine can raise issues related to a patient's capacity to consent to treatment. This relates primarily to therapies targeted at the brain, and it takes on particular importance with respect to regenerative medicine because of the newness of the technology, the complexity of the organ being targeted, and because many of the patients receiving such therapies will be suffering from neurodegenerative diseases that could compromise their decision-making capacity (Glannon, 2006).

Thirdly, clinicians could face issues regarding the appropriate application of regenerative medicine therapies given their potential dual use; that is, given their ability to be used as a therapeutic tool but additionally as a method of enhancing normal function (Daar, 2005). Precisely what constitutes "impaired" versus "normal" function, and thus what constitutes therapy or enhancement, remains undefined and will most likely be addressed on a case-by-case basis. Carrying out an intervention purely for enhancement purposes does not necessarily mean that it is unethical (Miller and Brody, 2005). Enhancements can, however, raise concerns that concepts of normalcy may be shifted, that the autonomy of children will not be respected, and that a person's sense of self may be affected, particularly when considering neurological enhancements (Wolpe, 2002; Sandel, 2004). One emerging neuroregenerative treatment, for instance, involves injecting self-assembling synthetic peptides into the brain, which form nanofiber scaffolds in vivo to stimulate brain tissue and nerve regrowth. This technique has been successfully used to restore sight in hamsters with severed optical nerves (Ellis-Behnke et al., 2006).

Finally, given that the application of many regenerative medicine therapies will involve the transplantation of cells, tissues, organs, or bioartificial constructs into the body, ethical issues similar to those faced by the field of traditional transplantation are raised. These issues include the ethics of procuring donor materials and compensating donors, respect for different cultural perspectives on organ transplantation, as well as protecting patient safety, particularly with respect to non-human animal-derived materials (Rizvi, 1999; Abouna, 2003). Unlike traditional transplantation, where organ procurement and transplantation occur within a relatively short time frame, it may be the case that cells donated for regenerative medicine therapies are preserved and used many months or even years after the time of donation. This raises the question of whether donors should be re-contacted to update their family history in the interests of protecting the safety of the recipient. Such re-contact would,

however, need to be weighed against the donor's right to privacy and confidentiality (Lo et al., 2005).

Law

The law relevant to regenerative medicine is primarily focused on the regulation of stem cell research. This legislation will affect the extent to which physicians will encounter regenerative medicine therapies in practice, and the kinds of therapy that are at their disposal. There is currently no international consensus on the regulation of stem cell research (Isasi et al., 2004). As such, legislation varies broadly worldwide, from permissive, to flexible, to restrictive policies (MBBNet, 2007).

Countries with permissive policies on stem cell research include China, India, and the UK (Human Fertilisation and Embryology (Research Purposes) Regulations, 2001; Greenwood et al., 2006). In these countries, stem cells may be derived from a wide variety of sources, including the derivation of human stem cells from embryos created specifically for research purposes through somatic cell nuclear transfer. Somatic cell nuclear transfer, also called therapeutic cloning, is a process in which the nucleus of an oocyte is removed and replaced with the nucleus of a somatic cell, and the oocyte is stimulated to divide. Once cell division has reached the blastocyst stage, approximately four to five days later, stem cells can be harvested from the inner cell mass of the embryo (Lanza et al., 1999).

Countries with flexible legislation limit the methods of acceptable stem cell procurement. In countries such as Canada (Assisted Human Reproduction Act, 2004) and Brazil (Biosafety Law of 2005 [Nelson, 2005]), human embryonic stem cells may be derived from unused embryos created for the purposes of in vitro fertilization given that proper consent procedures are followed. Embryos may not, however, be created specifically for research purposes using somatic cell nuclear transfer.

Countries with restrictive stem cell legislation vary widely. The USA, for instance, restricts federal funding for embryonic stem cell research to stem cell lines already in existence at the time of the

Presidential announcement on stem cell research in 2001. The ban on creating new embryonic stem cell lines, however, does not apply to research funded by private or state funding. A motion to loosen federal funding restrictions on human embryonic stem cell research, the Stem Cell Research Enhancement Act of 2005, passed both the House of Representatives and the Senate but was vetoed by President George W. Bush in July 2006 (Congress of the United States of America, 2006). In Italy, by comparison, all embryonic stem cell research is banned under legislation that regulates assisted human reproduction. A June 2005 referendum to amend this legislation failed because voter turnout was below the 50% required for quorum (UK Department of Health, 2005).

Policy

Distinct from legislation enacted to define what is and what is not legal with respect to regenerative medicine, several government agencies are creating policies to guide the development and use of regenerative medicine therapies. From a policy perspective, regenerative medicine presents new challenges in regulating emerging products to ensure quality control and patient safety (Daar, 2005). The case of tissue engineered products illustrates these challenges particularly well.

Traditionally, the regulatory route of a product depends on its principal purpose or mode of action. The primary mode of action of drugs is via chemical means, while medical devices act primarily through physical means (Jefferys, 2003). Tissue-engineered products, however, often integrate these two functions. A physical scaffold serves as the framework on which cells are seeded. Growth factors stimulate the growth of the cells on the scaffold, and the scaffold itself may release soluble molecules to encourage regeneration in vivo (Koh and Atala, 2004; Sohier et al., 2006). Many countries are still striving to create policy that can accurately and effectively regulate the development and application of tissue-engineered products (Jefferys, 2003). The European Union Commission to Regulate

Tissue Engineering Technologies released draft regulations for public comment in May 2005 (European Commission, 2005). In the USA, the Food and Drug Administration (2004) has created the Office of Combination Products to coordinate the regulation of tissue engineered products. Additionally, the current Good Tissue Practices Final Rule, released in the USA in May 2005 (US Food and Drug Administration, 2005), strives to regulate cell- and tissue-based products by focusing primarily on safety and the potential for communicable disease transmission rather than on product identity standards (Preti, 2005).

Empirical studies

Empirical studies on the ethics of regenerative medicine largely focus on public opinions regarding the appropriateness of embryonic stem cell research and their understanding of stem cell issues (Perry, 2000). These studies may provide some guidance for clinicians regarding the beliefs they are likely to encounter when discussing regenerative medicine therapies with their patients and the level of comprehension they can expect their patients to have.

A recent study of nine countries in the European Union, for example, showed that the majority of those surveyed supported using spare embryos from in vitro fertilization for stem cell research but not embryos derived via somatic cell nuclear transfer (Solter et al., 2003). Results released in a study involving 2212 Americans showed that two-thirds of respondents either approved or strongly approved of embryonic stem cell research (Hudson et al., 2005).

Public understanding of stem cell research has also been evaluated through empirical work. A study found that 60% of Americans surveyed felt that they had a "good understanding" of stem cell-related issues (Nisbet, 2004). A follow-up study, however, asked Americans to identify specific kinds of stem cells that came to mind when discussing stem cell issues. More than half of the respondents replied that they did not know, and only 17% identified embryonic stem cells (Nisbet, 2004). The Genetics and Public Policy Center in Washington DC tested public understanding of stem cell and cloning issues among Americans and revealed incomplete or incorrect knowledge among Americans regarding stem cells and cloning; 45% of the 4834 Americans surveyed believed that is was currently possible to clone a human baby (Burton, 2005).

How should I approach regenerative medicine in practice?

Regenerative medicine will present issues for a range of clinicians, including family physicians, transplant surgeons, neurologists, and other health-care practitioners providing care to patients seeking and undergoing regenerative medicine therapies.

Clinicians faced with the question of whether they should recommend patients for clinical trials of regenerative medicine therapies should take extra care to ensure that informed consent is a top priority. Clinicians should disclose all areas of potential risk, including any cases in which unforeseen risks have occurred (Kimmelman, 2005). Any areas of uncertainty with respect to emerging therapies should be openly acknowledged. Time for in-depth discussion with patients should be allotted and should include the specific purpose of the clinical trial in order to avoid any therapeutic misconception on the part of the patient (McKneally and Daar, 2003; Kimmelman, 2005). Clinicians should also inform the patient of any standard treatments available (McKneally and Daar, 2003). Throughout this process, clinicians should be sensitive to the fact that patients seeking experimental therapy may be particularly vulnerable because of severe illness or because they have exhausted all other treatment options.

The high level of media attention around regenerative medicine may result in clinicians facing frequent requests for information from patients about specific regenerative medicine therapies. Clinicians should attempt to provide a reliable source of information independent of what their patients may have heard through the media. The complexity of emerging treatments along with potential preconceived ideas based on media hype will require that they take extra time to engage in in-depth discussions with their patients regarding potential therapeutic options. They should attempt to explain treatment options clearly and simply, asking frequent questions of the patient to ensure full comprehension of the risks and benefits of treatment. Asking patients what they have heard regarding a particular therapy and what their expectations are will help clinicians to ascertain their level of understanding, their source of knowledge, and any assumptions and beliefs regarding regenerative medicine that they may hold.

Patients under consideration for neuroregenerative therapies should be carefully monitored to assess their capacity to consent for treatment. In cases of uncertainty, a formal decision-making capacity assessment should be undertaken. It may be the case that a substitute decision maker will be required to consent to treatment for the patient. A more detailed discussion of these issues is contained in Ch. 3.

The cases

The clinician should obtain a full explanation from the patient in the first case of what he has heard about the therapy in order to assess his preconceived assumptions and expectations regarding new blood vessel growth. She should clearly explain the nature of clinical trials, emphasizing that participation does not necessarily entail placement in the treatment group and that many trials are not testing for direct therapeutic benefit to the patient. The clinician should clearly explain the details of the trials, openly acknowledging any information of which she is unclear. Given that the treatment is experimental, the clinician should take extra time to explain in detail the risks and benefits, emphasizing that they are currently unknown and that there have been cases where gene therapy has resulted in unforeseen consequences. Throughout this discussion, the clinician should take steps to verify that the patient has fully understood the information and that he is properly informed of standard treatments available. As a final step, the clinician should refer the patient to the coordinators of the clinical trial to receive additional information and clarification.

The clinical problems of spina bifida are well known to clinicians and the potential regenerative medicine application is easy to comprehend. Literature that has already been published on the outcomes of a few patients can help to inform the clinician's discussion with his patient. In seven patients with spina bifida aged 4 to 19 years who received tissue-engineered autologous bladders, clinical outcomes were excellent and renal function was preserved. No adverse side effects such as metabolic consequences, urinary calculi, or abnormal mucus production were noted. Upon biopsy, the engineered bladders showed adequate structural architecture and phenotype (Atala *et al.*, 2006). Given that the results for this therapy are early and few, clinicians will have an ethical obligation to keep abreast of the current literature in order to monitor the relative risks and benefits of the procedure and to communicate these to their patients. By the time of publication of this book, there are likely to be additional studies on which clinicians can base their advice. The importance of this breakthrough and the media attention surrounding it could lead to many more patients who wish receive such therapy.

REFERENCES

Abouna, G. M. (2003). Ethical issues in organ and tissue transplantation. *Exp Clin Transplant* **1**: 125–38.

Assisted Human Reproduction Act 2004. Ottawa: Department of Justice.

Atala, A., Bauer, S. B., Soker, S., Yoo, J. J., and Retik, A. B. (2006). Tissue-engineered autologous bladders for patients needing cystoplasty. *Lancet* **367**: 1241–6.

Attorney General of California (2004). *Stem Cell Research. Funding. Bonds. State of California.* Sacramento, CA: Secretary of State of California.

Burton, K. W. (2005). Cloning in America: the Genetics and Public Policy Center surveys the nation. *Genewatch* **18**: 13–18.

Commission on Life Sciences (2002). *Stem Cells and the Future of Regenerative Medicine.* Washington, DC: National Academy Press.

Congress of the United States of America (2006). *Stem Cell Research and Enhancement Act of 2005.* Washington, DC: Library of Congress.

Cortesini, R. (2005). Stem cells, tissue engineering and organogenesis in transplantation. *Transplant Immunol* **15**: 81–9.

Daar, A. S. (2005). Regenerative medicine: a taxonomy for addressing ethical, legal and social issues. In *Ethical, Legal and Social Issues in Organ Transplantation*, ed. T. Gutmann, A. S. Daar, R. A. Sells, and W. Land. Munich: PABST, pp. 368–77.

Ellis-Behnke, R. G., Liang, Y. X., You, S. W., *et al.* (2006). Nano neuro knitting: peptide nanofiber scaffold for brain repair and axon regeneration with functional return of vision. *Proc Natl Acad Sci USA* **103**: 5054–9.

European Commission (2005). *Consultation Paper: Human Tissue Engineering and Beyond: Proposal for a Community Regulatory Framework on Advanced Therapies.* Brussels: European Commission, Enterprise and Industry Directorate-General.

Glannon, W. (2006). Neuroethics. *Bioethics* **20**: 37–52.

Greenwood, H. L., Thorsteinsdóttir, H., Perry, G., *et al.* (2006). Regenerative medicine: new opportunities for developing countries. *Int J Biotechnol* **8**: 60–77.

Haseltine, W. A. (2001). The emergence of regenerative medicine: a new field and a new society. *J Regen Med* **2**: 17.

Haseltine, W. A. (2003). Regenerative medicine 2003: an overview. *J Regen Med* **4**: 15–18.

Hudson, K. L., Scott, J., and Faden, R. (2005). *Values in Conflict: Public Attitudes on Embryonic Stem Cell Research.* Washington, DC: Genetics and Public Policy Center.

Human Fertilisation and Embryology (Research Purposes) Regulations (2001). London: The Stationery Office for the Office of Public Sector Information.

Isasi, R. M., Knoppers, B. M., Singer, P. A., and Daar, A. S. (2004). Legal and ethical approaches to stem cell and cloning research: a comparative analysis of policies in Latin America, Asia, and Africa. *J Law Med Ethics* **32**: 626–40.

Jefferys, D. B. (2003). An overview of recent developments in the European regulation of medicine/medical device combination products. *Drug Inform J* **37**: 39–43.

Kimmelman, J. (2005). Recent developments in gene transfer: risks and ethics. *BMJ* **330**: 79–82.

Koh, C. J. and Atala, A. (2004). Tissue engineering, stem cells, and cloning: opportunities for regenerative medicine. *J Am Soc Nephrol* **15**: 1113–25.

Kuntzman, G. (2004). Stem cell gal's miracle steps. *New York Post*, 29 November.

Lanza, R. P., Cibelli, J. B., and West, M. D. (1999). Prospects for the use of nuclear transfer in human transplantation. *Nat Biotechnol* **17**: 1171–4.

Lo, B., Zettler, P., Cedars, M. I., *et al.* (2005). A new era in the ethics of human embryonic stem cell research. *Stem Cells* **23**: 1454–9.

MBBNet (2007). http://mbbnet.umn.edu/scmap.html.

McKneally, M. F. and Daar, A. S. (2003). Introducing new technologies: protecting subjects of surgical innovation and research. *World J Surg* **27**: 930–5.

Miller, F. G. and Brody, H. (2005). Enhancement technologies and professional integrity. *Am J Bioethics* **5**: 15–17.

Mironov, V., Visconti, R. P., and Markwald, R. R. (2004). What is regenerative medicine? Emergence of applied stem cell and developmental biology. *Expert Opin Biol Ther* **4**: 773–81.

Nelson, L. (2005). Biosafety law brings stem-cell research to Brazil. *Nature* **434**: 128.

Nisbet, M. C. (2004). Public opinion about stem cell research and human cloning. *Pub Opin Q* **68**: 131–54.

Perry, D. (2000). Patients' voices: the powerful sound in the stem cell debate. *Science* **287**: 1423.

Petit-Zeman, S. (2001). Regenerative medicine. *Nat Biotechnol* **19**: 201–6.

Press, A. (2006). Stem cell proposal splits Missouri GOP. *New York Times*, 12 March.

Preti, R. A. (2005). Bringing safe and effective cell therapies to the bedside. *Nat Biotechnol* **23**: 801–4.

Rizvi, S. A. H. (1999). Ethical issues in transplantation. *Transplant Proc* **31**: 3269–70.

Sandel, M. J. (2004). The case against perfection: what's-wrong with designer children, bionic athletes, and genetic engineering. *Atlantic Month* **292**: 50–4, 56–60, 62.

Sohier, J., Vlugt, T. J., Cabrol, N., *et al.* (2006). Dual release of proteins from porous polymeric scaffolds. *J Contr Release* **111**: 95–106.

Solter, D., Beyleveld, D., Friele, M. B., *et al.* (2003). *Embryo Research in Pluralistic Europe*. Berlin: Springer.

UK Department of Health (2005). *UK Stem Cell Initiative*. London: Government Printing Office (http://www.advisorybodies.doh.gov.uk/uksci/global/italy.htm).

US Food and Drug Administration (2004). *Overview of the Office of Combination Products*. Rockville, MD: US Food and Drug Administration (http://www.fda.gov/oc/combination/overview.html).

US Food and Drug Administration (2005). *Good Tissue Practices Final Rule*. Rockville, MD: US Food and Drug Administration.

US Presidential Address (2001). *Stem Cell Research*. Washington, DC: Government Printing Office (http://www.whitehouse.gov/news/releases/2001/08/20010809-2.html).

Wagner, J. (2006). Stem cell bill could face filibuster. *Washington Post*, 8 March, B06.

Wolpe, P. R. (2002). Treatment, enhancement, and the ethics of neurotherapeutics. *Brain Cogn* **50**: 387–95.

22

Genetic testing and screening

Ruth Chadwick

Mr. and Mrs. A have recently had a baby son. They are both carriers of cystic fibrosis, although neither has the condition. Although they knew the risks of producing a child with cystic fibrosis, they decided to proceed with a pregnancy and now wish to know not only if their son has cystic fibrosis but also if he is a carrier.

Mrs. B attends her general practitioner wanting to be referred for a test for predisposition to breast cancer. Her mother had breast cancer and died at the age of 41. She is convinced that because of this family history she also may die prematurely, and she wishes to know the facts in planning her future life.

What is genetic testing and screening?

Although genetic testing and screening have a number of issues in common, they are different in their scope. Genetic "testing" applies to the determination of some genetic factor in an individual, whereas screening aims to ascertain the prevalence of such a factor in a population or population group where there is no evidence in advance that any particular individual has it (Danish Council of Ethics, 1993; Nuffield Council on Bioethics, 1993, 2006; Chadwick, 1998). Genetic testing is normally an issue when either an individual requests it, for example because of knowledge of a family history, or is referred by a medical practitioner. Screening programs, although they will involve actual testing of individuals, are typically part of a public health

program, for example in response to a government-determined need to address a given health issue. Screening may take place at different stages of life – neonatal, childhood or adult – and may raise different associated questions. Context is also important: reproductive testing and screening, for example, are linked with particular sensitivities, especially in light of the history of genetics and its use and abuse in the form of eugenics. It is important to note, however, that genetic testing and screening may also form part of medical research protocols, for example to establish links between genetic factors and predisposition to disease or adverse responses to drugs.

The term "genetic test" is not entirely transparent. It has been defined as "a test to detect the presence or absence of, or change in, a particular gene or chromosome" (Nuffield Council on Bioethics, 2006), but it may or may not involve analysis of DNA. In some cases, examination of other substances such as the proteins produced in the body can indirectly provide genetic information. The term "genetic information," however, also has a wider scope than that in the above definition of genetic test: it may include "data from the pedigree, the name of a genetic disorder, the genetic status of a family member (e.g., carrier/affected) or the result of a clinical or laboratory test" (Royal College of Physicians, 2006).

In the aftermath of the completion of the Human Genome Project, genetic testing and screening have,

The author gratefully acknowledges the support of the Economic and Social Research Council; the work described was part of the programme of its Research Centre for Economic and Social Aspects of Genomics.

at least potentially, acquired much more power and taken on a new degree of complexity, increasing the likelihood of obtaining more useful genetic information in the testing and screening not only for presence of single gene disorders, but also for susceptibility to common disease, for behavioral traits (Nuffield Council on Bioethics, 2002), for propensity to suffer adverse drug responses (Nuffield Council on Bioethics, 2003; Roses, 2004), and to respond well or badly to foodstuffs (Chadwick, 2004; Food Ethics Council, 2005).

Why is genetic testing and screening important?

As more is discovered about the relationship between genetic factors and common disease, genetics will become more important to specialties apart from clinical genetics itself. Healthcare professionals in a wide variety of areas of medicine, although not conducting research themselves, may find themselves dealing with genetic information and its associated ethical issues, and they may have patients enrolled in research projects that have a genetic element or are participating in bio-banks (collections of biological samples, such as blood samples, for the purpose of establishing associations between genetic factors and health status such as susceptibility to disease, and/or to study variation in a population).

Ethics

The ethical issues arising in relation to genetic testing and screening largely depend on the view that there is something special about genetic information which makes it different from other kinds of medical information. The features that make it special are that it has implications for family members other than the individual in question and that it is predictive and not specific to time. Although other kinds of medical information may share one or more of these features to some degree, and so it might be claimed that genetic information

is not one of a kind, nevertheless these features are important in addressing the ethical issues and they are relevant to both testing and screening.

The fact that genetic information is shared with family members gives rise to issues about confidentiality and sharing of information (Human Genetics Commission, 2003). An individual may wish his/her test results to be confidential, whereas the health professional may consider it important that a relative has access to the information if it is relevant to the relative's future health. There is, therefore, an issue for the health professional as to whether to disclose or not, if the patient is unwilling to share the information.

The predictive nature of genetic information indicates that there is an important distinction between types of testing; whereas some diagnose an existing condition, others may be predictive of future health status. Testing an individual for whether he or she has a particular disorder can be helpful either for identifying a course of action or simply for offering relief where anxiety has been caused by not knowing. Where predictive testing is concerned, however, whether for predisposition to a late-onset disorder or for susceptibility to common disease, the issues are more complicated. Uncertainty over the accuracy of the test results and how they are to be interpreted is an issue, as people may make life-changing decisions on the basis of test results, perhaps becoming fatalistic although it is not certain that they will actually develop a condition (e.g., heart disease) or how severe it will be. Where children are concerned, testing them for a late-onset disorder, especially one for which there is currently no treatment available (e.g., Huntington's disease), may cause them positive harm such as stigmatization (Clarke, 1998). There has also been concern that predictive information might be used by third parties such as insurance companies or employers to the detriment of individuals: for example raising premiums or denying insurance or employment to people on the basis of a higher risk of developing a particular disorder (Nuffield Council on Bioethics, 1993; European Group on Ethics in Science and New Technologies,

2003; UK Government and Association of British Insurers, 2005).

The third feature of genetic information mentioned, that it is not specific to time, facilitates its long-term storage for future analysis, as new associations and testing techniques are discovered. This has led to the setting up of bio-banks in different countries as research tools to enable associations to be made between genetic factors and health status, providing information about variation within the population (Häyry *et al.*, 2007). These initiatives are not typically justified on the basis of benefit to the individual donor of a sample but on the basis of public good or public health, as is the case in screening programs. Practice varies, however, on the extent to which an individual participant may expect to receive information revealed about their own genetic constitution.

Because of the disadvantages that might accrue to people on the basis of genetic test results, some have argued for the individual's "right not to know" information about their genetic constitution, and consent to have a sample taken for testing is thus a central ethical issue (Chadwick *et al.*, 1997). Questions arise both as to who may consent (e.g., in the case of childhood testing) and as to what information is provided and how (e.g., is some form of genetic counseling necessary?) (Nuffield Council on Bioethics, 1993). Where long-term storage is an issue, there are further questions about narrow or broad consent to future uses of the sample: whether recontacting of the donor is necessary at different stages.

Law

The range of possible applications of genetic information is vast, and there will be national differences in the ways in which different countries regulate in this area (Cutter *et al.*, 2004). For example, whereas in some countries (e.g., Iceland) national bio-banks are rooted in legislation, in others they are not (e.g., UK). As regards clinical practice, preexisting common law and/or legislation concerning consent and the use and disclosure of medical information will apply unless there has been specific legislation concerning genetic information and its applications. There are also some international instruments that have to be taken into consideration.

The *Universal Declaration on the Human Genome and Human Rights* (UNESCO, 1997), although it has no legal force, lays down certain principles such as the right of everyone to respect for their dignity and rights regardless of their genetic characteristics, and it provides that genetic data must be held in conditions of confidence. The *Convention for the Protection of Human Rights and Dignity of the Human Being with Regard to the Application of Biology and Medicine* (Council of Europe, 1997) also enunciates some general principles. It provides, for example, that tests which are predictive of genetic disease or which serve to identify a person as a carrier of a gene responsible for disease or to detect a genetic predisposition or susceptibility to a disease may be performed only for health purposes or for scientific research linked to health purposes and should be subject to appropriate counseling.

In some jurisdictions preexisting law relating to consent has been deemed to be insufficient. For example in the UK, under the Human Tissue Act 2004, a new offence of non-consensual analysis of DNA has been established. Although the intention is not to prevent use of DNA for medical or research purposes, it addresses concerns over the possibility of its malicious use. The Act does not apply to all material from the human body (it excludes, for example, gametes and embryos outside the body and dried blood spots), but it provides a legal framework for the removal and use of tissue, including the requirements of consent such as who can give "qualifying consent" for analysis of DNA in cellular tissue. Consent is not required for use of cellular material in the diagnosis and treatment of the donor, and this has led to concern that this could facilitate future use of screening without consent, although the Nuffield Council on Bioethics (2006) noted that the requirements of consent for use of personal data as laid down in the Data Protection Act 1998 apply. This Act regulates the obtaining, holding, use, or disclosure of personal information.

In both the UK and the USA, there is specific legislation concerning disabilities and discrimination, the Disability Discrimination Act 1995 and the Americans with Disabilities Act 1990, respectively, which may be relevant in the context of genetics. The question arises and debate continues as to how disability is defined, specifically as to whether it could or should include persons with a presymptomatic genetic disorder.

Policy

In a field where scientific knowledge tends to advance very rapidly, legislation is not always the governance mode of choice, and a variety of policy-making bodies and advisory committees have emerged. At international level, for example, the Human Genome Organisation (HUGO) Ethics Committee has issued a number of statements dealing with issues in genetics, starting with the *Statement on the Principled Conduct of Genetic Research* in 1996 (Human Genome Organisation, 1996). The statements are largely concerned with research, although they have wider relevance in so far as they touch on issues such as the collection of DNA samples (Human Genome Organisation, 1998). This is a field, however, in which ethical frameworks develop and change as well as the science, and in its recent statements the HUGO Ethics Committee has tended to emphasize considerations such as solidarity and equity, in addition to the long-standing concerns of individual consent and confidentiality (Knoppers and Chadwick, 2005). The move away from the centrality of the individual, however, has also made its mark on practice, with the suggestion of models such as the "joint account" to represent the family's shared ownership of genetic information (Parker and Lucassen, 2004).

In the light of the complexity of the issues, some committees or commissions have produced major and influential reports on topics such as genetic screening. For example, the Nuffield Council on Bioethics, which issued its report *Genetic Screening:*

Ethical Issues in 1993, has produced a supplement on developments since then (Nuffield Council on Bioethics, 2006). The supplement noted the danger of overexaggerating the promises of genetics and takes the view that some of the purported benefits are still some way off, including screening for polygenic diseases and realizing the benefits of pharmacogenomics, which studies links between genetic factors and drug response to facilitate genetically informed drug prescribing and to reduce the number of adverse drug responses. Also in the UK, the National Screening Committee (2003) has developed criteria for the introduction of genetic screening programs, which include considerations related to the nature of the condition screened for and what can be done in the light of a positive result. General guidelines have also been issued relating to consent, where the prevailing principles reflect the need for consent both to obtain a DNA sample and to disclose the information contained therein (Royal College of Physicians, 2006).

Empirical studies

In genetics, different kinds of empirical study are at issue, such as different association studies to establish links between genetic factors and disease and other characteristics of individuals. Association studies may be disease specific or concerned with human variation with a population, as in the UK bio-bank.

In the ethical context, however, empirical studies within the social sciences have taken on special importance because of concerns about public perception of genetics. Worries that opposition to genetically modified food might be mirrored by unwillingness to accept genetically informed medicine such as pharmacogenomics has led to the perceived need to undertake a wide range of initiatives in public engagement. While this might be viewed from an instrumental point of view, as designed to achieve public acceptance, it is now widely recognized that a one-way process of "informing" is inadequate, and listening to people's concerns is equally if not more important so that public policy can be appropriately shaped by awareness of these. Work on attitudes towards pharmacogenomics in the north west of England, for instance, has shown appreciation of its potential benefits, including faster access to a suitable drug, in place of trial and error, and more personalized side effect profiles, while there is concern among health professionals about the possible withholding of a drug on the basis of pharmacogenomic information (Fargher *et al*, 2006).

How should I approach genetic testing and screening in practice?

In the context of clinical genetics, the above issues have received a high degree of discussion and debate over the last 10 years in particular. It is arguably outside this context where guidance is needed. While there is an abundance of detailed guidance on approaching the issues, there are some common themes that need to be borne in mind.

Firstly, best practice on consent suggests that obtaining consent to donate a sample should be documented, along with information as to what current and future uses the consent covers (Royal College of Physicians, 2006). Secondly, with regard to confidentiality of the information, while there is a view that in some exceptional cases a healthcare professional should have discretion to disclose to family members where there may be risk of a serious condition and treatment is possible (e.g., in the case of colon cancer; Genetic Interest Group, 1998), such cases would be very rare, the balance of harms test is not an easy one to assess. The importance of confidentiality has been reiterated in recent discussions (see Nuffield Council on Bioethics, 2006; Royal College of Physicians, 2006).

Thirdly, there is a set of issues arising from the uncertainty of much of the information, the perception of risk information, and the hype surrounding genetic information (as well as the exaggeration of possible disadvantages). These

considerations lead to the need in practice to have effective communication aiming to generate realistic expectations.

The cases

In the first case, there is an issue as to who has authority to consent to the genetic testing of a child, and whether that testing is in the child's interests. There is an important distinction to be made between diagnostic and predictive testing here. It is widely accepted that children should only be tested where it is in their interests and some treatment can be offered, and that they should not be tested for a late-onset disorder. It is far from clear that it is in the interests of the child that it be disclosed to the parents whether or not he/she is a carrier. While this will be important to the child on reaching adulthood, in making his or her reproductive decisions, there is no obvious scope for immediate appropriate action and so the testing should not be carried out. In cases of testing of children, an additional complication may be that the test result will show that the male partner of the couple is not in fact the genetic parent, and then there will be issues of confidentiality of the mother versus the father's right to know, although this is not an issue in this case.

In the second case, Mrs. B may be a good candidate for testing for the *BRCA1* and *BRCA2* mutations, which confer a higher risk of breast cancer. More information about the family history needs to be obtained. It may be that she is being overfatalistic in thinking that her life path will have the same outcome as that of her mother. Interpretation of information is important. It needs to be made clear to her that a negative result does not mean that she will be free from risk of breast cancer, as the majority of breast cancers are not caused by *BRCA1* and *BRCA2*. What the options are in the light of a positive result also need to be discussed, in terms of types of therapy or preventive action available, including preventive mastectomy. The potential implications for other family members in the light of a positive result need to be considered, for example the interest her sister might have in this information. Mrs. B should be encouraged to discuss the situation with her sibling.

REFERENCES

Chadwick, R. (1998). Genetic screening. In *The Concise Encyclopedia of the Ethics of New Technologies*, ed. R. Chadwick. San Diego, CA: Academic Press, pp. 193–8.

Chadwick, R. (2004). Nutrigenomics, individualism and public health. *Proc Nutr Soc* **63**: 161–6.

Chadwick, R., Levitt, M., and Shickle, D. (eds.) (1997). *The Right to Know and the Right not to Know*. Aldershot: Avebury.

Clarke, A. (ed.) (1998). *The Genetic Testing of Children*, Oxford: Bios Scientific.

Council of Europe (1997). *The Convention for the Protection of Human Rights and Dignity of the Human Being with Regard to the Application of Biology and Medicine.* Brussels: Council of Europe.

Cutter, A. M., Wilson, S., and Chadwick, R. (2004). Balancing powers. *J Int Biotechnol Law* **1**: 187–9.

Danish Council of Ethics (1993). *Ethics and Mapping of the Human Genome.* Copenhagen: Danish Council of Ethics.

European Group on Ethics in Science and New Technologies (2003). *Ethical Aspects of Genetic Testing in the Workplace.* Brussels: European Commission.

Fargher, E. A., Eddy, C., Payne, K., *et al.* (2006). Exploring patients' and healthcare professionals' views of pharmacogenetic testing. In *From Genes to Patients: New Perspectives on Personalised Medicines*. Warwick University, 5 July, symposium poster.

Food Ethics Council (2005). *Getting Personal.* Brighton: Food Ethics Council.

Genetic Interest Group (1998). *Confidentiality Guidelines.* London: Genetic Interest Group.

Häyry, M., Chadwick, R., Arnason, V., and Arnason, G. (eds.) (2007). *The Ethics and Governance of Human Genetic Databases: European Perspectives.* Cambridge: Cambridge University Press, pp. 11–13, 43–87.

Human Genetics Commission (2003). *Inside Information: Balancing Interests in the Use of Personal Genetic Data.* London: Department of Health.

Human Genome Organisation (HUGO) Ethics Committee (1996). *Statement on the Principled Conduct of Genetic Research.* London: HUGO.

Human Genome Organisation (HUGO) Ethics Committee (1998). *Statement on DNA Sampling, Control and Access.* London: HUGO.

Knoppers, B. and Chadwick, R. (2005). Human genetic research: emerging trends in ethics. *Nat Rev Genet* **6**: 75–9.

Nuffield Council on Bioethics (1993). *Genetic Screening: Ethical Issues.* London: Nuffield Council on Bioethics.

Nuffield Council on Bioethics (2002). *Genetics and Human Behaviour: The Ethical Context.* London: Nuffield Council on Bioethics.

Nuffield Council on Bioethics (2003). *Pharmacogenomics: Ethical Issues.* London: Nuffield Council on Bioethics.

Nuffield Council on Bioethics (2006). *Genetic Screening: A Supplement to the 1993 Report by the Nuffield Council on Bioethics.* London: Nuffield Council on Bioethics.

Parker, M. and Lucassen, A. (2004). Genetic information: a joint account? *BMJ* **329**: 165–7.

Roses, A. D. (2004). Pharmacogenetics and drug development: the path to safer and more effective drugs. *Nat Rev Genet* **5**: 645–56.

Royal College of Physicians with the Royal College of Pathologists and the British Society for Human Genetics (2006). *Consent and Confidentiality in Genetic Practice: Guidance on Genetic Testing and Sharing Genetic Information. A Report of the Joint Committee on Medical Genetics.* London: Royal College of Physicians of London.

UK Government and Association of British Insurers (2005). *Concordat and Moratorium on Genetics and Insurance.* London: Department of Health.

UK National Screening Committee (2003). *Criteria for Appraising the Viability, Effectiveness and Appropriateness of a Screening Programme.* London: The Stationery Office.

UNESCO (1997). *The Universal Declaration on the Human Genome and Human Rights*, 11 November. New York: United Nations.

23

Bio-banking

Bartha Maria Knoppers and Madelaine Saginur

For many years, physicians at a cancer clinic have been storing biological samples left over after being used for diagnosis in clinical testing. Prior to 2000, no consent for storage or research was obtained. In 2000, the clinic changed its policy and began to systematically request consent for the use and storage of leftover biological samples "for future cancer research." From that point on, the clinic has been storing samples only when the patient consented. It discards samples when the patient does not consent. Many of the sample donors are still alive (some are still patients at the clinic), while others have died. The clinic now has over 4000 samples, with comprehensive clinical data. Two groups of geneticists would like to use the samples for research, one examining the genetic basis of certain cancers, and the other examining the genetic basis of ethnicity and drug response in a randomized, heterogeneous population study.

What is bio-banking?

Our knowledge of genetics has largely transformed the manner in which biomedical research takes place. From the Human Genome Project and the International HapMap Consortium, we now know the sequence of the human genome, and we have created a haplotype map of the human genome, describing the common patterns of haplotype ancestry. While in the past genetic research tended to focus more on the identification of single genes that follow a Mendelian pattern of inheritance (i.e., presence of single gene being both necessary and sufficient to cause the disease in question), there has been a shift in interest to the search for genetic risk

factors in common diseases (e.g., cardiovascular disease, cancer, diabetes), as well as to pharmacogenomics research (understanding the role of genetic variation in individual drug response) and to studies of normal genetic variation across entire populations (Knoppers and Sallée, 2005).

Researchers need access to systematic collections of tissue or fluid samples and related clinical data (bio-banks) to maximize their research progress in such areas, ultimately leading to better understanding of the role genes play in health, disease, and interactions with the environment (World Health Organization, 2003; Canadian Biotechnology Advisory Committee, 2004). Despite some controversy regarding their scientific utility, most believe that bio-banks are both important and extremely useful (Barbour, 2003; Finkelstein *et al.*, 2004; Foster and Sharp, 2005). Bio-banks differ in a number of respects, including the number of samples collected, the types of sample collected (disease specific/general, prospective/archival, individual or family/populations), the degree of identifiability of the samples, the range of possible or permitted uses, the status of the institution(s) in charge of their constitution and management (public/private), and the sector in which the samples were collected (clinical, research, forensic, etc.).

In this chapter, we discuss a key ethical issue that, although important for all research, has particular considerations in the context of bio-banking for clinicians, namely consent. We cover the general situation plus that applicable to deceased individuals and approach the issue from a variety of national and international perspectives. Related topics such as return of research results and commercialization are beyond the scope of this chapter.

Why is bio-banking important?

Ethics

Since the Nuremberg trials following World War II, international ethics protocols have been designed to protect human subjects who take part in medical research. The Nuremberg Code, the first international instrument on the ethics of medical research, established that, "voluntary consent of the human subject is absolutely essential" (Nuremberg Code, 1947; World Medical Association, 1964; Council of Europe, 2005). Voluntary consent requires the free (i.e., uncoerced) decision of a legally capable individual who has "sufficient knowledge and comprehension of the elements of the subject matter involved as to enable him to make an understanding and enlightened decision."

Informed consent is now the touchstone of ethical biomedical research and is codified in many policy documents, including those of the World Medical Association, the United Nations Educational, Scientific and Cultural Organization (UNESCO), the Council for International Organizations of Medical Sciences (CIOMS), the Human Genome Organisation (HUGO), the World Health Organization (WHO), and the Council of Europe. This principle is equally applicable in the context of genetic research (UNESCO, 2003, 2005; Canadian Institutes of Health Research, 2005; Council of Europe, 2005), as in the even more specific context of bio-banking (HUGO, 1998; WHO, 2003; Council of Europe Steering Committee on Bioethics, 2006). In each case, the underlying values that informed consent serves to protect are the same, and include dignity, autonomy and privacy. However, because of factual differences between the different types of research, how these values are weighted against the competing value of facilitating research that benefits humanity does change. For research on biological samples, as

opposed to research on a human subject directly, there are minimal, if any, physical risks to the research subjects; the potential harms relate to human dignity (e.g., unconsented use of specimens that goes against religious or personal beliefs) and individual (e.g., insurance) or group-based discrimination (Rothstein, 2005). For populational bio-bank research, the paradigm shifts even further: traditional research on biological specimens generally involves a single researcher or group of researchers obtaining and using samples in defined ways to research a discrete area. In contrast, population bio-banks often involve entities that obtain the sample but are not directly engaged in research, who supply specimens to other researchers. The purpose of a population bio-bank is to develop a "resource" that can be used for many research protocols, often in numerous scientific areas and in ways that cannot be foreseen at the time of collection (Canadian Biotechnology Advisory Committee, 2004). The movement towards population-based genetic research (requiring infrastructures such as bio-banks) has led to a concurrent movement to rethink the "paramount position of the individual in ethics" (WHO, 2003; Knoppers and Chadwick, 2005).

Law and policy

General issues

In general, consent requirements will vary with the degree of identifiability of the sample and the associated data. This makes sense: the weaker the link between sample and donor, the lower the chance of harm to the donor. It must be noted that there is considerable confusion in the terminology used to describe the identifiability of genetic samples (Knoppers and Saginur, 2005; US National Bioethics Advisory Committee, 1999). For the purpose of clarity, we use the term anonymized to refer to samples that were originally identified or coded but are then stripped of all possible identifiers. Coded is used to refer to samples that are identifiable only through breaking the unique (single coded) or the two unique (double coded) codes given the sample.

Double coding involves a keyholder who can link the two codes when necessary for research or clinical purposes.

After over a decade of inconsistency and uncertainty, certain trends are beginning to emerge in this area. First is the increasing recognition of the validity of waiver of consent for secondary research on double-coded specimens and data, and second is the increasing acceptability of broad consent for population projects.

At the international level, HUGO, CIOMS, WHO and UNESCO all advocate similar approaches. Consent may be waived for secondary uses of samples if the samples are anonymized or if they are double coded provided certain conditions are met: there is a general notification of such a policy and the patient has not objected (HUGO, 1998), patient confidentiality is protected and research ethics board approval is obtained (CIOMS, 2002), no future identification is possible of the sample source (WHO, 2003), and the data has medical or scientific significance and research ethics committee approval has been obtained (UNESCO, 2003).

At the regional (European) level, the Council of Europe allows waiver of consent for research uses of coded samples if an independent evaluation finds that the research addresses an important scientific interest, the aims of the research could not reasonably be achieved using biological materials for which consent can be obtained, and the individual did not expressly oppose such research use (Council of Europe Steering Committee on Bioethics, 2006). The European Society of Human Genetics (2001) considers that the consent requirement can be waived when samples are anonymized (rec. 9), and, provided it is approved by an ethics committee, in situations where the collection can be considered as abandoned (rec. 14). For collections of coded information, while in principle re-consent of participants for new studies is necessary, ethics review committees can waive the requirement for such consent when re-contact is impracticable and the study poses minimal risks (rec. 12).

At the national level, different countries have taken different approaches to regulating consent requirements, yet the actual content of the norms are beginning to converge. The UK (Human Tissue Act, 2004; Parry, 2005), France (Loi du 6 août, 2004), the USA (US Department of Health and Human Services, 2003a), Canada (Tri-Council Policy Statement, 1998), and Germany (Nationaler Ethikrat, 2004), for example, all hold that re-consent is not required when samples are anonymized. With respect to coded samples, the UK allows research on samples that are not anonymized where reasonable efforts have been made to obtain the consent of the donor (Human Tissue Act, 2004). In France, the secondary use of samples removed during medical care is permissible provided the donors have been notified of the secondary use and have not objected to such use (Code de la santé public, 2004). Further, the obligation to inform individuals can be waived if it is impossible to find the person, or when an ethics committee is consulted by the research investigator, and concludes that such information is not necessary (Code de la santé public, 2004; L. 1123–1). In the USA, consent is not required for secondary research uses of double-coded samples, if there are assurances (either through private agreement, institutional review board policies, or other legal requirements) that the keyholder will not under any circumstances release the key to the investigators until the individuals are deceased, as once deceased this is no longer considered "human subject research" (US Office for Human Research Protections, 2004). For identifiable samples, an institutional review board may alter or waive the requirement of informed consent if the research involves no more than minimal risk, the waiver or alteration will not affect the individual's rights and welfare, and the research could not be carried out without waiver or alteration of consent requirements (US Department of Health and Human Services, 2005).

In Canada, research ethics boards may waive some or all consent requirements if the research poses no more than minimal risk to the subject, the waiver is unlikely to adversely affect the rights and welfare of the subjects, and the research could not practicably be carried out without the waiver

(Tri-Council Policy Statement, 1998). In the context of secondary use, when determining whether consent may be waived in a given circumstance, a research ethics board must consider the following factors: the necessity of the personal data, whether potential harm to individuals is minimized and potential benefits of the research outweigh potential harms, whether seeking consent is inappropriate (e.g., psychological harm, risk of threat to privacy, or contact with individuals not permitted under a previous data-sharing agreement, law or policy) or impracticable, what the individuals' expectations are (no previous objections to the secondary use and expectations of a reasonable person), and what the views of relevant groups or communities are (Canadian Institutes of Health Research, 2005). Finally, in Germany, the balancing of patients' rights and freedom of research was addressed in the 2004 opinion of the German National Ethics Council. It concluded that an ethics committee can waive consent requirements when samples and data are double coded provided researchers do not have access to the code (Nationaler Ethikrat, 2004). Further, consent can be waived for research on identified data and samples when donors' interests are outweighed by the scientific importance of the research and the research cannot proceed otherwise or can proceed only at too high a cost, and disproportionate efforts (regulatory proposals 3 and 4).

Bio-bank research is moving beyond the one study/one informed consent model to a format of obtaining general or broad consent to participate in the research activities of a bio-bank (Rothstein, 2005). Allowing for broad consent eliminates the need to determine whether a waiver of consent should be granted in a specific instance. HUGO, in its *Statement on Human Genomic Databases* (2002) held that "[i]nformed consent may include notification of uses (actual or future) … or, in some cases, blanket consent. The CIOMS (2002) implied an acceptance of broad consent by stating "the original consent process [must] anticipate, to the extent that this is feasible, any foreseeable plans for future use of the records or specimens for research."

The Council of Europe similarly allowed for broad consent, yet emphasized that the individual "may place restrictions on the use of his or her biological materials" (Council of Europe Steering Committee on Bioethics, 2006).

While not all laws or policy documents address the issue of broad consent, those that do tend to endorse it. For example, the Canadian Biotechnology Advisory Committee (2004) held that, for bio-bank research to be most beneficial, consideration should be given to establishing an "authorization model" of informed consent specifically for prospective population genetic research. This model would require consent for the initial collection of the biological sample. Authorization of subsequent research would be given (or denied) by the donor at the time of the initial sample collection. Individuals must be able to specify which uses of their biological material and associated data are permitted or excluded as well as the degree of subsequent decision-making authority they want to retain; and individuals must have the option to give general or "broad consent" to any and all future uses. The German National Ethics Council went further. It recognized the necessity for archived samples (obtained during diagnosis and treatment) to remain available for further use and held that a "form-based" broad consent should be obtained at the time of collection and would be sufficient and so it would not take the "option" approach (Nationaler Ethikrat, 2004).

Despite this general trend towards more permissive rules governing secondary use of biological samples and consent, there remain jurisdictions that require a specific consent. For example, (though being re-evaluated), Sweden holds that "[t]issue samples preserved in a bio-bank may not be used for other purposes than those indicated in information submitted previously for which consent has been granted. In the event of a new purpose, the person who previously granted consent must be informed about the new purpose and grant new consent" (Swedish Ministry of Health and Social Affairs, 2002). However, overall there has been a gradual understanding by national policy makers of the difference between the degrees of identifiability of samples and data and corresponding levels of research access for secondary uses. There is also a move away from requiring an explicit re-consent for all secondary uses provided other safeguards are in place (i.e., through double coding, anonymization, data steward, research ethics board approval, etc.).

Postmortem issues

It is widely held that the death of a person does not extinguish the interests of that individual. Family members, and others who have physical possession or access to an individual's body, tissue or cells, have to respect certain obligations and rights following the death of the individual. The WHO (2003) does hold though that death affects the primacy of this interest and allows for the possibility, through appropriate ethical approval, of readjusting the balance of interests in light of death.

At the regional level, the European Society of Human Genetics (2001; rec. 13) holds that postmortem uses of samples are subject to the advance wishes of the donors. In the absence of any known wishes, use of those samples should be regulated, a policy of unfettered use not being ethically justified. The Council of Europe Committee of Ministers (2006) did not explicitly differentiate between research on archived human biological materials based on whether the sample source is living or not. It simply stated that postmortem uses have to meet satisfactory information and consent measures. Finally, the European Commission (2004) recommended allowing samples from the deceased to be used for research provided the sample is anonymized.

At the national level, there is variation with respect to whether, and if so under what circumstances, research can be performed on biological samples from deceased individuals. National positions cover the range from the theoretically unlimited power of officials to "deem" consent from the deceased to the restrictive position that essentially disallows research on identifiable samples from the deceased

unless the deceased previously consented to that research use (Genetic Privacy and Nondiscrimination Act, US Department of Energy, 2003). Yet, these differences have few practical consequences. Equally notable is the number of documents that do not address the issue at all.

In the UK, the Human Tissue Act 2004 s.4(a)–(e) provides for powers to dispense with the need for consent by providing a mechanism for "deeming" there to be appropriate consent for a research use. In theory, therefore, there are wide powers to perform research on biological material from the deceased. In France, while in principle biomedical research on a deceased individual can take place only if the individual had expressed consent to such research while alive, or if family members testify to the existence of such wishes (Code de la santé publique 2004; art. L. 1121–14), there is a key exception to this principle: the postmortem collection of cells, tissues, and human body products is allowed for therapeutic or scientific purposes if there is no prior opposition (art. L.1241–6). In the USA, research on tissue samples of deceased persons is not considered human subject research, and, consequently, consent is not required (US Department of Health and Human Services, 2003b). Therefore, legally, research is permissible on tissue samples from deceased individuals. In Canada, with the exception of Quebec (Sallée and Knoppers, 2006) in the case of deceased donors, "free and informed consent shall be expressed in a prior directive or through the exercise of free and informed consent by an authorized third party" (10.1(c)). Germany imposes identical conditions on collection and subsequent use in research whether the individual is alive or deceased. Next of kin can provide consent, as long as this is not inconsistent with the deceased's wishes (express or presumed), and there are broad provisions allowing for waiver (Nationaler Ethikrat, 2004).

Yet, all of these countries allow for waiver of consent when samples are anonymized. Since no further downloading of data from medical records is possible after the death of the sample source, it is, in fact, permissible to perform research on anonymized samples, as long as this is not inconsistent with the wishes of the deceased.

Empirical studies

Bio-banking is not of trivial scope or significance. As of 1998 in the USA alone, over 282 million archived and identifiable pathological specimens from more than 176 million individuals were being stored. At least 20 million are added each year (US National Bioethics Advisory Committee, 1999).

Yet, the scientific community identifies the limited availability of carefully collected and controlled human tissue samples annotated with essential clinical data as a major obstacle to progress in post-genomics research (US National Institutes of Health, 2006). Thus, whether or not broad consent has been obtained, and whether or not consent can be waived for a given research use, can have a profound impact on whether a particular project is possible (Kaiser, 2006).

Allowing for broad consent options is consistent with empirical evidence of the views of individuals. Most patients do want their tissues to be used for research. Indeed, a recent review (Wendler, 2006) of studies involving in total more than 33 000 persons, specifically examining secondary research uses of leftover samples from medical care, found that the vast majority of individuals (83–99%) were willing to donate their samples for research; those unsure about donation were often concerned about spreading their disease. Further, most people (79–95%) were willing to provide a sample for research in general (i.e., broad consent for research), as long as ethics committees would determine which research their samples would be used for and would ensure that those uses pose no more than minimal risk to the sample donor (Wendler, 2006).

How should I approach bio-banking in practice?

Before contributing clinical samples for research or starting a new collection, a policy for future uses should be set. The policy should outline the consent process and the necessary information to be given to patients. One fact that must be emphasized in a clinical setting is that patients' decisions regarding future research uses of their samples will in no way affect their care (US National Institutes of Health, 2006). As much as possible, future uses of biological samples should be anticipated and consent obtained. Not mentioning this possibility at the time of collection during care constitutes a lack of transparency (Cambon-Thomsen, 2004). According to "tick in the box" consent forms, allowing individuals to specify which uses of their biological material and associated data are permitted or excluded as well as the degree of subsequent decision-making authority they want to retain "strikes a reasonable balance that is supportive of individual autonomy and of genetic research" (Canadian Biotechnology Advisory Committee, 2004). This approach may not be practical however. Moreover, it would not be feasible for patients wishing to contribute their tissues or medical data to longitudinal studies in population genetics as the same data must be collected from a large number of individuals over time.

The case

The geneticist should contact the primary physician to ascertain the conditions under which the samples were obtained. Did the general consent signed upon admission or a more specific one prior to surgery or biopsy describe the policy of further uses of removed tissue? If so, was it for quality assurance programs or specifically for research? If the latter, was it limited in any way? The absence of a specific consent for research may be covered by a notification of the research policy in the general consent form signed at admission. In any event, the researcher will have to obtain the approval of a research ethics committee for the protocol. The committee may require a more specific consent from those patients that are still living. Tort laws vary on the access requirements for tissues of deceased persons. The same holds for access to the medical records, if needed for such research. The fact that the research is in the same field – cancer – may facilitate such research use but genetics raises issues of its own.

A randomized study of genetic variation to determine drug response would involve using only certain samples as representative of the general population. In all likelihood, such a study would not be foreseen in the admission consent. Access to the medical record for data on drugs prescribed would probably form part of the protocol. Therefore, while the study would not use any patient identifiers, the data collection stage would need to retrieve information from the randomly selected charts and then remove all identifiers before analysis. Usually, such studies only publish aggregate data, which serve as a resource for later, more specific disease protocols. Again, a research ethics board and local laws would determine whether a specific consent would be required. Anonymization may, however, obviate any consent and a waiver may be granted or even foreseen by law. The fact that ethnicity and relation drug response are under study, while no doubt helpful to the communities concerned, could also have untoward results such as insurance difficulties or no drugs at all being available to certain subpopulations.

REFERENCES

Barbour, V. (2003). Biobank: a project in search of a protocol? *Lancet* **361**: 1734–38.

Cambon-Thomsen, A. (2004). The social and ethical issues of post-genomic human biobanks. *Nat Rev Genet* **5**: 866–72.

Canadian Biotechnology Advisory Committee (2004). *Genetic Research and Privacy: Advisory Memorandum.* Ottawa: Canadian Biotechnology Advisory Committee (http://cbac-cccb.ca/epic/internet/incbaccccb.nsf/vwapj/genetic_research_privacy.pdf/$FILE/genetic_research privacy.pdf) accessed 24 February 2005.

Canadian Institutes of Health Research (2005). *Best Practices for Protecting Privacy in Health Research.* Ottawa: Supply and Services Canada (http://www.cihr-irsc.gc.ca/documents/et_pbp_nov05_sept2005_e.pdf).

CIOMS (2002). *International Ethical Guidelines for Biomedical Research Involving Human Subjects.* Geneva: Council for International Organizations of Medical Sciences (http://www.cioms.chlframe_guidelines_nov_2002.htm) accessed 27 March 2006.

Code de la santé publique (2004). Paris: Government of France.

Council of Europe (2005). *Additional Protocol to the Convention on Human Rights and Biomedicine concerning Biomedical Research.* CETS No. 195, art. 14. Strasbourg: Council of Europe.

Council of Europe Committee of Ministers (2006). *Recommendation Rec(2006)4 of the Committee of Ministers to Member States on Research on Biological Materials of Human Origin.* Strasbourg: European Commission (http://www.coe.int/t/e/legal_affairs/legal_co-operation/bioethics/activities/biomedical_research/Rec%20biomat%20CM.pdf) accessed 26 May 2006.

Council of Europe Steering Committee on Bioethics (2006). *Draft Recommendation on Research on Biological Materials of Human Origin.* Strasbourg: Council of Europe (http://www.coe.int/T/E/Legal affairs/Legal co-operation/Bioethics/News/Misc%20_2005_%203e%2OREV%20final.pdf) accessed 29 March 2006.

European Commission (2004). *The 25 Recommendations on the Ethical, Legal and Social Implications of Genetic Testing.* Brussels: European Commission (http://ec.europa.eu/research/conferences/2004/genetic/pdf/recommendations_en.pdf) accessed 26 May 2006.

European Society of Human Genetics (2001). *Data Storage and DNA Banking for Biomedical Research: Technical, Social and Ethical Issues.* Birmingham: European Society of Human Genetics (http://www.eshg.org/ESHGDNAbankingrec.pdf) accessed 28 March 2006.

Finkelstein, S. N., Sinskey, A. J., and Cooper, S. M. (2004). Biobanks: will they help promote the genomics revolution? *Pharm Disc* **4**: 20–4.

Foster, M. W. and Sharp, R. R. (2005). Will investments in large-scale prospective cohorts and biobanks limit our ability to discover weaker, less common genetic and environmental contributors to complex diseases? *Environ Health Persp* **113**: 119–22.

HUGO (1998). Statement on DNA sampling: control and access. *Genome Digest* **6**: 8. (http://www.hugo-international.org/statement_on_DNA_sampling.htm) accessed 2 October 2007.

HUGO Ethics Committee (2002). *Statement on Human Genomic Databases.* London: Human Genome Organization (http://www.hugo-international.org/Statement_on_Human_Genomic_Databases.htm) accessed 2 October 2007.

Human Tissue Act 2004. c. 30, s. 1(7–9), Schedule 5 paragraph 10 (http://www.opsi.gov.uk/acts/acts2004/20040030.htm).

Kaiser, J. (2006). Rule to protect records may doom long-term heart study. *Scientist* **311**: 1547–58.

Knoppers, B. M. and Chadwick, R. (2005). Human genetic research: emerging trends in ethics. *Nat Rev Genet* **6**: 75–9.

Knoppers, B. M. and Saginur, M. (2005). The Babel of genetic data terminology. *Nat Biotechnol* **23**: 925–7.

Knoppers, B. M. and Sallée, C. (2005). Ethical aspects of genome research and banking. In *Handbook of Genome Research: Genomics, Proteomics, Metabolomics, Bioinformatics, Ethical and Legal Issues*, Vol. 2, ed. C. W. Sensen. Chichester, UK: John Wiley, pp. 507–536.

Loi du 6 août 2004. Paris: Government of France.

Nationaler Ethikrat (2004). *Biobanks for Research-Opinion*. [Nationaler Ethikrat] regulatory proposal 3. Bonn: Nationaler Ethikrat (http://www.ethikrat.org/_english/publications/Opinion_Biobanks-for-research.pdf) accessed 24 February 2005.

Nuremberg Code (1947). *Article 1*. Washington, DC: Government Printing Office (http://www.ushmm.org/research/doctors/Nuremberg_Code.htm).

Parry, B. (2005). The new Human Tissue Bill: categorization and definitional issues and their implications. *Genom Soc and Pol* **1**: 74–85.

Rothstein, M. A. (2005). Expanding the ethical analysis of biobanks. *J Law Med Ethics* **33**: 154–9.

Sallée, C. and Knoppers, B. M. (2006). Secondary research use of biological samples and data. *Can Bar Rev* 137–51.

Swedish Ministry of Health and Social Affairs (2002). Biobanks in Medical Care Act. [Unofficial translation.] Stockholm: Government of Sweden.

Tri-Council Policy Statement (1998). *Ethical Conduct for Research Involving Humans*. Ottawa: Medical Research Council, Natural Sciences and Engineering Research Council, Social Sciences and Humanities Research Council (http://www.pre.ethics.gc.ca/english/pdf/TCPS%20June2003_E.pdf) accessed 30 March 2005.

UNESCO (2003). *International Declaration on Human Genetic Data*. Paris: UNESCO (http://portal.unesco.org/shs/en/file_download.php/6016a4bea4c293a23e913de638045ea9Declaration_en.pdf) accessed 2 October 2007.

UNESCO (2005). *Universal Declaration on Bioethics and Human Rights*. Paris: UNESCO (arts. 5 and 6. (http://portal.unesco.org/en/ev.php-URL_ID=31058&URL_DO=DO_TOPIC&URL_SECTION=201. html) accessed 2 October 2007.

US Department of Energy (2003). *Genetic Privacy and Nondiscrimination Act*, s.131 and s.133. Washington, DC: Government Printing Office.

US Department of Health and Human Services (2003a). *Code of Federal Regulations Title 45*, Volume 46.101(b)(4). Washington, DC: Government Printing office.

US Department of Health and Human Services (2003b). *Code of Federal Regulations Title 45*, Volume 46.102(f). Washington, DC: Government Printing Office.

US Department of Health and Human Services (2005). *Code of Federal Regulations Title 45*, Volume 46.116(d). Washington, DC: Government Printing Office.

US National Bioethics Advisory Committee (1999). *Research Involving Human Biological Materials: Ethical Issues and Policy Guidance*, Table 2.2, p. 18. Rockville, MD: National Bioethics Advisory Committee (http://bioethics.georgetown.edu/nbac/hbm.pdf) accessed 4 October 2005.

US National Institutes of Health, National Cancer Institute, Office of Biorepositories and Biospecimen Research (2006). *First-generation Guidelines for NCI-supported Biorepositories*. Bethesda, MD: National Institutes of Health. (NB First iteration document, revised and renamed the *NCI Best Practices for Biospecimen Resources* in June 2007.)

US Office for Human Research Protections (2004). *Guidance on Research Involving Coded Private Information or Biological Specimens*. Washington, DC: Department of Health and Human Services (http://www.hhs.gov/ohrp/humansubjects/guidance/cdebiol.pdf) accessed 23 March 2005.

Wendler, D. (2006). One-time general consent for research on biological samples. *BMJ* **332**: 544–7.

WHO (2003). *Genetic Databases: Assessing the Benefits and the Impact on Human and Patient Rights*. Geneva: World Health Organization (http://www.law.ed.ac.uk/ahrb/publications/online/whofinalreport.pdf) accessed 27 March 2006.

World Medical Association (1964). *Declaration of Helsinki: Ethical Principles for Medical Research Involving Human Subjects* [revised 1975, 1983, 1989, 1996, 2000]. Washington, DC: World Medical Association (http://www.wma.net/e/policy/b3.htm).

24

Behavioral genetics

Jason Scott Robert

Ms. C, a 32-year-old woman with no history of mental disorder, visits her family physician exhibiting mild symptoms of depression. She has been listless and riddled with guilt since her long-time boyfriend moved out the previous month, along with their golden retriever. They had been having money problems since her shifts at work had been cut back, and she missed her boyfriend and their dog. She had been having trouble sleeping and had spent her sleepless nights scouring the Internet for hints about her state of mind and how to "snap out of it." Ms. C tells her physician that she read a website about the serotonin transporter gene, 5-HTT or something, and that mutant versions of this gene make people more susceptible to depression. She asks for the physician to administer a test for this genetic mutation and warns that if he won't order it she will just find another doctor who will.

Mr. and Mrs. D have recently moved to the area. They have an 11-year-old son, E, who has been acting like "a child they don't even know anymore" since making friends with older kids in the new neighborhood. He won't listen to them around the house, refuses to clean his room, always breaks his curfew, acts up in class, and sometimes smells like cigarette smoke. The same thing happened with Mrs. D's brother at that age, and he wound up in a juvenile facility by age 14. She and her husband are concerned that maybe this kind of behavior runs in the family, and so they make an appointment with an internist to run a battery of genetic tests on E.

What is behavioral genetics?

Behavioral genetics is the statistical and, more recently, the molecular study of normal and pathological behaviors, their heredity, and their

development. Behavioral genetics is usually understood to comprise psychiatric genetics plus the genetics of other behaviors and behavioral traits (Schaffner, 2006a). Behavioral traits include aggressiveness, criminality, fearfulness, homosexuality, intelligence, novelty seeking, political affiliation, and xenophobia, whereas psychiatric traits include depression, mood disorders, and schizophrenia. Behavioral genetics has a long history; some of the earliest family and twin studies began over a century ago, and the field has been under critical scrutiny for approximately 40 years (since Jensen's [1969] controversial claims about race and intelligence). Until recently, most of the findings of behavioral genetics, while suggestive of genetic etiologies, have not borne fruit in terms of clinical or social application. The result is a well-justified and widespread skepticism about this field of inquiry. However, the recent history of behavioral genetics, characterized by advances in molecular genetics and genomics, suggests a more hopeful future for the field. In particular, the hopes of behavioral geneticists are buoyed by recent advances in the genetics of psychiatric disorders, which may translate into clinical applications for a range of conditions, including schizophrenia and depression. As a whole, though, behavioral genetics is not yet ready for the clinic. It is poorly understood, faces significant methodological challenges, and, by focusing on variation in the normal range, may strain the proper limits of the domain of medicine.

Behavioral geneticists employ a variety of methods, including so-called classical, quantitative, or epidemiological methods (family, twin, and adoption studies) as well as molecular techniques (such as linkage and association studies), to explore individual differences in behaviors. The individual differences approach helps to distinguish behavioral genetics from other enterprises, such as evolutionary psychology or developmental psychobiology, where the focus is not on *differences* in traits but rather on the traits themselves. Evolutionary psychologists study putatively universal traits, while developmental psychobiologists study developmental pathways within individuals. In contrast, behavioral geneticists attempt to understand why some individuals exhibit a trait while others (especially closely related others) do not. Why do some people have schizophrenia while others do not? Why are two diagnoses of schizophrenia more likely in twin pairs than in other sibling pairs, and more likely still in identical twins than in fraternal twins? These are the kinds of question that motivate behavioral genetics.

The logic of the individual differences approach helps to explain why behavioral genetics has not (yet) had an impact in the clinic: answers to questions about individual differences tell us nothing about why *this particular individual* has schizophrenia or another behavioral trait or disorder. This means that behavioral geneticists may be able to explain what makes a trait (say, aggressiveness) vary in a population without being able to explain why Johnny is aggressive and Jill is not. Put more technically, using the individual differences approach, behavioral geneticists try to explain how much of the total variance in a trait in a population can be explained by genetic variance, by environmental variance, and by the "interaction" between these two sources of variance. Yet, to explain variance is not to explain causation – the phenotypic variance may correlate with (be explained by) genetic variance even where genes are only one of many important causal factors. That is, it may be that the differences in a population with regard to political affiliation correlate with genetic differences, even if no genes are involved in actually causing one political affiliation or another.

Explanations of total variance in terms of genetic variance may, however, be suggestive of causation.

For instance, the three classical study designs in behavioral genetics – family, twin, and adoption studies – produce increasingly compelling data about the heritability of traits. ("Heritability" is a term of art in genetics, referring to the percentage of the total variance in a trait that can be accounted for by genetic variance.) Individuals within families have more genes in common than between families, and so a trait that runs in families may correlate well with genetic inheritance patterns. Of course, families share much more in common than genes, and so family study designs are subject to significant confounding. Consequently, adoption studies have been employed to eliminate some of these confounding factors. In an adoption study, siblings reared apart, and their biological and social families, are compared for the presence or absence of some trait. If the trait is shared by biological parents and offspring, but not by adoptive parents or adoptive siblings, then a genetic explanation may be inferred. By contrast, if a trait is shared by adopted children and their adoptive parents, but not by the biological parents, then an environmental explanation may be inferred. Again, confounders may be present, including selective placement of adopted children in homes and with adoptive parents (environments) that are significantly similar to their initial environments.

Twin study designs may be able to reduce confounding further. Twin study designs depend on the fact that twins have more of their genes in common than they share with other siblings. On average identical (monozygotic [MZ]) twins have 100% of their genes in common, while fraternal (dizygotic [DZ]) twins, like any other siblings, have only 50% of their genes in common. On the assumption that the family environment related to a trait is equally correlated between MZ and DZ twins (the "equal environments assumption"), behavioral geneticists explain differences in traits between MZ and DZ twins by appeal to genetics. A standard pattern, under the equal environments assumption, is that traits are shared more often between MZ twins than between DZ twins (that is, MZ twins are more concordant than DZ twins for a trait). Where that pattern does not hold, genetic variance is held to be less important than environmental variance in explaining variance in the trait. The equal environments assumption is controversial. It challenges the commonsense intuition that parents treat their identical twins more alike than they treat fraternal twins. Therefore, many behavioral geneticists, and many critics of behavioral genetics, are skeptical of this assumption that environments do not vary between MZ and DZ twins in any interesting way related to the trait in question.

Even where family, adoption, and twin studies lead to consistent results about the role of genetic variance in explaining phenotypic variance with regard to a trait in a population, these results remain, at best, suggestive of causal factors. With advances in molecular genetics, the suggestive results of quantitative studies may help to lead to the identification of specific causal factors – and thus to clinically relevant strategies for prevention and treatment. Molecular genetic techniques include genetic linkage and allelic association studies. In a family with a disproportionate number of members exhibiting a behavioral trait, a genetic linkage study may be used to identify a gene of major effect. Success in a linkage study depends on three conditions: that there really is a gene of major effect involved in the genesis of the trait, that there is only one gene of major effect segregating in a family, and that we know the mode of inheritance of the gene. For a complex trait, none of these conditions is likely to be met, and so despite successes with single-gene disorders (such as Huntington disease), linkage studies have not been particularly fruitful in behavioral genetics (Robert, 2000). Allelic association studies work in the opposite direction: rather than starting with individuals manifesting a trait and searching for candidate genes, association studies begin with a candidate genetic variant and investigators test individuals with that trait to see whether they have the same genetic variant. If so, then behavioral geneticists will infer that the candidate allele really is involved, and they may conduct biochemical or other analyses to determine the mode of action. Again, allelic association studies may reveal spurious correlations – if an

allele is in linkage disequilibrium with another allele, and only one of the alleles is involved in the genesis of the trait, an allelic association study may reveal association with the wrong allele.

Having knowledge of a correlation between genetic variance and variation in traits may sometimes suffice to design an intervention. For instance, if there is good evidence that a particular genotype is often associated with aggressive behavior, and if aggressive behavior may be prevented by a behavioral intervention, such evidence may guide school psychologists or social workers to direct their efforts at high-risk subgroups. But the surest route to the general and clinical utility of behavioral genetics is to take suggestive results (about individual differences) from quantitative, linkage, and association studies and then to explore causation (within individuals), so as to enable, where appropriate, prevention and treatment of the manifestation of certain behavioral traits.

Why is behavioral genetics important?

Behavioral genetics aims to study what makes human beings behave differently from each other. Accordingly, advances in behavioral genetics may threaten or reinforce long-cherished personal and social values and stereotypes, perceptions of group differences, and even perceptions of ourselves and our human nature. Moreover, findings in behavioral genetics may have broad applicability – for instance, in medical, legal, educational, and policy contexts – and so understanding the status and limits of behavioral genetics knowledge is imperative.

As with any studies of human behavior, and of human genetics, studies in behavioral genetics are prone to media hype. We have been bombarded by provocative stories in the popular press asking questions about whether babies are born gay or criminal, whether aggression or hyperactivity are in the genes, and whether propensity to get divorced is a genetic trait. These stories are not *made up* by the media; rather, journalists *play up* the more sensationalistic elements of actual research programs in behavioral genetics. As with other media reports about advances in genetics research, such stories result in patient inquiries for genetic services, from preconception, prenatal, and postnatal tests to genotyping and genetic interventions. Sometimes these requests will be entirely inappropriate, whether because of the test itself (e.g., there is no indication for ordering it) or the target of the test (e.g., there are ethical concerns about testing children for "gay genes"). But even in easier cases, behavioral genetic findings will raise a number of important ethical, legal, and policy considerations.

Consider highly publicized findings that the combination of a particular genotype with an early childhood experience of abuse can result in very bad outcomes (e.g., antisocial behaviors, including criminal charges and convictions; Caspi *et al.*, 2002). Though these findings referred specifically to an *interaction* between genotype and environment (as the mutation alone does not result in antisocial behaviors), the study was widely reported as having revealed "criminal genes," genes that lead to criminal behavior (Wilson, 2002). Thus a kind of genetic determinism was inappropriately read into the study, with significant implications for social policy – and potentially legal implications, too, if some defense attorney were to argue that a mutant gene made her client commit a crime, thereby abolishing criminal responsibility.

Clinicians must be especially attuned to interpretive challenges and the specter of genetic determinism in behavioral genetics. One helpful way to think about this issue was proposed by behavioral geneticist Eric Turkheimer (2000), who claimed that there are three laws of behavioral genetics: (i) that all human behavioral phenotypes are heritable (heritability $\neq 0$); (ii) that the effect of genes on phenotypic outcome is greater than the effect of being raised in the same family; and (iii) that, despite the second law, a significant amount of phenotypic variation cannot be accounted for by either genetic or familial effects. In his assessment of what these three laws actually mean, Turkheimer noted that, though well established, the first two laws are largely artifacts of the statistical techniques employed, and

so not particularly informative of biological explanations of (differences in) traits. They do not, for instance, suggest that nature prevails over nurture, except in a methodological sense, as there is no environmental equivalent of identical twins – the fiction of identical environment twins (both MZ and DZ). The major problem with this state of affairs is the likelihood of overestimating the meaning – the significance – of behavioral genetic findings. Heritability calculations must be properly contextualized, for they may be as much artifactual as genuine estimates of the genetic influence on traits.

With significant progress in human genetics and genomics enabled by the Human Genome Project, and with the refinement of molecular and developmental methods, there is every expectation that behavioral genetic explanations of differences in traits will continue to increase. While not yet ripe for clinical integration, clinicians can expect to see an increase in patient requests for behavioral genetic tests and, possibly, interventions in the coming decade. As indicated below, such requests will often be sensitive, and understanding the limitations of current methods, and the genuine prospects of the field, will be important for clinicians. For it is clinicians who will be required to discern the propriety of patient requests for behavioral genetic tests and interventions.

Ethics

Difference and discrimination

Behavioral genetics is the study of individual differences. In many social contexts, the identification of such differences may be used as the basis for discrimination (whether justifiable or not). The most controversial studies in behavioral genetics involve criminality and general intelligence (IQ or intelligence quotient), not only because the phenotypes are so poorly understood, but also because behavioral genetics findings with respect to these traits have been used to mark hierarchical distinctions between racial groups. For instance, in *The Bell*

Curve, Herrnstein and Murray (1994) claimed that genetics explains the performance gap between whites and blacks on standardized educational exams such as IQ tests and scholastic aptitude tests. On the basis of this behavioral genetic evidence, they argued that investment in social programs to narrow this gap is unwise. While Herrnstein and Murray did not explicitly argue that whites are superior to blacks, and so deserve their elevated social standing, such a conclusion has indeed been drawn by many others – however confounded the data may be. In most societies, the politics of difference are fraught, and behavioral genetics promises to exacerbate the problem. Additionally, where behavioral genetic findings are used to justify (rather than simply to help to explain) the status quo, the potential for societal harm is increased.

Normality and medicalization

Behavioral genetics studies a full range of behaviors, from the normal to the pathological. But how to draw the line between normal variation and pathology remains an open question. This is a generic problem, not one particular to behavioral genetics, but this does not make it any less important to address in this context. For, as some critics have argued, many of the traits explored by behavioral geneticists lack *construct validity*; that is, the traits (constructs) under study are not particularly robust and are thus inconstant and open to wide variation in interpretation (Press, 2006). Within behavioral genetics, these traits may be pathologized, or medicalized – stipulated as pathological and so as falling within the purview of medicine. As Press (2006, p. 141) argued, "the reification of a fluid, continuous, and essentially normal part of the human behavioral repertoire as a bounded entity is a necessary precondition for a behavioral genetics investigation." One of her examples is shyness, once a normal part of human behavior, now categorized in the American Psychiatric Association's *Diagnostic and Statistical Manual* (1994) and subject to treatment with powerful pharmaceuticals. A recurring theme in bioethics is the ever-expanding scope of medicine,

well beyond the historical limits of the field. Sometimes such expansions are entirely appropriate, as the trait in question clearly varies well beyond acceptable norms; other times, though, medicine overreaches, with significant social and ethical sequelae.

Eugenics

Eugenic considerations are not specific to behavioral genetics, though they are certainly germane. Whether and how behavioral genetics findings may be used to achieve eugenic goals is the subject of ongoing discussion and debate (e.g., Nuffield Council on Bioethics, 2002). The eugenics movement was founded by Sir Francis Galton in England in the 1860s. Eugenic means "well-born." Inspired by the success of plant and animal breeders, Galton wondered whether the human race might be similarly improved through a program of eugenics: we could, he thought, decrease the number of "undesirable" humans and increase the number of "desirable" ones (Galton, 1869). Eugenics is usually divided into positive and negative varieties. Negative eugenics involves discouraging or preventing those deemed unfit from reproducing. Involuntary sterilization is an instance of negative eugenics. Positive eugenics is the encouragement of those deemed fit to reproduce in abundance, and to give birth only to the most perfect offspring. Though there was considerable social and scientific support for eugenics in the late nineteenth and early twentieth centuries, the technologies for achieving positive eugenics were not yet available. It is only in the past few decades that some of these technologies (such as prenatal and preimplantation diagnostic technologies) have been developed. Combined with findings in behavioral genetics, and especially with creeping medicalization, we may witness increasing social pressure to improve humankind by eugenic means. Indeed, some have argued (controversially) that it is morally imperative to use genetic selection technologies in support of eugenic enhancement (e.g., Savulescu *et al.*, 2006).

Law

A different kind of concern raised by behavioral genetics – and, indeed, by any inquiry into human biology and especially the human brain – is the problem of free will. While human genetics and genomics have always raised issues of free will (Weir *et al.*, 1994) – for instance, whether a genetically influenced disease is avoidable via behavioral modification – these issues are more acute where what is at stake is the genetics of behavior itself. In investigating the relationship between human behaviors and genes, behavioral geneticists may generate results relevant to our conceptions of ourselves, our choices, and our freedom to act. Such issues are important to our understanding of *moral* responsibility and accountability, but also to our understanding of *legal* responsibility and accountability.

Claims about free will and determinism – "my genes made me do it" – are not only the stuff of courtroom dramas on television. Behavioral genetics has made its way into the real-world criminal justice system in attempts to exonerate defendants or at least to mediate the severity of their punishment. Consider another finding regarding the monoamine oxidase A isoform. A particular mutation in the allele for this isoform eliminates all enzyme activity, thus dramatically altering metabolism of monoamines (e.g., serotonin, dopamine, epinephrine [Brunner *et al.*, 1993a, b]. The behavioral outcome associated with this mutation is aggressive behavior. Lawyers attempted a legal defense on the basis of these "bad genes" in a murder trial in Georgia, and commentators have suggested that screening for mutations affecting monoamine oxidase A might be a good strategy for detecting potential criminals (Beckwith, 2006 [citing Morell, 1993; Felsenthal, 1994]). While the defense failed and no such genetic screening programs are (yet) in place, we can expect similar escapades in relation to genes correlated with impulsive and antisocial behavior of all sorts (e.g., Wasserman and Wachbroit, 2001; Edgar, 2006). Kenneth Schaffner (2006a, b) has written a terrifically clear imagined dialogue between a judge and a

behavioral geneticist to help to shed light on the science and its implications.

Policy

One excellent policy-related report is that of the UK Nuffield Council on Bioethics. Their 2002 report, *Genetics and Human Behaviour: The Ethical Context*, lays out the historical, ethical, legal, and policy dimensions of behavioral genetics in clear, accessible terms. Focusing on behaviors in the "normal" range (rather than behaviors that fall clearly in the domain of psychiatry), their recommendations include the need for heightened awareness (and possibly government or professional oversight) of the possibility of inappropriate medicalization; that clinicians and policy makers evaluate proposed behavioral genetic enhancement interventions mindful of the prospect of furthering social inequalities; that any direct-to-consumer marketing of behavioral genetic tests be regulated and monitored as appropriate; that the legal system should not be persuaded by defendants' claims that information about their genes (within the normal range) absolves them of legal responsibility for their actions (although behavioral genetic evidence may be useful in determining sentencing for crimes); that prescreening programs to identify potential criminals based on behavioral geneticss are entirely premature; that employers, educators, and insurers should have no special claim on behavioral genetic information; and that progress in public understanding of behavioral genetics begins with behavioral geneticists themselves, who should take particular care to communicate clearly their research findings and not to inflate their significance.

Empirical studies

There are very few empirical studies of the significance of behavioral genetics. One recent study, though, helpfully attempted to discern the beliefs and attitudes of healthcare providers and parents toward genetic tests for violent behaviors in children (Campbell and Ross, 2004). While such tests do not exist, Campbell and Ross based their study on plausible (though imaginary) tests and used the method of focus groups to study beliefs and attitudes toward these hypothetical tests. Particularly interesting results from the healthcare providers included that they tended to medicalize behaviors, that they would be reluctant to order tests in the absence of available treatments, and that they were concerned about the potential misuse of information from behavioral genetics. Parents, by contrast, tended not to medicalize behaviors and were not as concerned about testing in the absence of therapies. Yet parents may be ambivalent about testing their own children, and some in this study were concerned that behavioral genetic research may be detracting from political and environmental interventions that could be expected to yield socially beneficial outcomes.

How should I approach behavioral genetics in practice?

Given the methodological and ethical challenges discussed above, it is evident that behavioral genetics, as a science, is not entirely ready for clinical integration. Yet advances in the field, and especially in psychiatric genetics, will no doubt soon appear in clinical contexts, suggesting that clinicians would be well advised to anticipate potential clinical applications and prepare accordingly. Two exceptionally useful resources for clinicians are by Catherine Baker (2004) and Erik Parens, Audrey Chapman, and Nancy Press (2006). Both books were produced as part of a National Institutes of Health-funded collaboration between the Hastings Center and the American Association for the Advancement of Science to develop "tools for talking" about behavioral genetics, and they should help clinicians to be prepared for the safe, effective, and appropriate clinical integration of behavioral genetics.

As with genetics more generally, it is important for clinicians to understand the relevant science and, especially, the limits of the science of genetics for explaining development. Additionally, it is imperative that clinicians appreciate the scientific, social, and ethical complexity of genetic information; these issues of data management and counseling of patients are addressed in other chapters, particularly Ch. 22.

The cases

Ms. C is clearly exhibiting affective, somatic, and possibly cognitive symptoms of major depression. Whether she has a mutation in the serotonin transporter gene is moot from both a diagnostic and a therapeutic perspective. But just initiating treatment, whether with pharmaceuticals or talk therapy or both, will likely not satisfy Ms. C, who is adamant that she wants a finding of genetic susceptibility. A caring physician will want to explore Ms. C's desire for genetic self-knowledge, but also to explain to her that her current symptoms are perfectly understandable given the range of negative events she has recently experienced. There is no shame in a diagnosis of depression, and there are many different therapeutic approaches that can help relieve her symptoms. Bringing behavioral genetics findings to bear in this case is entirely unnecessary and may even be more debilitating than helpful if, for instance, Ms. C learns that she does not have the mutation (she may feel shame as a result) or if a positive test result is eventually used by a third party in ways unfavorable to Ms. C's interests. If Ms. C really does plan to find another physician to order the genetic test, her family physician should simply step aside. In this case, the physician explained some of these details to Ms. C and she was satisfied. She began anti-depression therapy (drugs and talk therapy) and her condition improved within a few weeks.

As with Ms. C, Mr. and Mrs. D's desire for genetic knowledge is understandable. Though they know full well that their son's environment has changed, the personality changes are so dramatic that they feel a chemical imbalance must be involved – especially given their familial history. This case is an especially difficult one, inasmuch as a minor is involved, the parents want specifically genetic tests, the parents are clearly worried that they are responsible for these negative personality changes in their son because they moved to a new town, and this is the first visit with a new clinician. The clinician had to work hard to establish the trust not only of the parents but also of E himself. While it is possible that E was at genetic risk of antisocial behavior and that the new environment has functioned as a stressor to trigger the manifestation of these behavioral problems, it is not clear what additional value genetic tests would have for diagnostic or therapeutic purposes. On the basis of current knowledge, genetic tests are simply not indicated. Instead, the clinician assessed the family's willingness to meet with a psychologist or other therapist and to work with teachers and school administrators to help to provide appropriate social supports for E. They agreed with the clinician's advice that adolescence is not a medical condition, or a condition necessarily requiring medical treatment. But insofar as E was experiencing performance difficulties, and insofar as Mr. and Mrs. D were having trouble coping, it was appropriate for the clinician and other healthcare providers to help this family to adjust to their new circumstances. Though he still spends time with the older kids, E is now fitting in better with his peers and is doing just fine.

REFERENCES

American Psychiatric Association (1994). *Diagnostic and Statistical Manual*, 4th edn. Washington, DC: American Psychiatric Press.

Baker, C. (2004). *Behavioral Genetics: An Introduction to How Genes and Environments Interact Through Development to Shape Differences in Mood, Personality, and Intelligence*. Washington DC: American Association for the Advancement of Science, Directorate for Science Policy Programs.

Beckwith, J. (2006). Whither human behavioral genetics? In *Wrestling with Behavioral Genetics: Science, Ethics, and Public Conversation*, ed. E. Parens, A. R. Chapman, and N. Press. Baltimore MD: Johns Hopkins University Press, pp. 74–99.

Brunner, H. G., Nelen, M., Breakefield, X. O., Ropers, H. H., and van Oost, B. A. (1993a). Abnormal behavior associated with a point mutation in the structural gene for monoamine oxidase A. *Science* **262**: 578–80.

Brunner, H. G., Nelen, M. R., van Zandvoort, P., *et al.* (1993b). X-linked borderline mental retardation with prominent behavioral disturbance: phenotype, genetic localization, and evidence for disturbed monoamine metabolism. *Am J Hum Gen* **52**: 1032–9.

Campbell, E. and Ross, L. F. (2004). Attitudes of healthcare professionals and parents regarding genetic testing for violent traits in childhood. *J Med Ethics* **30**: 580–6.

Caspi, A., McClay, J., Moffitt, T. E., *et al.* (2002). Role of genotype in the cycle of violence in maltreated children. *Science* **297**: 851–4.

Edgar, H. (2006). Impulsivity, responsibility, and the criminal law. In *Wrestling with Behavioral Genetics: Science, Ethics, and Public Conversation*, ed. E. Parens, A. R. Chapman, and N. Press. Baltimore MD: Johns Hopkins University Press, pp. 176–98.

Felsenthal, E. (1994). Man's genes made him kill, his lawyers claim. *Wall Street Journal*, 15 November, B1.

Galton, F. (1869). *Hereditary Genius*. London: Macmillan.

Herrnstein, R. J. and Murray, C. (1994). *The Bell Curve: Intelligence and Class Structure in American Life*. New York: Free Press.

Jensen, A. R. (1969). How much can we boost IQ and scholastic achievement? *Harv Ed Rev* **39**: 1–123.

Morell, V. (1993). Evidence found for a possible ''aggression gene.'' *Science* **260**: 1722–3.

Nuffield Council on Bioethics (2002). *Genetics and Human Behaviour: The Ethical Context*. London: Nuffield Council on Bioethics.

Parens, E., Chapman, A. R., and Press, N. (eds.) (2006). *Wrestling with Behavioral Genetics: Science, Ethics, and Public Conversation*. Baltimore MD: Johns Hopkins University Press.

Press, N. (2006). Social construction and medicalization: behavioral genetics in context. In *Wrestling with Behavioral Genetics: Science, Ethics, and Public Conversation*, ed. E. Parens, A. R. Chapman, and N. Press. Baltimore MD: Johns Hopkins University Press, pp. 131–49.

Robert, J. S. (2000). Schizophrenia epigenesis? *Theor Med Bioethics* **21**: 191–215.

Savulescu, J., Hemsley, M., Newson, A., and Foddy, B. (2006). Behavioural genetics: why eugenic selection is preferable to enhancement. *J Appl Philos* **23**: 157–71.

Schaffner, K. F. (2006a). Behavior: its nature and nurture, Part 1. In *Wrestling with Behavioral Genetics: Science, Ethics, and Public Conversation*, ed. E. Parens, A. R. Chapman, and N. Press. Baltimore MD: Johns Hopkins University Press, pp. 3–39.

Schaffner, K. F. (2006b). Behavior: its nature and nurture, Part 2. In *Wrestling with Behavioral Genetics: Science, Ethics, and Public Conversation*, ed. E. Parens, A. R. Chapman, and N. Press. Baltimore MD: Johns Hopkins University Press, pp. 40–73.

Turkheimer, E. (2000). Three laws of behavior genetics and what they mean. *Curr Direct Psychol Sci* **9**: 160–4.

Wasserman, D. and Wachbroit, R. (eds.) (2001). *Genetics and Criminal Behavior: Methods, Meanings, and Morals.* New York: Cambridge University Press.

Weir, R. F., Lawrence, S. C., and Fales, E. (eds.) (1994). *Genes and Human Self-Knowledge: Historial and Philosophical Reflections on Modern Genetics.* Iowa City IA: University of Iowa Press.

Wilson, J. (2002). Criminal genes. *Popular Mech* **179**: 46–7.

SECTION V

Research ethics

Introduction

Richard E. Ashcroft

The efficacy of modern medicine depends very largely on scientific research into the causes of disease, innovative therapies, and methods of organizing and delivering healthcare services. Interestingly, modern bioethics can also be considered to have developed from the articulation of standards for the ethical conduct of medical research. Discussion of the ethics of research in the aftermath of the violations of human life and dignity not only in the Third Reich and Imperial Japan but also in the Western liberal democracies before and after the World War II provoked more general discussions of the ethical basis of medical care. For instance, modern discussions of the role of patient autonomy in bioethics owe much to the analysis of this concept in the Belmont Report of 1979 (p. 195), which was concerned with the protection of human subjects of research.

Until relatively recently, medical research was considered to be an area of special ethical risk, involving, as it often did, exposing patients to risks of harm that could be serious, and that could involve doctors in treating their people more as "research subjects" than as patients who should under no circumstances be harmed. This way of thinking about research ethics remains important. However, more recent thinking about research ethics has pointed out that patients can be harmed by exposing them to untested or unevaluated medical interventions, and that there is far more continuity between research ethics and "ordinary" bioethics than had been thought. In addition, debate is currently continuing about whether very strongly protective (perhaps "risk averse") approaches to patient welfare undermine attempts to improve population health overall by blocking the sharing of data and by making certain kinds of research with children or members of other vulnerable groups *unnecessarily* difficult. At the same time, there is growing public concern over whether medical research is always as disinterested and beneficial as most of its practitioners would hope: controversy continues over conflict of interest in research, underreporting or misreporting of research findings, and the commercialization of medical research.

This section reviews the main areas of medical research ethics that affect working clinicians today. The opening chapter (Ch. 25) surveys the principal issues. Chapter 26 considers the boundary between innovation in medicine and surgery and formal research. While medical practice is modified piecemeal all the time, both to respond to specific features of individual patients' needs and to respond to innovative ideas of individual practitioners, formal research imposes specific requirements on doctors and may be quite tightly regulated. When does an innovation become a research project? Should ethical standards for innovation be different from those for research? The following chapters (27 and 28) concern the two most important forms of clinical research: clinical trials and epidemiology, respectively. Each describes the main ethical issues in each form of research methodology. Chapter 29 moves on to discuss the dual role of physician and researcher: do doctors who involve their patients in research projects face a conflict of roles and of moral obligations? Or can enrolling your patients in research projects be seen as entirely consistent with the requirements of "ordinary" bioethics? Chapter 30 considers another kind of conflict of role or conflict of interest. Do doctors who conduct research have obligations to the public or to their patients that conflict with their obligations to the sponsors of their research? How should such conflicts be minimized and regulated? The final chapter in this section (Ch. 31) concerns a form of research that is of growing importance, embryo research. Can such research be considered simply immoral? Whose interests need to be considered? Should the state intervene to regulate such research?

There are many types of research that could not be covered in the space available. Nor have we been able to give more than a passing mention to some of the wider issues of scientific integrity, the relationship between medical research and evidence-based medicine, the impact of medical innovation on public health, and the global health context of research. Nonetheless, this section sets out the chief issues of current importance, and the general principles that can be applied to these related problems.

Several of these other topics are taken up in Sections IV, VI, and VIII.

25

Research ethics

Eric M. Meslin and Bernard M. Dickens

Dr. A is a family practitioner with a special interest in the treatment of chronic obstructive pulmonary disease. He receives a letter from the coordinator of a study to evaluate a promising new treatment for this condition. The letter invites Dr. A to submit the names of potentially eligible patients. He will be paid $100 for each name provided.

Dr. B, a psychiatrist in private practice, is approached by a pharmaceutical company to assist with a clinical trial to test the efficacy of a new drug in the treatment of acute psychosis. The study will enroll acutely psychotic patients with no history of psychosis (or of treatment with antipsychotic drugs) through physicians' offices and emergency departments. Patients enrolled in the study will be randomly assigned to receive the new medication or a placebo and will remain in hospital for eight weeks. During this time, they will not be permitted to receive antipsychotic medications other than the study drug. Informed consent will be obtained from each participant or a proxy. Patients may be withdrawn from the study if their medical condition worsens substantially.

What is research ethics?

Research involving human subjects can raise difficult and important ethical and legal questions. The field of research ethics is devoted to the systematic analysis of such questions to ensure that study participants are protected and, ultimately, that clinical research is conducted in a way that serves the needs of such participants and of society as a whole.

Why is research ethics important?

Many of the ethical issues that arise in human experimentation – such as those surrounding informed consent, confidentiality, and the physician's duty of care to the patient – overlap with ethical issues in clinical practice. Nevertheless, important differences exist between research activities and clinical practice. In clinical practice, the physician has a clear obligation to the patient; in research, this obligation remains but may come into conflict with other obligations – and incentives (Hellman and Hellman, 1991). The researcher has an obligation to ensure that the study findings are valid and replicable, and this has implications for the design and execution of the study. For example, the study must be designed in such a way that the research question is answered reliably and efficiently; sufficient numbers of subjects must be enrolled in a reasonable period, and study participants must comply with their allocated treatment. Substantial rewards can accrue to the successful completion of a research project, such as renewed funding, academic promotion, salary increases, respect from colleagues, and, in some cases, fame. Unfortunately, in a number of research studies, including some conducted in the world's leading research institutions, the welfare of individual subjects has been sacrificed to these competing interests (Elliott and Weijer, 1995; Weijer, 1995).

An earlier version of this chapter has appeared: Weijer, C., Dickens, B., and Meslin, E. M. (1997). Research ethics. *CAMJ* **156**: 1153–57.

Various ethical principles, legal requirements, and policy statements have been formulated at national, international, and intergovernmental levels in an attempt to ensure that clinical research is conducted in accordance with the highest scientific and ethical standards.

Ethics

The predominant ethical framework for human experimentation was set out by the US National Commission for the Protection of Human Subjects of Biomedical and Behavioral Research (1979) in the *Belmont Report*. This report articulated three guiding principles for research: respect for persons, beneficence, and justice. These principles are also found in leading international formulations of research ethics. Respect for persons requires that the choices of autonomous individuals be respected and that people who are incapable of making their own choices be protected. This principle underlies the requirement to obtain informed consent from study participants and to maintain confidentiality on their behalf (Levine, 1988). The principle of beneficence requires that participation in research be associated with a favorable balance of potential benefits and harms (Levine, 1988). In the articulation of the *Belmont Report*, beneficence included non-maleficence – the principle commonly understood as the injunction to "do no harm." The principle of justice entails an equitable distribution of the burdens and benefits of research. Researchers must not exploit vulnerable people or exclude without good reason eligible candidates who may benefit from participation in a study (Levine, 1988).

There is an ongoing and important discussion about the sufficiency and continuing relevance of the *Belmont Report* and its principles (Childress *et al.*, 2005), since the principles it set out do not exhaust the ethical requirements for clinical research (Meslin *et al.*, 1995). Conditions such as the following must also be met.

- A study must employ a *scientifically valid design* to answer the research question. Shoddy science

is never ethical (Freedman, 1987a; Sutherland *et al.*, 1994).
- A study must address a *question of sufficient value* to individuals and/or population groups to justify the risk posed to participants. Exposing subjects even to low risk to answer a trivial question is unacceptable (Freedman, 1987a).
- A study must be *conducted honestly*. It should be carried out as stated in the approved protocol, and research ethics boards have an obligation to ensure that this is the case (Weijer *et al.*, 1995).
- Study findings must be *reported accurately and promptly*. Methods, results, and conclusions must be reported completely and without exaggeration of benefits or minimization of harmful effects to allow practicing clinicians to draw reasonable conclusions (World Medical Association, 2000; International Committee of Medical Journal Editors, 1997). Whenever possible, study results should be reported quickly to allow physicians timely access to potentially important clinical information (Meslin, 1994).

Law

The researcher's duty to have informed consent from research subjects is established in almost all of the world's legal systems. The legal doctrine often described as "informed consent" is better understood as "informed choice," since a physician's legal duty is to inform the subject so that he or she may exercise *choice* – which does not always result in *consent*. The physician's duty to disclose information relevant to the choice that the subject is asked to make falls under an aspect of civil (that is, non-criminal) law: the law of negligence. A physician may be found negligent if a subject's choice (including the choice to forgo medically indicated treatment) is inadequately informed and results in harm (*Truman* v. *Thomas*, 1980). Accordingly, subjects who are invited to enter a study must be informed of, among other things, the nature and extent of the known risks of participation, the possibility that participation may present unknown risks, and the intended benefit of the study to participants and others. A subject's treatment in a trial without consent may be grounds for legal action on the basis of "unauthorized touching," which is dealt with in two domains in the UK: assault in criminal law and battery in civil law.

The duty to ensure confidentiality is usually implicit in the physician–patient contract, fiduciary duty, and legislation, and it is now equally applicable to research subjects. Confidentiality is a usually implicit term of the physician–patient contract (that is, the tacit agreement between physician and patient on the rendering of care), and its violation is, therefore, a basis for legal action against the physician. Increasingly, however, as physicians move from fee-for-service payment to salaries or other remuneration systems, confidentiality is addressed under the law of fiduciary duty (Dickens, 1994). Fiduciary duty – the highest standard of duty implied by law – requires that physicians disclose information about a patient only in the patient's best interests and that they avoid any conflict of interest in the disclosure of patient information (even if that information is contained in records physicians lawfully hold). Unauthorized disclosure is actionable as a breach of fiduciary duty. It may also violate a duty of confidentiality enacted in legislation. For example, in the Canadian province of Quebec, the Civil Code is so protective of patient information that some have claimed that anonymous epidemiological studies may be unlawful without the consent of each person whose medical record is used (Deleury and Croubau, 1994).

Policy

A number of international policies guide the conduct of research. Although the Nuremberg Code (1947) and the UN International Covenant on Civil and Political Rights (1958) remain important early statements, the World Medical Association's *Declaration of Helsinki*, as amended most recently in October 2000, with clarifications in 2002 and 2004, is probably the most influential document governing research worldwide (World Medical Association, 1964). Many of the requirements set out under

"Ethics" in this article reflect the *Declaration of Helsinki*. The Declaration highlights an important additional requirement: subjects' participation in research should not put them at a disadvantage with respect to medical care.

Researchers conducting studies funded by the US National Institutes of Health must do so in accordance with the regulations of the US Department of Health and Human Services (1991), and where the studies involve drugs, biological products, or devices that are to be licensed or marketed in the USA, the research must be conducted in accordance with additional regulations from the Food and Drug Administration (US Department of Health and Human Services, 1991). Researchers conducting research in other countries should consult the guidelines of the Council for International Organizations of Medical Sciences (CIOMS) (CIOMS, 2002). Similarly, geneticists, for instance, should consult the guidelines developed by the Human Genome Organization (1996).

Both the Nuremberg Code and the *Declaration of Helsinki* address how medical research should be conducted, but neither offers a definition or description of what is medical research (Levine, 1988) as opposed to other medical interventions such as therapeutic innovation. The CIOMS 2002 *International Ethical Guidelines for Biomedical Research Involving Human Subjects* stated:

The term "research" refers to a class of activity designed to develop or contribute to generalizable knowledge. Generalizable knowledge consists of theories, principles or relationships, or the accumulation of information on which they are based, that can be corroborated by accepted scientific methods of observation and inference. In the present context "research" includes both medical and behavioural studies pertaining to human health. Usually "research" is modified by the adjective "biomedical" to indicate its relation to health.

The CIOMS guidelines go on to note that:

Research involving human subjects includes: studies of a physiological, biochemical or pathological process, or of the response to a specific intervention – whether physical, chemical or psychological; in healthy subjects or patients;

controlled trials of diagnostic, preventive or therapeutic measures in larger groups of persons, designed to demonstrate a specific generalizable response to these measures against a background of individual biological variation; studies designed to determine the consequences for individuals and communities of specific preventive or therapeutic measures; and studies concerning human health-related behavior in a variety of circumstances and environments.

Research that is not intended to result in generalizable knowledge, such as quality-assurance studies for internal institutional use, and audits of departmental safety and efficacy of care, is generally not considered research. Proposals for research involving human subjects must be submitted to a relevant research ethics review board. Whether a proposal requires review by such a board is a decision for the board itself, which may find a proposal to fall outside its mandate or jurisdiction. Investigators should not decide for themselves not to submit their proposals for review, except in self-evident cases such as department audit not intended for publication.

Empirical studies

Empirical studies have much to contribute to our understanding of informed consent and the risks and benefits of participation in research. For example, if the principle of respect for persons is to be upheld, it follows that research subjects must not only be *informed* of the purpose, nature, risks, benefits, and alternatives associated with their participation but must also *understand* this information. But how well *do* research subjects understand information presented to them in the consent process? The answer seems to be "Not well at all" (Reicken and Ravich, 1982). Indeed, because of a phenomenon that Appelbaum and colleagues (1987) referred to as "therapeutic misconception," patients commonly believe that experimental projects are tailored to optimize their individual care. In its final report, the White House Advisory Committee on Human Radiation Experiments (1995) detailed the results of a survey of 1900 research participants and

concluded that serious deficiencies remain in the current system of protecting human subjects of research.

Two lessons follow from the empirical studies on informed consent to participation in research. Firstly, researchers need to establish and maintain effective strategies to ensure that research subjects comprehend the information they are given during the consent process. In an elegant review of this topic, Silva and Sorrell (1988) listed a wide range of methods available to improve participants' understanding. Secondly, although such additional measures are important, the empirical data highlight the inadequacy of consent alone to protect study participants. Consent is a necessary component of this protection, but not sufficient. A research study also must present an acceptable balance of risks and benefits (US Department of Health and Human Services, 1991).

Empirical studies on the risks and benefits of research participation have also made an important contribution to research ethics. For many years, participation in research was viewed as a risky endeavor, one from which people ought to be protected (Levine, 1994). However, a number of studies in the late 1970s and early 1980s showed that the risks associated with study participation were, in reality, relatively small (Weijer, 1996). Indeed, recent empirical work in oncology suggests that patients with cancer who participated in clinical trials received – apart from the specific study treatment – a *net benefit*, namely, improved survival (Hjorth *et al.*, 1992; Freedman and Shapiro, 1994; Weijer *et al.*, 1996). If further study establishes conclusively that trial participation *in itself* is associated with a higher probability of benefit, it may be that prospective study participants should be informed of this fact.

How should I approach research ethics in practice?

Ethical issues in research must not be addressed by researchers as an afterthought. Ethical issues permeate research and must guide research design. What should be used as a control treatment? Who should be included or excluded from a study? How large should the sample be? All of these questions have an ethical component (Freedman and Shapiro, 1994). Researchers ought, therefore, to consider ethical issues from the first stages of planning.

A critical component in assuring the protection of human subjects in research is the prior review and approval of any study by an ethics review committee. Although these institutional committees are referred to by different names–in the USA they are institutional review boards, in Canada they are research ethics boards, and in other countries they are ethics review committees – they have a common commitment to ensuring the protection of the rights and welfare of subjects. These committees are increasingly being consulted *prior* to the design and conduct of research and have expertise in research ethics.

What resources are available to researchers to guide them in ethical matters? Clearly, all physicians involved in research ought to be familiar with the key documents outlined above, particularly the *Declaration of Helsinki*, CIOMS guidelines, and comparable guidelines. Though directed primarily toward an American audience, a number of excellent reference texts are available (Levine, 1988; US Office for Protection from Research Risk, 1993). Many peer-reviewed journals now discuss ethical issues in research, and two in particular focus exclusively to research ethics: *IRB: Ethics and Human Research*, which has been available many years (formerly as *IRB: A Review of Human Subjects Research*), and a new journal, the *Journal of Empirical Research on Human Research Ethics*. Both are excellent sources for the researcher in an ethical quandary. Finally, and perhaps most important, clinicians should routinely consult with colleagues who have expertise in the ethics of research, particularly where relevant in developing countries (Benatar, 2002), including members of research ethics boards.

The cases

Dr. A is offered a financial reward if he will provide the names of patients to a third party who is coordinating a research study. Such "finders' fees" are ethically and legally objectionable (Lind, 1990). Physicians act in breach of fiduciary duty and in conflict of interest if they use their professional knowledge of a patient's medical or other circumstances for their personal benefit. Firstly, names may not be given to third parties without patient consent. A physician who believes that entry in a study may benefit an eligible patient should inform that patient and let the patient decide whether his or her name may be given to the investigator. Secondly, physicians must not accept a fee based on the number of names provided. If a physician is asked to consult patients' records or to do other searches, he or she may be remunerated for the time required to perform that service, whether or not any patients are identified and consent to participate.

Dr. B is invited to enroll his patients in a placebo-controlled study of a new antipsychotic drug. Is it ethical for him to recommend the study to his patients? No. As we have discussed, consent alone is an insufficient ethical basis for enrolling patients in a study: the study must present a favorable balance of benefits and harms. A physician may recommend participation in a study only if the treatments being studied are in a state of "clinical equipoise," that is, if there is "genuine uncertainty" within "the expert clinical community about the comparative merits of the alternatives to be tested" (Freedman, 1987b). In other words, genuine uncertainty must exist in the community of expert practitioners as to the preferred treatment (Freedman, 1987b). When effective standard treatment exists for a disease, as it does for schizophrenia (Kane, 1996), it is unethical (since placebo is an inferior "treatment") to expose patients to the risk of "treatment" with placebo alone. Practicing physicians may be told that placebo controls are necessary in clinical research for scientific, ethical, or regulatory reasons. Freedman and colleagues have reviewed these claims comprehensively and concluded that practitioners should regard them with skepticism (Freedman *et al.*, 1996a, b).

REFERENCES

Appelbaum, P., Roth, L., Lidz, C., Benson, P., and Winslade, W. (1987). False hopes and best data: consent to research and the therapeutic misconception. *Hastings Cent Rep* **2**: 20–4.

Benatar, S. R. (2002). Reflections and recommendations on research ethics in developing countries. *Soc Sci Med* **54**: 1131–41.

Childress, J. F., Meslin, E. M., and Shapiro, H. T. (eds.) (2005). *Belmont Revisited: Ethical Principles for Research with Human Subjects*. Washington, DC: Georgetown University Press.

CIOMS (2002). *International Ethical Guidelines for Biomedical Research Involving Human Subjects*. Geneva: Council for International Organizations of Medical Sciences.

Deleury, E. and Croubau D. (1994). *Le droit des personnes physiques*. Cowansville, QC: Éditions Yvon Blais, pp. 119–20.

Dickens B. M. (1994). Medical records – patient's right to receive copies – physician's fiduciary duty of disclosure: *McInerney* v. *MacDonald. Can Bar Rev* **73**: 234–42.

Elliott, C. and Weijer C. (1995). Cruel and unusual treatment. *Saturday Night* **110**: 31–4.

Freedman, B. (1987a). Scientific value and validity as ethical requirements for research: a proposed explanation. *IRB, Rev Hum Subj Res* **17**: 7–10.

Freedman, B. (1987b). Equipoise and the ethics of clinical research. *N Engl J Med* **317**: 141–5.

Freedman, B. and Shapiro, S. (1994). Ethics and statistics in clinical research: towards a more comprehensive examination. *J Stat Plann Inference* **42**: 223–40.

Freedman, B., Weijer, C., and Glass, K. C. (1996a). Placebo orthodoxy in clinical research. I: Empirical and methodological myths. *J Law Med Ethics* **24**: 243–51.

Freedman, B., Glass, K. C., and Weijer, C. (1996b). Placebo orthodoxy in clinical research. II: Ethical, legal and regulatory myths. *J Law Med Ethics* **24**: 252–9.

Hellman, S. and Hellman, D. (1991). Of mice but not men: problems of the randomized clinical trial. *N Engl J Med* **324**: 1584–9.

Hjorth, M., Holmberg, E., Rodjer, S., and Westin, J. (1992). Impact of active and passive exclusions on the results of a clinical trial in multiple myeloma. *Br J Haematol* **80**: 55–61.

Human Genome Organization (1996). Statement on the principled conduct of genetic research. *Genome Dig* **3**: 2–3.

International Committee of Medical Journal Editors (1997). Uniform requirements for manuscripts submitted to biomedical journals. *Can Med Assoc J* **156**: 270–7.

Kane, J. M. (1996). Schizophrenia. *N Engl J Med* **334**: 34–1.

Levine R. J. (1988). *Ethics and Regulation of Clinical Research*. New Haven; CT: Yale University Press.

Levine, R. J. (1994). The impact of HIV infection on society's perception of clinical trials. *Kennedy Inst Ethics J* **4**: 93–8.

Lind, S. E. (1990). Finder's fees for research subjects. *N Engl J Med* **323**: 192–5.

Meslin, E. M. (1994). Toward an ethic in dissemination of new knowledge in primary care research. In *Disseminating Research/Changing Practice: Research Methods for Primary Care*, ed. E. V. Dunn. Vol. 6, Thousand Oaks, CA: Sage, pp. 32–44.

Meslin, E. M., Sutherland, H. J., Lavery, J. V., and Till, J. E. (1995). Principlism and the ethical appraisal of clinical trials. *Bioethics* **9**: 399–418.

National Commission for the Protection of Human Subjects of Biomedical and Behavioral Research (1979). *The Belmont Report: Ethical Principles and Guidelines for the Protection of Human Subjects of Research*. Washington, DC: *Office for Protection from Research Risks*.

Nuremberg Code (1947). *Article 1*. Washington, DC: Government Printing Office (http://www.ushmm.org/research/doctors/Nuremberg_Code.htm).

Reicken, H. W. and Ravich, R. (1982). Informed consent to biomedical research in Veteran's administration hospitals. *JAMA* **248**: 344–50.

Silva, M. C. and Sorrell J. M. (1988). Enhancing comprehension of information for informed consent: a review of empirical research. *IRB, Rev Hum Subj Res* **10**: 1–5.

Sutherland, H. J., Meslin, E. M., and Till, J. E. (1994). What's missing from current clinical trials guidelines? A framework for integrating science, ethics and the community. *J Clin Ethics* **5**: 297–303.

Truman v. *Thomas* (1980), 611 Pacific (2d) 902 (Sup Ct Calif).

United Nations (1958). *International Covenant on Civil and Political Rights*. New York: United Nations.

US Department of Health and Human Services (1991). *Code of Federal Regulations Title 45 part 46: Protection of Human Subjects*, revised 1991. Washington, DC: Government Printing Office.

US Office for Protection from Research Risk (1993). *Protecting Human Subjects: Institutional Review Board Guidebook*. Washington, DC: Office for Protection from Research Risk.

Weijer, C. (1995). The breast cancer research scandal: addressing the issues. *CMAJ* **152**: 1195–7.

Weijer, C. (1996). Evolving ethical issues in selection of subjects for clinical research. *Camb Q Healthc Ethics* **5**: 334–45.

Weijer, C., Shapiro, S. Fuks, A., Glass, K. C., and Skrutkowska, M. (1995). Monitoring clinical research: an obligation unfulfilled. *CMAJ* **152**: 1973–80.

Weijer, C., Freedman, B., Fuks, A., *et al.* (1996). What difference does it make to be treated in a clinical trial? A pilot study. *Clin Invest Med* **19**: 179–83.

White House Advisory Committee on Human Radiation Experiments (1995). *Final Report* [doc no 061-000-00-848-9]. Washington, DC: Government Printing Office.

World Medical Association (1964). *Declaration of Helsinki: Ethical Principles for Medical Research Involving Human Subjects* [revised 1975, 1983, 1989, 1996, 2000]. Washington, DC: World Medical Association (http://www.wma.net/e/policy/b3.htm).

26

Innovation in medical care: examples from surgery

Randi Zlotnik Shaul, Jacob C. Langer, and Martin F. McKneally

C, a newborn infant, develops persistent vomiting on the second day of life. X-rays show midgut volvulus, a condition in which the intestines have twisted around their blood supply. Surgical exploration reveals necrosis of all but 15 cm of his small bowel. The necrotic bowel is removed and total parenteral nutrition (TPN) is initiated. At one year of age, he is taking half of his nutritional needs through his intestinal tract; the other half is given intravenously. Blood chemistry tests show that he is starting to develop significant liver damage from the TPN. C's remaining small bowel has become dilated and dysfunctional. You have recently read about a new operation called the serial tapering enteroplasty (STEP), an innovative technique, which may be able to lengthen the remaining intestine and permit it to function more effectively. A surgical stapler in common use is deployed to segment the dilated bowel into a tapered, lengthened tube more closely resembling the shape of the small intestine (Kim et al., 2003). This operation, first developed in dogs, has been undertaken in a small number of infants with short bowel syndrome. It is considered a non-validated innovation by most pediatric surgeons and is not yet accepted as part of standard surgical practice. You would like to offer the procedure to your patient, but you do not think that there is time to go through the full Research Ethics Board approval process at your hospital. Your intention is to try to help, and perhaps other patients like him. You do not have a formal research protocol, but will develop your approach to treatment of this problem as you gain experience with this new procedure.

You struggle to manage your patient, a young soldier with severe respiratory failure caused by a blast injury. Conventional ventilation, at the high levels of positive pressure now required to maintain adequate gas exchange, is further damaging the lungs. An innovative lung assist device (ILA) has been proven in the laboratory and in preliminary human trials to remove carbon dioxide directly from the bloodstream, permitting ventilation at lower pressure and reducing treatment-related injury, but it is not yet approved for use in the institution. You contact the manufacturer, who agrees to supply the device on a compassionate basis at no charge. The company will provide a professional support team to instruct and assist you and your team in introducing and managing the ILA.

What is innovation?

Innovation is a notional concept: there are many notions of its meaning and no widely accepted definition. For the purpose of this chapter, we will define innovation as "a new evolving intervention whose effects, side effects, safety, reliability, and potential complications are not yet generally known in the community of practitioners" (McKneally and Daar, 2003). As a practical matter, we also include cost, convenience, and impact on institutional resources and personnel among the important aspects of innovation that should be taken into consideration when an innovation is introduced.

We will exclude from this discussion incremental improvements in established procedures and evolutionary variations, such as stapled instead of sutured anastamoses. Such variations and refinements are generally accepted as implicit components of improving standard practice. They fit well within professional and institutional practice and policies for quality improvement. An informal process of collegial oversight of practice and its innovative variations is already in effect, as operating rooms, hospitals, and clinics form moral communities of caregivers who share a commitment to safeguard their patients, colleagues, and institutions from unnecessary risks. Accreditation, "credentialing" (validating qualifications), peer review, and quality improvement practices strengthen this protection. When an innovation introduces unknown risks, potential side effects, complications, resource requirements, or costs, the protection of the patients, innovators, institutions, and device manufacturers can be enhanced by collegial review (McKneally and Kornetsky, 2003; Morreim *et al.*, 2006).

Innovation is not formal research as defined by the *Belmont Report* (National Commission for the Protection of Human Subjects of Biological and Behavioral Research, 1979), which designates research as "an activity designed to test an hypothesis, permit conclusions to be drawn and thereby to develop or contribute to generalizable knowledge (expressed, for example, in theories, principles, and statements of relationships). Research is usually described in a formal protocol that sets forth an objective and a set of procedures designed to reach that objective." Under the current regulatory ethics paradigm, "innovative treatments are regarded as questionable until they are framed in a research protocol with formal mechanisms of informed consent" and innovators participate in the exploratory phase that precedes formal research, working "in the borderland outside the regulatory ethics paradigm" (Agich, 2001). Hypotheses and protocols can only be developed after exploration by innovators to stabilize techniques and identify appropriate patients for study.

Why is innovation important?

Most of the important advances in medical practice, from anesthesia and appendectomy to heart surgery and transplantation, were introduced through an informal process we will call the *innovation pathway*. This pathway has become the major driver of increasing medical costs, as expensive innovative technologies for diagnosis and treatment are added to healthcare budgets. Generally motivated by strong financial incentives, biotechnology and medical device companies are constantly pushing out the boundaries of medical treatment. Since the passage of the Bayh-Dole Act (1980), clinicians, hospitals, and universities in the USA have had similar incentives to pursue patents and equity shares in industry. The biotechnology industry's growth has been further accelerated by venture capitalists seeking investment opportunities in this volatile, high-stake market (Leaf, 2005). In this setting of dynamic growth in medical innovation, traditional safeguards may be overwhelmed. Research ethics boards (REB) and institutional review boards (IRB) utilize mechanisms to review protocols that are designed to systematically generate generalizable data rather than strategies uniquely tailored to individual patients. There is a clear need for a nimble, informed, flexible mechanism of collegial oversight to protect the interests of patients, innovators, and institutions.

Ethics

According to Wilton *et al.* (2000, p. 49), "Continued innovation is necessary if there are to be future gains in our ability to serve patients." Improvements in clinical care are dependent upon the development and integration of safe and effective innovations. The clinician's ethical responsibility to act in the best interests of patients, and continue to improve his or her knowledge and skills, is consistent with the pursuit of innovation (Canadian Medical Association, 2004; American Medical Association, 2005). Establishing a pathway that minimizes risk to patients while facilitating the pursuit of innovation is consistent with these values as well as the principles of beneficence and non-maleficence.

In most ethical formulations of the issues that arise in health research involving human subjects, research is defined by its ends: that is, what is to be learned (Lantos, 1994). Research is generally considered an activity designed to test a hypothesis systematically, permit conclusions to be drawn, and thereby develop or contribute to generalizable knowledge. By contrast, "[i]nnovation is focused solely on the benefit of the individual being cared for. If at any point it appears that any aspect of what is being done is not in that person's best interest, the physician must change course" (Morreim, 2005, p. 42). These formulations have some overlap but they help to distinguish which frameworks should apply to a given intervention. In some cases, new practices should be introduced through the protective framework of research ethics and in others it is appropriate to have new or innovative practices governed by traditional medicolegal standards combined with professional and institutional policies.

The threshold at which innovation becomes accepted standard practice is not sharply defined. Many widely accepted procedures remain unvalidated, despite their acceptance (Levine, 1988). A commitment to accountability grounds the clinician's ethical responsibility to evaluate innovative healthcare interventions. Conducting good research not only protects patients from unevaluated, potentially harmful interventions, it also fosters and maintains the integrity of clinical knowledge (Frader and Flanagan-Klygis, 2000).

Law

The fact that there may be unexpected harms resulting from innovative procedures does not in and of itself qualify them for the same type of review and oversight as research, but it does justify an increase in the level of safeguards to protect patients. The challenge is to delineate methods that offer protection to patients without stifling innovation (Strasberg and Ludbrook, 2003).

Canadian case law, for example, provides an articulation of standards clinicians will be expected to meet when providing innovative treatment. A clinician's standard of care is often described as "the degree of care and skill which could reasonably be expected of a normal, prudent practitioner of the same experience and standing in the similar circumstances" (*Lyne* v. *McClarty*, 2001). When treating a patient, whether the treatment is innovative or standard practice, the clinician "...owes a duty to the patient to use diligence, care knowledge, skill and caution in administering the treatment..." (*Lyne* v. *McClarty*, 2001). In terms of reasonable precautions, it would be expected that a clinician using an innovative treatment would be able to show that others in the same field would have considered the precautions taken to be sufficient, that the clinician "...could not have learnt how to avoid the accidents by example of another, that most probably no other practical precautions could have been taken" (*Lyne* v. *McClarty*, 2001).

While many forms of oversight for the introduction of innovative procedures have been proposed in the literature (Reitsma and Moreno, 2005), the best options are those mechanisms that are consistent with standards that have been generated through the law in the relevant jurisdiction and that operationalize the values of fiduciary responsibility and accountability.

The legal standard of informed consent requires that patients and substitute decision makers not only understand and appreciate the potential risks and benefits of a procedure but also the innovative nature of the procedure (*Coughlin* v. *Kuntz*, 1987). The law of informed consent requires that the consent be voluntary; that the patient be capable of understanding and appreciating the potential risks, benefits and impact of the intervention in his or her own life situation; and that the patient be informed – must be told and comprehend all that a reasonable person would want to know about the risks, benefits, and impact of the proposed treatment. In the consent discussion, clinicians need to discuss the kind of information that a "reasonable patient" might consider material information for making an informed decision about whether or not to consent to the innovative procedure (*Coughlin* v. *Kuntz*, 1987).

Professional standards are developed within professional bodies and healthcare institutions and are relevant to innovative practices. Maintenance of professional standards through continuing education and examinations are intended to help to ensure that clinicians have the skill level and knowledge to meet the challenges of rapidly changing technology and scientific information.

Policy

Surgeons are constantly exposed to new procedures and devices through medical journals, conversations with colleagues at meetings, and through advertising and promotion by representatives from the companies making new products. Most hospitals do not have a specific policy in place for surgeons to follow when introducing innovative procedures, other than the REB, which is infrequently used for this purpose (Reitsma and Moreno, 2002). A policy for the introduction of innovative procedures and devices should have a number of attributes if it is going to be used by surgeons. These include ease of use and a short timeline between application and approval or rejection. The policy should provide transparent accountability, patient protection, and legal protection for the surgeon and the hospital.

We have developed a policy at The Hospital for Sick Children, Toronto, for the introduction of innovative procedures and devices that attempts to address as many of the relevant issues as possible, and have implemented and carried out a preliminary evaluation of the policy. At the time of this writing, the policy addresses only procedures or devices that have been introduced previously at other institutions but are new to this hospital. An on-line form contains 10 points about the proposed innovation (Table 26.1) that the surgeon must address and then submit to the surgeon-in-chief, who has three options: approve of the proposal, request for expert advice, or recommend submission to the REB/IRB. The process is evaluated using structured interviews and a compliance review as part of the hospital's quality assurance program.

Table 26.1. Ten points to be addressed and submitted to the surgeon-in-chief by a surgeon who is hoping to use an innovative procedure or device

1. Description of the innovative procedure or device
2. Evidence of effectiveness/rationale for request
3. Evidence of collegial endorsement and suggestion of advisers (internal or external) with whom The surgeon-in-chief may consult
4. Potential risks and benefits to patient
5. Special consent considerations
6. Initial number of patients to be treated
7. Expected impact (positive or negative) on resources, for example for procedure time, device costs, postoperative care
8. Assurance of device safety and approval (may include "special" approval) for use in the jurisdiction
9. Evidence of necessary skill or training on the part of the surgeon and the interdisciplinary team
10. Plans for collecting and reporting quality assurance and outcome data

Over a one-year period, 14 applications to perform innovative procedures were submitted through this policy. All were approved, two after expert consultation, and 23 procedures were performed. Case review revealed perceived benefit to the patient in 78% of the cases, and lower cost in 56% of the cases compared with the standard approach. Surgical innovators strongly supported the process. Compliance review indicated incomplete written documentation of the innovative nature of the procedure/device in 10% of the cases. Experience with this policy suggests that innovative procedures and devices can be introduced through a user-friendly process that promotes accountability and responsible resource utilization, intending to protect patients, surgeons, and hospitals, but that the evolving consent process needs further improvement.

Empirical studies

Reitsma and Moreno (2002) identified 59 published papers that described surgical innovations, then surveyed the corresponding authors: 15 of 21 authors did not submit their protocol to an REB/IRB; seven mentioned the innovative nature of the procedure on the consent form. Although 14 authors described their work as research, only six sought prior REB/IRB review.

In a subsequent study, Reitsma and Moreno (2005) surveyed surgeons for their definitions of innovative surgery and research, and for their attitudes toward regulation, the need for specific informed consent, and IRB review of surgical innovations. The surgeons' responses differentiated routine surgical variation from research requiring IRB review by two criteria: a formal protocol and prior consent regarding the experimental nature of the procedure. Suggestions regarding oversight for significant innovations that are not formal research include clearance with the chief of surgery or a hospital committee, registries, tracker trials, and review by experts in a particular field.

Strasberg and Ludbrook (2003) analyzed experience with the introduction of laparoscopic cholecystectomy, live donor liver hemitransplantation, radiofrequency tumor ablation, and coronary artery angioplasty. They emphasized the value of registries of early experience for detecting new or unexpected problems that were not discovered in randomized trials of the same procedures. Hazelrigg *et al.* (1993) reported a registry of early experience with 1820 video-assisted thoracic surgical procedures. The early publication of this collective experience helped to identify the problems encountered during the learning phase, and to establish safe limits to the application of this innovative technology.

At the time of writing, the Children's Hospital in Boston (Kornetsky, 2001) and the Massachusetts General Hospital had similar effective policies that emphasized expert collegial review, and consultation with the REB/IRB when appropriate. The Hospital for Sick Children and the University Health Network in Toronto have both adopted a somewhat similar model, as described in the policy section of this chapter.

How should I approach innovation in practice?

Innovation should be encouraged and facilitated in a supportive setting that includes collegial oversight, full patient consent that is explicit about the fact that the consent is for an innovative procedure, attention to effects on institutional personnel and resources, and responsible reporting of outcomes. Innovators should participate in registries of early experience to teach and learn from colleagues about the effects, side effects, useful modifications, and complications of the new procedures or devices. Where doubt exists as to whether an innovation should be the subject of an REB/IRB review, consultation should be pursued.

Innovations should improve healthcare because of greater convenience, less disability or pain, reduced cost, improved accuracy and safety, or better treatment outcomes. Claims to these advantages should be validated before the innovations are widely accepted. Expensive innovations should be held to a high standard of validation before they alter the allocation of institutional resources, and healthcare budgets should include an allocation for innovations to protect standard services from destabilization. While collaboration with industry can accelerate progress toward technological solutions, clinicians should give highest priority to their fiduciary obligation to their patients.

The cases

C's parents should be informed of the novelty of the STEP procedure, the rationale and experience at other centers, and the fact that C will be the first patient in your hospital to be treated using this innovative technique. Collegial review and support should be sought from a well-informed pediatric surgeon and the surgeon-in-chief, who should ensure that responsible members of the healthcare team who will be involved in C's care have the appropriate skills and endorse the treatment plan. A specific pre-agreed number of the serial tapering enteroplasties should then be evaluated, including their cost, outcome, and impact on the institution. Information on the experience with C should be shared with the registry (T. Jaksic, personal communication, 2006). A formal research protocol to establish the scientific validity of the procedure should then be developed in collaboration with the REB/IRB and other clinical scientists. This might include a formal protocol to measure the absorptive capacity of the newly formed intestine and the quality of life of the patient before and after the innovative procedure.

Emergency approval to use the innovative lung assist device (ILA) should be sought from the authorities responsible for evaluating medical devices in human patients. The surgeon-in-chief should be provided with a summary of the evidence supporting the use of the ILA in this young soldier, a summary of the potential risks and benefits, and the endorsement of the planned procedure signed by an informed colleague. All relevant team members should have the necessary skill or training to perform the procedure. The consent process should clearly disclose the innovative nature of the procedure. The experience gained should be carefully evaluated and reported in a registry of ILA applications. This experience and the advice of the innovating team should be shared with the manufacturer to help to improve the effectiveness and safety of the innovative device to enable their research. When the technical and procedural details of the treatment and the most appropriate patients have been identified, a formal research study should be developed working with the REB/IRB to validate the innovation.

REFERENCES

Agich G. J. (2001). Ethics and innovation in medicine. *J Med Ethics* **27**: 295–6.

American Medical Association (2005). *Code of Ethics*. Washington, DC: American Medical Association (http://www.ama–assn.org/ama/pub/category/2498.html) accessed 21 July 2006.

Bayh-Dole Act 1980. PL 96–517, Patent and Trademark Act Amendments of 1980.

Canadian Medical Association (2004). *Code of Ethics*. Ottawa: Canadian Medical Association (http://www.cma.ca/index.cfm/ci_id/2419/la_id/1.htm) accessed 21 July 2006.

Coughlin v. *Kuntz* (1987). 17 B.C.L.R. (2d) 365.

Frader, J. E. and Flanagan-Klygis, E. (2000). Innovation and research in pediatric surgery. *Semin Pediatr Surg* **10**: 198–203.

Hazelrigg, S. R., Nunchuck, S. K., and LoCicero, J., III (1993). Video Assisted Thoracic Surgery Study Group data. *Ann Thorac Surg* **56**: 1039–43.

Kim, H. B., Fauza, D., Garza, J., *et al.* (2003). Serial transverse enteroplasty (STEP): a novel bowel lengthening procedure. *J Pediatr Surg* **38**: 425–9.

Kornetsky, S. (2001). *Guidelines, Concepts and Procedures for Differentiating Between Research and Innovative Therapy*. Boston, MA: Children's Hospital Committee on Clinical Investigation.

Lantos, J. (1994). Ethical issues: how can we distinguish clinical research from innovative therapy? *Am J Pediatr Hematol/Oncol* **16**: 72–5.

Leaf, D. (2005). The law of unintended consequences. *Fortune Magazine* **152**: 250.

Levine R. F. (1988). *Ethics and Regulation of Clinical Research*, 2nd edn. New Haven, CT: Yale University Press, p. 4.

Lyne v. *McClarty* [2001] 155 Man. R (2d) 191.

McKneally, M. F. and Daar, A. S. (2003). Introducing new technologies: protecting subjects of surgical innovation and research. *World J Surg* **27**: 930–4.

McKneally, M. F. and Kornetsky, S. (2003). Protecting participants in surgical innovation: Ideas and experiments from Canada and the United States. In *Joint Meeting of the American Society for Bioethics and Humanities and the Canadian Bioethics Society*, 25 October 2003.

Morreim, H. (2005). Research versus innovation: real differences. *Am J Bioethics* **5**: 42–3.

Morreim, H., Mack, M. J., Sade, R. M. (2006). Surgical innovation: too risky to remain unregulated? *Ann Thorac Surg* **82**: 1957–65.

National Commission for the Protection of Human Subjects of Biomedical and Behavioral Research (1979). *The Belmont Report: Ethical Principles and Guidelines for the Protection of Human Subjects of Research.* Washington, DC: *Office for Protection from Research Risks.*

Reitsma, A. M. and Moreno, J. D. (2002). Ethical regulations for innovative surgery: the last frontier? *J Am Coll Surg* **194**: 792–801.

Reitsma, A. M. and Moreno, J. D. (2005). Ethics of innovative surgery: US surgeons' definitions, knowledge, and attitudes. *J Am Coll Surg* **200**: 103–10.

Strasberg, S. M. and Ludbrook, P. A. (2003). Who oversees innovative practice? Is there a structure that meets the monitoring needs of new techniques? *J Am Coll Surg* **196**: 938–48.

Wilton, H., Brunch, V., and Dyonch, M. (2000). Moral decisions regarding innovation. *Clin Orthopaed Relat Res* **378**: 44–9.

27

Clinical trials

Richard E. Ashcroft and A. M. Viens

Dr. D, a clinical investigator, is conducting a clinical trial on a recently developed therapy for the treatment of a progressive neurodegenerative disorder. While initial results in a previous study generally appeared promising, the therapy has been associated with fatal bone marrow suppression in approximately 1% of patients. A colleague pediatrician, who has a patient with this neurodegenerative disorder, asks Dr. D if the child can be enrolled in the clinical trial. There are no data in the literature about this therapy having ever been used or tested in children with this condition, and Dr. D wonders whether the child should be included in the trial.

What are clinical trials?

Clinical trials are scientific evaluations of medical interventions for the treatment of somatic or psychological conditions that provide an analysis of the quality, safety, and efficacy of particular products, or a method of evaluating two products for their comparative value. While clinical trials are most often used to test therapeutic pharmaceutical products, they can also be utilized to evaluate medical devices or surgical procedures, plus other preventive, screening, detection, and non-pharmacological therapeutic products/methods.

Clinical trials influence clinical practice by providing vital information to clinicians and patients to use in assessing appropriate treatment options. Clinical trials allow for the generation of sound empirical evidence that individuals can use to address important questions concerning the benefits and harms of particular therapies in a scientifically rigorous and ethical way.

At the planning stage of a clinical trial, investigators produce a research protocol that specifies the procedures and methods to be performed throughout the course of the trial. An appropriately constituted research ethics committee – be it an institutional research ethics board or a multicenter research ethics board – must approve this protocol for scientific thoroughness and ethical appropriateness. This may include, amongst other considerations, ensuring that the experimental design is sound, the number of research subjects will accurately represent an adequate statistical sample, there is a suitable informed consent process, if there is compensation being provided it is not unduly coercive, and that the proposed research is in accordance with current scientific practices and ethical/legal regulations (Chow and Liu, 2003).

Clinical trials can be randomized (RCT) and non-randomized. An RCT comprises two (or possibly more) experimental or treatment groups/arms in which trial subjects are randomly assigned into different groups to ensure internal validity. If there are two groups, one group receives the product being studied and the other group receives the standard therapy/product, or a placebo. Where possible, the highest standards for RCTs include blinding, where the trial subjects (single-blind trial) or the trial subjects and investigators (double-blind trial) do not know which product is being tested. Non-randomized trials are sometimes conducted where randomization is impossible for ethical or pragmatic reasons. They face greater problems of bias, although these can sometimes be limited by careful design (Reeves *et al.*, 2001).

When new therapies are tested in humans, especially in the case of pharmaceutical therapies, RCTs generally comprise four progressive phases. The successful completion of each phase provides further evidence that the product may demonstrate to be safe and efficacious. Not all therapies will complete all four phases; for instance, RCTs may be stopped prematurely if the results show great potential, or if there are safety concerns for trial subjects. At any time during the course of the trial if adverse results arise that suggest possible risk or harm to trial subjects, these findings should be reported to current trial subjects, potential future subjects, other clinicians involved in the subjects' medical care, institutional research ethics board, study sponsor(s), and possibly national bodies responsible for research regulation and licensing (Piantadosi, 1997; Levine, 1998). The different types of clinical trials are as follows (with phase III trials usually being RCTs).

Phase I. In this phase, products are tested on a small number of subjects to collect data on considerations such as toxicity and best method of administration. These subjects may be healthy volunteers or patients with specific conditions, depending on the type and nature of the product. Testing in this stage seeks to collect data on the pharmacokinetic action of products in humans, possible risks or side effects associated with products at different dosages, amongst other consideration. The number of subjects participating in this phase is usually under 100. If sufficient and appropriate data are collected in this preliminary phase, it is used to design phase II studies.

Phase II. In this phase, products continue to be tested on a larger number of subjects to collect further data on pharmacological and pharmacokinetic activity, particularly in patients with the condition the product is proposed to treat. It is also at this stage that the new product is measured against the standard treatment or placebo for its comparative efficacy. The number of subjects participating in this phase is usually no more than several hundred. If sufficient and appropriate data are collected in this secondary phase, it is used to design phase III studies.

Phase III. In this phase, the product is tested on an even larger number of subjects in a continued effort to evaluate the product's safety and efficacy, especially in relation to standard treatments or placebos. At this stage, the product is generally dispensed as it would when it is to be marketed, and it is evaluated for its overall risk–benefit relationship and clinical labeling profile. The number of subjects participating in this phase is usually several hundred to several thousand. When this stage is complete, the study sponsors usually make an application to the appropriate national regulatory and licensing bodies for approval to market the product as safe and efficacious.

Phase IV. In this phase, which occurs only after the product has been approved and licensed for use, the product is evaluated for potential long-term side effects associated with the drug. This postmarketing surveillance phase could also include studies concerning how different dosages, schedules, or length of administration of the product affect patients, or how different patient populations react to the product.

While clinical trials are valuable for testing safety and efficacy, it is also important that other research methods of validating products are not forgotten (Fried, 1974; Freireich and Gehan, 1979; Reeves *et al.*, 2001).

In addition to the important exchange of information between study investigators, sponsors, and institutional/regulatory bodies, it is essential that the dissemination of results from clinical trials – positive, negative, and inconclusive results – occurs through peer-reviewed conferences and peer-reviewed journals; even if the results are unpublished, it is important that they are registered in a clinical trials registry. This ensures that clinicians and patients have access to the best information possible to make responsible decisions about what medical interventions are worthwhile undertaking (Simes, 1986; Horton and Smith, 1999; Rennie, 2004; International Committee of Medical Journal Editors, 2006).

Why are clinical trials important?

Ethics

The ethical importance of clinical trials is sometimes underestimated. Yet the need to evaluate treatments for their safety and efficacy, so as to minimize harm to patients, reduce clinical uncertainty, and improve the efficiency of resource allocation, is great, as has been recognized since Archie Cochrane's (1972) lectures on *Effectiveness and Efficiency* and the rise of the evidence-based medicine movement (Daly, 2005). Much more attention has been paid to the ethics of the conduct of clinical trials. The standard principles of research ethics apply to clinical trials, such that the avoidance of coercion and undue inducement, the properly informed consent of the patient, the proportionality of risk and benefit, and the scientific and clinical competence of the investigators all need to be assured. In recent years, attention has focused on the need to warrant randomization in clinical trials. The principal theory of the ethics of randomization is the "equipoise" theory (Freedman, 1987; Ashcroft, 1999; Miller and Weijer, 2003). On this theory, clinicians discharge their responsibilities to do their best for their patients if, faced with genuine uncertainty as to which one of the available treatments is most effective (or safest) in treatment of a condition, they allocate the patient treatment by randomization, thereby giving the patient an equal chance of receiving the treatment which is actually most effective. On the equipoise theory, clinicians may have a preference for one or other treatment, but where the clinical community is uncertain or divided, clinicians should submit their judgements to that of the clinical community at large, and enter a patient

into a properly conducted clinical trial. At issue is the question of whether the uncertainty is genuine, and whether the patient understands this. Some patients can experience the "therapeutic misconception," according to which they believe that the treatment they are receiving must be the treatment that is best for them, when this is actually not certain and the treatment is in a broader or narrower sense "experimental" (see Ch. 29). Current best practice is that uncertainty should be underwritten by the conduct of an appropriately rigorous systematic review of the existing clinical evidence before a trial is initiated; and a stronger claim is sometimes advanced, that where uncertainty exists a trial *ought* to be initiated.

In practice, not all clinical trials exist to resolve clinical uncertainty, since many trials are run in order to establish the safety and licensure credentials of a new treatment, rather than to assess the merits of a new or established treatment in the light of the alternatives. This has provoked some controversy when it came to light in the context of trials run in the developing world. There is a heated controversy about the choice of controls in many such trials (but also in some trials in the developed world). Many commentators argue that use of a placebo control where a proven effective treatment exists is unethical, since trial lists are failing to act in the best interests of their patients. Some would go further and say that such trials exploit poor patients by taking advantage of their inability to purchase or access treatments known to be effective in the developed world. Critics of this position hold that duties of beneficence do not extend to providing treatments to trial participants that would otherwise be unavailable, and further that imposition of this standard as an ethical norm would make much medical research unaffordably expensive, thus limiting possible benefit to future patients in the developed and developing world alike (Schüklenk and Ashcroft, 2000). Ethical controversy also exists about the extent to which patients' preferences should be allowed in what treatment they receive, and about the way to make resource-allocation decisions in order to prioritize which trials are conducted in the public sector. A large proportion of trials are conducted by the private sector for largely commercial or regulatory reasons, rather than scientific or clinical reasons (insofar as these are distinct). Finally, early phase clinical trials, which are conducted with little prospect of benefit to the patient, can be ethically challenging for that reason, especially where the trial may be seen by the patient as their last hope, or where the risks of the new treatment are genuinely uncertain (Ashcroft, 2004). Often there can be moral conflict in clinical trials between an investigator's scientific duty and protective duty – with the predominant view being that, when in conflict, the protective duty must override scientific duty. Merritt (2005) has recently argued that, in such conflicts, we need not choose one duty over the other; instead, in hard cases, investigators should proceed by taking into consideration the interests that research subjects have in achieving their personal goals for participation in research.

Law

Clinical trials are now strictly regulated throughout the developed world, for example under the European Clinical Trial Directive (European Union, 2001) in the European Community (adopted as the Clinical Trials Regulations [2004] in the UK, for instance), the relevant part of the *Code of Federal Regulations* in the USA (US Department of Health and Human Services, 2005), the International Committee on Harmonization (1996), and the relevant medicines licensing law and regulations. There is little case or statute law in most jurisdictions relating to the consent of patients, or the assessment of risk and benefit in trials. However, most developed countries have extensive legislation relating to conduct and registration, and oversight of trials is now fairly detailed (Plomer, 2005).

Policy

Alongside the law on clinical trials, there exists an extensive body of policy and guidelines.

Internationally, the key documents are the *Declaration of Helsinki* (World Medical Association, 1964), the Council of the International Organizations of Medical Sciences (2002) guidelines on biomedical research, and the International Committee on Harmonization (1996) *Good Clinical Practice* guidelines. At national level, guidance is available from both professional regulators and from research sponsors. In the UK, for example, the General Medical Council, which licenses doctors, has guidance on the ethical conduct of research by doctors, as does the Medical Research Council (the major public funder of medical research), and the Central Office for Research Ethics Committees (the government office responsible for the oversight of ethical review of research) (Medical Research Council, 1998; General Medical Council, 2002; Central Office for Research Ethics Committees, 2006). The organizing principle for clinical trials research in the early years of the twenty-first century is "good clinical practice" or "research governance," which is designed to ensure that clinical trials are conducted with methodological rigor, in accordance with predetermined protocols, and with appropriate oversight and ethical standards.

Empirical studies

Considerable efforts have been made in recent years to investigate empirically different features of the ethics of clinical trials. For example, studies have investigated patients' recall of randomization concepts, the quality of informed consent to participation in trials, the methods doctors use to explain trial methods to patients, patients' preferences about access to different treatments in trials and how to incorporate these into different designs, and so on. This literature has been thoroughly reviewed in a number of systematic reviews sponsored by the UK National Health Service (Ashcroft *et al.*, 1997; Edwards *et al.*, 1998; Bartlett *et al.*, 2005; Robinson *et al.*, 2005). The review by Bartlett *et al.* (2005) is of particular importance because it focuses on the justice of clinical trial recruitment in theory and practice, and on the impact on trial quality of formal and informal exclusion criteria. Given that the evidence base is built out of the trials that are done, not those that ought to be done, this issue is of growing importance not only for research ethics but also for healthcare equity more generally.

How should I approach clinical trials in practice?

A reasonably logical approach is available. Firstly, one should assess what is already known, ideally through conducting or consulting a well thought out systematic review of the evidence. Secondly, one should assess whether the proposed trial is methodologically adequate to resolve the key uncertainties regarding the effectiveness, efficacy, or safety of the interventions under trial. Thirdly, one should consider whether the trial is being conducted in accordance with the general principles of research ethics (Weijer and Miller, 2004). Are the consent arrangements adequate? Is the risk–benefit ratio fair and appropriate? Has the burden on research participants been minimized? Are recruitment policies fair to the population at large and to those recruited? Finally, one should assess whether the trial will be conducted in a disinterested fashion. Are inducements to researchers appropriate (not excessive or inappropriate in kind) and properly declared? Will the trial data be published in a timely way and made available for meta-analysis by other qualified researchers? Are measures in place to stop the trial early if overwhelming evidence of effectiveness or of harm to patients comes to light? A key check in this process is review by the research ethics committee, but the final responsibility lies with the doctor involved with the trial.

The case

Since the neurodegenerative disorder the drug under study was meant to treat is extremely rare in children, Dr. D did not think to exempt children from the trial in the enrollment criteria. The ability of Dr. D to enroll the child as a trial subject will depend on a number of factors. Firstly, whether Dr. D has any experience treating or investigating children (or whether Dr. D can identify collaborators who can become co-investigators). Secondly, the ability to secure proper consent from a minor and their parents for enrollment into such research. Thirdly, whether the inclusion of children can be scientifically justified; for instance the number of children with this disorder makes it unlikely that there will be sufficient numbers for a meaningful examination of either separate or pooled analysis of data at Dr. D's institution. It may be possible that the investigator could collaborate with other sites to obtain a sufficient number of eligible child study participants. Barring that prospect, it may be possible for the child to be given the study drug on compassionate grounds but not be formally entered into the study. Fourthly, whether the inclusion of children can be ethically justified, for instance given the rarity of the disease in the pediatric population, limited treatment options, and the mortality and morbidity associated with the disease the potential benefits would likely outweigh the risks and could justify enrolling the child (or finding alternative provisions for the drug).

REFERENCES

Ashcroft, R. (1999). Equipoise, knowledge and ethics in clinical research and practice. *Bioethics* **13**: 314–26.

Ashcroft, R. (2004). Gene therapy in the clinic: whose risks?. *Trend Biotechnol* **22**: 560–3.

Ashcroft, R. E., Chadwick, D. W., Clark, S. R. L., *et al.* (1997). Implications of socio-cultural contexts for ethics of clinical trials. *Health Technol Assess* **1**: 1–66.

Bartlett, C., Doyal, L., Ebrahim, S., *et al.* (2005). The causes and effects of socio-demographic exclusions for clinical trials. *Health Technol Assess* **9**: 1–152.

Central Office for Research Ethics Committees (2006). Website (http://www.corec.org.uk/applicants/index.htm) accessed 14 July 2006.

Chow, S. C. and Liu, J. P. (2003). *Design and Analysis of Clinical Trials: Concepts and Methodologies*. New York: John Wiley.

Cochrane, A. (1972). *Effectiveness and Efficiency: Random Reflections on Health Services*. London: Nuffield Provincial Hospitals Trust.

Council of the International Organizations of Medical Sciences (CIOMS) (2002). *International Ethical Guidelines for Biomedical Research Involving Human Subjects*. Geneva: CIOMS.

Daly, J. (2005). *Evidence-Based Medicine and the Search for a Science of Clinical Care*. Berkeley, CA: University of California Press.

Edwards, S. J. L., Lilford, R. J., Braunholtz, D. A., *et al.* (1998). Ethical issues in the design and conduct of randomised clinical trials. *Health Technol Assess* **2**: 1–128.

European Union (2001). *Clinical Trials Directive*, 2001/20/EC. Brussels: European Communities Press.

Freedman, B. (1987). Equipoise and the ethics of clinical research. *N Engl J Med* **317**: 141–5.

Freireich, E. J. and Gehan, E. A. (1979). The limitations of randomized clinical trials. In *Methods in Cancer Research: Cancer Drug Development*, ed. V. T. DeVita and H. Busch. New York: Academic Press, pp. 277–310.

Fried, C. (1974). *Medical Experimentation: Personal Integrity and Social Policy*. New York: Elsevier.

General Medical Council (2002). *Research: The Role and Responsibilities of Doctors*. London: General Medical Council.

Horton, R. and Smith, R. (1999). Time to register randomised trials. The case is now unanswerable. *BMJ* **319**: 865–6.

International Committee of Medical Journal Editors (2006). *Uniform Requirements for Manuscripts Submitted to Biomedical Journals: Writing and Editing for Biomedical Publication*. Philadelphia, PA: American College of Physicians.

International Committee on Harmonization (1996). *Tripartite Guideline E6(1): Good Clinical Practices*. Geneva: International Committee on Harmonization (http://www.ich.org/LOB/media/MEDIA482.pdf) accessed 17 July 2006.

Levine, R. J. (1998). *Ethics and Regulation of Clinical Research*, 2nd edn. New Haven, CT: Yale University Press.

Medical Research Council (1998). *MRC Guidelines for Good Clinical Practice in Clinical Trials*. London: Medical Research Council.

Merritt, M. (2005). Moral conflict in clinical trials. *Ethics* **115**: 306–30.

Miller, P. B. and Weijer, C. (2003). Rehabilitating equipoise. *Kennedy Inst Ethics J* **13**: 93–118.

Piantadosi, S. (1997). *Clinical Trials: A Methodologic Perspective*. New York: John Wiley.

Plomer, A. (2005). *The Law and Ethics of Medical Research: International Bioethics and Human Rights*, Oxford: Cavendish.

Reeves, B., MacLehose, R., Harvey, I. M. *et al.* (2001). A review of observational, quasi-experimental and randomised study designs for the evaluation of the effectiveness of healthcare interventions. In *The Advanced Handbook of Methods in Evidence Based Healthcare*, ed. A. J. Stevens, K. Abrams, J. Brazier, R. Fitzpatrick, R. J. Lilford. London: Sage, pp. 116–35.

Rennie, D. (2004). Trial registration: a great idea switches from ignored to irresistible. *JAMA* **292**: 1359–62.

Robinson, E. J., Kerr, C. E. P., Stevens, A. J., *et al.* (2005). Lay public's understanding of equipoise and randomisation in randomised controlled trials. *Health Technol Assess* **9**: 1–178.

Schüklenk, U. and Ashcroft, R. E. (2000). International research ethics. *Bioethics* **14**: 158–72.

Simes, R. J. (1986). Publication bias: the case for an international registry of clinical trials. *J Clin Oncol* **4**: 1529–41.

US Department of Health and Human Services (2005). *Code of Federal Regulations, Title 45*. Washington DC: US Government Printing Office.

US Health Insurance Portability and Accountability Act of 1996, Public Law 104–191, 104th Congress (http://aspe.hhs.gov/admnsimp/p1104191.htm) accessed 7 October 2005.

Weijer, C. and Miller, P. B. (2004). When are research risks reasonable in relation to anticipated benefits? *Nat Med* **10**: 570–3.

World Medical Association (1964). Declaration of Helsinki. Ethical principles for medical research involving human subjects. *JAMA* **284**: 3043–3046.

28

Epidemiological research

Richard E. Ashcroft

Dr. E is a primary care physician (general practitioner) with an extensive patient list. He is approached by researchers leading a large epidemiological study into the association between asthma and heart disease. He is asked for de-identified patient data on all his patients with a history of asthma concerning their age, sex, age at first diagnosis with asthma, current medication, and cardiovascular history. He is assured that the research ethics committees of both his local university hospital and the researchers' own institution has approved the study. He is offered payment for the administrator's time required to prepare this data.

What is epidemiological research?

Epidemiology may be defined as "the study of the distribution and determinants of disease in human populations" (Dunn, 2003, p. 34). There is no very tight distinction between epidemiology and other data collection and analysis practices in public health, but for practical purposes epidemiology can be considered a research activity, which is to say that it is concerned with producing generalizable scientific knowledge. A standard textbook of epidemiology (Farmer *et al.*, 1996, p. 6) defined the principal uses of epidemiology as:

The investigation of the causes and natural history of disease, with the aim of disease prevention and health promotion.

The measurement of health care needs and the evaluation of clinical management, with the aim of improving the effectiveness and efficiency of health care provision.

Both of these can be read as service objectives (What caused this disease outbreak? How can we assess the health needs of this group of patients?) and as research objectives. For the purposes of this chapter, we are interested mainly in epidemiological research. Epidemiological research has a number of different approaches, which include experimental methods (principally randomized controlled trials) and observational methods (principally cohort studies, case–control studies, cross-sectional studies, ecological studies, and analyses of routine data). The ethical issues involved in experimental methods in epidemiology are discussed in Ch. 27. This chapter will be concerned mainly with observational methods in epidemiological research.

Classical examples of epidemiological research include John Snow's identification of the waterborne nature of the cause of cholera in the early nineteenth century, Richard Doll and colleagues' establishment of the causal link between smoking and lung cancer in the late 1940s, and the definition of acquired immunodeficiency syndrome in the early 1980s.

Why is epidemiological research important?

Ethics

Because epidemiological research is concerned with the causes and management of disease and ill-health in populations, there is an associated generic risk that it may place community interests in conflict with the interests of individual patients and citizens. Because epidemiological research is concerned with characteristics of populations, a central methodological preoccupation of epidemiologists is with bias. In particular, epidemiologists are concerned with biased sampling from populations, which would produce inaccurate representations of the variables of interest in a population, and false or misleading interpretations of associations between such variables. In a cohort study, for instance, if significant numbers of the participants in a cohort were "lost to follow-up" or withdrew their consent to the use of their records in a study, this could fatally undermine the study. For this reason, many epidemiologists are keen to use designs that minimize the risk (as they see it) that their sample will be biased in construction or in operation. Two ways that bias can arise are that a significant number of people might refuse to participate or that a significant number of people might drop out during the course of a study. The major ethical debates in epidemiology have, therefore, concerned consent and methods of recruitment and retention in studies (Hart *et al.*, 1997).

Other ethical issues do arise. In epidemiological studies that involve collecting new data from study participants (such as by measuring blood pressure or collecting genetic samples), an important question arises when person-specific data are collected that indicate that the person may have a health problem or risk which was not foreseen by the person or the researcher – so-called "incidental findings." Does the researcher or research team have a duty of care to the patient that would require disclosure of this information? What if there is nothing that can be done about this information? What if this information represents a risk to third parties? This problem can arise across the study as a whole once the findings of the study are interpreted (Richards, 2003). For instance, in genetic epidemiology, it can happen that a gene is identified that seems to raise the risk of heart disease in those that have a given allele. Should all those people in the study with this allele be informed? Do they have a right to this information? (Sharp and Orr, 2004).

Aside from individual-level ethical challenges, there may also be population-level challenges. While epidemiological research can be a powerful tool for identifying inequities in healthcare, epidemiological research can reinforce inequities both through study design and through the (mis)interpretation of results. For instance, an epidemiological study may be constructed to investigate a health issue in a particular ethnic group, where there is no particularly good reason to think that this ethnic group is different from the population at large from a health or medical point of view. The interpretation of the results of such a study (either by the researchers themselves or by some audience of the research) may then be used to reinforce stigma against this ethnic group (Singer *et al.*, 2003). Although epidemiology is at least as much a social science as a medical and natural science, it is relatively unusual for the social impact of epidemiological research to be considered.

The most notorious example of unethical epidemiological research is probably the Tuskegee Syphilis Study. This study, initiated in 1932, was a study in a cohort of African-American men of the natural history of syphilis. The men were not told or were misled about the nature of the disease they had; they were denied treatment, discouraged from seeking alternative medical advice or treatment, even when effective treatment for syphilis became available in the 1940s, and were followed up until 1972 when the study was closed owing to the outcry when the study came to public attention (Reverby, 2000). Although this study is an extreme example, which is hardly representative of modern epidemiological research, it does illustrate in a salutary way the ethical issues described in this section.

Law

To this author's knowledge, no jurisdictions have specific laws or regulations for epidemiological research as such. In this respect, epidemiological research may be considered less regulated than clinical trials. However, many activities that form central parts of epidemiological research do fall under regulation: either relating to research in general or framed with other purposes in mind. An example will suffice to explain this. Firstly, many epidemiological studies involve the collection of new data from research participants. For example, participants in a study of blood pressure and mortality may be asked to undergo blood pressure measurements and blood samples, in addition to giving their consent for access to their medical records for long-term follow-up. These blood samples may be processed for DNA analysis in the context of a search for genetic factors that may partially explain health outcome variations over the course of the study. The additional measurements and invasive procedures to collect data and blood samples would fall under relevant law and regulations relating to research with human subjects in general (the *Declaration of Helsinki* [World Medical Association, 1964], *Code of Federal Regulations* [US Department of Health and Human Services, 2005], the common law of consent and applicable professional guidance in the UK, and so on). The processing of patient data for research purposes would fall under data protection legislation and confidentiality law in Europe, or the US Health Insurance Portability and Accountability Act (1996) and associated regulations in the USA. In both Europe and the USA, this class of legislation was not framed with research purposes in mind, although both bodies of legislation make mention of research in passing. The archiving of human biological samples and their use for purposes known at the time of collection, or re-use for purposes determined subsequent to collection by the original research team or some other group, may be governed by common law provisions relating to consent, by novel legislation such as the UK Human Tissues Act (2004), or by regulations drafted pursuant to existing law and regulation ad hoc. (For more information on this issue, see Ch. 23.) It is arguable that the regulation of epidemiological research is somewhat unstructured and difficult to apply given the rapidity with which epidemiology

has developed since the early 1980s under the influence of new technology (both information and data-processing and biomedical research techniques) and the scaling up of research from studies based on single communities to large-scale multi-site projects.

Policy

In contrast to experimental methods in medical research, relatively little has been written about the ethics of epidemiological research. It is not a central focus of the *Declaration of Helsinki*, for instance, although the provisions of the Declaration relating to non-therapeutic research procedures would apply to epidemiological studies, which involve the collection of new data from research participants (World Medical Association, 1964). However, the Council of the International Organizations of Medical Sciences (1991) has issued international guidance on ethics in epidemiology (these are currently being revised). From the early 1990s onwards, a series of ethical guidelines were produced at national and international levels, most importantly the statement of *Good Epidemiological Practice* of the International Epidemiological Association (2002 [updated in 2004]). There have been a number of academic reviews of ethical principles in research, and several specialist epidemiological associations have produced guidance on ethical issues in their specific areas of epidemiological research (Coughlin, 2007).

Empirical studies

Given the complex situation regarding the regulation of epidemiological research, there has been a growth in empirical studies that seek to examine the awareness among researchers of existing guidance and ethical principles in epidemiological research, the development of consensus within the research community and in society at large about what guidance and principles are required, the specific ethical issues in research, and how best to make the trade off between individual patient, community, researcher, and societal interests in epidemiological research (Prineas *et al.*, 1998; Wynia *et al.*, 2001; Kessel, 2003). This growth in empirical research as a way of defining issues and generating consensus has been particularly notable in relation to research involving genetic databases and tissue sample collections, and to a lesser extent in relation to research involving the use of patient data without consent or with generic prospective consent (i.e., a consent to the future collection and use of data without the researcher returning to re-seek consent from participants in connection with each future use) (Richards *et al.*, 2003; Tutton and Corrigan, 2004; Eriksson and Helgesson, 2005; Matsui *et al.*, 2005; Stolt *et al.*, 2005).

Empirical research can be useful in a number of ways: it can identify the issues that are at stake in practice (as opposed to what theoreticians think they should be); it can evaluate the relative importance of different concerns; it can gauge how widely particular views are held; and it can act as a kind of surrogate for a poll on policy decisions to be made. Although this last use of empirical data is frequently regarded as disreputable, in the context of epidemiological research it may be important. Since such research may depend for its ethical justification on appeal to the public interest, it may be important to establish both the content of the public interest (what is it in this case?) and how far the public interest is consistent with the aggregate of individuals' interests (Ashcroft, 2004). The latter can be established by survey or polling, although this should be handled with care (Rose, 2001; Wendler, 2006).

No good systematic reviews have been conducted of empirical research in this area, so findings need to be handled with care. For example, Richards and colleagues (2003) established that research participants in a breast cancer epidemiology study would welcome feedback of the findings of research. Yet while acknowledging that individual feedback would be desirable, they recognise the problems this might create. In a later study, Dixon-Woods *et al.* (2006) found that participants wanted individual feedback and found

general feedback unhelpful. The current state of empirical research considering ethics in epidemiology is, therefore, rather inchoate. At its best, it can help researchers to frame their own thoughts. It is too early to suggest that empirical research can lead policy making in this area, but it can perhaps be a counsel of humility regarding how far we know the ethical answers.

How should I approach epidemiological research in practice?

It is clear that many practice and policy issues remain to be resolved in epidemiological research, and that guidelines and regulations may not be entirely helpful either in conducting epidemiological research or in setting good practice standards. Nonetheless, some basic principles apply generally. Firstly, the general principles of research ethics apply to epidemiological research as they do to any biomedical and public health research. Consequently, so far as is possible, research should be carried out with the voluntary and informed consent of the research participants, in such a way as to minimize harm, risk of harm, and inconvenience to them, while maximizing the benefits to science and society that could accrue from the successful conduct of the project. Epidemiological research will rarely directly benefit the research participant, although some recruitment and data-collection processes do involve what is effectively a health screen for the participant. In this case, it will be important to ensure that this is conducted with proper information to the participant, and to a clinically competent standard. It is necessary to have a policy on the feedback of unexpected findings of such a screening process to the participant (Illes *et al.*, 2006).

The main challenges lie where either it is not possible to adhere to the normal ethical standards in research or there is not yet a consensus on what those standards require. Examples of the latter include the as-yet-unresolved controversy on the scope of consent to future uses of research samples in genetic database research and the debate on feedback of individual test results from research where those results are not validated to clinical quality standards, their interpretation is as yet uncertain, or there is no clinical intervention to address any health problem they may indicate (Duncan et al., 2005).

The standard examples of research that may depart from the standard of informed voluntary consent are research projects that involve collection of patient data from records without the express prior consent of the patient. Most health systems contain a vast amount of useful clinical data, which can be a very valuable resource for epidemiologists. In some cases, data can be collected in an anonymized form, such that the researcher cannot, in principle or practice, identify any individual from the data collected. It can be argued that this does not, in fact, violate any privacy right of the patient. In other cases, the data can be collected in a form that could in principle be decoded to allow identification of the patient, although in practice this would be very difficult, and coding and firewalls can be put in place to make this as difficult as possible. Here, the justification might be based on the minimal risk of any actual harm to the patient even pursuant to their possible identification by a malign third party. This justification would essentially accept that a privacy right of the patient may have been violated but hold that this was at worst a technical breach only, outweighed by the value of the research and the minimal risk of harm to the patient. Some commentators would go further and argue that there is not even a technical breach of a patient's privacy right in such a case. There are standard arguments here. One is to hold that some breaches of confidence are only breaches of "prima facie" rights, since patient confidentiality can always be overridden in the face of a clear public interest, such as protection of third parties from serious harm or in the administration of justice (Gostin, 2000). Another is to hold that individual rights of privacy arise from communal interests, rather than the other way around: the "communitarian" approach

(Rubinstein, 1999). This type of justification may be applied where patient information is identifying but where there are privacy rules and safeguards to protect the patient's privacy from invasion by unauthorized external parties. In any case, it is clear that there is a very strong presumption in favor of patient confidentiality and privacy, and in favor of seeking patient's consent to participation even in minimal-risk database research. Part of the case for this presumption lies in the common interest in securing patient trust and support for medical research. This may, in turn, underwrite such practices as "broad" consent to re-use of tissue samples, by ensuring that the public at large understands and supports medical research as such and accepts that detailed "narrow consent" may be a costly and inefficient brake on an activity that is widely supported by the public (O'Neill, 2002). The present author's research suggests that most participants are less concerned with issues around consent than they are with governance. So long as they believe that the study is appropriately governed, and driven by a concern with patient welfare rather than political or commercial interests, they have a high level of trust in this type of research (Williamson et al., 2004).

The role of the research ethics committee or institutional review board here may be particularly important as it can act as an independent check on the claim that the research represents an appropriate balance between individual interests, the interests of the researcher, and the public interest.

The case

In the light of the above discussion, the main concerns of Dr. E will be as follows. Firstly, would passing on data collected from his patient's notes in this way be lawful and consistent with relevant professional guidance? The fine detail here may vary between jurisdictions. But in principle, although this information is not explicitly identifying, in that names and addresses are not collected, a third party could potentially identify one or more of the patients in the data table from the information given. So what the doctor needs to satisfy himself about would be the nature of the procedural and technical protections in place to prevent researchers or unauthorized third parties from using the information in that way. He would also need to satisfy himself that this is not a breach of confidence or, if it is, that it is a justified breach. For practical purposes, assurance by a research ethics committee that the study has their ethical approval may satisfy him on this point. Nonetheless, primary care physicians would normally be legally responsible for this decision, and liability in tort for a breach of confidence would not be removed by the fact of ethical approval from an ethical committee. The central issue, therefore, would be whether patient consent is required for this data processing. This is, in part, a legal question. So far as it is an ethical question, we are to consider first whether the patient has a right to be asked for his or her consent. Most would consider that it would be good practice to seek the patient's consent; however, this might introduce significant bias into the sampling, and moreover we have some research evidence to suggest that patients regard collection of their data for this sort of purpose as important and they are surprised by the request for their consent (Robling *et al.*, 2004). Thus Dr. E could be advised to take the following approach. Firstly, make it generally known to his patients that medical research studies using their data, subject to independent ethical review and careful information security controls, are carried out with his practice's cooperation. They can be asked to notify the practice if they do not wish their information to be used in this way, thus giving them an opt-out. However, the opt-out would be a generic opt-out, so that there is no risk (from the scientific point of view) of "consent bias" in recruitment to particular studies (Medical Research Council, 2000). Secondly, he should ensure that he is satisfied that the risk of patient identification has been minimized. On that basis, he can be satisfied that any breach of patient confidentiality and risk

to patients' interests has been minimized and he can agree with the request. The issue of whether paying his practice for the administrative work required in producing the data may raise a question of whether he is being induced to hand over this information, but since it is only a question of reimbursement for time spent on research at the expense of other practice activities, this is not a significant concern.

REFERENCES

Ashcroft, R. E. (2004). From public interest to political justice. *Camb Q Healthc Ethics* **13**: 20–7.

Coughlin, S. S. (2007). Ethical issues in epidemiology. In *Principles of Health Care Ethics*, 2nd edn, ed. R. E. Ashcroft, A. J. Dawson, H. J. A. Draper, J. McMillan. Chichester, UK: John Wiley, pp. 601–6.

Council of the International Organizations of Medical Sciences (1991). *International Guidelines for Ethical Review of Epidemiological Studies*. Geneva: Council of the International Organisations of Medical Science (http://www.cioms.ch/frame_1991_texts_of_guidelines.htm) accessed 13 July 2006.

Dixon-Woods, M., Jackson, C., Windridge, K. C., and Kenyon, S. (2006). Receiving a summary of the results of a trial: qualitative study of participants' views. *BMJ* **332**: 206–10.

Duncan, R. E., Delatycki, M. B., Collins, S. J., *et al.* (2005). Ethical in presymptomatic testing for variant considerations CJD. *J Med Ethics* **31**: 625–30.

Dunn, N. (2003). Observational and epidemiological research. In *Manual for Research Ethics Committee* 6th edn, ed. S. Eckstein. Cambridge, UK: Cambridge University Press, pp. 34–36.

Eriksson, S. and Helgesson, G. (2005). Keep people informed or leave them alone? A suggested tool for identifying research participants who rightly want only limited information. *J Med Ethics* **31**: 674–8.

Farmer, R., Miller, D., and Lawrenson, R. (1996). *Lecture Notes on Epidemiology and Public Health Medicine*, 4th edn, Oxford: Blackwell Scientific, p. 9.

Gostin, L. O. (2000). *Public Health Law: Power, Duty, Restraint*. Berkeley, CA: University of California Press, pp. 124–42.

Hart, J. T., Ebrahim, S., and Davey Smith, G. (1997). Response rates in south Wales 1950–96: changing requirements for mass participation in human research. In *Non-random Reflections on Health Services Research*, ed. A. Maynard and I. Chalmers. London: BMJ Books, pp. 31–57.

Human Tissues Act 2004. London: The Stationery Office.

Illes, J., Kirschen, M. P., Edwards, E., *et al.* (2006). Incidental findings in brain imaging research. *Science* **311**: 783–4.

International Epidemiological Association (2002). *Good Epidemiological Practice (GEP): Proper Conduct in Epidemiologic Research*. Dundee, UK: International Epidemiological Association (http://www.dundee.ac.uk/iea/Download/gep.pdf) accessed 13 July 2006.

Kessel, A. S. (2003). Public health ethics: teaching survey and critical review. *Soc Sci Med* **56**: 1439–45.

Matsui, K., Kita, Y., and Ueshima, H. (2005). Informed consent, participation in, and withdrawal from a population based cohort study involving genetic analysis. *J Med Ethics* **31**: 385–92.

Medical Research Council (2000). *Personal Information in Medical Research*. London: Medical Research Council (http://www.mrc.ac.uk/pdf–pimr.pdf) accessed 13 July 2006.

O'Neill, O. (2002). *Autonomy and Trust in Bioethics*. Cambridge, UK: Cambridge University Press.

Prineas, R. J., Goodman, K., Soskolne, C. L., *et al.* (1998). Findings from the American College of Epidemiology ethics survey on the need for ethics guidelines for epidemiologists. *Ann Epidemiol* **8**: 482–9.

Reverby, S. M. (ed.) (2000). *Tuskegee's Truths: Rethinking the Tuskegee Syphilis Study*. Chapel Hill: University of North Carolina Press.

Richards, M. P. M., Ponder, M., Pharoah, P., Everest, S., and Mackay, J. (2003). Issues of consent in a genetic epidemiological study of women with breast cancer. *J Med Ethics* **29**: 93–6.

Robling, M., Hood, K., Houston, H., *et al.* (2004). Public attitudes toward the use of primary care record data in medical research without consent: a qualitative study. *J Med Ethics* **30**: 104–9.

Rose, H. (2001). *The Commodification of Bioinformation: The Icelandic Health Sector Database*. London: Wellcome Trust (http://www.wellcome.ac.uk/assets/WTD003281.pdf) accessed 13 July 2006.

Rubinstein, H. G. (1999). If I am only for myself, what am I? A communitarian look at the privacy stalemate. *Am J Law Med* **25**: 203–31.

Sharp, H. M. and Orr, R. D. (2004). When "minimal risk" research yields clinically significant data, maybe the risks aren't so minimal. *Am J Bioethics* **4**: w32–6.

Singer, P. A., Benatar, S. R., Bernstein, M., *et al.* (2003). Ethics and SARS: lessons from Toronto. *BMJ* **327**: 1342–4.

Stolt, U. G., Helgesson, G., Liss, P. E., Svensson, T., and Ludvigsson, J. (2005). Information and informed consent in a longitudinal screening involving children: a questionnaire survey. *Eur J Hum Genet* **13**: 376–83.

Tutton, R. and Corrigan O. (eds.) (2004). *Genetic Databases: Socio-ethical Issues in the Collection and use of DNA*. London: Routledge.

US Department of Health and Human Services (2005). *Code of Federal Regulations Title 45*, Vol. 46.116(d). Washington, DC: Government Printing Office.

US Health Insurance Portability and Accountability Act of 1996, Public Law 104–191, 104th Congress (http://aspe.hhs.gov/admnsimp/pl104191.htm) accessed 7 October 2005.

Wendler, D. (2006). One-time general consent for research on biological samples. *BMJ* **332**: 544–7.

Williamson, E., Goodenough, T., Kent, J., and Ashcroft, R. E. (2004). Children's participation in genetic epidemiology: consent and control. *In Genetic Databases: Socio-ethical Issues in the Collection and use of DNA*, ed. R. Tutton and O. Corrigan. London: Routledge, pp. 139–60.

World Medical Association (1964). *Declaration of Helsinki: Ethical Principles for Medical Research Involving Human Subjects* [revised 1975, 1983, 1989, 1996, 2000]. Washington, DC: World Medical Association (http://www.wma.net/e/policy/b3.htm).

Wynia, M. K., Coughlin, S. S., Alpert, S., *et al.* (2001). Shared expectations for protection of identifiable health care information. Report of a national consensus process. *J Gen Intern Med* **16**: 100–11.

29

Clinical research and the physician–patient relationship: the dual roles of physician and researcher

Nancy M. P. King and Larry R. Churchill

Dr. F, an oncologist in a small community practice, has been asked by a pharmaceutical company to conduct early-phase clinical trials involving several new investigational chemotherapeutic agents that do not yet have FDA approval. These would be very small phase I trials, with the possibility of conducting some phase I/II and phase II trials in the future as well. The reimbursement he will receive for the research will substantially increase the income of his practice, provided that he is able to recruit and retain a sufficient number of subjects. "More importantly, though," Dr. F thinks to himself, "I have so little to offer many of my sickest patients now. The best thing about doing clinical research is being able to offer them something new, that just might be their best hope."

Dr. G treats patients with hemophilia. Although treatments have improved dramatically in recent years, hemophilia is a devastating, and devastatingly expensive, chronic disease. Because she has high hopes about promising experimental technologies, she also conducts research. She prides herself on the research partnerships she develops with patient–subjects who seek to contribute to the development of better treatments. Recently, however, she has received inquiries from patients with hemophilia from around the world who want to enroll in her research because the experimental interventions are provided free of charge. These patients tell her that they cannot afford standard therapies, and that enrolling in her research is their only hope for treatment. Dr. G is troubled by this reasoning, and discusses it with a colleague, who responds, "Lots of people enroll in research to get treatment. Almost all pediatric cancer patients are enrolled in research. And when HIV-positive patients can't afford the drugs, my colleagues in the ID clinic immediately look to see what trials they might qualify for – even before they look for a free drug program they could use. Why are you worried about patients who want to be in research to get treated?"

What is the dual role of clinician and researcher?

The differences between the role of physician and that of researcher become readily apparent in the definitions of "clinical research" and "medical practice." The *Belmont Report* distinguished between these activities as follows: "For the most part, the term 'practice' refers to interventions that are designed solely to enhance the well-being of an individual patient ... and that have a reasonable expectation of success .... By contrast, the term 'research' designates an activity designed to test an hypothesis, permit conclusions to be drawn, and thereby to develop or contribute to generalizable knowledge ..." (National Commission for the Protection of Human Subjects of Biomedical and Behavioral Research, 1979). Clinical research enrolling patients as research subjects is essential for the efficient development of safer and more effective treatments, but because of the differences between research and clinical practice, clinical research is given special regulatory oversight and research subjects are afforded special protections.

When physicians who treat patients also engage in clinical research, they take on a dual role, because the activities in which they engage have elements of both the clinician and the researcher. These roles have important differences that can conflict or become blurred. The differences in the conduct and goals of clinical research and medical practice can affect informed consent, alter the rights and duties of patient–subjects and clinical investigators, and give rise to conflicts of interest.

Why is the dual role of clinician and researcher important?

It is increasingly common for physicians in private practice as well as in academic medicine to find themselves in the dual role. Failure to understand and appreciate the differences between research and treatment can have adverse effects on patients' understanding and safety, and it could compromise the value and validity of research. It is, therefore, increasingly important for physicians to recognize and manage the dual role, both in order to conduct scientifically and ethically sound research and to avoid confusion, harm, and exploitation of patients and research subjects.

There are several key issues for clinicians considering involvement in research: (i) understanding the scientific justification for conducting clinical research and what counts as an acceptable balance of risks of harm and potential benefits in clinical research; (ii) avoiding exploitation of patient–subjects and promoting justice in recruitment, enrollment, and the post-trial care of patients; (iii) ensuring that patients' participation in research is voluntary and adequately informed; and (iv) properly managing the dual roles of physician and researcher.

There is a great deal of ethical, legal, regulatory, and policy guidance addressing both clinical research and medical practice. However, little of this guidance addresses the particular challenges of the physician's dual role.

Ethics

A small number of scholarly articles directly addresses the problem of managing the dual roles of physician–investigator (Churchill, 1980; Glass and Waring, 2002; Lemmens and Miller, 2002;

Brody and Miller, 2003). A much larger body of scholarly literature addresses the physician's moral role and responsibilities in conducting clinical research. Most of this discussion focuses on phase III randomized controlled clinical trials (RCTs). How can physicians' moral obligation of beneficence – the obligation to do the best for their patients – be compatible with conducting research that involves their patients? For phase III research – the last step in determining whether an experimental intervention is sufficiently safe and effective to be considered a treatment – if a researcher believes that the experimental intervention is better than standard treatment, her duty as a physician seems to be to provide the experimental intervention. If the researcher believes that standard treatment is better, her duty is to provide the standard treatment. Either way, the physician should not be doing the research.

This conundrum centers on the concept of "equipoise." Research should develop evidence that answers questions about an unproven intervention; the novel intervention has to look promisingly safe and effective, but the evidence for its safety and effectiveness relative to the alternatives must be lacking. That is, the research itself should be necessary in order to "disturb" equipoise and cause the scientific community to say, "Yes, now we know that intervention A is/is not a better treatment for X disease." Because individual physician–researchers cannot easily both be in equipoise and fulfill their duties to their patients, the philosopher Benjamin Freedman advocated for the concept of "clinical equipoise" (Freedman, 1987) – meaning that in order for RCTs to go forward there must be a collectively held equipoise within the field. Individual clinical researchers need not have equipoise themselves; they need only recognize that there is disagreement within medicine about whether standard treatment or the unproven intervention is really better. Importantly, proponents of clinical equipoise oppose the use of placebo controls in clinical research except in very limited circumstances (Freedman, 1990; Freedman *et al.*, 1996a,b).

Recently, debate has emerged about whether equipoise is the right concept to employ when distinguishing clinical research from medical practice. Some bioethics scholars argue that focusing on clinical equipoise, because it addresses the question of which is the better treatment, makes the moral mistake of blurring research and treatment. These scholars reason that research should be viewed as a distinct enterprise, which does not, cannot, and should not in itself serve the goal of providing treatment to patients. "Which is the better treatment?" is a question that cannot be answered until the research is completed; therefore, clinical equipoise is a misleading moral compass for clinical research. The alternative proposed by these scholars is a shift away from the norm of beneficence to non-maleficence, that is, an effort to minimize or eliminate where possible harms from research participation. The failure to reduce or eliminate such harms results in exploitation of patient–subjects (Miller and Brody, 2002, 2003; Miller and Rosenstein, 2003).

Although adhering to the norm of non-maleficence and a goal of "non-exploitation" may promote clear distinctions between clinical research and medical practice, clinical equipoise appears to be a richer and more satisfying moral standard for physician–researchers, who often view themselves as treating patients through clinical research (Miller and Weijer, 2003). Whether clinical equipoise provides adequate guidance for physicians' decision making about whether research participation can maximize potential benefit to particular patient–subjects is currently the subject of debate (Hellman, 2002; Evans and London, 2006). Clinical equipoise does not, however, adequately address the issues raised by the enrollment of patients in early-phase clinical trials, as its focus is on RCTs.

Related to the challenge of appropriately distinguishing research from medical practice is the problem of the "therapeutic misconception." This name was coined by Paul Appelbaum and colleagues (Appelbaum *et al.*, 1982, 1987; Appelbaum, 1996, 2002) to describe the observation that some patients enrolled as subjects in clinical research failed to recognize that they were participating in research and misinterpreted some key features of research protocols. For example, subjects might not understand that they could be randomized to receive standard treatment, an unproven intervention, or a placebo, believing instead that the intervention they received was selected by their physician as the best treatment for them. Another aspect of therapeutic misconception, according to at least some definitions, is an unrealistic expectation of direct benefit from the experimental intervention. For instance, subjects may expect to be cured of their disease if they take an unproven drug, even though the research goal is to determine a safe dose of the drug in the short term (Horng and Grady, 2003).

Although Appelbaum and colleagues posited that both patients and physician–researchers could be affected by therapeutic misconception, it has most often been described as a characteristic of research subjects. However, when researchers have great hope in an unproven intervention, or are excited by the promise of new science, their own misconception may not only blur their sense of the differences between research and medical practice but also affect the informed consent process, inappropriately influencing patients' decisions about research participation (Churchill *et al.*, 1998; Dresser, 2000, 2002; Miller, 2000).

Another moral tension in the dual roles of the physician–researcher becomes evident when physicians approach their own patients about research participation. The patient may be reluctant to say no, out of a sense of indebtedness to the physician or out of concern that a refusal could impair the relationship and adversely affect future treatment. When there is confusion between research and treatment, or about the role and responsibilities of the physician–investigator, these perceived pressures could also affect subjects' understanding of the research, or unduly influence their enrollment or continued participation. This may be true whether the confusion is the patient's or the physician's (Kass *et al.*, 1996; Levinsky, 2002; Chen and Miller, 2003).

Law

There are relatively few court decisions about clinical research. Many of those decisions address plaintiffs' claims that they were unaware they were participating in research or were led by researchers to believe that they were being treated when in fact they were enrolled in research (*Toth* v. *Community Hospital at Glen Cove*, 1968; *Estrada* v. *Jacques*, 1984; *Re Cincinnati Radiation Litigation*, 1995). Several recent decisions involving research with vulnerable populations have suggested that researchers have physician-like obligations of beneficence toward their subjects and would restrict research participation by vulnerable subjects to circumstances where benefit to them is expected (*TD* v. *New York State Office of Mental Health*, 1996; *Grimes* v. *Kennedy Krieger Institute*, 2001). Such a stringent standard may protect vulnerable patients at the expense of maintaining a meaningful distinction between clinical research and medical practice.

A recent and controversial decision by the US Court of Appeals has further reinforced a treatment-oriented perspective on clinical research by finding that, under some circumstances, terminally ill patients may have a constitutional right of non-trial access to experimental interventions that have been shown to be safe enough in phase I trials to proceed to further testing (*Abigail Alliance* v. *Eschenbach*, 2006). It remains to be seen whether these legal developments will make it more difficult for patients and physicians to distinguish research from treatment.

Policy

The precise nature and significance of the difference between clinical research and medical practice has been debated as a matter of policy since the creation of the Nuremberg Code, the document that emerged from the Doctors' Trial at Nuremberg describing the duties of researchers conducting human experimentation (Nuremberg Code, 1949). In 1964, the World Medical Association promulgated the *Declaration of Helsinki* specifically to address medical research enrolling patients as subjects, to which many physicians believed the Nuremberg Code did not apply. The Declaration addresses the challenges of combining clinical research with medical care, framed in terms of the duties of physicians "to promote and safeguard the health of the people."

Another important policy perspective on the dual role comes from the legal literature on clinical research. A key legal characteristic of the physician–patient relationship is its fiduciary character: patients repose trust in their physicians, who make recommendations based on the patients' best interests, as mutually determined. It has recently been persuasively argued by several scholars that the researcher–subject relationship has at least some characteristics of a fiduciary relationship (Coleman, 2005; Miller and Weijer, 2006). Although the two relationships are not the same, clinical researchers have some duties that are similar to those of physicians: for example, to protect patient–subjects from undue harm, and to support their informed decision making about research participation. Precisely how to characterize the differences between the roles of physician and researcher and the duties that follow from them remains to be determined; nonetheless, the fiduciary model offers a promising way to think about dual-role problems in clinical research.

Empirical data

There has been a great deal of empirical research addressing "therapeutic misconception." Each study employs a somewhat different definition of the concept, as well as different questions to measure it in research subjects, but all the literature acknowledges that many patients who are research subjects appear to lack an adequate understanding of the difference between clinical research and medical treatment (Gray, 1975; Daugherty *et al.*, 2000; Joffe *et al.*, 2001; Appelbaum *et al.*, 2004; Henderson *et al.*, 2006). Recently, some scholars have begun examining in more depth the views of physician–investigators and research coordinators, in addition to patient–subjects, in order to assess whether therapeutic misconception in other participants involved in research is related to that in patient–subjects (Daugherty *et al.*, 1995; Joffe and Weeks, 2002; Henderson *et al.*, 2004a,b). Some of this research also examines how both patient–subjects and clinical researchers view the dual roles of physician and researcher (Henderson *et al.*, 2004b; Easter *et al.*, 2007). Other research examines how research consent forms describe clinical trials and their potential benefits for patient–subjects. There is agreement that the consent form and process can be a source of misconception in patient–subjects, but consensus does not exist regarding recommendations and guidance based on these data (Horng *et al.*, 2002, 2003; King *et al.*, 2005).

How should I approach the dual roles of physician and researcher in practice?

It is essential that physicians think of clinical research as distinguishable from, and complementary to, medical treatment. All clinical research is essentially future oriented: after the research is completed, the data gathered from it will inform medical treatment for future patients. In contrast, the physician's duty to act in the best interests of the patient is immediate. Yet the clinical researcher also has immediate duties to research subjects: to protect them from harm insofar as possible, to ensure that they are provided with adequate information about research participation, and sometimes – depending on the design of the research – to maximize the possibility of benefit to them.

A great deal of guidance exists to assist clinical researchers in addressing research ethics questions, but there are few resources specifically focused on the problem of dual roles. Some have suggested maintaining a clear demarcation between the roles, for example by donning a red coat instead of a white coat in research settings (Dresser, 2002) or explaining to patients "I have two hats; a doctor hat and a researcher hat. I'm going to take off my doctor hat now and put on my researcher hat, so I can talk to you about a research study."

Regardless of how physician–investigators emphasize the distinction to patients and research subjects, the best opportunities for clarifying the differences lie in the consent form and process. As a classic article in the legal literature notes, informed consent "encourages self-scrutiny by the physician–investigator" (Capron, 1974): meaning that the duty to explain the research to potential subjects also provides physician–researchers with an opportunity to make their own views clear to themselves, through articulating them to others.

It is important to recognize that delineating the characteristics of clinical research and the differences between participating in clinical research and receiving medical treatment is an exercise that is ultimately specific to each research protocol as well as to the treatments available to patients who may become subjects. Physician–researchers, and physicians who refer patients to clinical researchers, should take the time necessary to consider the ethical implications of their roles and to undertake clear and careful discussion about the differences between research and treatment with patients.

To manage the dual role, physician–researchers should:
- discuss the differences between research and medical practice with patients
- disclose both physician and researcher roles to patients, and distinguish them ("switch hats") as needed
- consistently use "research" terminology, not "treatment" language, when referring to investigators, subjects, and experimental interventions
- present benefit to society as the sole or primary goal of research
- explain that benefit to research participants, while often hoped for, is always uncertain and may be unlikely or impossible, depending on the design and phase of the trial
- when clinical benefit from the experimental intervention in a study is not possible or not likely, say so

- when clinical benefit from the experimental intervention in a study is reasonably possible, describe it clearly, including its nature, magnitude, duration, likelihood, and limits
- remember that, even though clinical research is not medical practice, researchers can, do, and should care about and for their research subjects.

The cases

Dr. F wants very much to be able to help his patients but has little to offer that can meaningfully extend the lives of many of them. As a result, he believes, as many oncologists do, that experimental agents hold more promise of safety and efficacy than do standard treatments. If Dr. F's research goal is to treat his patients through a trial, then he may have a therapeutic misconception. Although it is appropriate for him to consider experimental agents promising, in early-phase oncology trials the genuine potential for subjects to experience meaningful benefit is often very small (Horstmann et al., 2005). In addition, because research participation is not the only way to care for patients with advanced cancer, Dr. F should also discuss and offer palliative care and other support services to his patients and their families. It is important that Dr. F recognizes his mixture of motivations for conducting early-phase research. If he decides to proceed with a research program, his desire to recruit and retain subjects to improve his income could bias the information he provides to them, and he and his research colleagues will have to work hard to avoid that (Klanica, 2005).

Dr. G has become aware of some of the pressures on the healthcare system that can blur the distinction between research and treatment and affect patients' willingness to become research subjects. Patients who enroll in research because they do not have access to standard treatments may or may not have TM, but because their goal is to maximize their chances of benefit, they may not have the same view of their participation as Dr. G hopes for. They may resist randomization, or try to break a study

blind, or drop out of the research at the end of the intervention period, avoiding follow-up data-gathering visits as not beneficial to them. If Dr. G continues to enroll these patients in her studies, she must work especially hard to educate them about research participation and to develop research partnerships with them. Once they have completed participation in her research, many of these patients will continue to lack access to treatment. Asking whether clinical research, and clinical researchers, can or should ameliorate inequities in access to healthcare opens up a significant global social policy question. There are other avenues Dr. G could pursue for improving healthcare access for patients both at home and abroad.

REFERENCES

Abigail Alliance v. *Eschenbach* [2006] US App. LEXIS 10874 (D.C. Cir. 2006).

Appelbaum, P. S. (1996). Commentary: examining the ethics of human subjects research. *Kennedy Inst Ethics J* **6**: 283–7.

Appelbaum, P. S. (2002). Clarifying the ethics of clinical research: a path toward avoiding the therapeutic misconception. *Am J Bioethics* **2**: 22–3.

Appelbaum, P. S., Roth, L. H., and Lidz, C. (1982). The therapeutic misconception: informed consent in psychiatric research. *Int J Law Psychiatry* **5**: 319–29.

Appelbaum, P. S., Roth, L. H., Lidz, C. W., Benson, P., and Winslade, W. (1987). False hopes and best data: consent to research and the therapeutic misconception. *Hastings Cent Rep* **17**: 20–4.

Appelbaum, P. S., Lidz, C. W., and Grisso, T. (2004). Therapeutic misconception in clinical research: frequency and risk factors. *IRB, Ethics Hum Res* **26**: 1–5.

Brody, H. and Miller, F. G. (2003). The clinician–investigator: unavoidable but manageable tension 13. *Kennedy Inst Ethics J* **13**: 329–36.

Capron, A. M. (1974). Informed consent in catastrophic disease research and treatment. *U Penn Law Rev* **123**: 340–61.

Chen, D. and Miller, F. (2003). Clinical research and the physician–patient relationship. *Ann Int Med* **138**: 669–72.

Churchill, L. R. (1980). Physician–investigator, patient–subject: exploring the logic and the tension. *J Med Philos* **5**: 215–24.

Churchill, L. R., Collins, M. L., King, N. M. P., Pemberton, S. G., and Wailoo, K. A. (1998). Genetic research as therapy: implications of "gene therapy" for informed consent. *J Law Med Ethics* **26**: 38–47.

Coleman, C. (2005). Duties to subjects in clinical research 58. *Vand Law Rev* **58**: 387–449.

Daugherty, C., Ratain, M. J., Grochowski, E., *et al.* (1995). Perceptions of cancer patients and their physicians involved in phase I trials. *J Clin Oncol* **13**: 1062–72.

Daugherty, C., Banik, D., Janish, L., *et al.* (2000). Quantitative analysis of ethical issues in phase I trials: a survey of 144 advanced cancer patients. *IRB, Ethics Hum Res* **22**: 6–14.

Dresser, R. (2000). *When Science offers Salvation.* New York: Oxford University Press.

Dresser, R. (2002). The ubiquity and utility of the therapeutic misconception. *Soc Philos Pol* **19**: 271–94.

Easter, M. M., Henderson, G. E., Davis, A. M., Churchill, L. R., and King, N. M. P. (2007). The many meanings of care in clinical research. In *The View from Here: Social Science and Bioethics*, ed. R. DeVries, L. Turner, K. Orfali and C. Bosk. Oxford: Blackwell for Sociology of Health and Illness.

Estrada v. *Jacques* (1984) 321 S.E.2d 240 (N.C. Ct. App. 1984).

Evans, E. E. and London A. J. (2006). Equipoise and the criteria for reasonable action. *J Law Med Ethics* **34**: 441–50.

Freedman, B. (1987). Equipoise and the ethics of clinical research. *N Engl J Med* **317**: 141–5.

Freedman, B. (1990). Placebo-controlled trials and the logic of clinical purpose. *IRB, Rev Hum Subj Res* **12**: 1.

Freedman, B., Weijer, C., and Glass K. C. (1996a). Placebo orthodoxy in clinical research. I. Empirical and methodological myths. *J Law Med Ethics* **24**: 243–51.

Freedman, B., Weijer, C., and Glass K. C. (1996b). Placebo orthodoxy in clinical research. II. Ethical, legal and regulatory myths. *J Law Med Ethics* **24**: 252–9.

Glass, K. C. and Waring, D. (2002). Effective trial design need not conflict with good patient care. *Am J Bioethics* **2**: 25.

Gray, B. (1975). *Human Subjects in Medical Experimentation: A Sociological Study of the Conduct and Regulation of Clinical Research.* New York: John Wiley.

Grimes v. *Kennedy Krieger Institute* (2001) 782 A.2d 807 (Md. 2001).

Hellman, D. (2002). Evidence, belief, and action: the failure of equipoise to resolve the ethical tension in the randomized clinical trial. *J Law Med Ethics* **30**: 375–9.

Henderson, G. E., Davis, A. M., King, N. M. P., *et al.* (2004a). Uncertain benefit: investigators' views and communications in early phase gene transfer trials. *Mol Ther* **10**: 225–31.

Henderson, G. E., Davis, A. M., and King, N. M. P. (2004b). Vulnerability to influence: a two-way street. *Am J Bioethics* **4**: 50–2.

Henderson, G. E., Easter, M. M., Zimmer, C., *et al.* (2006). Therapeutic misconception in early phase gene transfer trials. *Soc Sci Med* **62**: 239–53. [Epub 5 July 2005.]

Horng, S. and Grady, C. (2003). Misunderstanding in clinical research: distinguishing therapeutic misconception, therapeutic misestimation, and therapeutic optimism. *IRB, Ethics Hum Res* **25**: 11–16.

Horng, S., Emanuel, E. J., Wilfond, B., *et al.* (2002). Descriptions of benefits and risks in consent forms for phase 1 oncology trials. *N Engl J Med* **347**: 2134–40.

Horng, S., and Emanuel, E. J., Wilfond, B., *et al.* (2003). Authors reply. *N Engl J Med* **348**: 1497.

Horstmann, E., McCabe, M. S., Grochow, L., *et al.* (2005). Risks and benefits of phase 1 oncology trials, 1991 through 2002. *N Engl J Med* **352**: 895–904.

Joffe, S., and Weeks J. C. (2002). Views of American oncologists about the purposes of clinical trials. *J Natl Cancer Inst* **94**: 1847–53.

Joffe, S., Cook, E. F., Cleary, P. D., *et al.* (2001). Quality of informed consent in cancer clinical trials: a cross-sectional survey. *Lancet* **358**: 1772–7.

Kass, N. E., Sugarman, J., Faden, R. *et al.* (1996). Trust: the fragile foundation of contemporary biomedical research. *Hastings Cent Rep* **26**: 25–9.

King, N. M. P., Henderson, G. E., Churchill, L. R., *et al.* (2005). Consent forms and the therapeutic misconception: the example of gene transfer research. *IRB, Ethics Hum Res* **27**: 1–8.

Klanica, K. (2005). Conflicts of interest in medical research: how much conflict should exceed legal boundaries? *J Biolaw Bus* **8**: 35–45.

Lemmens, T. and Miller P. B. (2002). Avoiding a Jekyll-and-Hyde approach to the ethics of clinical research and practice. *Am J Bioethics* **2**: 14–17.

Levinsky, N. G. (2002). Nonfinancial conflicts of interest in research. *N Engl J Med* **347**: 759–61.

Miller, F. G. and Brody, H. (2002). What makes placebo-controlled trials unethical? *Am J Bioethics* **2**: 3.

Miller, F. G. and Brody, H. (2003). A critique of clinical equipoise: therapeutic misconception in the ethics of clinical trials. *Hastings Cent Rep* **33**: 19–28.

Miller, F. G. and Rosenstein D. L. (2003). The therapeutic orientation to clinical trials. *N Engl J Med* **348**: 1383–6.

Miller, M. (2000). Phase I cancer trials. A collusion of misunderstanding. *Hastings Cent Rep* **30**: 34–43.

Miller, P. B. and Weijer, C. (2003). Rehabilitating equipoise. *Kennedy Inst Ethics J* **13**: 93–118.

Miller, P. B. and Weijer, C. (2006). Fiduciary obligation in clinical research. *J Law Med Ethics* **34**: 424–40.

National Commission for the Protection of Human Subjects of Biomedical and Behavioral Research (1979). *The Belmont Report: Ethical Principles and Guidelines for the Protection of Human Subjects of Research.* Washington, DC: *Office for Protection from Research Risks.*

Nuremberg Code (1949). *Trials of War Criminals before the Nuremberg Military Tribunals under Control Council Law No. 10,* Vol. 2. Washington, DC: US Government Printing Office, pp. 181–2. (http://www.hhs.gov/ohrp/references/nurcode.htm).

Re Cincinnati Radiation Litigation [1995] 874 F. Supp. 796 (S.D. Ohio 1995).

TD v. *New York State Office of Mental Health* (1996) 650 N.Y.S.2d 173.

Toth v. *Community Hospital at Glen Cove* [1968] 22 N.Y.2d 255; 239 N.E.2d 368; 292 N.Y.S.2d 440 (N.Y. Ct. App.1968).

World Medical Association (1964). *Declaration of Helsinki: Ethical Principles for Medical Research Involving Human Subjects* [revised 1975, 1983, 1989, 1996, 2000]. Washington, DC: World Medical Association (http://www.wma.net/e/policy/b3.htm).

30

Financial conflict of interest in medical research

Trudo Lemmens and Lori Luther

Dr. H is an expert on the treatment of depression. A pharmaceutical company, Calaxy Inc. signed a contract with Dr. H and his institution for a multisite three-year study on the efficacy and safety of a new antidepressant, Xanadu, for use in pregnant women. The contract stipulates that Dr. H will have access to all data for final analysis and that all publications based on the study will be submitted for final approval to the sponsor before public disclosure. Dr. H's budget includes money for finder's fees for clinicians who recruit patients into the trial and rewards for clinician–researchers whose patients remain in the trial for the duration of their pregnancy. In the course of the trial, Dr. H becomes worried about potential negative effects of Xanadu on newborns. He reveals his concern to the company, requests immediate access to all the data, and indicates that he will reveal his concerns at an upcoming international meeting. The company refers to a contradictory opinion of an internal data-monitoring committee set up by the sponsor, refuses to provide full access to the data, and points out that researchers have to obtain final approval of the sponsor before any public discussion of the results. Shortly after, Dr. H receives from Calaxy an abstract discussing the interim results of the study, accepted for presentation at an international conference. Dr. H is first author on the abstract, which does not contain any reference to his concerns. Dr. H contacts the chair of his department, Dr. I, who is a remunerated board member of Calaxy. She points out that Calaxy is a trusted and transparent partner in research, that it has its own data-monitoring committee, that it is ultimately responsible for the safety and efficacy of its products, and that contractual obligations have to be *respected. She mentions also in passing that Calaxy provides close to 20% of the research funding of the institution and that discussions are underway for the funding of a Calaxy research chair, for which Dr. H would be an excellent candidate.*

What is financial conflict of interest in research?

Thompson (1993) defined a conflict of interest as "a set of conditions in which professional judgment concerning a primary interest tends to be unduly influenced by a secondary interest." When clinician–researchers engage in research, tensions can exist between their interests as researchers and their primary obligations as clinicians. While Ch. 29 considers these divergent roles, we will focus specifically on financial conflicts of interest (COIs).

Several reasons justify the focus on financial COIs. Firstly, financial interests in research have exponentially increased in the last decades as a result of legislative (Bayh-Dole Act, 1980; Eisenberg, 2003; Lemmens, 2004) and funding agency initiatives that promote commercial matching funding (Downie *et al.*, 2002; Atkinson-Grosjean, 2006; Downie, 2006; Lemmens, 2006). Medical research is increasingly submerged in the competitive context of a lucrative biotechnology industry. Secondly, many significant

This chapter was funded by Genome Canada through the Ontario Genomics Institute, by Génome Québec, the Ministère du Développement Économique et Régional et de la Recherche du Québec and the Ontario Cancer Research Network.

recent controversies that have affected the public trust in the medical research enterprise are associated with financial COIs (Silberner, 2000; Healy, 2002; Krimsky, 2003, 2006; Angell, 2004; Viens and Savulescu, 2004; Revill, 2005; Armstrong, 2006a; Gelsinger, 2006). Thirdly, an array of reports, initiatives, and regulations emanating from official organizations and governmental agencies reflect an awareness that the potential negative impact of financial interests is a serious cause for concern (Office of the Inspector General, 2000; American Association of Medical Colleges, 2001, 2002; Canadian Institutes for Health Research, 2001, 2005; Institute of Medicine, 2001; US Department of Health and Human Services, 2004; UK House of Commons Health Committee, 2005). Fourthly, the tensions described in Ch. 29 are an inherent part of research while financial interests are more objective, tangible, and measurable, and can in theory be separated from the conduct of research itself (Thompson, 1993).

Types of financial interests of clinician–researchers

Researchers can have various financial interests. Some have stock in the company whose product they are testing or significant interests in spin-off companies set up for the purpose of commercializing research results. The controversy surrounding the death of Jesse Gelsinger, for example, revealed that the director and lead investigator of the Human Gene Therapy Institute, several of its researchers, and the University of Pennsylvania all had substantial equity stakes, reportedly in the millions of dollars, in a company that had invested in the genetically altered virus used in the experiment (Gelsinger, 2006; Krimsky, 2006).

Others are consultants for sponsoring companies or are remunerated members of advisory boards. Many receive significant payment for conference presentations or as members of speaking bureaus set up by pharmaceutical companies to promote their products at academic, educational, and promotional venues.

Financial rewards are also offered to researchers for research recruitment, as described in the case study (Lemmens and Miller, 2003). Financial recruitment incentives can be offered as finder's fees (i.e., per capita payments for every research subject recruited) or as bonuses for speedy recruitment, recruiting extra subjects, or keeping subjects in a trial (Office of the Inspector General, 2000). Finder's fees are often part of more general compensation for the costs of being involved in research, making it hard to identify whether and how much researchers receive for the mere recruitment of research subjects.

Even when clinician–researchers have nothing to gain from being involved in a research project, their institutions can be financially dependent on, or have close relations with, commercial sponsors, creating institutional COIs (Emanuel and Steiner, 1995). This may have an influence on institutional policies and behavior and create pressure on individual researchers. Financial interests of individuals with decision-making authority within institutions (e.g., departmental chairs, heads of research) can transform an individual COI into an institutional one (American Association of Medical Colleges, 2002).

The mere sponsorship of a clinical trial may create financial COIs that impact on research. The conflict resides then in the fact that commercial sponsors have a direct interest in obtaining commercially favorable results, while the goal of research is to obtain reliable and scientifically accurate information that benefits patient care.

Why is it important to deal with financial conflict of interest in research?

Ethics

Safety and well-being of research subjects

Financial interests in research may influence how researchers recruit subjects and how they treat them in the course of a clinical trial. When significant amounts of money can be gained by recruiting more subjects, or for recruiting them faster, researchers may be tempted to be more lenient with inclusion criteria. Financial interests in the results of a study or in keeping subjects enrolled can negatively impact on the decision to withdraw research subjects or to halt a trial when this is in the subjects' best interests.

Integrity of research

Commercial interests may threaten the integrity of the research process in two ways. Firstly, financial interests may impact on the design of the study, the conduct of the study itself, the interpretation of research data, and the presentation of the results in publications. Empirical studies establish a statistically significant link between source of funding and research outcome. Industry-sponsored research is more likely than research sponsored by non-commercial sources to lead to a conclusion that a new therapy is better than the standard therapy (Bekelman *et al.*, 2003; Lexchin *et al.*, 2003; Bhandari *et al.*, 2004; Chalmers, 2004). Commentators have pointed out that positive results are more likely to be published than negative ones and that industry-organized studies in which adverse effects of new drugs are discovered often remain unreported (Chan *et al.*, 2004; Chan and Altman, 2005; Chalmers, 2006).

Secondly, recent controversies have indicated how pharmaceutical sponsors and academic investigators have participated in the conscious control over, or even manipulation of, research questions and dissemination of results. Research is increasingly coordinated by specialized contract research organizations, which either conduct research in specialized research centers or involve a multitude of clinicians. Sponsors increasingly control the design of the study, the recruitment of subjects, the collection and analysis of data, and the publication of the results. The final results are often written by ghost authors, offered as easy publications to established academics and

published in the most prestigious medical journals (Healy and Cattell, 2003; Tereskerz, 2003; Angell, 2004; Lemmens, 2004). Academic authors are accustomed to giving credibility to publications. Instances of such practices are documented, for example, in a 2004 lawsuit of the Attorney General of New York against GlaxoSmithKline, which was settled out of court (*AG New York* v. *GlaxoSmithKline*, 2004; Lemmens, 2004).

Particularly when companies have already invested significantly in product development and expect to market a blockbuster drug in the near future, they have significant financial interest in emphasizing benefits more and harms less. Careful selection of comparators and overemphasis of positive findings is a tempting business strategy (Aronson, 2006). Concerns about biased reporting, lack of transparency, and research manipulation are not limited to commercially sponsored research, yet ample empirical evidence combined with various reports suggest that the problem is more prevalent in this area. This creates reasonable doubts about the validity of clinical treatment recommendations based only on publicly available data (Bhandari *et al.*, 2004; Marshall, 2004).

Distortion of the research agenda

The increase of industry funding and the growing commercial focus of funding agencies also has an impact on the health research agenda. Researchers funded to conduct research with a commercial focus are not available for other research endeavors. Since commercial sponsors are able to offer higher recruitment incentives to researchers and research subjects, it may become harder to launch other studies. Commercial interests also create incentives for pharmaceutical companies to conduct research that contributes to the creation of new categories of disease or that influence the level of diagnosis of existing illnesses (Lexchin, 2006; Moynihan and Henry, 2006; Tiefer, 2006).

It is less likely that research will be conducted on diseases affecting only few people ("orphan diseases'') or poor people (e.g., uninsured people in industrialized countries or the majority of people in developing countries). Proportionally less research funding is available to study the impact of other health factors, non-commercial products, or drugs that are no longer protected by patents.

Another cause for concern is that pharmaceutical sponsors are currently not required to conduct research on the long-term health effects of their products (Editorial, 2004; Lemmens, 2004). Indeed, they may have significant financial interests in avoiding long-term follow-up studies. If no one else is conducting these studies, significant adverse effects may remain undetected for a long period.

Policy

The nature of conflict of interest regulations

Clearly, commercial interests of research cannot justify exposing research subjects to direct harm. Researchers who include non-eligible subjects in a clinical trial because of the financial rewards involved clearly violate widely accepted ethical norms of research. In the same vein, those who participate in the falsification of research, or who misrepresent research findings, are guilty of research misconduct or fraud (Anon., 2002; Holden, 2005; Couzin and Unger, 2006; Cyranoski, 2006). In these cases, it is clear that moral culpability is associated with behavior that is per se reprehensible, whether it is stimulated by financial greed or not.

In reality, it is hard to determine whether and to what extent financial interests are the primary motive behind reprehensible behavior. It is impossible to enter into the mind of investigators. In the Gelsinger case, there is no direct evidence that the investigators acted because of financial gain. We can only identify the fact that there were huge financial interests at stake, and that there was research misconduct. Subtle influence of commercial funding of research is also possible. Involved

researchers may simply be unaware of the extent to which they are influenced by commercial interests in the research.

This explains the growing interest for precautionary approaches. They are based on the presumption that financial interests are likely to influence some to behave in ways that may expose people to risks or that may affect the integrity of research. Rules for COIs do not suggest that all those who are in COI situations are necessarily morally culpable. However, they reflect a growing awareness of the impact of COIs and of the need to set regulatory standards. A violation of these standards becomes an issue of professional misconduct. The sanctions associated with these rules are imposed not because subjects *are* directly harmed, or because the research they are involved with *is* fraudulent or bias, but because we know that this *can be* the result.

Regulatory remedies

Many universities, professional organizations, and medical journals have established guidelines that reflect the precautionary approach. Regulations for COIs are further introduced by drug regulatory and healthcare agencies. There is also growing attention for the use of criminal law and professional misconduct rules to deal with COIs (Kalb and Koehler, 2002; Lemmens and Miller, 2003). The procedural mechanisms introduced by these organizations and agencies include disclosure of COIs, review by research ethics committees (REC) or specialized COI committees, increased monitoring, and outright prohibition.

Disclosure is the most basic requirement. The idea behind disclosure is that people who have been informed of the existence of COI can make a well-informed judgement about its potential impact. Many medical journals have clear disclosure policies in place, obliging authors to reveal financial relations with sponsors (International Committee of Medical Journal Editors, 2006), although some established journals are still struggling to impose disclosure or to enforce their policies (Editorial, 2003; Brownlee, 2004; Armstrong, 2006a, b, c, d; Waters, 2006).

Disclosure is also a core component of respect for research subjects. Indeed, it seems crucial to disclose to those who accept at times significant risks in research the various interests that may impact on research. Yet some guidelines, such as those issued by the American Association of Medical Colleges (2001, 2002) and the US Department of Health and Human Services (2004), remain surprisingly vague about the requirement of disclosure and do not endorse a strict disclosure obligation. Instead, they give institutional authorities, such as RECs, leeway in determining when and to what extent financial interests ought to be disclosed (Lemmens and Miller, 2003). In our opinion, disclosure is a necessary although clearly not always sufficient condition for dealing with COI.

Disclosure is also the basis of other procedures. Academic institutions, journals, and funding agencies submit COI situations to a review process. Based on this review process, researchers can be told to disclose the conflicts, or to make required changes to, for example, the informed consent procedure. Such COI committees or RECs may further recommend that independent investigators be added to a research project, or that an independent data-monitoring committee be established to monitor the safety of clinical trials, analysis of data, and presentation of findings.

The financial COI may be deemed so significant that a prohibition is warranted. The American Association of Medical Colleges (2001, 2002), for example, recommends that institutions introduce in their COI policies a rebuttable presumption that researchers with significant financial interests ought not to be involved in the research, and that institutions with significant interests ought not to have research take place in their establishments.

Finally, COIs may be the subject of specific prohibitions. Various academic centers, for example, have issued guidelines prohibiting the use of finder's fees (Lemmens and Miller, 2003). Researchers who violate these guidelines can be held accountable by their institution for these violations.

Novel approaches

Many of these remedies have been in place for some time without preventing major controversies. Several authors have called for more radical and stricter COI approaches. For example, to counter the overall impact of financial interests on the focus of research, some have suggested that public funding for research should be significantly increased (Downie, 2006; Lemmens, 2006), or even that research on healthcare products should be fully publicly funded (Brown, 2000, 2006).

To deal with the phenomenon of ghost authorship (Flanagin et al., 1998), stricter sanctions have been proposed. Two medical journals have announced that they would ban those who have been involved in submitting a ghost-authored article from submitting new articles for several years (Brownlee, 2004). Others have recommended that more details ought to be provided as to who contributed to a study and that academic institutions ought to diminish the focus on quantity of publications in the assessment of academic performance and ought to recognize better other contributions to research (Davidoff, 2000).

Commentators and official reports have pointed out that the regulatory structures set up to deal with COIs are themselves affected by COIs and are in need of significant reform (Office of the Inspector General, 2000; Institute of Medicine, 2001; Lemmens, 2004; Viens and Savulescu, 2004; Ferris and Naylor, 2006). For example, REBs are increasingly expected to deal with COIs while they are themselves affected by COIs and are in need of significant reform. It is also not clear that internal COI committees are independent enough to curb significant institutional COIs.

The idea of mandatory registration of clinical trials has also been gaining ground. This would track trials before they begin, which would avoid secrecy and ensure full reporting of results. Registration is already a regulatory requirement in the

USA for all clinical trials involving serious and life-threatening diseases. It has been recommended by the International Committee of Medical Journal Editors (2006; see also De Angelis *et al.*, 2005) a group of international experts (Krleža-Jerić *et al.*, 2005), and the World Health Organization (2006a,b,c). Participation in clinical registration is a major step toward transparency and accountability (Horion, 2006; Sim *et al.*, 2006) but should not be regarded as a panacea to COI concerns (Lemmens, 2004).

Another more drastic suggestion is to separate those who conduct medical research from those who have a financial interest in the outcome of the research through the establishment of a new drug-testing agency (Krimsky, 2003; Angell, 2004; Lemmens, 2004). The agency, in dialogue with the submitting company, would determine the appropriate design of clinical trials aimed at testing efficacy and safety of the new compound and would rely on independent accredited drug-testing centers to conduct the trials and analyze the results.

How should I approach financial conflict of interest in research in practice?

The mounting evidence and exposures of the impact of financial COIs should alert for clinician researchers. Disclosure of financial interests to RECs, COI committees, research subjects, and in publications is necessary although not sufficient. Clinician–researchers should help to promote in their institutions a system of oversight that incorporates regulation, includes assessment and analysis independent of commercial interests, protects patients from harm, improves transparency in clinical research, and contributes to restoring public trust.

Clinician–researchers should obviously respect institutional COI policies and procedures. They should consult with professional organizations and institutions when they are in doubt about how to deal with COIs. They should refuse to be involved in research fully controlled by sponsors and should insist on full access to the data before accepting to sign on to any publications reporting the results

of the study. Institutions should develop more stringent COI policies and should have the courage to prohibit research projects when personal or institutional financial interests may impact or appear to impact on the integrity of the research. They should also be willing to sanction those who violate COI policies. It is, for example, remarkable that so many instances of ghost authorship have been documented, yet that no significant sanctions have been enacted.

Clinician–researchers ought not to rely on institutional policies and initiatives alone. Increased vigilance, informing oneself about the empirical evidence on COIs, and educational initiatives to explore and resolve financial COIs may all help in the long run to create a new research culture and to restore integrity in research. Clinician–researchers ought to critically determine how they can best contribute to promote independent and socially relevant medical research. Finally, clinical investigators ought to ensure that clinical trials in which they participate are registered, even if it is rarely a legal requirement at this point in time.

The case

The research contract signed by the institution and Dr. H gives the sponsor too much control over future publications. Although it is common to allow the sponsors to see the results before final publication and provide time for the potential filing of patent applications, sponsors ought not to be given the power to prevent publications. Dr. H should refuse to sign this stipulation and the institutional review should also screen out these clauses. In addition, clinician–researchers have a primary ethical and professional obligation to ensure the well-being of research subjects. When in their professional opinion, safety is at stake, they have to disclose this to research subjects and to their colleagues regardless of contractual clauses (Thompson *et al.*, 2001; Viens and Savulescu, 2004).

Dr. H is in a difficult position to enforce his obligations. Clearly, he should not be swayed by

Dr. I's assertions and promises. He should contact the chair of the REC over his concerns related to the safety of the product tested and people higher up in the hierarchy of the institution with respect to the pressure put on him. Dr. I's personal interests and the relationship between the institution and the sponsor reveal a significant institutional COI. The potential impact of these institutional interests ought to have been evaluated by the REC or a COI committee before the research started.

At a minimum, the institution ought to investigate what happened and ought to support Dr. H fully in pressing for access to the full data and withdrawal of the abstract. If the conference is organized by a professional organization, that organization ought also to investigate allegations of ghost authorship and misrepresentation. If no support is forthcoming and institutional support is lacking, Dr. H has an ethical obligation to go public. This may come at a high personal and professional cost, as indicated by several recent controversies (Thompson *et al.*, 2001; Viens and Savulescu, 2004; Revill, 2005). In an increasingly commercialized research context, professional organizations, academic institutions, and governments ought to develop adequate procedures to evaluate allegations of misconduct and appropriate remedies to protect whistle-blowers.

Dr. H ought not to have accepted the finder's fees and competitive enrollment fees provided for in the budget and the REC ought to also have spotted these. Although it is appropriate to remunerate clinicians for the work they perform for the study – these services ought not to be covered as a clinical service by the healthcare system – financial perks for mere recruitment are unacceptable.

REFERENCES

AG New York v. *GlaxoSmithKline* (2004). http://www4. dr-rath-foundation.org/pdf-files/nyglaxo21303cmp.pdf (accessed 19 July 2006).

American Association of Medical Colleges (2001). *Task Force on Financial Conflicts of Interest in Clinical Research. Protecting Subjects, Preserving Trust, Promoting Progress: Policy and Guidelines for the Oversight of Individual Financial Conflict of Interest in Human Subjects Research*. Washington, DC: American Association of Medical Colleges (http://www.aamc.org/research/coi/start.htm) accessed 17 July 2006.

American Association of Medical Colleges (2002). *Task Force on Financial Conflicts of Interest in Clinical Research. Protecting Subjects, Preserving Trust, Promoting Progress II: Principles and Recommendations for Oversight of an Institution's Financial Interests in Human Subjects Research*. Washington, DC: American Association of Medical Colleges (http://www.aamc.org/research/coi/start.htm) accessed 17 July 2006.

Anon. (2002). Scientific fraud. Outside the bell curve. A major scientific fraud has just been confirmed. *Economist*, 26 September.

Angell, M. (2004). *The Truth about the Pharmaceutical Industry; How They Deceive us and What To Do About It*. New York: Random House.

Armstrong, D. (2006a). Financial ties to industry cloud major depression study; at issue: whether it's safe for pregnant women to stay on medication. *JAMA* asks authors to explain. *Wall Street Journal* 11 July, A1 (http://online.wsj.com/article/SB115257995935002947.html) accessed 19 July 2006.

Armstrong, D. (2006b). *JAMA* to toughen rules on author disclosure. *Wall Street Journal* 12 July B2.

Armstrong, D. (2006c). Medical journal to issue correction on review of depression treatment. *Wall Street Journal*, 18 July (http://online.wsj.com/article/SB115322997681109756.html) accessed 19 July 2006.

Armstrong, D. (2006d). Medical reviews face criticism over lapses. *Wall Street Journal* 19 July, B1 (http://online.wsj.com/article/SB115322997681109756.html) accessed 19 July 2006.

Aronson, J. K. (2006). Industry-sponsored research: an editor's view. In *Proceedings of a Workshop on Patients, Physicians and Pharma: Divergent or Congruent Approaches to the Individual and Society*, April 2006, Haifa, Israel.

Atkinson-Grosjean, J. (2006). *Public Science Private Interests: Culture and Commerce in Canada's Networks of Centres of Excellence*. Toronto: University of Toronto Press.

Bayh-Dole Act 1980. Pub. L. No. 96–517, s.6(a), 94 Stat.3015, 3019–281980 (codified as amended at 35 U.S. C. ss.200-121994).

Bekelman, J. E., Li, Y., and Gross, C. P. (2003). Scope and impact of financial conflicts of interest in biomedical research. *JAMA* **289**: 462–3.

Bhandari, M., Busse, J. W., Jackowski, D., *et al.* (2004). Association between industry funding and statistically significant pro-industry findings in medical and surgical randomized trials. *CMAJ* **170**: 477–80.

Brown, J. R. (2000). Privatizing the university: the new tragedy of the commons. *Science* **290**: 1701–2.

Brown, J. R. (2006). Self-censorship. In *Law and Ethics in Biomedical Research: Regulation, Conflict of Interest, and Liability*, ed. T. Lemmens and D. R. Waring. Toronto: University of Toronto Press, pp. 82–94.

Brownlee, S. (2004). Doctors without borders. *Washington Monthly* **36**: 38–43.

Canadian Institutes for Health Research (2001). *Revolution – CIHR: Towards a National Health Research Agenda.* Ottawa: Canadian Institutes for Health Research (http://www.cihr-irsc.gc.ca/e/26539.html) accessed 17 July 2006.

Canadian Institutes for Health Research (2005). *Transforming Health Research in Canada.* Ottawa: Canadian Institutes for Health Research (http://www.cihr-irsc.gc.ca/e/documents/cbj_supplement_e.pdf) accessed 17 July 2006.

Chalmers, I. (2006). From optimism to disillusion about commitment to transparency in the medico-industrial complex. *J R Soc Med* **99**: 337–41.

Chalmers, I. (2004). In the dark. Drug companies should be forced to publish all the results of clinical trials. How else can we know the truth about their products? *New Scientist*, 19.

Chan, A.-W. and Altman, D. G. (2005). Identifying outcome reporting bias in randomized trials on *PubMed*: review of publications and survey of authors. *BMJ* **330**: 753–8.

Chan, A.-W., Krleža-Jerić, K., Schmid, I., and Altman, D. G. (2004). Outcome reporting bias in randomized controlled trials funded by the Canadian Institutes of Health Research. *CMAJ* **171**: 735–40.

Couzin, J. and Unger, K. (2006). Scientific misconduct. Cleaning up the paper trail. *Science* **312**: 38–43.

Cyranoski, D. (2006). Veredict: Hwang's human stem cells were all fakes. *Nature* **439**: 122–3.

Davidoff, F. (2000). Who's the author? Problems with biomedical authorship, and some possible solutions. *Report to the Council of Science Editors, Task Force on Authorship.* Reston, VA: Council of Science Editors (http://www.councilscienceeditors.org/publications/v23n4p111-119.pdf) accessed 17 July 2006.

De Angelis, C. D., Drazen, J. M., Frizell, F. A., *et al.* (2005). Is this clinical trial registered? A statement from the International Committee of Medical Journal Editors. *Lancet* **365**: 1827–9.

Downie, J. (2006). Grasping the nettle: confronting the issue of competing interests and obligation in health research policy. In *Just Medicare: What's In, What's Out, How We Decide*, ed. C. M. Flood. Toronto: University of Toronto Press, pp. 427–448.

Downie, J., Baird, P., and Thompson, J. (2002). Industry and the academy: conflicts of interest in contemporary health research. *Health Law J* **10**: 103–22.

Editorial (2003). Financial disclosures for review authors. *Nat Neurosci* **6**: 997.

Editorial (2004). Vioxx: An unequal partnership between safety and efficacy. *Lancet* **364**: 1288.

Eisenberg, R. (2003). The Robert L. Levine distinguished lecture series. Patents, product exclusivity and information dissemination: how law directs biopharmaceutical research and development. *Fordham Law Rev* **2**: 477.

Emanuel, E. J. and Steiner, D. (1995). Institutional conflict of interest. *N Engl J Med* **332**: 262–7.

Ferris, L. E. and Naylor, C. D. (2006). Promoting integrity in industry-sponsored clinical drug trials: conflict of interest issues for Canadian health science centers. In *Law and Ethics in Biomedical Research: Regulation, Conflict of Interest, and Liability*, ed. T. Lemmens and D. R. Waring. Toronto: University of Toronto Press, pp. 95–131.

Flanagin, A., Carey, L. A., Fontanarosa, P. B., *et al.* (1998). Prevalence of articles with honorary authors and ghost authors in peer-reviewed medical journals. *JAMA* **280**: 222–4.

Gelsinger, P. L. (2006). Uninformed consent: the case of Jesse Gelsinger. In *Law and Ethics in Biomedical Research: Regulation, Conflict of Interest, and Liability*, ed. T. Lemmens and D. R. Waring. Toronto: University of Toronto Press, pp. 12–32.

Healy, D. (2002). Conflicting interests in Toronto: anatomy of a controversy at the interface of academia and medicine. *Persp Biol Med* **45**: 250–63.

Healy, D. and Cattell, D. (2003). Interface between authorship, industry and science in the domain of therapeutics. *Br J Psychol* **183**: 22–7.

Holden, C. (2005). Stem cell research. Korean cloner admits lying about oocyte donations. *Science* **310**: 1402–3.

Horion, R. (2006). Trial registers: protecting patients, advancing trust. *Lancet* **367**: 1633–5.

Institute of Medicine (2001). Committee on Assessing the System for Protecting Human Research Participants.

Responsible Research: A Systems Approach to Protecting Research Participants. Washington, DC: National Academies Press.

International Committee of Medical Journal Editors (2006). *Uniform Requirements for Manuscripts Submitted to Biomedical Journals: Writing and Editing for Biomedical Publication.* Philadelphia, PA: American College of Physicians (http://www.icmje.org/) accessed 17 July 2006.

Kalb, P. E. and Koehler, K. G. (2002). Legal issues in scientific research. *JAMA* **287**: 85.

Krimsky, S. (2003). *Science in the Private Interest: Has the Lure of Profits Corrupted Biomedical Research?* Lanhan: Rowman and Littlefield.

Krimsky, S. (2006). The ethical and legal foundations of scientific ''Conflict of Interest.'' In *Law and Ethics in Biomedical Research: Regulation, Conflict of Interest, and Liability*, eds. T. Lemmens and D. R. Waring. Toronto: University of Toronto Press, pp. 63–81.

Krleža-Jerić, K., Chan, A.-W., Dickersin, K., *et al.* (2005). Principles for international registration of protocol information and results from human trials of health related interventions: Ottawa statement (part 1). *BMJ* **330**: 956–8.

Lemmens, T. (2004). Leopards in the temple: restoring scientific integrity to the commercialized research scene. *J Law Med Ethics* **32**: 641–57.

Lemmens, T. (2006). Commercialized medical research and the need for regulatory reform. In *Just Medicare: What's In, What's Out, How We Decide*, ed. C. M. Flood. Toronto: University of Toronto Press, pp. 396–426.

Lemmens, T. and Miller, P. B. (2003). The human subjects trade: ethical and legal issues surrounding recruitment incentives. *J Law Med Ethics* **31**: 398–418.

Lexchin, J. (2006). Bigger and better: how Pfizer redefined erectile dysfunction. *PLoS Med* **3**: 429–32 (e132).

Lexchin, J., Berg, L. A., Djulbegovic, B., and Clark, O. (2003). Pharmaceutical sponsorship and research outcome and quality: systemic review. *BMJ* **326**: 1167–77.

Marshall, E. (2004). Antidepressants and children; buried data can be hazardous to a company's health. *Science* **304**: 1576–7.

Moynihan, R. and Henry, D. (2006). The fight against disease mongering: generating knowledge for action. *PLoS Med* **3**: 425–8 (e191).

Office of Inspector General (2000). *Recruiting Human Subjects: Pressures in Industry-Sponsored Research.* Washington DC: Department of Health and Human Services.

Revill, J. (2005). How the drug giant and a lone academic went to war. *The Observer*, 4 December (http://education.guardian.co.uk/businessofresearch/story/0,1658042,00.html) accessed 17 July 2006.

Silberner, J. (2000). A gene therapy death. *Hastings Cent Rep* **30**: 6.

Sim, I., Chen, A.-W., Gulmezoglu, A. M., Evans, T., and Pang, T. (2006). Clinical trial registration: transparency is the watchword. *Lancet* **367**: 1631–3.

Tereskerz, P. M. (2003). Research accountability and financial conflicts of interest in industry-sponsored clinical research: a review. *Account Res* **10**: 137–58.

Thompson, D. F. (1993). Understanding financial conflicts of interest. *N Engl J Med* **8**: 573–6.

Thompson, J., Baird, P., and Downie, J. (2001). *The Olivieri Report.* Toronto: James Lorimer.

Tiefer, L. (2006). Female sexual disfunction: a case study of disease mongering and activist resistance. *PLoS Med* **3**: 436–40 (e178).

UK House of Commons Health Committee (2005). *Fourth Report of Session 2004–2005*, Vol. 1: *The Influence of the Pharmaceutical Industry.* London: The Stationery Office (http://www.publications.parliament.uk/pa/cm200405/cmselect/cmhealth/42/42.pdf) accessed 31 July 2006.

US Department of Health and Human Services (2004). *Financial Relationships and Interests in Research Involving Human Subjects: Guidance for Human Subject Protection.* [Federal Register 69, 26393–26397.] Washington, DC: Government Printing Office.

Viens, A. M. and Savulescu, J. (2004). Introduction to the Olivieri Symposium. *J Med Ethics* **30**: 1–7.

Waters, R. (2006). Medical journal to correct cyberonics device article. *Bloomberg News* 8 July.

World Health Organization (2006a). *International Clinical Trials Registry Platform. Open Comments.* [Series 2.1, 27 January.] Geneva: World Health Organization (http://www.who.int/ictrp/comments/en/index2.html) accessed 17 July 2006.

World Health Organization (2006b). *International Clinical Trials Registry Platform. Trial Registration Data Set.* Geneva: World Health Organization (http://www.who.int/ictrp/data_set/en/index1.html) accessed 17 July 2006.

World Health Organization (2006c). *International Clinical Trials Registry Platform. Open Comments.* [Series 2.2, 5 April.] Geneva: World Health Organization (http://www.who.int/ctrp/comments/en/index3.html) accessed 17 July 2006.

31

Embryo and fetal research

Ronald M. Green

The year is 2016. J and K meet with their pediatrician to discuss whether their 11-year-old daughter, L, should undergo a newly available course of stem cell therapy to cure her type 1 juvenile diabetes. Left untreated, L's illness could lead to blindness, life-threatening circulation problems in her extremities, and, perhaps, early death. The therapy that L's parents and her pediatrician are contemplating requires careful HLA (immunological compatibility) matching with one of the thousands of human embryonic stem cell (hESC) lines identified in an international registry. These were created over the previous decade from frozen human embryos remaining from infertility procedures and were donated to research or therapy by their progenitors. A matching population of specially created pancreatic stem cells could be made from one of these lines and infused into L to remedy her insulin deficit. While many parents would leap at this life-saving opportunity, J and K – and their physician – face a moral quandary. They are all devout Roman Catholics and share their church's view that human life must be regarded as sacred from the moment of conception. They view the destruction of a human embryo for stem cell research or therapy as equivalent to killing a human being. The physician explains to J and K that the frozen human embryos used to create hESC lines were slated for destruction. Is it not better, he asks, that such embryos at least be used to save lives? But J and K are also aware of their church's moral teaching that "one should not do evil in order that good may result."

What is fetal and embryo research?

Any research that uses human embryonic or fetal tissues, or that implicates living human embryos or fetuses, comes under the heading of embryo or fetal research. Such research can be direct or indirect. The use of living human embryos to derive a line of embryonic stem cells is an example of direct research on the embryo, as is research on a non-viable fetus that has survived abortion or miscarriage. Research aimed at the healthcare needs of a pregnant woman that could inadvertently affect the embryo or fetus she is carrying is an example of indirect research.

Because different questions can arise depending on whether research involves embryos or fetuses, it is important to state what we mean by the fetus or embryo. For scientific purposes, the embryo is usually defined as the product of conception until eight weeks of gestation. From that point onward, the term fetus is used. However, these definitions are not pertinent to the major legal and ethical debates about research. The important distinction here is between entities produced by in vitro fertilization (IVF) and existing outside the womb and those that have implanted in a womb, where research necessarily implicates the gestational mother. Following

This chapter is adapted from: Green, R.M. (2008). Research with fetuses, embryos, and stem cells. In *The Oxford Textbook of Clinical Research Ethics*, ed. E.J., Emanuel, G., Grady, R., Lie, F., Miller, and D. Wendler. New York: Oxford University Press, in press.

Tauer (2004) and others (Gratton, 2002, p. 17), I will define the embryo as "the product of conception (whether produced in vitro or flushed from a uterus) as it exists in the laboratory and that has not undergone transfer to a woman." The fetus is "the product of conception existing in a womb" and comprises both in vivo embryos and fetuses. These definitions bypass the question of the organism's developmental stage. However, since it is not possible to culture an embryo in vitro for more than five or six days, a limit not likely to be exceeded soon, the term "embryo" as used here describes the early product of conception, a mass of largely undifferentiated cells with no bodily form or organs, while the term fetus usually refers to a more developed entity undergoing organogenesis and possessing an incipient nervous system.

A further question is when an embryo can be said to have come into being. Although many people speak of the "moment of conception," it is now well established that conception/fertilization is not a discrete event but a process that takes places over many hours or days (President's Council on Bioethics, 2004). There are at least several candidate "events" for conception/fertilization, ranging from sperm penetration of the egg to syngamy, the lining up of male and female pronuclei inside the egg, almost a day later. The choice among these can significantly alter our moral and legal conclusions with regard to specific research protocols. It is important to recognize that a biologically and morally informed choice is necessary here and that conception/fertilization is not the "bright line" that many people believe it is.

A different problem concerns the nature and moral status of the entities produced by nuclear transfer cloning technology. This approach, known as therapeutic cloning, is being researched for the production of immunologically compatible stem cell lines. It involves inserting a patient's own cell into an enucleated egg, and chemically or electrically stimulating the egg to divide like one that has been normally fertilized. The resulting embryo is then disaggregated to produce a stem cell line that can be used for tissue repair or organ replacement in the original cell donor without rejection (Lanza et al., 2000). Since the entity produced in this way has never been fertilized by a sperm, some ask whether it should even be regarded as a human embryo (Kiessling, 2001). Richard Hurlbut, an opponent of human embryonic stem cell research, has also recently proposed using cloning technology combined with genetic engineering to produce an embryo incapable of developing beyond the earliest stages of growth, an approach known as "altered nuclear transfer" (President's Council on Bioethics, 2005). Since this developmentally incompetent embryo could never become a human being, Hurlbut argues, its destruction for stem cell purposes would not be morally objectionable (Cook, 2004). Others have criticized these alternatives as definitionally inadequate or as not really eliminating the moral objections to human embryonic stem cell research (Melton et al., 2004).

Why is embryo and fetal research important and how should I approach it in practice?

Research directed primarily at the health needs of fertile or pregnant women is likely to implicate a developing fetus. In such cases, it is necessary to balance possible risks and benefits for the woman with risks or benefits to the fetus. This consideration has long made fetal research an important area of ethical inquiry, leading to regulations in many jurisdictions that seek to balance maternal and fetal claims. Direct research on the fetus has also been pursued in the effort to reduce the incidence of miscarriages or birth defects. Specific health problems affecting embryos or fetuses, such as the impacts of drugs, diagnostics, nutrition, or regimens of prenatal care have required direct fetal research with its attendant ethical questions. Recently, in utero fetal surgery for spina bifida has raised questions concerning how we should balance maternal and fetal claims in a research or clinical context (Howe, 2003; Bliton, 2005).

Fetal tissue transplantation research has also long been an object of medical interest. Fetal neural tissue has been used, with mixed results, in the treatment of Parkinson disease and other neurological disorders (Freed *et al.*, 2001). With the discovery that fetal germ cells are able to differentiate into a variety of other tissues (Shamblott *et al.*, 1998), the issues raised by fetal tissue transplantation research have reappeared in connection with embryonic stem cell research.

Today, the most intensely debated issues arise in connection with human embryonic stem cell research. The creation of stem cell lines for use in regenerative medicine research currently requires the destruction of human embryos. This raises questions about the moral status of the early human embryo and when, if ever, nascent human life may be sacrificed for the medical benefit of children and adults. Research is underway on non-destructive methods of stem cell derivation (Chung, 2006), and, as mentioned above, some theorists have offered controversial proposals for alternative ways of generating stem cells that they believe could reduce or eliminate the moral issues raised by embryo destruction (President's Council on Bioethics, 2005). However, the availability of tens of thousands of frozen embryos remaining from infertility treatments as a resource for stem cell research suggests that this issue will not go away. In addition, researching some of these alternatives may require the destruction of human embryos.

Ethics

Fetal research

Three distinct research areas come under the heading of fetal research: (i) direct research on the fetus itself, (ii) research directed toward pregnant women or the condition of pregnancy (for which the fetus is an indirect subject of research), and (iii) fetal tissue transplantation research. For each of these research areas, current US regulations identify the major moral issues involved and, with one or two exceptions, also reflect the international moral consensus on these issues (Green, 2002a).

Where direct research on the fetus itself is concerned, the US *Code of Federal Regulations* distinguishes between research of medical benefit to a particular fetus and research not to its benefit. In the former case, the risks must be "the least possible for achieving the objectives of the research" (US Department of Health and Human Services, 2005). In the latter case, institutional review boards can approve a protocol if the risk to the fetus is not greater than minimal and the purpose of the research is the development of important biomedical knowledge that cannot be obtained by any other means. Examples are minor changes in maternal diet or the use of ultrasonography.

Regulations in the USA, and most other nations, do not distinguish between a fetus destined for abortion and one meant to be carried to term. At first sight, it might seem reasonable to permit some degree of increased risk when the termination of the pregnancy is in prospect and when useful research can be done. An example is an experiment to see whether an agent likely to cause birth defects passes through the placenta. However, endangering the fetus in such cases will either limit a woman's freedom to change her mind about the abortion or will result in harm to a born child if she should choose to continue the pregnancy. The unacceptability of either of these alternatives counsels a standard of similar treatment of all fetuses.

Direct research on the fetus can also take place on the fetus outside the womb following a spontaneous or induced abortion. A viable fetus is treated by existing US regulations as a premature infant and comes under the protections of regulations governing research on children or newborns. A non-viable fetus (or neonate) may be involved in research only if (i) the vital functions of the neonate will not be artificially maintained, (ii) the research will not terminate the heartbeat or respiration of the neonate, (iii) there will be no added risk to the neonate resulting from the research, and (iv) the purpose of the research is the development of important biomedical knowledge that cannot be obtained by other means (US Department of Health and Human Services, 2005).

Since fetuses normally have male and female progenitors, the question arises as to whose consent is required for such research. The need for the mother's consent is evident and is recognized in all jurisdictions. Perhaps reflecting heated debates in the USA on maternal–paternal consent for abortion, the father, as co-progenitor, is also required to consent on behalf of the fetus. However, federal regulations permit three exceptions to this rule: if the father is unavailable, incompetent or temporarily incapacitated, or the pregnancy resulted from rape or incest (US Department of Health and Human Services, 2005).

Research directed at women who are pregnant can also indirectly affect the fetus. The US federal regulations specify that no pregnant woman may be involved as a research subject unless either (i) the purpose of the activity is to meet the health needs of the mother, and the fetus will be placed at risk only to the minimum extent necessary to meet such needs; or (ii) the risk to the fetus is minimal (US Department of Health and Human Services, 2005). Since some procedures, drugs, or dosage levels may enhance maternal outcomes while increasing fetal risk, these regulations can require institutional review boards to weigh the mother's welfare against that of the fetus.

Fetal transplantation research is currently allowed in many jurisdictions, including the USA and UK. Since the mid 1990s, a strong international consensus has emerged about the conditions for good clinical practice regarding this (de Wert et al., 2002). These aim at separating the motives and timing for the abortion decision from the decision to donate fetal tissue, and they preclude commercialization of the tissue. There are voices that entirely reject this international consensus on the grounds that fetal tissue transplantation either encourages abortion or involves wrongful complicity in it. The Roman Catholic Church and some conservative Protestant groups hold these views (de Wert et al., 2002).

Embryo research

Public debate about embryo research began in earnest in 1978 with the birth of Louise Brown, the world's first "test tube" baby. The development of IVF made the early, ex utero embryo a possible research "subject," but, additionally, the rapid growth of infertility medicine created demand for more successful and less risky infertility treatments, intensifying the demand for embryo research (Green, 2001). The development of the first human embryonic stem cell lines by James Thomson and John Gearhart in 1998 (Thomson et al., 1998; Shamblott et al., 1998) opened up new uses for human embryos in the area of regenerative medicine research.

Unlike fetal research, where the welfare of born children and women complicates matters, embryo research unavoidably raises the question of how much protection nascent human life deserves. Two main ethical answers to this question have been proposed. One, strongly associated with the views of conservative religious groups, holds that human life deserves full moral protection from conception onward. This places the earliest embryo (and fetus) on a plane of equality with child and adult subjects and rules out embryo research that is not medically to the benefit of the embryo under study (Sacred Congregation for the Doctrine of the Faith, 1974; Pontifical Academy for Life, 2000).

Opposing this position is a range of views that can be termed "gradualist" or "developmental." Some views stress the moral importance of qualities like sentience, brain activity, the presence of substantial bodily form, or the ability to survive independently of the mother (viability). Others emphasize not one but a variety of considerations that, taken together, compel us to extend protections (NIH Human Embryo Research Panel, 1994; Warren, 1997). What all these views have in common is the belief that the moral weight of the embryo and fetus is not established once and for all, but rather it increases over the course of a pregnancy as additional morally significant features make their appearance. Most who hold this view are willing to permit embryo research, including research that destroys the embryo, up to 14 days of development. At that time, the primitive streak appears, organ formation begins, and further morally significant developmental events cannot be ruled out.

Law

Most legal jurisdictions permit carefully regulated direct or indirect research on the human fetus and many also permit fetal tissue transplantation research. The legal treatment of human embryo research is much more diverse. In 1990, the British Parliament passed the Human Fertilisation and Embryology Act, which led to the establishment of the Human Fertilisation and Embryology Authority, an official government agency that provides oversight and guidance for clinical and research programs in infertility medicine. In its current activities, the agency oversees and licenses all clinical infertility programs in the UK, as well as research on human embryos. Regulations in the UK are at once the most comprehensive and the most permissive in the world. Embryo research is permitted for a wide variety of reasons (Human Fertilisation and Embryology Authority, 2003), and therapeutic cloning research is allowed.

The situation in the USA is very different. Federal funding for any research requiring the destruction of human embryos is prohibited by law (Green, 2001). At the same time, except for some restrictive state laws, private sector research on embryos in the US is unregulated, unlike the UK where all research falls under the authority of the government agency. Despite this relative research freedom, the absence of federal support for human embryo research in the USA, a country with over 450 infertility programs, has contributed to the inefficiency and high cost of IVF (Neumann *et al.*, 1994; Chambers *et al.*, 2006). It has also increased the risks to women undergoing these procedures (Rossing *et al.*, 1994; Rebar, 2002) and the children produced by them (Jones and Schnom, 2001; Kovalesky *et al.*, 2003; Powell, 2003). The US regulations have blocked most federal funding for human embryonic stem cell research and slowed the pace of that research (Dreifus, 2006).

Similar diversity of legislation is also evident on the international scene. Some nations (for example, Israel, Singapore, China, and India) permit or even fund embryonic stem cell research, while others (Ireland, Italy, and Germany) forbid it (Hoffman, 2004). Religion is a driving force in these differences. Nations with large Roman Catholic or evangelical Christian populations tend to oppose human embryonic stem cell research, whereas nations with non-Christian populations or fewer conservative Protestants or Catholics tend to be more supportive (Walters, 2004).

Policy

Since it is unlikely that moral positions on fetal or embryo research will change in the near future, a resolution of these debates may partly hinge on a series of science and technology policy determinations. Among these is the possibility of developing alternatives to the use of human embryos or fetuses in regenerative medicine research. This might include the use of adult stem cells or alternatives to the derivation of stem cells from spare human embryos. Recently, there has been considerable debate about the viability of these alternatives as a way of bypassing the current stem cell impasse and, in the USA, legislation has been proposed to encourage these directions (Hulse, 2006).

A second policy issue raised by embryo research concerns which considerations should guide public policy. Is it possible to separate one's personal moral or religious views from the question of what should be appropriate public policy in a democratic society where citizens hold very different moral beliefs?

Finally, those who oppose research involving the destruction of embryos or fetuses will have to determine the extent to which they are prepared to benefit from the fruits of this research. Are they prepared to use stem cell lines derived from human embryos or vaccines made with fetal tissues? At what point does *use* become *complicity* and how does one form public policy in this area (Green, 2002b)? Germany and Italy currently ban the derivation of embryonic stem cell lines, but permit the clinical or research use of lines created before the dates that these bans went into effect. Although US President George Bush opposes research destroying human embryos, he authorized the use of stem cell lines created before the imposition of his restrictive policy. These and other cases reveal how complex are the issues raised by morally controversial but potentially beneficial research.

The case

Now that embryonic stem cells have demonstrated curative potential, J and K and their physician will have to re-examine the bases of their opposition to the medical uses of human embryonic stem cells. Does the privileging of early embryos over more developed human beings really make sense? The pediatrician can also play a useful role by making clear how pervasive and difficult is the question of the extent to which we are prepared to help ourselves or others by using the fruits of deeds we morally oppose. For example, versions of the polio vaccine, which most citizens hailed as a major advance in human health, were prepared from cell cultures grown on the tissues of aborted fetuses. Each individual must determine where he or she will draw the line between benefiting from wrongful deeds and complicity in them.

REFERENCES

Bliton, M. (2005). Parental hope confronting scientific uncertainty: a test of ethics in maternal–fetal surgery for spina bifida. *Clin Obstet Gynecol* **48**: 595–607.

Chambers, G. M., Ho, M. T., and Sullivan, E. A. (2006). Assisted reproductive technology treatment costs of a live birth: an age-stratified cost–outcome study of treatment in Australia. *Med J Aust* **184**: 155–8 (http://www.mja.com.au/public/rop/chambers/cha10890_fm.html).

Chung, Y. (2006). Embryonic and extraembryonic stem cell lines derived from single mouse blastomeres. *Nature* **439**: 216–19.

Cook, G. (2004). New technique eyes in stem-cell debate. *Boston Globe*, 21 November, A1.

de Wert, G., Berghmans, R. L., Boer, G. J., *et al.* (2002). Ethical guidance on human embryonic and fetal tissue transplantation: a European overview. *Med Health Care Philos* **5**: 79–90.

Dreifus, C. (2006). At Harvard's stem cell center, the barriers run deep and wide. *New York Times*, 24 January.

Freed, C. R., Greene, P. E., Breeze, R. E., *et al.* (2001). Transplantation of embryonic dopamine neurons for severe Parkinson's disease. *N Engl J Med* **344**: 710–19.

Gratton B, for the European Group on Ethics in Science and New Technologies to the European Commission. (2002). *Survey on the National Regulations in the European Union Regarding Research on Human Embryos.* Brussels: European Union. http://ec.europa.eu/european_group_ethics/publications/docs/nat_reg_en.pdf.

Green, R. M. (2001). *The Human Embryo Research Debates: Bioethics in the Vortex of Controversy.* New York: Oxford University Press.

Green, R. M. (2002a). Research involving fetuses and in vitro fertilization. In *Institutional Review Board: Management and Function*, ed. R. J. Amdur and E. A. Bankert. Sudbury, MA: Jones and Bartlett, pp. 373–9.

Green, R. M. (2002b). Benefiting from "evil"; an incipient moral problem in human stem cell research. *Bioethics* **16**: 544–56.

Hoffman, W. (2004). Stem cell policy: world stem cell map. Delaware, MN: MBBNet (http://mbbnet.umn.edu/scmap.html).

Howe, E. G. (2003). Ethical issue in fetal surgery. *Semin Perinatol* **27**: 446–57.

Hulse, C. (2006). Senate approves a stem-cell bill; veto is expected. *New York Times*, 19 July.

Human Fertilisation and Embryology Authority (2003). *Code of Practice*, 6th edn, 10.2. London: Human Fertilisation and Embryology Authority (http://www.hfea.gov.uk/HFEAPublications/CodeofPractice/Code%20of%).

Jones, H. W., Jr. and Schnom, J. A. (2001). Multiple pregnancies: a call for action. *Fert Steril* **75**: 11–17.

Kiessling, A. A. (2001). In the stem-cell debate, new concepts need new words. *Nature* **413**: 453.

Kovalesky, G., Rinaudo, P., and Coutifaris, C. (2003). Do assisted reproductive technologies cause adverse fetal outcomes? *Fert Steril* **79**: 1270–2.

Lanza, R. M., Caplan, A. L., Silver, R. M., *et al.* (2000). The ethical validity of using nuclear transfer In human transplantation. *JAMA* **284**: 3175–9.

Melton, D., Daley, G., and Jennings, C. G. (2004). Altered nuclear transfer in stem-cell research: a flawed proposal. *N Engl J Med* **351**: 2791–2.

Neumann, P. J., Gharib, S. D., and Weinstein, M. C. (1994). The cost of a successful delivery with in vitro fertilization. *N Engl J Med* **331**: 239–43.

NIH Human Embryo Research Panel (1994). *The Human Embryo Research Report*, Vols. I and II. Bethesda, MD: National Institutes of Health (http://ospp.od.nih.gov/pdf/volume1_revised.pdf).

Pontifical Academy for Life (2000). *Declaration on the Production and the Scientific and Therapeutic Use of Human Embryonic Stem Cells*. Rome: The Curia (http://www.vatican.va/roman_curia/pontifical_academies/acdlife/documents/rc_pa_acdlife_doc_20000824_cellule–staminali_en.html).

Powell, K. (2003). Seeds of doubt. *Nature* **422**: 656–8.

President's Council on Bioethics (2004). *Report of the President's Council on Bioethics: Monitoring Stem Cell Research*. Washington, DC: Government Printing Office (http://bioethics.gov/reports/stemcell/index.html).

President's Council on Bioethics (2005). *Alternative Sources of Pluripotent Stem Cells: A White Paper*. DC: Government Printing Office. http://www.bioethics.gov/reports/white_paper/index.html.

Rebar, R. (2002). ASRM statement on risk of cancer associated with fertility drugs. Available online at: http://www.inciid.org/article.php?cat=infertility&id=146.

Rossing, M. A., Daling, J. R., Weiss, N. J., *et al.* (1994). Ovarian tumors in a cohort or infertile women. *N Engl J Med* **331**: 771–6.

Sacred Congregation for the Doctrine of the Faith (1974). *Declaration on Procured Abortion*. Rome: The Curia (http://www.vatican.va/roman_curia/congregations/cfaith/documents/rc_con_cfaith_doc_19741118_declaration-abortion_en.html).

Shamblott, M. J., Axelman, J., Wang, S., *et al.* (1998). Derivation of pluripotent stem cells from cultured human primordial germ cells. *Proc Natl Acad Sci* **95**: 13726–31.

Tauer, C. A. (2004). Embryo research. In *Encyclopedia of Bioethics*, 3rd edn, ed. S. G. Post. New York: Macmillan Reference USA, pp. 712–22.

Thomson, J. A., Itskovitz-Eldor, J., Shapiro, S. S., *et al.* (1998). Embryonic stem cell lines derived from human blastocysts. *Science* **282**: 1145–7.

US Department of Health and Human Services (2005). *Code of Federal Regulations Title 45*, Vol. 46. 204(b,c,e), 46.203(b). Washington, DC: Government Printing Office.

Walters, L. (2004). Human embryonic stem cell research: an intercultural perspective. *Kennedy Inst Ethics J* **14**: 3–38.

Warren, M. A. (1997). *Moral Status: Obligations to Persons and Other Living Things*. New York: Oxford University Press.

Health systems and institutions

Introduction

Ross Upshur

As ethical reflection in healthcare evolves, the scope and range of issues of concern continues to grow. Early scholarship in ethics focused primarily on ethical issues arising from the care of individual patients in hospitals, such as end of life care, broad policy issues such as euthanasia and abortion, or the domain of research ethics. For the most part, the issues concerned analyzing ethical dilemmas arising from the extensive and well-described value conflicts that can arise between healthcare providers, patients, and families.

There is a transition occurring, with a new emphasis on issues emerging from intersection of the actions of healthcare providers, healthcare institutions, and broader social and community concerns. As well, there are new and emerging ethical issues arising at organizational levels. In terms of the level of reflection, the concerns are less with interactions between individuals as between individuals and collectives, and between collectives and collectives. Current efforts explicating the ethical challenges in planning for an influenza pandemic illustrate the interactions of ethical reflection at several levels of application and the complex set of values required for a coherent framework for analysis of these issues (Joint Centre for Bioethics Pandemic Influenza Working Group, 2005). For the most part, this level of ethical reflection has been neglected or underdeveloped in standard accounts of clinical ethics.

These issues fall, somewhat neatly, under the heading of health systems and institutions. The chapters in this section illustrate this transition.

While some chapters focus on the more classic issues arising in individual care, others explore the trade offs between collective goods and individual good.

Chapter 32 outlines the challenges of organizational ethics. This represents a new field of ethical reflection that explores issues arising in healthcare organizations as corporate citizens. Priority setting is a ubiquitous challenge in healthcare, occurs at all levels of health service provision, and raises difficult ethical issues requiring systematic deliberation. In Ch. 33, a framework is provided for analyzing these difficult issues. Error has similarly been shown to be a universal issue in healthcare provision and Hébert et al. in Ch. 34 survey recent initiatives in what can broadly be termed a revolution in the way in which error is conceived and managed. Rather than focusing on faulting individual agents, the emphasis is on seeing error as a system issue and error reduction as part of a transparent and collaborative effort.

Conflicts of interest are also a ubiquitous component of medical care. The extent to which they pervade every day practice is largely underestimated. Chapter 35 provides a succinct overview of the multiple ways in which conflicts of interest arise and provides guidance on their management. Ethical issues at the intersection of clinical care and public health are discussed in Ch. 36. The mission of public health is the protection and promotion of the health of communities. As such, the focus of practice is on populations, and the interests of communities may be at variance with the rights of individuals. How these conflicts are managed and the obligations of clinicians to public health are discussed in Ch. 36. In the aftermath of the tsunami, Hurricane Katrina, 9/11 and several notable terrorist acts against civilians, it has become evident that healthcare providers may find themselves drawn into disaster responses. The set of obligations for physicians in these contexts pose novel ethical challenges that are summarized in Ch. 37. The unique challenges faced by rural practitioners are described in Ch. 38 while Ch. 39 focuses on the provision of community healthcare – both drawing awareness to the lack of attention that these topics have received in the literature.

The chapters in this section summarize the current issues and controversies in the various fields.

It is evident from each chapter that they are characterized by diverse and complex ethical challenges where some consensus exists but where further research and scholarship, both empirical and conceptual, are required.

REFERENCES

Joint Centre for Bioethics Pandemic Influenza Working Group (2005). *Stand on Guard for the Ethical Considerations in Pandemic Influenza Preparedness*. Toronto: University of Toronto's Joint Centre for Bioethics (http://www.utoronto.ca/jcb/home/documents/pandemic.pdf).

32

Organizational ethics

Jennifer L. Gibson, Robert Sibbald, Eoin Connolly, and Peter A. Singer

A hospital has faced significant resource constraints over the last five years. After making significant cuts in administrative costs, the hospital senior management team is exploring revenue-generating options to help fund its clinical programs. One option under consideration involves renting cafeteria space to a popular fast-food restaurant. In the past, hospital cardiologists and endocrinologists have opposed similar proposals on the grounds that offering fast food is inconsistent with the hospital's patient care mission and its national reputation in the treatment of cardiac disease and non-insulin-dependent diabetes. The Clinical Operations Committee, which includes clinical and administrative leaders from across the organization, considers whether it should support or oppose the current proposal.

Mr. A is a 62-year-old male, who presents at the emergency department with severe chest pain. Mr. A is stabilized and diagnostic tests indicate triple vessel coronary artery disease. Bypass surgery is recommended. Prior to admission, it is discovered that Mr. A is a non-resident on a short visit to his son, who immigrated four years ago. As a non-resident, Mr. A is not covered by the national public health insurance plan and he did not purchase medical insurance for his trip. Neither he nor his son has the financial resources to pay for the bypass surgery. Although Mr. A is sufficiently stable to survive a flight home, he would not have access to the necessary medical treatment in his home country. The treating clinician wonders if the hospital should cover the cost of the surgery.

What is organizational ethics?

Organizational ethics is concerned with the ethical issues faced by managers and governors in health-care organizations and the ethical implications of organizational decisions and practices on patients, staff, and the community. Organizational ethics can be defined as "the organization's efforts to *define* its core values and mission, *identify* areas in which important values come into conflict, *seek* the best possible resolution of these conflicts, and *manage* its own performance to ensure that it acts in accord with espoused values" (Pearson *et al.*, 2003, p. 32). Organizational mission and value statements describe how the organization proposes to conduct its activities and outline a set of standards according to which the organization's actions and decisions are to be judged (Spencer *et al.*, 2000; Boyle *et al.*, 2001). Thus, the mission and values are sometimes described as the "moral compass" of the organization (Pearson *et al.*, 2003).

Organizational ethics has been described as the next step in the evolution of bioethics, which has focused primarily on ethical issues in direct patient care (Potter, 1996; Bishop *et al.*, 1999). Organizational ethics focuses on the business aspects of healthcare, the multiple stakeholder interests (e.g., patients, staff, suppliers, other providers, the community) affected by organizational decisions and actions, and the organization's "total mission," which includes the goal of patient care as well as other important goals such as financial sustainability, staff wellbeing, and public accountability (Hall, 2000; Spencer *et al.*, 2000). There are three main categories of organizational ethics issues: (i) ethical issues emerging in clinical care as a result of decisions taken elsewhere in the organization, (ii) ethical issues in clinical care with wide-reaching organizational implications, and (iii) ethical issues related specifically to the business aspects of healthcare organizations. The goals of organizational ethics are to achieve a strong alignment between the organization's stated mission, vision, and values and the decisions and actions by individuals on behalf of the organization (Silverman, 2000) and to create an organizational climate where organizational ethics issues can be constructively addressed (Spencer *et al.*, 2000).

Why is organizational ethics important?

Ethics

Organizational ethics involves "the intentional use of values in [organizational] decision-making" (Potter, 1996, p. 4). Winkler *et al.* (2005) proposed four substantive principles of organizational ethics to guide decision making based on values inherent to the organization's relationships with key stakeholders (Table 32.1). Other values have also been argued to be important for creating an ethical organization: humaneness, reciprocal benefit, trust, gratitude, dignity, service, and stewardship (Reiser, 1994). Trust has been emphasized by several authors as a key to organizational ethics effectiveness in healthcare organizations (Buchanan, 2000; Goold, 2001; Pearson *et al.*, 2003). These and other values are often articulated in an organization's mission/vision/value statements, code of ethics, policies, and staff orientation and performance evaluation processes. Ethical decision-making processes are also essential to organizational ethics. Organizational decision making is often fraught with moral uncertainty about *what* ought to be done in the context of competing stakeholder interests, conflicting values, and limited information. Ethical decision-making processes help to establish the ethical legitimacy of organizational decisions by facilitating agreement around *how* decisions ought to be made. Key procedural values include openness, transparency, inclusiveness, empowerment, and reciprocal accountability (Buchanan, 2000; Emanuel, 2000;

Silverman, 2000; Spencer *et al.*, 2000; Boyle *et al.*, 2001; Gibson, *et al.*, 2005a). Ethical processes are important for establishing institutional trust and promoting constructive stakeholder engagement around organizational decisions (Goold, 2001; Gibson *et al.*, 2005b). Although an organizational decision may not favor a stakeholder's interests, the stakeholder may nevertheless be able to accept the decision if the decision-making process is (and is perceived to be) ethical. One prominent process model is Daniels and Sabin's (2002) accountability for reasonableness framework which is described in detail in ch. 33. described. When integrated into organizational mechanisms and structures, these substantive and procedural values can contribute to the establishment of a strong ethical climate and culture in the organization (Emanuel, 2000; Silverman, 2000; Spencer *et al.*, 2000; Boyle, *et al.*, 2001).

The field of business ethics offers additional concepts and tools to address the business aspects of healthcare, the importance of collective responsibility for mission fulfillment, and the unique value-creating activity of organizations as compared with individuals (Spencer *et al.*, 2000; Ells and MacDonald, 2002). For example, "stakeholder impact analysis" involves identifying all stakeholder groups and interests, ranking and weighting the stakeholders and their interests, and assessing the impact of a proposed action on each stakeholder group (Brooks, 2004). Several bioethicists have proposed stakeholder impact analysis as a tool to facilitate organizational ethics decision making in healthcare organizations (Hall, 2000; Spencer *et al.*, 2000; Werhane, 2000; Boyle *et al.*, 2001; Ells and MacDonald, 2002).

Law

Healthcare organizations are legal entities with corresponding rights and responsibilities defined by a range of common and civil law provisions. Although the specific legal responsibilities of healthcare organizations may differ from one jurisdiction to the next, common domains of legal responsibility include employment standards (e.g. occupational

Table 32.1. Principles of organizational ethics in healthcare

	Patients	Employees	Community	Resources
Normative principle	Provide care with compassion	Treat employees with respect	Act in a public spirit	Spend resources reasonably
Stakeholders	Patients	Employees	Community	Patients, public
Values	Competence, compassion, trust, shared decision making	Fairness, empowerment, participation	Common good, community, benefit	Quality, equity, efficiency, sustainability

From Winkler *et al.*, 2005, p. 113.

health and safety standards, human rights provisions), consumer protections, corporate governance requirements, tax regulations, privacy legislation, and so on. Faith-based healthcare organizations may have additional responsibilities defined by canon law related to the religious mission of the sponsoring organization (National Conference of Catholic Bishops, 1995; Catholic Health Corporation of Ontario, 2000).

Healthcare organizations can be held legally liable for decisions made on their behalf. For example, in *Darling* v. *Charleston Community Memorial Hospital* (1965), the US court ruled that hospitals and their governing bodies have a direct duty of care for patients and can be held liable for injury resulting from negligent supervision of medical staff. The doctrine of corporate negligence holds that "a hospital has a direct and independent responsibility to its patients over and above that of the physicians and surgeons participating therein" (*Johnson* v. *Misericordia Community Hospital*, 1981). The common law finding defines clinicians and administrators (including Board members) as legal cofiduciaries of patient care.

The law recognizes that an organization cannot control every action taken by an individual associated with it. However, the law expects healthcare organizations to act in good faith and to make reasonable efforts to create a workplace environment where illegal action is prohibited (Seay, 2004). Many healthcare organizations have instituted

corporate compliance programs, which are designed to mitigate organizational culpability through the implementation of strategies to prevent and detect illegal behavior, take corrective action in the case of a legal violation, and enforce compliance with legal standards among staff (Boyle *et al.*, 2001; Pearson *et al.*, 2003). However, recent corporate governance scandals (e.g., Enron) suggest that corporate compliance programs may not be sufficient alone to mitigate organizational culpability or to ensure corporate ethical conduct. As a result, some healthcare associations have developed education programs and policy guidance to clarify the legal and ethical obligations of corporate governance in healthcare organizations (Corbett and MacKay, 2005.)

Policy

With the advent of managed care in the USA and fiscal constraints elsewhere, concerns have been raised about the encroachment of financial considerations in patient care (Silverman, 2000; Pearson *et al.*, 2003). In 1994, the US Joint Commission for Accreditation of Healthcare Organizations incorporated organizational ethics into its accreditation standards (Joint Commission on Accreditation of Healthcare Organizations, 2006). Other accreditation bodies have followed suit (Canadian Council for Health Services Accreditation, 2004). In addition to requiring ethics in the delivery of direct patient care, accredited healthcare organizations are expected to include ethical considerations in decision making (e.g., resource allocation, risk management, human resource management), to develop mechanisms to address ethical issues as they emerge, and to align organizational decisions with the organization's mission and values (Joint Commission for International Accreditation, 2002; Canadian Council for Health Services Accreditation, 2004; Joint Commission on Accreditation of Healthcare Organizations, 2006).

Professional codes of ethics specify the ethical obligations of health services managers to patients, the organization, and the community (American College of Health Executives, 2003; Veteran's Health Administration, 2003; Canadian College of Health Service Executives, 2005; General Medical Council, 2006). In Canada, for example, an ethical healthcare executive "services the public interest in an ethical fashion, strives to provide quality services, communicates truthfully and avoids misleading or raising unreasonable expectations in others, uses sound management practices and ethical use of resources, promotes public understanding of health and health services, and conducts inter-organisational activities in a cooperative way that improves community health" (Canadian Council for Health Services Accreditation, 2004). There is an emerging consensus within the health sector that clinicians and managers are both accountable for the care and safety of patients (Bishop *et al.*, 1999; Chervenak and McCullough, 2003). The Australian Medical Association's *Code of Conduct for Corporations Involved in the Provision of Management and Administrative Services in Medical Centers in Australia* offers a concrete attempt to clarify this shared accountability (Australian Medical Association, 2001).

Clinician–managers may experience unique ethical challenges in situations where their ethical obligations as clinicians may conflict with their ethical obligations as managers, for example, providing high-quality care to individual patients versus ensuring high-quality care within available resources for the populations of patients served by the organization. In recent years, a number of professional organizations have developed specific policies in an effort to guide clinician–managers (Ozar *et al.*, 2000; Canadian Nursing Association, 2002; General Medical Council, 2006).

Empirical studies

Empirical studies of organizational ethics are limited. The vast majority of empirical research has focused on a single organizational ethics issue: resource allocation. Studies of institution-level resource allocation in hospitals and health authorities have highlighted the importance of fair decision-making processes to resolve these challenges (Hope *et al.*, 1998; Ham, 1999; Daniels and Sabin, 2002; Martin, *et al.*, 2003; Peacock *et al.*, 2006). Failure to resolve the tension between managing economic constraints and providing high-quality service was identified by nurses as the most pressing organizational ethics issue in their workplace (Cooper, *et al.*, 2002, 2004).

Recent studies of organizational ethics in healthcare organizations highlight a number of other key organizational ethics issues. Pearson *et al.* (2003) identified six domains of organizational ethics issues in managed care organizations based on interviews with senior executives and physicians: confidentiality, community benefits, vulnerable populations, medical necessity and appropriateness, end of life care, and consumer empowerment. A Canadian study found that clinician–managers faced ethical issues related to resource allocation, workplace safety, intraprofessional and interprofessional conflict, conflict of interest, and balancing the competing needs of the patient, the community, and the organization (Lemieux-Charles *et al.*, 1993; see also Sibbald and Lazar, 2005).

The ethical climate of the organization has been shown to be a significant factor in nurses' decisions to leave their positions or the nursing profession (Hart, 2005) and in nurses' self-reports of moral distress and burnout (Corley, 1995; Severinsson, 2003; Corley *et al.*, 2005). Perceived organizational fairness is associated with increased quality of care ratings, job satisfaction, and trust of management as well as decreased emotional exhaustion among nurses (Aiken *et al.*, 2001; Laschinger, 2004), while perceptions of unfairness are correlated with increased psychological distress among physicians (Sutinen *et al.*, 2002) and increased absenteeism among hospital staff generally (Kivimaki *et al.*, 2003).

How should I approach organizational ethics in practice?

Organizational ethics effectiveness depends on, firstly, knowing what ethical issues your organization is facing, and secondly, ensuring there are effective mechanisms in place to address these issues. In 2005, we interviewed 150 Board members, senior executives, clinical and administrative managers, and senior clinical leaders in 13 publicly funded healthcare organizations in Toronto, Canada to find out what ethical issues their organizations were facing and what strategies were being used to address them. The key ethical issues and strategies are summarized in Table 32.2 and these serve as a good "roadmap" for approaching organizational ethics in practice.

Organizational ethics effectiveness is reflected in the degree to which an organization's stated mission and values are expressed in the choices and actions of the organization's agents, including staff, managers, and board members. Ethical guidelines, policies, and decision-making frameworks are important mechanisms for realizing the organization's mission and values, guiding ethical conduct, and resolving value conflicts. However, experience shows that ethical leadership from the board and senior management, including senior clinical leaders, is important for setting the ethical tone of an organization (Spencer *et al.*, 2000; MacRae *et al.*, 2005). Each of the 13 organizations we surveyed had at least one full-time ethicist, who provided expert leadership in ethics. The ethicist can play a key role in helping to resolve organizational ethics issues as well as building ethics capacity across the organization through staff education and policy development (Godkin *et al.*, 2005). Given the complexity of many organizational ethics issues,

consultation with affected stakeholders is a key strategy for clarifying the impact of alternative organizational decisions. Finally, the effectiveness of organizational ethics requires evaluation of these strategies to ensure that organizational decisions reflect the organization's stated mission and values, individual actions of staff embody these values, organizational ethics issues are identified and resolved constructively, and together these actions contribute to a positive ethical climate.

The cases

The Clinical Operations Committee is faced with determining whether or not the proposed business opportunity is consistent with the mission and values of the organization. The financial benefits of the commercial partnership would certainly generate revenue to support clinical programs. However, these benefits may undermine the patient care mission, particularly in the eyes of stakeholders. The Clinical Operations Committee should engage in a candid and cooperative discussion with the senior management team about alternative solutions to address the funding gap. Funding alternatives should be assessed on the basis of the organization's mission and values, their impact on key stakeholder groups, and other relevant factors (e.g., clinical data, legal considerations, professional obligations). If the organization does not already have a policy guiding business development decision making, a key recommendation of the Clinical Operations Committee should be that the organization should develop such a policy, based on broad range of stakeholder input, which outlines explicit criteria and processes for making business-development decisions and includes an evaluation component.

Healthcare professionals have an ethical obligation to advocate for their patients. However, they should also be good stewards of societal resources. A physician's professional autonomy allows for the physician to donate his or her services, but it does not necessarily give the physician the authority to

Table 32.2. Organizational ethics in publicly funded organizations

Issues	Strategies
End of life care	Mission/vision/values
Disclosure of risk	Ethics guidelines, e.g., organizational code of conduct,
Treatment of uninsured patients	professional codes of ethics, accreditation standards
Resource allocation	Organizational policies, e.g., conflict of interest, access to care
Human resources management	for the uninsured, end of life care, fund raising, disclosure,
Commercialization of research	intellectual property
Fund-raising ethics (e.g., event sponsorship)	Ethical decision-making frameworks, e.g., accountability for
Business development	reasonableness
Governance ethics (e.g., conflict of interest)	Ethical leadership, e.g., board ethics committee, senior
	management champion, ethicist
	Ethics consultation, e.g., ethicist, ethics committee,
	legal counsel, stakeholders
	Evaluation, e.g., accreditation standards, staff performance
	evaluation, quality review

donate hospital resources such as medical devices and costly medication. These dual obligations may create a conflict for the healthcare professional involved in the care of Mr. A. The healthcare professional can fulfill both obligations by bringing Mr. A's case forward to the decision makers within the organization who are directly responsible for allocating hospital resources. Decision makers should consider (i) the gravity of Mr. A's clinical and financial need, (ii) the impact on other stakeholder groups (e.g., access to care), (iii) the professional obligations of the healthcare professional, and (iv) the mission and values of the healthcare organization. Consultation with an ethicist may facilitate decision making in this case. Although availability of resources may be a limiting factor on the ability of an organization to provide the surgery to treat Mr. A, it may be possible to fulfill the hospital's patient care mission and the healthcare professional's obligations in other ways, for example by securing access to care for Mr. A through another provider or by seeking alternative funding sources. As in the previous case, an organizational policy would be helpful to guide decision making in future cases.

REFERENCES

Aiken, L. H., Clarke, S. P., Sloane, D. M., *et al.* (2001). Nurses' reports on hospital care in 5 countries. *Health Affairs* **20**: 43–53.

American College of Health Executives (2003). *Code of Ethics.* Washington: American College of Health Executives (http://www.ache.org) accessed 14 March 2006.

Australian Medical Association (2001). *Code of Conduct for Corporations Involved in the Provision of Management and Administrative Services in Medical Centres in Australia.* Canberra, ACT: Australian Medical Association (http://www.ama.com/au/web.nsf/doc/SHED-5G2D8H) accessed 5 May 2006.

Bishop, L. J., Cherry, M. N., and Darragh, M. (1999). Organizational ethics and health care: extending bioethics to the institutional arena. *Kennedy Inst Ethics J* **9**: 189–208.

Boyle, P. J., DuBose, E. R., Ellingson, S. J., Guinne, D. E., and McCurdy, D. B. (2001). *Organizational Ethics in Health Care: Principles, Cases, and Practical Solutions.* San Francisco, CA: Jossey-Bass.

Brooks, L. J. (2004). *Business and Professional Ethics for Directors, Executives, and Accountants*, 3rd edn. Mason, OH: Thomson Learning.

Buchanan, A. (2000). Trust in managed care organizations. *Kennedy Inst Ethics J* **10**: 189–212.

Canadian College of Health Services Executives (2005). *Code of Ethics*. Ottawa: Canadian College of Health Service Executives (http://www.cchse.org/Standeng.htm) accessed 14 March 2006.

Canadian Council for Health Services Accreditation (2004). *The Canadian Health Accreditation Report 2004*. Ottawa: Canadian Council for Health Accreditation (http://www.cchsa.ca/pdf/2004report.PDF) accessed 14 March 2006.

Canadian Nursing Association (2002). *Code of Ethics*. Ottawa: Canadian Nursing Association (http://www.cna/nurses.ca/cna/documents/pdf/publications/CodeofEthics2002_3.pdf) accessed 5 May 2006.

Catholic Health Corporation of Ontario (2000). *CHCO Indicators for Catholic Hospitals*. Toronto: Catholic Health Corporation (document available upon request: http://www.chco.ca/index.php?section=3).

Chervenak, F. A. and McCullough, L. B. (2003). Physicians and hospital managers as cofiduciaries of patients: rhetoric or reality? *J Healthcare Manag* **48**: 172–80.

Cooper, R. W., Frank, G. L., Gouty, C. A., and Hansen, M. C. (2002). Key ethical issues encountered in healthcare organizations: perceptions of nurse executives. *J Nurs Admin* **32**: 331–7.

Cooper, R. W., Frank, G. L., Hansen, M. C., and Gouty, C. A. (2004). Key ethical issues encountered in health care organizations: the perceptions of staff, nurses, and nurse leaders. *J Nurs Admin* **34**: 149–56.

Corbett, A. and MacKay, J. (2005). *Guide to Good Governance*. Toronto: Ontario Hospital Association.

Corley, M. C. (1995). Moral distress of critical care nurses. *Am J Crit Care* **4**: 280–5.

Corley, M. C., Minick, P., Elswick, R. K., and Jacobs, M. (2005). Nurse moral distress and ethical work environment. *Nurs Ethics* **12**: 381–90.

Daniels, N. and Sabin, J. E. (2002). *Setting Limits Fairly: Can We Learn to Share Medical Resources?* Oxford: Oxford University Press.

Darling v. *Charleston Community Memorial Hospital* (1965). 33 Ill 2d 326 [211 N. E. 2d 253, 14 A. L. P. 3d 860] (http://biotech.law.lsu.edu/cases/Medmal/darling.htm) accessed 14 March 2006.

Ells, C. and MacDonald, C. (2002). Implications of organisational ethics to health care. *Healthcare Manag Forum* **15**: 32–8.

Emanuel, L. (2000). Ethics and the structure of healthcare. *Camb Q Healthc Ethics* **9**: 151–68.

General Medical Council (2006). *Guidance: Management for Doctors*. London: General Medical Council (http://www.gmc-uk.org/guidance/library/management_for_doctors.asp) accessed 5 May 2006.

Gibson, J. L., Martin, D. K., and Singer, P. A. (2005a). Priority setting in hospitals: fairness, inclusiveness, and the problem of institutional power differences. *Soc Sci Med* **61**: 235–6.

Gibson, J. L., Martin, D. K., and Singer, P. A. (2005b). Evidence, economics, and ethics: resource allocation in health services organizations. *Healthcare Quart* **8**: 50–9.

Godkin, M. D., Faith, K., Upshur, R. E. G., on behalf of the PEECE Group of Investigators (2005). Project examining effectiveness in clinical ethics (PEECE): phase 1– descriptive analysis of nine clinical ethics services. *J Med Ethics* **31**: 505–12.

Goold, S. D. (2001). Trust and the ethics of health care institutions. *Hastings Cent Rep* **31**: 26–33.

Hall, R. T. (2000). *An Introduction to Health Care Organizational Ethics*. Oxford: Oxford University Press.

Ham, C. (1999). Tragic choices in health care: lessons from the Child B case. *BMJ* **319**: 1258–61.

Hart, S. E. (2005). Hospital ethical climates and registered nurses' turnover intentions. *J Nurs Scholar* **37**: 173–7.

Hope, T., Hicks, N., Reynolds, D., Crisp, R., and Griffiths, S. (1998). Rationing and the health authority. *BMJ* **317**: 1067–9.

Jennings, B., Gray, B. H., Sharpe, V. A., and Fleischman, A. R. (2004). *The Ethics of Hospital Trustees*. Washington, DC: Georgetown University Press.

Johnson v. *Misericordia Community Hospital* (1981). 301 N. W.2d 156, (Supreme Court, Wisconsin) (http://www.estesparkinstitute.com/docs/con_materials/archive/1981/pdf/HortySpringer_Johnson.PDF) accessed 14 March 2006.

Joint Commission for International Accreditation (2002). *International Standards for Hospitals*, 2nd edn. Oakbrook Terrace, IL: Joint Commission for International Accreditation (http://www.jointcommissioninternational.com/docViewer.aspx) accessed 5 March 2006.

Joint Commission on Accreditation of Healthcare Organizations (2006). *Overview of 2007 Leadership Standards*. Oakbrook Terrace, IL: Joint Commission on Accreditation of Healthcare Organizations (http://www.jointcommission.org/NR/rdonlyres/A55ACEC4-E027-4FE0-8532-C023E8817A30/0/07_bhc_ld_stds.pdf) accessed 5 March 2006.

Kivimaki, M., Elovainio, M., Vahtera, J., and Ferrie, J. E. (2003). Organizational justice and health of employees: prospective cohort study. *Occup Environ Med* **60**: 27–33.

Laschinger, S. (2004). Nurses' perceptions of respect and organizational justice. *J Nurs Admin* **34**: 354–64.

Lemieux-Charles, L., Meslin, E. M., Aird, C., Baker, R., and Leatt, P. (1993). Ethical issues faced by clinician/ managers in resource allocation decisions. *Hosp Health Serv Admin* **38**: 267–85.

Mackie, J. E., Taylor, A. D., Finegold, D. L., Daar, A., and Singer, P. A. (2006). Lessons on ethical decision making from the bioscience industry. *PLoS Medi* **3**: 605–10.

MacRae, S., Chidwick, P., Berry, S., *et al.* (2005). Clinical bioethics integration, sustainability, and accountability: the hub and spokes strategy. *J Med Ethics* **31**: 256–61.

Martin, D. K., Shulman, K., Santiago–Sorrell, P., and Singer, P. A. (2003). Priority setting and hospital strategic planning: a qualitative case study. *J Health Serv Res Policy* **8**: 197–201.

National Conference of Catholic Bishops (2001). *The Ethical and Religious Directives for Catholic Health Care Services*, 4th edn. Washington, DC: National Conference of Catholic Bishops (http://www.usccb.org/bishops/ directives.shtml) accessed 14 March 2006.

Ozar D., Berg J., Werhane P. H., for the Institute for Ethics National Working Group on Organizational Ethics (2000). *Organizational Ethics in Health Care: Toward a Model for Ethical Decision Making by Provider Organizations*. Washington, DC: American Medical Association (http://www.ama-assn.org/ama/upload/mm/369/ organizationalethics.pdf) accessed 6 February 2005.

Peacock, S., Ruta, D., Mitton, C., *et al.* (2006). Using economics to set pragmatic and ethical priorities. *BMJ* **332**: 482–5.

Pearson, S. D., Sabin, J. E., and Emanuel, E. (2003). *No Margin, No Mission: Health Care Organizations and the Quest for Ethical Excellence*. Oxford: Oxford University Press.

Potter, R. L. (1996). From clinical ethics to organizational ethics: the second stage of the evolution of bioethics. *Bioethics Forum* **12**: 3–12.

Reiser, S. J. (1994). The ethical life of health care organizations. *Hastings Cent Rep* **24**: 28–35.

Seay, J. D. (2004). The legal responsibilities of voluntary hospital trustees. In *The Ethics of Hospital Trustees*, ed. B. Jennings, B. H. Gray, V. A. Sharpe, and A. R. Fleischman. Washington, DC: Georgetown University Press, pp. 41–57.

Severinsson, E. (2003). Moral stress and burnout: qualitative content analysis. *Nurs Health Serv* **5**: 59–66.

Sibbald, R. W. and Lazar, N. M. (2005). Bench-to-bedside review: ethical challenges for those in direct roles in critical care units. *Crit Care* **9**: 76–80.

Silverman, H. J. (2000). Organizational ethics in health care organizations: proactively managing the ethical climate to ensure organizational integrity. *HEC Forum* **12**: 202–15.

Spencer, E. M., Mills, A. E., Rorty, M. V., and Werhane, P. H. (2000). *Organization Ethics in Health Care*. New York: Oxford University Press.

Sutinen, R., Kivimaki, M., Elovainio, M., and Virtanen, M. (2002). Organizational fairness and psychological distress in hospital physicians. *Scand J Pub Health* **30**: 209–15.

Veterans Health Administration (2003). *VHA Code of Ethics*. Washington, DC: Veterans Health Administration (http://www.index.va.gov/search/va/va_search. jsp?QT=Code+of+ethics) accessed 14 March 2006.

Werhane, P. H. (2000). Business ethics, stakeholder theory, and the ethics of health care organizations. *Camb Q Healthc Ethics* **9**: 169–81.

Winkler, E. C., Gruen, R. L., and Sussman, A. (2005). First principles: substantive ethics for healthcare organizations. *J Healthcare Manag* **5**: 109–20.

33

Priority setting

Douglas K. Martin, Jennifer L. Gibson, and Peter A. Singer

Dr. B is on the seventh day of his rotation as medical director of the intensive care unit (ICU) when he receives a referral call about a patient in emergency who needs ICU admission for ventilation support. Dr. B examines his ICU census and notes that not only are there no ICU beds available but there is also a request from a thoracic surgeon for an ICU bed for a patient currently in the observation room, and there is a request from a nearby hospital to transfer one of their patients to Dr. B's ICU.

Dr. C, a pediatrician, has been asked to chair her hospital drug formulary committee to examine new drugs and determine which ones should be provided from the hospital budget. She is aware that these decisions are complex and often controversial and is unsure how to proceed.

What is priority setting?

Priority setting involves deciding which resources to allocate to competing needs. It is a key component of every health system because, whether wealthy or poor, no system can afford to provide every service that it may wish to provide. Both publicly and privately funded systems have the challenge of delivering quality care within the limits of government budgets or enrollee and employer contributions.

Within health systems, priority setting occurs at each decision level: micro (at the bedside or in clinical programs), meso (in hospitals or regional institutions), and macro (at the system-wide level). Clinicians are directly involved in priority setting at the micro level and often involved at other levels; however, decisions at each of these levels are inter-related. In the context of clinical programs, such as in the first case opening this chapter, the ICU director must decide which patient gets an ICU bed. This decision itself is related to decisions in the critical care program about how many beds to keep open and how many nurses to maintain on staff, and these are related to the hospital level decision about the importance of critical care in that institutions and how much of the hospital's budget flows there, and these are related to both funding for that hospital and system-wide funding for critical care.

Why is priority setting important?

Health system sustainability is related to the effectiveness of the priority setting decision making within the system. The costs of health-related services are constantly increasing, with drug costs leading the rise. Demands for health services are increasing as a result of new technologies; increased public awareness fueled by the Internet; aging populations in Western democracies; pandemics such as HIV/AIDS, malaria and tuberculosis; and an alarming increased prevalence of non-communicable diseases, such as cancer and cardiac disease, in the developing world. The current growth in healthcare expenditures is unsustainable and is limiting the ability of governments to fund education, infrastructure, and other priorities. Therefore, setting priorities regarding what we will and will not provide is vital to the sustainability of any and all health systems.

Ethics

Justice requires that like cases should be treated alike and that the benefits and burdens of health services be allocated equitably across patients. Knowing what decisions to make would be quite simple if we could agree on the criteria to guide equitable allocation of resources. However, at the crux, priority setting decisions involve choosing among a complex cluster of criteria (e.g., clinical factors, patient values, system goals) that may be morally relevant to any one specific decision. Moreover, reasonable people may disagree about how these criteria should be applied and which values should be emphasized, particularly in the context of clinical uncertainty; competing patient, program, or system goals; and multiple stakeholder interests. For example, when deciding which patient gets the bed in the intensive care unit (ICU), should the ICU director emphasize benefit, and give the bed to the patient with the longest most productive life ahead, or emphasize need, and give the bed to the patient who is the most vulnerable? The conflict widens when the choice involves cost differences. For example, should patients be given a very costly drug that may keep them out of the ICU? Or, in the context of drug-funding decisions, such as in the second case opening this chapter, should we prefer a very costly drug that would provide a large benefit to a few patients or a less costly drug that will provide a lesser benefit to many patients?

No consensus exists about an overarching moral theory to help to resolve differences between conflicting values. Therefore, the goal must be to make these decisions in an environment where the conflicting values can be explicitly identified and deliberated upon in a morally acceptable manner. In other words, the goal is fairness.

One of the most helpful advances in priority setting has been the development of "accountability for reasonableness," an explicitly ethical framework that provides guidance for decision makers who want to implement fair priority setting (Daniels and Sabin, 1997; Daniels, 2000; Daniels and Sabin, 2002). It is theoretically grounded in justice theories emphasizing democratic deliberation (Rawls, 1993; Cohen, 1994). "Accountability for reasonableness" specifies conditions that operationalize the ethical concept of fairness. A fair priority setting process meets four conditions: relevance, publicity, revisions/appeals, and enforcement (Table 33.1). Recently, we proposed a fifth condition – empowerment – arguing that power differences between individuals within healthcare institutions, which prevent some from fully participating in decision making, may negatively influence the fairness of priority setting and so must be attenuated by leaders within the institution (Gibson et al., 2005).

Other approaches, such as economic evaluations, may be helpful: for example, cost-effectiveness analysis when setting priorities among new technologies or drugs, or program budgeting and marginal analysis when deciding among programs. However, these approaches emphasize a narrow range of values (e.g., efficiency), and not the full range of relevant values. Therefore, economic evaluations, like any other technical approach, must be considered within the context of a fair priority setting process (as described above). For example, recent work in Canada and the UK has shown how program budgeting and marginal analysis may be used in conjunction with "accountability for reasonableness" framework (Gibson et al., 2006; Peacock et al., 2006).

Law

Legal frameworks are not clinically precise and are more often helpful in identifying what decision makers may *not* do, rather than what they should do. In general, the law focuses on the reasonableness of allocation decisions in light of existing legal standards and the salient facts. Legally, physicians have a fiduciary relationship with their patients and are expected to meet a reasonable standard of care. Similarly, as fiduciaries of the hospital corporation, hospital board directors have a duty to act honestly and in the best interests of the corporation and its members as a whole, to exercise due diligence in making decisions on the basis of

Table 33.1. The four conditions of "accountability for reasonableness"

Condition	Characteristics
Relevance	Priority setting decisions must rest on reasons that "fair-minded" people can agree are relevant in the context; "fair-minded" people seek to cooperate according to terms they can justify to each other
Publicity	Priority setting rationales must be publicly accessible
Revision	There must be a mechanism for challenge, including the opportunity for revising decisions in light of considerations that stakeholders may raise
Enforcement	Leaders within the organization are responsible for ensuring that the other conditions of fairness are met

information reasonably available, and to meet an expected standard of care in discharging these duties. Therefore, in some jurisdictions, the courts have been reluctant to become involved in judicial review of how physicians or hospitals use their resources (e.g., *R.* v. *Cambridge Health Authority*, 1995.) To use Canada as an example, the Canada Health Act mandates reasonable access to medically necessary services but does not specify what those services should be, nor does it specify a mechanism for making these difficult and contentious decisions. The Canadian Charter of Rights and Freedoms and provincial human rights codes prohibit discrimination on grounds of race, ethnicity, religion, age, sex, sexual orientation, and physical or mental disability. In case law, a British Columbia judge noted that physicians' primary duty is to their patients, and that financial considerations cannot play a decisive role in clinical decisions (*Law Estate* v. *Simice*, 1994).

Empirical studies

At the micro level, healthcare professionals decide which individuals are cared for first, which patients receive which diagnostic tests and which drugs, which patients are admitted to a hospital bed, and which patients are taken to the operating theater. Micro-level priority setting (also known as bedside rationing) is inevitable because of the increasing gap between the possibilities of effective medical interventions and the available resources (Pearson,

2000). Klein *et al.* (1998) described six forms of bedside rationing: denial, deflection, deterrence, delay, dilution, and termination. They stated that denial and termination were the most severe forms of bedside rationing and they rarely occurred in industrialized countries with publicly financed healthcare systems.

However, broad characterizations often cover context-specific practices, which often vary. In emergencies, triage conventions require that life-threatening situations be addressed first. But in non-emergency clinical programs, such as critical care, neurosurgery, cardiac surgery, and general medicine, the allocation conventions are unclear and variable and should be examined in context. A number of professional associations have also developed detailed allocation policies for non-emergency clinical programs such as critical care (e.g., Council on Ethical and Judicial Affairs of the American Medical Association, 1995; Carlet *et al.*, 2004). However, the allocation conventions are often variable across policies and it is not always clear how they should be applied in context.

Critical care studies by Mielke *et al.* (2003), Martin *et al.* (2003a), and Cooper *et al.* (2005) determined that ICU admission decisions varied from clinician to clinician. Some prioritized great need, others the potential for benefit. Some prioritized the young, others the elderly; often, referring physicians who pushed the hardest and loudest "found" a bed for their patient. Even in contexts where admission policies exist, the policies only distinguished between broad categories of patients and not between specific patients. Moreover, where ICU admission policies exist, they are typically not well known.

Severe funding cuts and an increased prevalence of severe head injuries challenged neurosurgeons at Groote Schuur Hospital in South Africa. Unsure about what to do and troubled by the enormous moral consequences of these decisions, the clinicians initiated a collaborative effort with the University of Cape Town Bioethics Centre to develop a morally defensible allocation policy. A key feature of the policy was that it allowed all head-injured patients to be fully resuscitated and admitted to the ICU, followed by a full assessment by a neurosurgical team 24 hours later with a view to withdrawing aggressive treatment from those with the worst prognosis (Benatar *et al.*, 2000)

Walton *et al.* (2007) examined the selection of patients for elective cardiac surgery and described the clinical reasons (e.g., pathology and anatomy) and non-clinical reasons (e.g., social supports, clinician-specific experiences, and remuneration schemes) that surgeons used to decide which patient to take to surgery. Even in jurisdictions where standardized urgency rating scores had been developed to help cardiac surgeons to prioritize patients on waiting lists, the scores were used for record-keeping purposes only, not for allocation decisions; decisions were based on "clinician judgement," which varied from clinician to clinician.

In general medicine, Kapiriri and Martin (2007) found that in Uganda, where drugs are extremely scarce, publicly funded drugs were routinely denied to patients with sufficient resources to purchase them privately. In addition, those patients who received a first course of treatment often did not receive a second course, so that the drug could be given to another patient who had not yet received any treatment.

In a hospital drug formulary in Canada, funding decisions were based on a complex cluster of factors, including benefit, quality of evidence, toxicity, number of patients requiring the drug, comparison with alternatives, cost, and an informal assessment of cost effectiveness (Martin *et al.*, 2003b). Significantly, though often perceived as the accepted

approach to drug evaluation, several studies of actual practice provide evidence that cost effectiveness analysis plays a relatively minor role in drug formulary decisions (Luce and Brown, 1995; Sloan *et al.*, 1997; Foy *et al.*, 1999; Martin *et al.*, 2001; PausJenssen *et al.*, 2003).

How should I approach priority setting in practice?

At the micro level, clinicians are forced to act as gatekeepers for the health system, though they are neither trained nor inclined to perform this burdensome task (Carlson and Norheim, 2005). Consequently, they often fall back on clinical guidelines. But guidelines are typically based on the narrow range of values inherent in "evidence-based medicine" and not on the entire range of values relevant to these difficult allocation decisions (Norheim, 1999). Clinicians often struggle with these complex allocation decisions without support or guidance. They find themselves torn between the position that "physicians are required to do everything that they believe may benefit each patient without regard to costs or other societal considerations" (Levinsky, 1984), and the view that "the physician's obligations to the patient ... [must] be weighed against the legitimate competing claims of other patients, of payers, of society as a whole, and sometimes even of the physician himself" (Morreim, 1995). Sabin (2000) argued that the ethical physician should embrace both the values of fidelity and stewardship. Moreover, the role of clinician expertise has been viewed by the public as essential to priority setting (Cookson and Dolan, 1999).

Ultimately, the way forward for clinicians making priority setting decisions at the micro level is to form collaborations with supportive managers, patients, and others to develop admissions policies and elective treatment guidelines (as was described in the South African situation above). Such decisions can be made using a fair process guided by "accountability for reasonableness" that encompasses the views of all relevant stakeholders and makes the policies/ guidelines accessible and known. In addition, the experiences of clinicians are vital to priority setting at other decision points in the health system, including the meso (institutional) and macro (system) levels.

This usually involves determining the substantive criteria for allocation decisions, as well as the processes that will be followed in such decisions. An example of criteria and processes for priority setting, in the context of hospital strategic planning, is provided in Box 33.1 (Gibson *et al.*, 2004). Analogous criteria and processes could be developed for other types of priority setting decision.

Box 33.1 Priority setting

Criteria

- Strategic fit
- Alignment with external directives
- Academic commitments: education, research
- Clinical impact
- Community needs
- Partnerships with external institutions or organizations
- Interdependency between programs within the same institution
- Resource implications

Process elements

1. Confirm the strategic plan
2. Clarify program architecture, including program groupings and definitions
3. Clarify board/management roles and responsibilities
4. Determine who will make priority setting decisions and what they will do
5. Engage internal/external stakeholders
6. Define priority setting criteria and collect data/information
7. Develop an effective communication strategy
8. Develop a decision review process
9. Develop process monitoring and evaluation strategies
10. Support the process with leadership development and change management strategies

---

The cases

Deciding which patient to admit, or not admit, without support is "a damned if I do, damned if I don't" distressing situation. Dr. B should evaluate the alternatives and clearly articulate the criteria being used; discuss the criteria with others for feedback and transparency; make a decision; communicate the decision and the reasons to all relevant staff and the patients involved; then be open to responding to new information or different arguments. Once the presenting situation is dealt with, Dr. B should immediately initiate a process to develop an admission policy that meets the conditions of "accountability for reasonableness," and which includes a dissemination strategy to ensure that all critical care staff participate, buy-in, and use the policy. A regularly scheduled policy review that examines people's experiences with the policy, which acts as a quality-control mechanism, will help to ensure that the policy is "fairness in action."

Dr. C must develop an environment of fair deliberation concerning decisions about which drugs should be included in the formulary, guided by the four conditions of accountability for reasonableness (Table 33.1). This priority setting process should be characterized by inclusiveness (i.e., seeking honest deliberation about competing values advanced by different types of people, including managers, clinicians, and patients), transparency (i.e., ensuring that decision criteria are communicated throughout the hospital, and even to the hospital's community), and responsiveness (i.e., providing a vehicle for others to contribute to, or even challenge, the committee's reasoning, as a quality improvement mechanism).

REFERENCES

Benatar, S. R., Fleischer, T. E., Peter, J. C., Pope, A., and Taylor, A. (2000). Treatment of head injuries in the public sector in South Africa. *S Afr Med J* **90**: 790–3.

Carlet, J., Thijs, L. G., Antonelli, M., *et al.* (2004) Challenges in end-of-life-care in the ICU. Statement of the Fifth

International Consensus Conference in Critical Care, Belgium, April 2003. *Intens Care Med* **30**: 770–84.

Carlson, B. and Norheim, O. F. (2005). "Saying no is no easy matter" a qualitative study of competing concerns in rationing decisions in general practice. *BMC Health Serv Res* **5**: 70.

Cohen, J. (1994). Pluralism and proceduralism. *Chicago–Kent Law Rev* **69**: 589–618.

Cookson, R. and Dolan, P. (1999). Public views on health care rationing: a group discussion study. *Health Policy* **49**: 63–74.

Cooper, A. B., Joglekar, A. S., Gibson, J. L., Swota, A. H., and Martin, D. K. (2005). communication of bed allocation decisions in a critical care unit and accountability for reasonableness. *BMC Health Serv Res* **5**: 67.

Council on Ethical and Judicial Affairs of the American Medical Association (1995). Ethical considerations in the allocation of organs and other scarce medical resources among patients. *Arch Intern Med* **155**: 29–40.

Daniels, N. (2000). Accountability for reasonableness. *BMJ* **321**: 1300–130.

Daniels, N., and Sabin, J. E. (1997). Limits to health care: fair procedures, democratic deliberation and the legitimacy problem for insurers. *Philos Publ Aff* **26**: 303–502.

Daniels, N. and Sabin, J. E. (2002). *Setting Limits Fairly: Can we Learn to Share Medical Resources?* Oxford: Oxford University Press.

Foy, R., So, J., Rous, E., and Scarffe, H. (1999). Perspectives of commissioners and cancer specialists in prioritizing new cancer drugs: impact of the evidence threshold. *BMJ* **318**: 456–91.

Gibson, J. L., Martin, D. K., and Singer, P. A. (2004). Setting priorities in health care organizations: criteria, processes, and parameters of success. *BMC Health Serv Res* **4**: 25.

Gibson, J. L., Martin, D. K., and Singer, P. A. (2005). Priority setting in hospitals: fairness, inclusiveness, and the problem of institutional power differences. *Soc Sci Med* **61**: 2355–62.

Gibson, J. L., Mitton, C., and Martin, D. K., Donaldson, C. Singer, P. A. (2006). Ethics and economics: does programme budgeting and marginal analysis contribute to fair priority setting? *J Health Serv Res Pol* **11**: 32–7.

Kapiriri, L. and Martin, D. K. (2007). Bedside rationing by health practitioners in a context of extreme resource constraints: the case of Uganda. *Med Decision Making* **27**: 44–52.

Klein, R., Day, P., and Redmayne, S. (1998). *Managing Scarcity: Priority Setting and Rationing in the National Health Service*, 2nd edn. Buckingham, UK: Open University Press.

Law Estate v. *Simice* (1994). 21 CCCT (2d)228 (BCSC), affd [1996] 4 WWR 672 (BCCA).

Levinsky N. G. (1984). The doctor's master. *N Engl J Med* **311**: 1575.

Luce, B. R. and Brown, R. E. (1995). The use of technology assessment by hospitals, health maintenance organizations and third-party payers in the United States. *Int J Technol Assess Health Care* **11**: 79.

Martin, D. K., Pater, J. L., and Singer, P. A. (2001). Priority setting decisions for new cancer drugs: what rationales are used. *Lancet* **358**: 1676–81.

Martin, D. K., Bernstein, M., and Singer P. A. (2003a). Neurosurgery patients' access to ICU beds: priority setting in the ICU: a qualitative case study and evaluation. *J Neurol Neurosurg Psychiatry* **74**: 1299–1303.

Martin, D. K., Hollenberg, D., MacRae, S., Madden, S., and Singer, P. A. (2003b). Priority setting in a hospital formulary: a qualitative case study. *Health Pol* **66**: 295–303.

Mielke, J., Martin, D. K., and Singer, P. A. (2003). Priority setting in critical care: a qualitative case study. *Crit Care Med* **31**: 2764–8.

Morreim, E. H. (1995) *Balancing Act: The New Medical Ethics of Medicine's New Economics*. Washington, DC: Georgetown University Press, p. 2.

Norheim, O. F. (1999) Health care rationing: are additional criteria needed for assessing evidence based clinical practise guidelines? *BMJ* **319**: 1426–9.

Peacock, S., Ruta, D., Mitton, C., *et al.* (2006). Using economics to set pragmatic and ethical priorities. *Br Med J* **332**: 482–5.

Pearson, S. D. (2000), Caring and cost: the challenge for physician advocacy. *Ann Int Med* **133**: 148–53.

PausJenssen, A. M., Singer, P. A., and Detsky, A. S. (2003). How a formulary committee makes listing decisions. *Pharmacoeconomics* **21**: 285–94.

Rawls, J. (1993). *Political Liberalism*. New York: Columbia University Press.

Sabin, J. E. (2000). Fairness as a problem of love and the heart: a clinician's perspective on priority setting. In *The Global Challenge of Health Care Rationing*, ed. C. Ham and A. Coulter. Buckingham, UK: Open University Press, pp. 117–22.

Sloan, F. A., Whetten-Goldstein, K., and Wilson, A. (1997). Hospital pharmacy decisions, cost containment, and the use of cost effectiveness analysis. *Soc Sci Med* **45**: 523–33.

Walton, N., Martin, D. K., Peter, E., Pringle, D., and Singer, P. A. (2007) Priority setting in cardiac surgery: a qualitative study. *Health Pol* **80**: 444–8.

34

Disclosure of medical error

Philip C. Hébert, Alex V. Levin, and Gerald Robertson

A 77-year-old farmer with recurring kidney stones visits his urologist for an annual examination. Prior to seeing the patient, the physician is taken aside by her nurse, who tells her the patient had been in the emergency department the previous night with hematuria. A CAT scan had been done, which indicated that the renal tumor seen on last year's CAT scan was larger and there were now lung metastases. The physician cannot remember ever seeing the radiology report from last year. To her complete surprise, it is found filed in the patient's chart. There is no record in the chart that the results were ever shared with the patient. She considers herself extremely meticulous and has never had such an oversight before. The urologist considers what she should tell the patient.

A 12-year-old boy has cataract surgery at a large teaching hospital. At a critical moment the surgeon's hand slips, severely rupturing the lens capsule. The planned implant-ation of an intraocular lens has to be abandoned. Instead, the patient will have to use a contact lens. The physician wonders what he should tell the patient and his family about the surgery.

What is medical error?

Well-publicized reports of harm occurring to patients as a result of their medical care in the USA (Patient Safety Foundation, 1998), Canada (Sinclair, 1994) and the UK (Smith, 1998) have raised public concerns about the safety of modern healthcare. The US Institute of Medicine report (Kohn *et al.*,

2000). *To Err is Human* encouraged efforts to prevent patient harm as did the UK Department of Health (2000). In Canada, the release of the Canadian Adverse Events Study (Baker *et al.*, 2004) resulted in the first tangible federal funding for a national Canadian Patient Safety Initiative. Similar initiatives are underway in Spain, Australia, and many other countries.

Adverse medical incidents are by definition injurious or cause a setback to someone's interests (Davies *et al.*, 2003). Harmful effects of healthcare include recognized natural complications causing some injury to patients, such as a wound infection following an appendectomy. Failure to manage illness according to best practices, such as improper hand-washing techniques or poor instrument sterilization prior to patient contact, are other forms of error, not so much events as harmful processes of care. Errors are considered "preventable" and not primarily a result of the disease process. One definition states that an error occurs when there is "failure to complete a planned action as it was intended, or when an incorrect plan is used in an attempt to achieve a given aim" (Leape, 1994a).

Negligence is established only in a court of law and should be distinguished from "honest mistakes," the latter being typically errors of judgement (Sharpe, 1987). For example, careful and capable practitioners may make a mistake in diagnosis

An earlier version of this chapter has appeared. Hébert, P. C., Levin, A. V., and Robertson, G. (2001). Disclosure of medical error. *CMAJ* **164**: 509–13.

despite having done everything correctly up to that moment. Such acts may not be considered liable. Perfection is not the standard as "even reasonable doctors make mistakes" (Picard and Robertson, 1996). If a mistake could be made by a reasonably careful and knowledgeable practitioner acting in a similar situation, then the mistake may not be negligent (Kapp, 1997; Wu *et al.*, 1997).

Why is disclosure of medical error important?

Ethics

Most obviously, further harm to a patient may be caused by a clinician's non-disclosure. For example, a patient who is not told that he was given a wrong medication will not know what side effects to look for and might suffer avoidable injury as a consequence.

Failing to disclose errors to patients undermines public trust in medicine because it potentially involves deception (Bok, 1979). Non-disclosure is, potentially, a breach of the physician's fiduciary responsibilities, a lapse in the commitment to act solely out of concern for the patient's welfare (Robertson, 1987).

Disclosure of error and adverse events is also consistent with recent trends in healthcare toward more openness with patients and the involvement of patients in their own care (Etchells *et al.*, 1999; Hébert, 2008). Patients are due information about errors out of respect for them as persons. They also cannot properly consent to further treatment unless they know what went wrong.

By the principle of justice (fairness), patients or families, when harmed, should be able to seek appropriate restitution. This may involve seeking monetary recompense or pursuing professional regulatory misconduct hearings. Although some people sue solely for financial reasons, many are disturbed, as Vincent *et al.* (1994) and others have written, by the absence of explanations, a lack of honesty, the reluctance to apologize, or being

treated as a neurotic. Where serious harm occurs to a patient through the egregious and/or willful violation of safe and reliable healthcare practices or through deliberate dishonesty about the incident, families may gain some solace from knowing that the issues are treated seriously and that violators are identified and receive appropriate professional sanction (Shore, 2004).

Finally, non-disclosure of error may also undermine efforts to improve the safety of medical practice in general (Lansky, 2002). If practitioners are unable to be honest with patients or families regarding the untoward event, they are unlikely to be entirely candid in reporting the incident to the appropriate authorities within the healthcare setting. This will retard efforts to identify the faults and weaknesses in our healthcare processes and procedures.

Physicians sometimes argue that non-disclosure may be justified out of concern about needlessly increasing patient anxiety or confusing the patient with complicated information, thus obscuring true choice (Lantos, 1997). This perspective, called "therapeutic privilege," has not been viewed positively in recent years by Anglo-American courts and should be invoked only in extraordinary circumstances (Kent, 2005). With regards to complex procedures, suggesting that the information would only be confusing to a patient is in direct contradiction to the initial assumption that the patient was capable enough such that the physician accepted his/her informed consent to proceed. Those who support the concept of therapeutic privilege argue most strongly in cases of "harmless" error or "near misses," and in relation to contentious aspects of the incident, such as "who did it." It has also been suggested that requiring disclosure of harmless "almost incidents" would threaten to overwhelm the disclosure process with "noise." Requiring disclosure of "who did it" simplifies what are usually complicated incidents and might result in poisonous finger-pointing, interfering with efforts to improve patient safety. That said, professionals must be prepared to share some of the burden of the incident and not always attribute blame to the "system."

Law

The law recognizes that physicians may make mistakes without negligence. Indeed it frowns less on the mistakes than on dishonesty and attempts to conceal error – such concealment being incompatible with the doctor's fiduciary role (Robertson, 1987; Picard and Robertson, 1996). In *Stamos* v. *Davies* (1985), a respirologist mistakenly biopsied the patient's spleen in attempting a lung biopsy. When the patient asked for the results, rather than honestly admitting the error, the doctor replied he had "got something else." The judge found that the respirologist had breached a duty of disclosure owed to the patient "as a matter of professional relations."

Punitive damages of $20 000 were awarded in a 1999 British Columbia case in which a surgeon left an abdominal roll in the patient's abdomen during a laparotomy and presacral neurectomy. The surgeon waited over two months before telling the patient. During that time, he took active steps to cover up the mistake (e.g., by telling the nurses not to make any written record of it). The court described the surgeon's delay in informing his patient and his deliberate attempts to cover up his mistake as demonstrating "bad faith and unprofessional behavior deserving of punishment" (*Shobridge* v. *Thomas*, 1999).

These decisions and similar cases (*Vasdani* v. *Sehmi*, 1993; *Gerula* v. *Flores*, 1995) suggest that, in Canada at least, a doctor who makes an error in treating a patient has a positive legal duty to inform the patient. We recognize that the adversarial legal climate may be perceived as a disincentive for clinicians to be honest about error. However, the reality of this threat is often exaggerated and misplaced. The Harvard Medical Practice Study found that only 2% of negligent adverse events ever led to actual malpractice claims (Localio *et al.*, 1991). In one study, aggressive error disclosure by a Veteran's Administration Hospital in Kentucky led to a significant reduction in total dollars devoted to lawsuits (Kraman and Hamm, 1999).

In order to improve patient safety, certain jurisdictions currently have legislation requiring the reporting of incidents to the appropriate health authorities (Oklahoma State Legislature, 2004). More far-reaching examples of such legislation also require disclosure to patients and/or families (Legislative Assembly of Quebec, 2006) and also makes the admissions of error or adverse events safe from legal discovery (Illinois 93rd General Assembly, 2005). Lacking such addendums, legislative efforts to improve the quality of care and encourage reporting may falter.

Policy

Since the publication of the earlier version of this chapter in 2001, there has been a proliferation of professional policies addressing disclosure of adverse healthcare events. Disclosure of error is now explicitly addressed in Codes of Ethics for physicians in Canada (Canadian Medical Association, 2004) and the USA (American College of Physicians and Surgeons, 2005). Many professional and regulatory bodies or licensing authorities for physicians have, or are in the process of adopting, policies requiring physicians to disclose adverse events to patients (College of Physicians and Surgeons of Ontario, 1994). In the past, insurers of medical professionals were traditionally too liability-shy to openly advise candor with patients when adverse events occur. This is now changing. For example, the insurance organization for Canadian physicians, the Canadian Medical Protective Association, well aware of new trends in this area, advises honesty, seeing it as the best way to strengthen the doctor–patient relationship and so lessen the sting of any potential malpractice (Canadian Medical Protective Association, 2000).

Hospitals often have policies encouraging the reporting and disclosure of "medical incidents" as part of quality-assurance programs (VA Healthcare Network, 1998; Lamb *et al.*, 2003). Efforts to develop policies of disclosure in the USA have been fueled, in particular, by the requirement of their national hospital accrediting body that all hospitals must have in place a way of disclosing "unanticipated outcomes of care" to patients and/or to families

(Leape *et al.*, 1998). Guidelines for and articles addressing the "open disclosure" of untoward medical incidents may be found in the USA (ECRI, 2002), UK (Vincent *et al.*, 1999), Canada (Ontario Hospital Association, 2005), and Australia (Walton and the Clinical Practice Improvement Unit, 2001).

Empirical studies

Medical care causing harm is a very significant problem. The Harvard Medical Practice Study from the mid 1980s showed that 3.7% of patients in hospital suffered an adverse event. Approximately half of these events were considered preventable (Brennan *et al.*, 1991; Leape *et al.*, 1991). The Quality in Australian Health Care Study, conducted in the mid 1990s, found that 17% of admissions were associated with an adverse event, with 51% of these considered preventable (Wilson *et al.*, 1995). In Utah and Colorado, 1992 data revealed a rate of injury from medical care of 2.9% (Gawande *et al.*, 1999). Recent studies in the UK, Denmark, France, New Zealand, Canada (Canadian Institute for Health Information, 2004), and Spain (ENEAS, 2005) all show similar rates of adverse events (3–16% of hospitalized patients) and for preventability (20–50% of all such events).

However, inconsistencies in definitions of error and study methodology (Goldman, 1992; Rubin *et al.*, 1992; Smith *et al.*, 1997) should make us question claims that tens of thousands of patient deaths per year result from physician error (Leape, 1994b). The studies cannot say that the patient would be alive today were it not for this or that error. These are not studies of causality.

The real situation might be better (Brennan *et al.*, 1991; Wilson *et al.*, 1992). It also might be worse – hospital records are notorious for underreporting adverse events (Cullen *et al.*, 1995) and there are many barriers for accurate reporting by staff (Vincent *et al.*, 1999). As well, there are other dimensions of error that are not explored by these studies. For example, ambulatory care, the site of many healthcare encounters, remains largely not subjected to monitoring and study. Error studies are limited in

that up to half of all US healthcare interventions can be shown to be "inappropriate," although perhaps not always unsafe (McGlynn *et al.*, 2003).

Regardless of the precise magnitude of harmful medical events, each event raises the issue of disclosure. In one study in which patients of primary care physicians were given hypothetical situations, 98% wanted honest acknowledgement of errors, even if minor (Witman *et al.*, 1996). If not so informed, the surveyed patients indicated that they would be more likely to sue the physician. A recent survey, also of patients in the USA, bears this out: without full disclosure of an error, 34% of those surveyed would seek legal advice; 19.6% stated they would do so even with full disclosure, if the error was life threatening (Mazor *et al.*, 2004).

The Kentucky experiment shows that hospitals can be honest with patients about unanticipated care outcomes and not increase their legal risks. It did not address whether openness either eliminated or reduced lawsuits directed against physicians in particular.

Patients and physicians often differ in what should happen to the erring physician. In a study by Blendon *et al.* (2002), one-quarter of patient responders favored more lawsuits; 40% wanted the erring doctor to be fined, and 50% favored suspension of licenses. These options were chosen by a very small number of surveyed doctors. In a 2005 study, health plan members were prepared to forgive an erring doctor if the patient withheld critical information from the doctor (93%) but would not do so if the doctor was simply tired (32%), lacked knowledge (24%), or failed to follow up (15%) (Mazor *et al.*, 2005).

One problem with these studies is the assumption of a ready distinction of error – a term suggesting moral failure and fault to some – from other adverse events: if something bad happens, it must be somebody's fault. Study subjects are asked to respond to a simplified scenario, drained of the complexity the participants experienced at the time of the event. When harm to a patient occurs because of medical care, it is important, where possible, to be sure about what happened, yet it is often difficult to distinguish different classes of event or where fault may or may not lie. Whereas some adverse events are the result of individual error or even negligence, other events arise because of systemic issues (e.g., two medicine bottles with a similar appearance) or the errors and oversights of multiple members of the healthcare team.

How should I approach the disclosure of medical error in practice?

Frankly disclosing error can be challenging for practitioners (Hilfiker, 1984; Newman, 1996). Medical professionals have high expectations of themselves and, not surprisingly, find it difficult to acknowledge their errors openly before patients and colleagues (Finkelstein *et al.*, 1997). Clinicians who have observed a colleague disclosing an error to a patient are more likely to do so themselves (Hobgood *et al.*, 2006). This ethical "see-one, do one" is a nice variation on an old medical pedagogical technique and clearly needs a little refinement. It is reassuring as it suggests that disclosure is enabled by seeing that your fellow clinicians have done so and have survived. Disclosing such events may be less traumatic if practitioners follow practical guidelines for breaking bad news (Buckman *et al.*, 1998). If uncertain about how to talk to a patient concerning an error, clinicians would be wise to seek advice from their peers, mentors, or skilled hospital representatives before doing so. In any case, early notification of the clinician's professional insurers is recommended.

In general, it should be assumed that the patient would want full disclosure of errors and adverse events. The professional duty to disclose error is a proportionate duty: as the harm or risk of harm from an event to the patient increases, so increases the duty to disclose (Bogardus *et al.*, 1999). When an error is made but there is no obvious harm, the requirement to disclose error diminishes. For example, minor deviations from a plan of care should not necessarily trigger disclosure; major deviations clearly should. Everything between is subject to discussion and needs to be addressed, but the focus should always be on what is best for the patient as seen from someone in the patient's position. Clinicians might consider asking themselves: "if you (or a loved one) were the patient, what would you want to be told?"

Disclosure should take place at the right time, when the patient is medically stable enough to absorb the information, and in the right setting. Physicians should take the lead in disclosing error to patients and their families (Levinson *et al.*, 1997). They should try not to act defensively or evasively but, rather, explain what happened in an objective and narrative way, trying to avoid reacting to the charged response that such disclosure might generate. A physician may say "I'm sorry this has happened." Patients may appreciate this form of acknowledgement and empathy. This may strengthen, rather than undermine, the physician–patient relationship.

If the adverse outcome requires medical attention, practitioners should disclose this and seek prompt help for the patient. Patients may be reassured by knowing that the physician is not only remorseful but also dedicated to rectifying the harm and preventing further harm by a clearly defined course of action. It may be wise to offer to get a second opinion or the option of transferring care to another physician if the physician–patient relationship no longer seems viable.

Meeting with patients, and their families if necessary, in a timely way after an error can help to avoid suspicions about a "cover-up." Although worrisome and uncomfortable to most clinicians, having lawyers present, if desired by the patient or the family, may help to ensure that all their concerns are expressed and addressed. A healthcare team meeting in advance of a conference with the patient and family should establish that all relevant information regarding the sequence of events leading to the adverse outcome is at hand, mutually understood, and presented as clearly and openly as possible. It will also be important to say what, if anything, will be done to prevent the recurrence of such errors in the future. Patients and families may better accept what has happened to them if they can be reassured that medical care will be improved in the future.

Willful violations of safe healthcare practices and procedures are rare but must not be tolerated (Goldmann, 2006). When practitioners witness errors made by other healthcare providers, they have an ethical, if not legal, obligation to act on that information. Errors causing serious medical harm are ignored to the peril of the profession as well as the public (Irving *et al.*, 1998).

An emphasis on the faults of the system does not abrogate individual responsibility for untoward events. Individuals who exhibit poor judgement and show no signs of insight into their conduct ought to be reported by their peers to the appropriate authorities. Depending on the circumstances and the magnitude of the error, options range from encouraging disclosure by the erring practitioner to discussing the situation with the hospital unit director, department chief, risk manager, a professional insurer, or a representative from a regional health authority. The goal of reporting is not necessarily punitive. Where appropriate, reporting of error may lead to therapeutic attempts to identify treatable causes of error such as substance abuse or psychiatric illness (Shapiro, 2003). Hospitals and healthcare regions should have policies in place to protect such reporters from retaliation.

Medical harm and error are complex and multifaceted problems for practitioners, patients, families, and society. Adequate responses and solutions to them will depend on heightened personal, professional, and cultural commitments to honesty and truthfulness.

The cases

Assuming the report of renal cell cancer is accurate and in the right chart, the urologist should first find out what the patient now knows. If the patient is indeed unaware, the urologist needs to tell the patient, at this visit, about the findings on both the initial and current studies. She must be prepared for anger, shock, and disbelief. She should empathically acknowledge that emotion as well as her own upset. The patient may ask about the consequences for his health and his farming business. False reassurances, blame placed on the patient for failed follow-up or on office staff or fellow health professionals (radiology, trainees) will not be helpful. Neither, however, should the urologist shoulder the entire blame as there may be other contributing factors such as systems issues. If the patient wishes, he should be offered immediate referrals that week, if not that day, to another urologist and to an experienced oncologist. The physician should re-evaluate her office procedures and inform the patient of what will be done to prevent similar errors in the future. As serious error is typically emotionally difficult for healthcare professionals, appropriate support should be sought for the consultant through peers, family, friends, and, if needed, helping professionals (Shapiro, 2003).

In the second case, the surgeon should inform the patient and his family about the intraoperative event and the inability to achieve the intended outcome. Although the incident may not have a bad visual outcome for the patient, the surgeon must warn them of the possibility. He should arrange for appropriate follow-up surveillance and tell them what, if anything, can be done should the bad outcome occur. Hopefully, the possibility of the bad outcome was addressed in the initial informed consent. If so, the surgeon is not responsible for contact lens expense. However, he may offer to provide help by making appropriate referrals (e.g., to social work) to address the issues of contact lens cost and management.

REFERENCES

American College of Physicians and Surgeons (2005). Ethics manual, 5th edn, *Ann Intern Med* **142**: 560–82.

Baker G. R., Norton P. G., Flintcroft, V., *et al.* (2004). The Canadian Adverse Events Study: the incidence of adverse events among hospital patients in Canada. *CMAJ* **170**: pp. 1678–86 (http://www.ncbi.nlm.nih.gov/entrez/query.

fcgi?cmd=Retrieve&db=PubMed&dopt=Citation&list_uids=15159366).

Blendon, R. J., DesRoches, C. M., Brodie, M., et al. (2002). Views of practicing physicians and the public on medical errors. N Engl J Med 347: 1933–40.

Bogardus, S. T., Jr., Holmboe, E., Jekel, J., et al. (1999). Perils, pitfalls, and possibilities in talking about medical risk. JAMA 281: 1037–41.

Bok, S. (1979). Lying: Moral Choice in Public and Private Life. New York: Vintage Books, p. 71.

Brennan, T. A., Leape, L. L., Laird, N., et al. (1991). Incidence of adverse events and negligence in hospitalized patients. Results of the Harvard Medical Practice Study I. N Engl J Med 324: 370–6.

Buckman, R., Korsch, B., Baile, W., et al. (1998). A Practical Guide to Communication Skills in Clinical Practice. [CD–ROM set.] Toronto: Medical Audio Visual Communications.

Canadian Institute for Health Information (2004). Health Care in Canada. Ottawa: Statistics Canada.

Canadian Medical Association (2004). Code of Ethics. Ottawa: Canadian Medical Association. (http://www.cma.ca/index.cfm/ci_id/2419/la_id/1.htm) accessed 31 July 2006.

Canadian Medical Protective Association (2000). Disclosing Adverse Events to Patients: CMPA Information Sheet. Ottawa: Canadian Medical Protective Association.

College of Physicians and Surgeons of Ontario (1994). Policies. Professional Misconduct. Toronto: College of Physicians and Surgeons (http://www.cpso.on.ca/Policies/profmisc.htm) accessed 22 December 2000.

Cullen, D., Bates, D., Small, C., et al. (1995). The incident reporting system does not detect adverse drug events: a problem for quality improvement. Jt Comm J Qual Improv 21: 541–8.

Davies, J., Hébert, P., and Hoffman, C., (2003). The Canadian Patient Safety Dictionary. Ottawa: Royal College of Physicians and Surgeons of Canada.

ECRI (2002). Disclosure of unanticipated outcomes. Healthc Risk Contr RA:IRM 5 (Suppl A): 1–27.

ENEAS (2005). Report. National Study on Hospitalisation-Related Adverse Events. Madrid: Ministry of Health and Consumer Affairs Madrid (http://www.who.int/patientsafety/research/RESUMEN.ENEAS_INGLES.pdf) accessed 22 August 2006.

Etchells E., Sharpe G., Walsh, P., et al. (1999). Consent. In Bioethics at the Bedside, ed. P. Singer. Ottawa: Canadian Medical Association pp. 1–7.

Finkelstein, D., Wu, A. W., Holtzman, N., et al. (1997). When a physician harms a patient by a medical error: ethical, legal, and risk–management considerations. J Clin Ethics 8: 330–5.

Gawande, A. A., Thomas, E. J., Zinner, M., et al. (1999). The incidence and nature of surgical adverse events in Colorado and Utah in 1992. Surgery 126: 66–75.

Gerula v. Flores (1995). 126 DLR (4th) 506, 128 (Ont CA).

Goldman, R. L. (1992). The reliability of peer assessments of quality of care. JAMA 267: 958–60.

Goldmann, D. (2006). System failure versus personal accountability: the case for clean hands. N Engl J Med 355: 121–3.

Hébert, P. (2008). Doing Right. A Practical Guide to Ethics. Toronto: Oxford University Press.

Hilfiker, D. (1984). Facing our mistakes. N Engl J Med 310: 118–22.

Hobgood, C., Weiner, B., and Tamayo-Sarver, J. H. (2006). Medical error identification, disclosure, and reporting: do emergency medicine provider groups differ? Acad Emerg Med 13: 443–51.

Illinois 93rd General Assembly (2005). Patient Safety Act. Bill HB4245. (http://www.ilga.gov/legislation/BillStatus_pf.asp?DocNum=4245&DocTypeID=HB&LegID=8461&GAID=3&SessionID=3&GA=93) accessed 6 July 2006.

Irving, M., Berwick, D. M., Rubin, P., et al. (1998). Five times: coincidence or something more serious. BMJ 316: 1736–40.

Kapp, M. B. (1997). Legal anxieties and medical mistakes: barriers and pretexts. J Gen Intern Med 12: 787–8.

Kent, C. (2005). Medical Ethics: The State of the Law. Toronto: LexisNexis Butterworths.

Kohn, L., Corrigan, J., and Donaldson, M. S. (eds.) (2000). To Err is Human: Building a Safer Health System. Washington, DC: National Academy Press.

Kraman, S. S. and Hamm, G. (1999). Risk management: extreme honesty may be the best policy. Ann Intern Med 131: 963–7.

Lamb, R. M., Studdert, D. M., Bohner, R. M., et al. (2003). Hospital disclosure practices: results of a national survey. Health Aff (Millwood) 22: 73–83.

Lansky, D. (2002). Improving quality through public disclosure of performance information. Health Aff (Millwood) 21: 52–62.

Lantos, J. (1997). Do We Still Need Doctors? New York: Routledge, pp. 116–32.

Leape, L. L. (1994a). Error in medicine. JAMA 272: 1851–7.

Leape, L. L. (1994b). The preventability of medical injury. In *Human Error in Medicine*, ed. M. S. Bogner. Hillsdale, NJ: Erlbaum, pp. 13–25.

Leape, L. L., Brennan, T. A., Laird, N., *et al.* (1991). The nature of adverse events in hospitalized patients. Results of the Harvard Medical Practice Study II. *N Engl J Med* **324**: 377–84.

Leape, L. L., Woods, D. D., Hattie, M., *et al.* (1998). Promoting patient safety by preventing medical error. *JAMA* **280**: 1444–7.

Legislative Assembly of Quebec (2006). R.Q., c. M–9, r.4.1. Section 56.

Levinson, W., Roter, D. L., Mulloly, J., *et al.* (1997). Physician–patient communication. The relationship with malpractice claims among primary care physicians and surgeons. *JAMA* **277**: 553–9.

Localio, A. R., Lawthers, A. G., Brennan, T., *et al.* (1991). Relation between malpractice claims and adverse events due to negligence. Results of the Harvard Medical Practice Study III. *N Engl J Med* **325**: 245–51.

Mazor, K. M., Simon, S. R., Yood, R. A., *et al.* (2004). Health plan members' views about disclosure of medical errors. *Ann Intern Med* **140**: 409–18.

Mazor, K. M., Simon, S. R., Yood, R. A., *et al.* (2005). Health plan members' views on forgiving medical errors. *Am J Manag Care* **11**: 49–52.

McGlynn, E. A., Asch, S. M., Adams, T., *et al.* (2003). The quality of health care delivered to adults in the United States. *N Engl J Med* **348**: 2635–45.

Newman, M. C. (1996). The emotional impact of mistakes on family physicians. *Arch Fam Med* **5**: 71–5.

Oklahoma State Legislature (2004). *Act Relating to Public Health and Safety.* SB 1592. Oklahoma City: State Printing Office.

Ontario Hospital Association (2005). *Patient Safety in Ontario: An Overview of Patient Safety Policies in Select Ontario Academic Hospitals.* Toronto: Ontario Hospital Association.

Patient Safety Foundation (1998). *Tale of Two Stories: Contrasting Views of Patient Safety.* North Adams, MA: Patient Safety Foundation (*http://www.npsf.org/exec/report.html*).

Picard, E. and Robertson, G. (1996). *Legal Liability of Doctors and Hospitals in Canada*, 3rd edn. Toronto: Carswell, pp. 170–2.

Robertson, G. (1987). Fraudulent concealment and the duty to disclose medical mistakes. *Albert Law Rev* **25**: 215–23.

Rubin, H. R., Rogers, W. H., Robertson, L., *et al.* (1992). Watching the doctor-watchers. How well do peer review organization methods detect hospital care quality problems? *JAMA* **267**: 2349–54.

Shapiro, D. (2003). *Delivering Doctor Miranda: The Story of a Gifted Young Obstetrician's Mistake and the Psychiatrist who Helped Her.* New York: Harmony Books.

Sharpe, G. (1987). *The Law and Medicine in Canada*, 2nd edn. Toronto: Butterworths, pp. 15–16.

Shobridge v. *Thomas* (1999). BCJ no. 1747 (SC. online: QL (BCJ).

Shore, S. (2004). *No Moral Conscience: The Hospital for Sick Children and the Death of Lisa Shore.* Toronto: Trafford.

Sinclair, M. (1994). *The Report of the Manitoba Pediatric Cardiac Surgery Inquest: An Inquiry into Twelve Deaths at the Winnipeg Health Sciences Centre in 1994.* Winnipeg: Manitoba Health (http://www.pediatriccardiacinquest.mb.ca).

Smith, M. A., Atherly, A. J., Kane, R., *et al.* (1997). Peer review of the quality of care. Reliability and sources of variability for outcome and process assessments. *JAMA* **278**: 1573–8.

Smith, R. (1998). All changed, changed utterly. British medicine will be transformed by the Bristol case. *BMJ* **316**: 1917–18.

Stamos v. *Davies* (1985). 21 DLR (4th) 507 (Ont HC).

UK Department of Health (2000). *An Organisation with a Memory: Report of an Expert Group on Learning from Adverse Events in the NHS.* London: The Stationery Office (http://www.dh.gov.uk/assetRoot/04/06/50/86/04065086.pdf) accessed 31 July 2006.

VA Healthcare Network (1998). *Integrated Patient Safety/Risk Management Program.* New York: Veterans Health Administration (http://www.va.gov) accessed 22 December 2000.

Vasdani v. *Sehmi* (1993). OJ no. 44 (Gen Div) online: QL (OJ).

Vincent, C., Young, M., and Phillips, A. (1994). Why do people sue doctors? A study of patients and relatives taking legal action. *Lancet* **343**: 1609–13.

Vincent, C., Stanhope, N., Crowley-Murphy, P. I., *et al.* (1999). Reasons for not reporting adverse incidents: an empirical study. *J Eval Clin Pract* **5**: 13–21.

Walton, M. For the Clinical Practice Improvement Unit (2001). *Open Disclosure to Parents or Families After an Adverse Event. A Literature Review.* Sydney: Clinical Practice Improvement Unit (http://www.nsh.nsw.

gov.au/teachresearch/cpiu/CPIUwebdocs/Webversion
LiteratureReview.pdf) accessed 31 July 2006.

Wilson, D. S., McElligott, J., Fielding, L., *et al.* (1992). Identification of preventable trauma deaths: confounded inquiries? *J Trauma* **32**: 45–51.

Wilson, R. M., Runciman, W. B., Gibbard, R. W., *et al.* (1995). The Quality in Australian Health Care Study. *Med J Aust* **163**: 458–71.

Witman, A. B., Park, D. M., Hardin, S., *et al.* (1996). How do patients want physicians to handle mistakes? A survey of internal medicine patients in an academic setting. *Arch Intern Med* **156**: 2565–9.

Wu, A. W., Cavanaugh, T. A., McPhee, S. J., *et al.* (1997). To tell the truth: ethical and practical issues in disclosing medical mistakes to patients. *J Gen Intern Med* **12**: 770–5.

35

Conflict of interest in education and patient care

Ann Sommerville

A company producing drugs for the management of common conditions including asthma and diabetes has offered to pay the salary of a nurse in a doctor's practice. The nurse's role is to audit patients' records, ensuring that those with conditions such as asthma and diabetes are regularly examined and receive up-to-date medication. The doctor thinks this enhances patient care. The nurse provides anonymized patient data to the company and is barred from promoting its products. Information about the company's drugs is regularly provided by a sales team who visit the practice and pay for working lunches with the doctor. A good relationship exists and the company provides occasional gifts and invites the doctor's staff to dinner.

A well-referenced and user-friendly handbook on the medical care of a range of allergies in babies and children has been issued without charge to medical students and practicing doctors. Distribution has been funded by a leading charity whose remit is to raise awareness in society and the profession about childhood allergies. Prescribing advice is included in the handbook and two specific anti-allergy drugs are recommended. They are described as being particularly suitable for babies and young children. Various companies market variations of the same products but the brands named in the free book are glowingly described as effective even in difficult childhood cases. Parents who have also seen the book are starting to request them by name for their children's allergies. Both named brands are produced by the same pharmaceutical company. Student leaders have contacted local doctors and university colleagues urging them to lobby for the book to be withdrawn and to avoid prescribing these products. This is because the pharmaceutical company that produces the two named drugs previously donated $50 000 to the

allergy charity that is distributing it. It is not obvious that the donation was specifically for this handbook, however, and many students are reluctant to reject a free learning tool, arguing that they are sensible enough not to be unduly influenced by the prescribing advice (Jack, 2006).

What are conflicts of interest in education and patient care?

A conflict of interest has been described as "a set of conditions in which professional judgment concerning a primary interest tends to be unduly influenced by a secondary interest" (Thompson, 1993). Medical research is notorious for giving rise to significant conflicts of interest and these are discussed in Ch. 30. Here the focus is on the influence exercised by the pharmaceutical industry's promotional activities on medical education and patient care, which is also highly controversial. Sixteen compromising but common ways have been identified in which health professionals become entangled with drug companies (Moynihan, 2003). More potentially arise as the industry seeks new marketing methods. Such measures include the provision of hospitality or gifts for prescribers, company funding for clinical audit or research, paid meetings with company representatives, sponsored travel to conferences in exotic locations, inordinately high fees for conference speakers, and publishing opportunities for industry-friendly reports. Some of these activities are acceptable but only if on a modest level and open to scrutiny. Some are unacceptably compromising but seen by those involved as merely "the entwinement of individuals from different backgrounds and value sets who get to know each other and therefore want to reciprocate friendships and favours" (Smith, 2003). The result is that boundaries are blurred. As evidence mounts that prescribing patterns are seriously affected by such marketing strategies, prescribers often seem unwilling to acknowledge the excessive influence of venal interests (gifts and hospitality), clever advertising, or the apparently reassuring company information sheets.

Conflicts of interest occur in medical education in several ways. Educational meetings may be subsidized or feature sponsored speakers who only provide a pro-industry picture. Participants' travel or lavish accommodation may be subsidized so that they feel well disposed towards the sponsor. Educational materials or journal articles may be provided by a sponsoring company to reflect its views. More subtle influence may be exercised by the sponsor's views being incorporated into educational material published by an apparently independent third party. The media spotlight is increasingly turning, for example, on to the way in which charitable donations by drug manufacturers to patient support groups can result in an indirect but still very powerful influence on prescribing patterns (Jack, 2006). As a proportion of the overall funding of postgraduate medical education, the sums spent by pharmaceutical and biomedical companies frequently rival that of independent funders, including governments. The industry also exerts an enormous influence on practitioners' prescribing and treatment patterns, not least because its drug information is often more readily available and more reassuringly worded than other sources of prescribing advice. Drug advertising often associates brands with attributes designed to appeal to prescribers, particularly inexperienced ones. Despite reams of analysis about how such conflicts can be minimized or avoided, they appear undiminished.

More crucial than ever, therefore, is the need for practicing health professionals and students to raise their awareness of them.

Why are conflicts of interest in education and patient care important?

Ethics

While there is nothing inherently unethical in the occurrence of conflicts of interest in medicine, there may well be in the manner in which they are addressed. Society expects particularly high standards of the caring professions, whose advice should be independent, evidence based, and motivated by altruistic concern for patient welfare. These same expectations apply to doctors working within the pharmaceutical industry, who may feel pressured by product loyalty or colleagues' drive to maximize profits. Pharmaceutical and allied industries are well aware of the common public perception that they are disproportionately profit orientated and are increasingly try to address the range of ethical issues raised by their work (Mackie *et al.*, 2006). For doctors working for pharmaceutical companies, the conflicts of interest can be acute, but their ethical obligations to be truthful, maintain professional integrity, and put patient safety first are no less than those of any other doctor. Public trust can be seriously undermined if self-regarding interests supersede in medicine, even though they may be endemic in other sectors of society. Public confidence is also compromised if it appears that prescribing and treatment decisions are influenced more by pharmaceutical promotional materials than objective evidence. Professional and regulatory bodies acknowledge that even the unfounded *perception* of undue influence can be as damaging to public trust as corrupt practice. A common emphasis found in the guidance is that prescribers must be wary when any pecuniary or other incentive is offered. They must be as alert to perceived conflicts of interest as well as to actual ones since patients' erroneous belief that doctors' judgement is skewed towards personal advantage undermines trust as much as real corruption.

Law

Legal provisions vary in different jurisdiction. Nevertheless, there is a generally shared recognition that certain professionals, including doctors, are in a privileged position in the community in terms of the power and knowledge they acquire. The trust and societal status given to them requires them to avoid acting solely in their own interests when in a professional relationship with patients or clients. In some societies, this is covered by the concept of "fiduciary duties" obliging doctors to act conscientiously to maintain patient trust and public confidence. In jurisdictions that lack explicit reference to fiduciary duties, the same obligation is expressed in other terms. It is usually covered by the codes of professional bodies that may have the force of law. In the UK, for example, the General Medical Council is the regulatory body for medicine. Its powers are derived from the Medical Act 1983 and its guidance has binding force on doctors who are registered. The guidance reminds doctors of their legal and ethical obligation to act in patients' best interests and warns them against accepting any inducement, gift, or hospitality that may either affect or be seen to affect their judgement (General Medical Council, 2001). In addition in many jurisdictions, pharmaceutical and biomedical industries are bound by a range of regulations that similarly require them to exercise social responsibility. Not only do these regulations govern the conduct of clinical trials, pharmacovigilance, and the reporting of adverse events but they also cover marketing and product promotion. For example, the advertising of drugs in the UK is controlled by a combination of statutory measures such as the Medicines Act 1969, with both criminal and civil sanctions, and the pharmaceutical industry's own self-regulatory codes. Nevertheless, the law sometimes needs interpretation in the context of new scenarios, such as the situation described in the second case opening this chapter.

Policy

Public policy requires that patients be able to have confidence in healthcare services. The professional codes for both doctors and the pharmaceutical industry proscribe activities that might undermine patient or public trust. National pharmaceutical codes focusing on marketing activities are published, for example, by the Association of the British Pharmaceutical Industry (ABPI) in the UK, Medicines Australia and the Pharmaceutical Research and Manufacturers of America. Promotional activities are also covered in international guidance, such as those published by the International Federation of Pharmaceutical Manufacturers and Associations (2003), the European Federation of Pharmaceutical Industries and Associations (2006), and the World Health Organization (1988). What is less clear is how widely these are known and how rigorously enforced. In the UK, a survey of doctors (ABPI, 2006) found that few were aware of the rules governing pharmaceutical representatives' relations with them and even fewer knew how to make a complaint under the pharmaceutical code. Yet the complaints procedure can be an effective tool in enforcing standards and drawing public attention to breaches by the industry.

Empirical studies

The enormous influence of the pharmaceutical industry is an issue of concern in many countries. A growing literature has examined it in different contexts and eminent bioethicists have summarized it (Lemmens and Singer, 1998). Medical journals have produced thematic issues devoted to it (e.g., the *British Medical Journal*; Anon., 2003). In the UK, a Parliamentary committee (House of Commons Health Committee, 2005) investigated it, finding that the industry's marketing affects all sectors of society – not only prescribers, but patients, regulators, managers, medical charities, researchers, academics, the media, and politicians. Pharmaceutical industry influence is particularly crucial for current and future prescribers of medicinal products and devices. The parliamentary report described how doctors become tainted by their association with industry and recommended measures to curb marketing excesses. This echoes concerns long expressed in other countries including the USA, Canada, and Australia. All have experienced calls for stricter control on the way that drugs are advertised, particularly to young health professionals.

In fact, since the 1980s, attention has been repeatedly drawn to the way in which medical education and prescribing are influenced by pharmaceutical companies, whose advertising also constitutes a large percentage of the revenue of many medical journals. In the UK, the problem was highlighted and guidelines published in the mid 1980s (Royal College of Physicians, 1986). As concern grew internationally, more guidance followed. In 1990, the American College of Physicians published *Physicians and the Pharmaceutical Industry*, followed in 1998 by guidance from the Canadian Medical Association and in 1999 by the Australian (Royal Australasian College of Physicians, 2005). Such guidelines expose common quandaries in the way in which industry influences the structure and function of medical education at all levels. Codes provide guidance on the handling of conflicts of interest that need to be addressed from both the perspective of health professionals and from that of the pharmaceutical industry. They forbid doctors from accepting – and companies from offering – significant gifts, including lavish travel, expensive hospitality, or extravagant meals. Any funding must be modest and open to scrutiny.

Detailed international guidance for medical practitioners working in the field of pharmaceutical medicine is also available. It recognizes that they experience an understandably strong interest in the drugs they have been involved in developing. They must recognize, in turn, their ethical responsibility to stand aside from product loyalty and other pressures stemming from their employment and ultimately put the protection of patients' interests first. Just as prescribers must seek independently verified data, doctors employed in the pharmaceutical industry must seek to ensure that only reliable and accurate information is used in marketing. They have difficult conflicts of interest that demand considerable determination and doctors should be supported by their professional bodies when they make a stand.

Conflicts of interest in education

Pharmaceutical representatives have been described as the "stealth bombers of medicine: they swoop in, change practice, better than any journal article or formal educator" (Shaughnessy and Slawson, 1996). Drug companies' interaction with doctors and academia has also been compared to porcupine quills – numerous and harmful if approached the wrong way (Lewis *et al.*, 2001). Scholarships, grants, or other educational funds are provided by biomedical industries. Over half of all UK postgraduate medical education and much nurse education are funded by the pharmaceutical industry from its marketing budget (House of Commons Health Committee, 2005). This is not unique to the UK but is representative of a general trend. The powerful effect of such influence on medical students was the focus of a Finnish study (Vainiomaki *et al.*, 2004), which found that students' reliance on pharmaceutical promotions as an educational source increased over the course of their studies. It does not disappear after graduation. Former *New England Journal of Medicine* editor Arnold Relman (2003) commented that practicing doctors "are taught about drugs by agents of the pharmaceutical industry, which works hard to persuade them to select the newest and most expensive medication – even in the absence of scientific evidence that they are any better than older, less costly ones." Even when aware that marketing was likely to affect their later prescribing, the Finnish students did not favor reducing it. This may be because the importance of avoiding undue industry influence is insufficiently emphasized in medical ethics teaching in most countries. Even in the USA, where awareness of the power of pharmaceutical marketing is probably highest, only one in four medical schools provide courses to prepare students in this respect (Black, 2004).

The need to inculcate good prescribing habits in young doctors has been the focus of a considerable literature, and some student organizations have taken on the task of awareness raising. In 2002, the American Medical Student Association started its nationwide "PharmFree" campaign urging an end to sponsored education, free lunches, and pharmaceutical advertising aimed at students. It encourages members to seek out independent, evidence-based sources of healthcare information and rejects all pharmaceutical advertisements and sponsorship. Its website highlights how "the practice of pharmaceutical gifting to students and physicians increases the costs of health care for patients and does not primarily serve patient interests" (American Medical Student Association, 2006). The topic of relationships with industry has also been a major issue in Australian and Canadian student groups, among others.

Conflicts of interest in patient care

Professional codes require prescribers to put the patient's interest first, but prescribing patterns are often influenced by drug companies through the provision of gifts, dinners, funding, financial assistance with travel for prescribing doctors and nurses, or accommodation at scientific meetings. Inexpensive gifts, limited hospitality and travel sponsorship are acceptable, and clear criteria are set out by professional associations. Professional codes ban lavish gifts or inducements from pharmaceutical companies and prohibit company representatives from offering them.

Traditionally, doctors and medical students have been the main targets of pharmaceutical advertising, but nurse prescribers are increasingly approached. All health professionals suffer information overload, but they have a responsibility to inform themselves independently about the drugs they prescribe. Professional organizations must also strive to help doctors working in pharmaceutical companies to exercise rigorous control over the marketing information. The dangers of not doing so were highlighted by a Scottish investigation into a child's death. Ten times the licensed dose of a common asthma drug had been prescribed, largely because of the reassurance provided by the manufacturer's marketing material about its safety (National Patient Safety Agency, 2005). Advertising slogans stressing the drug's benefits for children led doctors to prescribe high doses without checking evidence-based guidance.

How should I approach conflicts of interest in education and patient care in practice?

A number of strategies for individual and collective action have been identified. The most basic duty is for all health professionals to be vigilant about the kinds of circumstance in which temptation occurs and to familiarize themselves with their professional bodies' rules. Obviously, they need to be able to recognize the potential for conflicting interests, but this is not necessarily as easy as it sounds, as shown by the case examples at the start of the chapter.

Familiarity with regulatory codes and guidelines

Codes of practice must not only be taught and known but also enforced. Whereas the regulatory codes for medicine can result in doctors being banned from practice, one of the problems with pharmaceutical codes has generally been their voluntary nature and lack of enforceability. They are, however, backed up by a complaints procedure, which, in an increasingly image-conscious world, there seems to be growing willingness to implement and publicize. This means that people employed in healthcare and industry should understand how the relevant complaints procedures work.

Training and awareness raising

Regrettably, the provisions of professional codes and evidence of the strong influence of marketing on prescribing appear to be poorly appreciated by many practitioners. Internationally, few courses exist to help students and doctors to evaluate marketing campaigns, but general issues around pharmaceutical promotion and its influence on prescribing must be highlighted in undergraduate education for all health professionals. Such training should also guide them about where to find reliable non-industry sources of prescribing guidance. Undergraduate and continuing professional training need to highlight independently validated sources of data and international evidence-based clinical publications. In countries such as the UK, where nurse prescribing is growing, the lack of specific courses for nurses makes them particularly reliant on pharmaceutical company promotional information. Training is a key issue, not only for health professionals but also for pharmaceutical company employees, who need to be aware of the acceptable boundaries of their interaction with clinicians.

Alternative sources of funding

Despite the repeatedly stated desire of health organizations and professional groups to distance prescribing from the influence of marketing, finding acceptable alternative funders for education has remained a problem. This needs to be further addressed nationally and internationally.

Transparency

Openness and public disclosure are key factors in defusing many potential conflicts of interest. Speakers at conferences and authors of articles must declare any interest or links they have with industry when presenting their views. They should alert their audience to the possibilities of conscious or unconscious bias. The duty to disclose financial or professional interests is also recognized in the publishing rules of medical journals. Regulatory codes emphasize the importance of health professionals always declaring to patients or to institutional healthcare purchasers any personal or financial interests they (or close relatives) hold. Registers have been proposed in some countries for

all health workers to record all gifts and benefits given to them over a trivial sum, including travel and hospitality. Even where such registers exist, according to evidence from the pharmaceutical industry itself, many health professionals remain unaware of the requirement to declare their interests (ABPI, 2005). Cases undoubtedly still occur in which doctors accept significant benefits or cost-free opportunities to attend symposia in exotic locations with pharmaceutical sponsorship. Such offers are likely to be seen by the public as thinly disguised bribes. Only inexpensive tokens or modest hospitality at meetings with clear educational content are likely to be above suspicion. In any case of doubt, reference should be made to the local professional guidance. Even if prescribers themselves are convinced their independence will not be compromised, the perception that the industry is buying influence needs be avoided. Therefore, rigorous attention is needed in any situation that could be perceived as compromising.

The cases

The cases have been chosen because they are common and represent the borderline between what is clearly prohibited and what is deemed ethically acceptable. In the first case, it is unwise of the doctor to accept gifts or expensive meals. The services of the audit nurse represent a significant gift and, although it not clearly prohibited, any strings attached to it need to be carefully reviewed. If accepted, it should be declared if a local public register exists. Although company-sponsored nurses do not promote drugs, the data they research are used by the company sales teams to assess the practice's potential market. Nurses may also receive bonuses by identifying patients who could be transferred to costly new drug schemes and so pressure to transfer them builds up on the doctor. Any form of company-sponsored service must be handled with care and with a keen eye to the public's and patients' perceptions. Doctors' awareness of their own and colleagues' prescribing patterns needs to be high and in line with peer practice, with regular review if patterns change as a result of accepting the service.

The second case illustrates one of the subtle ways that medical education can be influenced when sponsored material is provided to medical students and practicing doctors as if it were completely independent, unbiased advice. Unfortunately, such material is often aimed at, and taken up by, the most inexperienced prescribers. In accepting such free books, students and doctors need to be aware that they are likely to be perceived as acting in a biased way if they subsequently prescribe the products recommended, unless they have clearly considered rival products. In the UK, regulators have forced the withdrawal of some sponsored information booklets for doctors (Jack, 2006). Similar educational materials to which patients have access and which mention specific drugs have also been ruled as violating the UK ban on advertising drugs directly to the public. While there is nothing unethical or illegal in companies donating to charities or patient groups or sponsoring their materials, all such donations must be open and transparent.

REFERENCES

ABPI (2005). *Health Select Committee Inquiry into the Influence of the Pharmaceutical Industry. Supplementary Submission.* London: Association of the British Pharmaceutical Industry.

ABPI (2006). *Press Release ABPI Code of Practice: Informing Doctors.* London: Association of the British Pharmaceutical Industry (www.abpi.org.uk/press/press_ releases_06/060306.asp).

American College of Physicians (1990). *Physicians and the Pharmaceutical Industry.* Washington, DC: American College of Physicians.

American Medical Student Association (2006). *Towards a PharmFree Profession.* Washington, DC: American Medical Student Association (www.amsa.org/prof/history.cfm).

Anon. (2003). Theme issue on time to untangle doctors from drug companies. *BMJ* **326**: 1155.

Black, H. (2004). Dealing in drugs. *Lancet* **364**: 1655–6.

Canadian Medical Association (1998). *Physicians and the Pharmaceutical Industry.* Ottawa: Canadian Medical Association.

European Federation of Pharmaceutical Industries and Associations (2006). *Code of Practice on the Promotion of Medicine.* Brussels: European Federation of Pharmaceutical Industries and Associations (http://www.efpia.org/6_publ/promotionofmedicinesq&a2006.pdf).

General Medical Council (2001). *Good Medical Practice*, paragraph 55. London: General Medical Council.

House of Commons Health Committee (2005). *The Influence of the Pharmaceutical Industry. Fourth Report of Session 2004–5.* London: The Stationery Office.

International Federation of Pharmaceutical Manufacturers and Associations (2003). *Code of Practice of Pharmaceutical Marketing Practice.* Geneva: International Federation of Pharmaceutical Manufacturers and Associations.

Jack, A. (2006). Too close for comfort? *BMJ* **333**: 13.

Leemens, T. and Singer, P. A. (1998). Bioethics for clinicians: conflict of interest in research, education and patient care. *CMAJ* **159**: 960–5.

Lewis, S., Baird, P., Evans, R. G., *et al.* (2001). Dancing with the porcupine: rules governing the university–industry relationship. *CMAJ* **165**: 783–5.

Mackie, J. E., Taylor, A. D., Finegold, D. L., *et al.* (2006). Lessons on ethical decision making from the bioscience industry. *PLoS Med* **3**: e129.

Moynihan, R. (2003). Who pays for the pizza? Redefining the relationships between doctors and drug companies. *BMJ* **326**: 1189–96.

National Patient Safety Agency (2005). *Lessons from a Fatal Accident Inquiry.* London: National Patient Safety Agency (www.saferhealthcare.org.uk/IHI/Topics/MedicationPractice/CaseStudies/lessonsfromafatalaccidentinquiry.htm).

Relman, A. S. (2003). Your doctor's drug problem. *New York Times*, 18 November.

Royal College of Physicians (1986). The relationship between physicians and the pharmaceutical industry. *J R Coll Physicians Lond* **20**: 235–42.

Royal Australasian College of Physicians (2005). *Ethical Guidelines in the Relationship Between Physicians and the Pharmaceutical Industry.* Canberra: Royal Australasian College of Physicians (http://www.racp.edu.au/public/Ethical_guide_pharm.pdf).

Shaughnessy, A. and Slawson, D. (1996). Pharmaceutical representatives. *BMJ* **312**: 1494.

Smith, J. (2003). Food, flattery and friendship. *BMJ* **326**: 1151.

Thompson, D. F. (1993). Understanding financial conflicts of interest. *N Engl J Med* **329**: 573–6.

Vainiomaki, M., Helve, O., Vuorenkovski, L., *et al.* (2004). A national survey on the effect of pharmaceutical promotion on medical students. *Med Teach* **26**: 630–4.

World Health Organization (1988). *Ethical Criteria for Medicinal Drug Promotion*. Geneva: World Health Organization.

36

Public health ethics

Halley S. Faust and Ross Upshur

A 42-year-old female sees her family physician for a vaginal discharge. She and her physician have a long-standing doctor–patient relationship, as well as a personal friendship. Three weeks previously, the patient had been to a sales convention in Reno and committed a "marital indiscretion." She is worried she may have a sexually transmitted disease (STD). She gives consent for her physician to do the appropriate diagnostic work-up and treatment, but states that if this is an STD she doesn't want her physician to report it to the public health authorities, nor to tell her husband, with whom she has had sexual intercourse since her return from the convention two weeks ago.

What is public health ethics?

Public health has been described as the science and art of promoting and protecting health, preventing disease, prolonging life and improving quality of life through the organized efforts of society (Last, 2001). It achieves these goals using community interventions, disease control, and principles of epidemiology and biometry. Public health ethics is concerned with the ethical issues raised by such community and population-based approaches to health problems.

While the goals of public health and clinical medicine are to increase well-being, the latter uses individual action and intervention for the good of *individual* well-being, while the former uses a social approach to improving the good of *communities*. The principles used in determining which programs are worthy of public health action and which are not have evolved over time; the

elaboration of these principles is now gaining currency in the fledgling field of public health ethics (Kass, 2001; Roberts and Reich, 2002; Nixon *et al.*, 2005). Ethical principles for consideration in planning for disaster responses to pandemic influenza have recently been proposed (University of Toronto Joint Centre for Bioethics, Pandemic Influenza Working Group, 2005). Most of these principles would also apply to the reasoning for requiring a reporting and surveillance system in the first place.

Various authors have proposed public health ethics frameworks that would uniquely appeal to one or more of utilitarianism, duty-based systems, or communitarianism. In all cases, the basic moral considerations are to produce benefits to the public as a whole, while minimizing harms, fairly distributing benefits and burdens, respecting individual autonomy and privacy, and honoring prior commitments and promises (Childress *et al.*, 2002). If a principles-based approach is used, the following principles have been proposed.

Effectiveness. A public health intervention or requirement should have been proven to be effective in preventing or mitigating specific health conditions. For example, reporting and early intervention are known to reduce the spread and impact of sexually transmitted disease (STD).

Proportionality. Any moral infringement that will be incurred with the effective intervention should be considerably outweighed by the benefits gained. In the case of STDs, the benefits are to prevent or alleviate harm to any sexual partners of the patient.

Necessity. The intervention proposed should produce an outcome that cannot be produced by another intervention that does not create a moral infringement. As STDs do not go away by themselves, suspected contacts need evaluation and treatment.

Least infringement. Only the least amount of restriction or disclosure of information should occur. The patient in our case, would not have any other non-STD-related information transmitted to the health department. Further, encouraging the patient to speak with her husband first would reduce the harm that might occur if the husband first hears about the exposure from a public health worker.

Public justification. Public health policies and the imposition of such policies/rules/regulations on individuals or families need to be justified through public debate. The need for a law for reporting of notifiable conditions has been debated in the public arena many times and deemed in nearly all political jurisdictions to be a necessity. When notification occurs with patient-identifying information, then discussions ensue with the patient by both the physician and the public health agency as to why disclosure is required, and then contacts are traced.

Reciprocity. Society has an obligation to mitigate the burdens imposed by public health regulations and actions by supporting an individual who is complying with public health mandates. Training physicians in counseling patients about STD case reporting and assisting patients in educating and informing partners are examples of reciprocity.

Transparency. Similar to public justification, this principle requires public deliberations on the determining of public health laws, rules, and regulations; public accountability for the imposition of those rules; and the assessment of their effectiveness. Public reporting of STD trends would be an example.

In this chapter, our specific focus is on the ethical issues raised by reporting and surveillance for communicable diseases. This is arguably the most important and most common interface between clinicians and public health agencies. We will review the ethical and legal aspects of when clinicians' duties to the public's health may supersede their duties to their patients, recognizing that, while reporting infectious disease cases to public health authorities may create a hardship on the part of patients, the clinician's role is not solely to that patient but also legitimately extends, in certain circumstances, to the public's welfare.

What is public health reporting and surveillance?

One of the great accomplishments in healthcare in the twentieth century has been the reduction of the impact of infectious diseases in the developed world (Figure 36.1; Centers for Disease Control and Prevention, 1999a). While sanitation and the advent of antibiotics and immunizations are two of the key factors in infectious disease control and prevention, a third important factor has been public health surveillance systems designed for tracking and reacting to trends in infectious disease incidence (Centers for Disease Control and Prevention, 1999b). Since the second half of the nineteenth century, surveillance has largely relied on the goodwill of physicians and healthcare institutions to report the diagnosis (or suspicion of a diagnosis) of diseases that have relevance for prevention and control in the population at large (Koo and Wetterhall, 1996).

While clinician reporting to public health authorities started out as voluntary (Fox, 1986), in the twenty-first century nearly all countries have laws that require clinicians to report incidents of an array of diseases. Which diseases are reportable is dependent on the jurisdiction and changes over time as the incidence, treatment, and control of diseases have changed. The World Health Organization through its International Health Regulations currently requires reporting of only three diseases: plague, cholera, and yellow fever (World Health Organization, 1998). In the

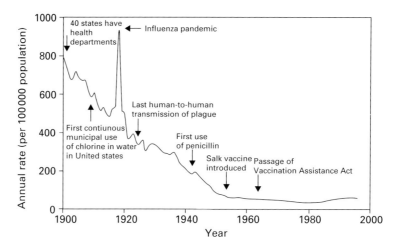

Figure 36.1. Crude death rate for infectious disease in the USA 1900–1996. (From Centers for Disease Control and Prevention, 1999a.)

USA and Canada, each state and province has its own list of reportable conditions (Roush *et al.*, 1999), often based upon recommendations from the Centers for Disease Control and Prevention (2006a). The case definitions are provided as well (Centers for Disease Control and Prevention, 2006b). Canada is the manager for the Global Public Health Intelligence Network, which searches the World Wide Web for communicable disease reports (Public Health Agency of Canada, 2004). Each province in Canada has its own list of reportable diseases in addition to a list of diseases under surveillance, carried out through its provinces in the Canadian Integrated Public Health Surveillance program.

Further, in some jurisdictions not only must clinicians report suspected or confirmed cases of some communicable diseases but laboratories are mandated to report as well. Therefore, even if the patient asks the clinician not to report her own case, the case will be reported to the relevant authorities if laboratory studies are done to confirm suspected diagnoses.

What criteria are used to determine which diseases/conditions need reporting?

Obtaining identifiable information about an individual poses serious concerns of privacy for the patient. Additionally, public health agencies recognize that reporting of diseases takes time and effort by practitioners, and also requires resources at the local public health level to review reports, trace contacts, collate data, and report surveillance information. Consequently, over the years, fairly strict criteria have evolved for determining which diseases to list as reportable.

Surveillance systems are designed to spot trends in incidence for diseases (i) that occur normally in the population (e.g., Lyme disease, pneumococcal pneumonia, chlamydial infection), (ii) that occur in regular outbreaks (e.g., influenza, gastroenteritis, hepatitis A), and (iii) that are not expected to occur – where one case could be a major problem (e.g., measles, meningococcal meningitis, hantavirus). In the first case, spotting increasing trends may encourage public health personnel to move available resources from one program to another to help to reduce the incidence over time. In the second case, contact tracing and source eradication or isolation would be important in a timely fashion. In the third case, immediate mobilization of all available resources might be necessary to limit any further spread, particularly for highly serious diseases like hantavirus, plague, Ebola virus, or severe acute respiratory syndrome (SARS). Reporting completeness is particularly important for this last category of diseases, where one case is cause for alarm.

The criteria used are related to seriousness of the disease, potential for transmission by either human-to-human or animal-to-human methods, and ability to control and/or treat the problem.

Unfortunately, we know that the norm is under-reporting by clinicians and institutions. Various studies have shown that, on average, only 63% of cases are reported, and, depending on the disease and jurisdiction, somewhere between 10% (giardiasis; Campos-Outcalt, *et al.*, 1991) and 99% (tuberculosis; Trepka *et al.*, 1999) of disease-specific cases are reported (Doyle *et al.*, 2002). A 2002 study in the USA (St Lawrence *et al.*, 2002) revealed that "The frequency of case reporting [by clinicians] was lowest for chlamydia (37% . . .), intermediate for gonorrhea (44%), and highest for syphilis, HIV, and AIDS (53–57%)." If the relative completeness of reporting does not change from time to time, then incidence trends are still good gauges of actual disease activity in the population, and public health authorities can respond accordingly.

Why is public health ethics important?

While public health functions have only been part of governmental activities in their current form since the mid 1800s, they originally evolved to protect the public broadly from the introduction or spread of communicable diseases. In the early years, public health activities were quite liberty restrictive and impacted mostly on immigrants and the lower classes: mandatory isolation through quarantine, rejection of diseased individuals attempting to migrate at national borders, enforced treatments. While we are not as heavy handed about these activities these days, in emergencies classic public health interventions are still used. For example during the SARS outbreak in 2003 in Toronto, isolation and quarantine of suspected cases and limited hospital access occurred (National Advisory Committee on SARS and Public Health, 2003). There was heightened surveillance of airline travelers and travel advice was issued (World Health Organization, 2003).

An example of the third principle, mandatory treatment, is invoked with tuberculosis, wherein directly observed therapy and sometimes police actions are undertaken to force individuals to comply with required treatment (Taylor *et al.*, 2005).

Lapses in mandatory compliance with case reporting are sanctioned in some jurisdictions by substantial fines. Courts have held that doctors may be liable if persons are infected by the doctor's patient if the doctor "... negligently fails to diagnose a contagious disease, or, having diagnosed the illness, fails to warn members of the patient's family ..." (Menikoff, 2001).

Clearly, when the condition of one patient has a potential for harming another, we are under legal imperative to minimize harm to others who are not our patients. Indeed, there are many legal mandates to violate our patient's confidentiality, or for which we have dual loyalties: suspected child and elder abuse, occupational injury, and insurance reimbursement are just three examples (R. E. G. Upshur and S. R. Benatar, unpublished observations).

Of course, legal imperatives are not necessarily coincident with moral imperatives. For, by divulging personal patient information, we violate our duty to maintain our patient's confidence and privacy. Whereas in health emergencies like SARS, where large numbers of individuals may be at risk, the physician's responsibility shifts from being primarily patient oriented to being public oriented (Lo and Katz, 2005), with individual patients for whom transmission of disease is likely to be more limited, why shouldn't we work hard to protect our patient's privacy and the key ongoing trust relationship we have?

Trust is not the only concern for violating the privacy pact in the doctor–patient relationship. We have concern for other types of harm patients may experience when certain types of disease are known to afflict them: stigmatization (HIV), embarrassment, ostracism, reduced insurability, discrimination in employment and housing, and even political retribution can be the consequences of private health information becoming public. How do we balance these individual concerns with the public's welfare? What are the key components of public health ethics decision making?

How should I approach public health ethics in practice?

The translation of public health ethics principles into daily medical practice is fairly straightforward for reporting notifiable conditions. All things considered, not only is reporting the correct ethical act to take but it is also the required act to take legally in virtually all political jurisdictions.

Firstly, the clinician needs to be familiar with the diseases required to be reported in their respective practice jurisdictions, as well as the mechanisms to be used to make full reports. Many jurisdictions make this information available through newsletters or on their websites (e.g., Connecticut Department of Public Health, 2006).

Secondly, clinicians need to appreciate the value of reporting diseases. By internalizing this appreciation, the hesitancy to comply with the requirement (or alternatively the willingness to comply with a patient's request *not* to report a disease, as in the case at the beginning of this chapter) will be reduced. Physicians should not consider this requirement unpleasant; instead it should be considered virtuous. Having personal conviction that taking an action is the right action helps in complying more completely with the reporting requirement. Additionally, it shows conviction during the discussion with the patient. This would be consistent with the effectiveness, necessity, and proportionality principles.

Thirdly, the clinician should practice discussing the need to report diseases with patients, including working on specific wording that is most effective for communicating the need with sympathy and care. Some reportable diseases, like cholera, measles, or tularemia, are not as sensitive to discuss with patients as STDs or diseases with social stigma

attached, such as tuberculosis or Hansen's disease (leprosy). As with other diseases that carry profound implications, there are various ways to communicate unpleasant information to patients (Epstein *et al.*, 2004). We spend a lot of time training oncologists to discuss the options of cancer treatment and prognosis, or palliative care with patients (Sutherland *et al.*, 1991; Hagerty *et al.*, 2005). Similar training and practice is appropriate for reporting discussions. Frank discussion and proposed actions are necessary to conform to a transparency approach.

Finally, in keeping with the principle of reciprocity, the clinician should be sure that the health department is supplying the patient with all of the emotional and treatment support appropriate for the situation. By entering into the reporting relationship, the clinician is, in a sense, now an arm of the government, which has responsibility for assuring that the burdens imposed by breaking confidentiality are offset as much as possible with support for minimizing the harm that may come of it.

The case

The clinician empathized with the patient's request and then discussed the importance of reporting for the good not just of the patient's husband but also so that the contacts from whom the patient had received her illness could also be traced for proper testing and treatment. In addition, the clinician made the patient aware that her clinician was not the only source of information to the public health authorities: for an accurate diagnosis some tests would have to be sent to the laboratory, which is also mandated by law to report information about positive test results. The clinician emphasized that the public health authorities are quite knowledgeable and sensitive about handling these situations, and that they try to keep contacts anonymous, though, of course, if contacts only had sex with one person the inference would be obvious. The patient nervously consented to testing and reporting, but asked that she be allowed to speak with her husband before the physician reported to the public health authorities. The clinician agreed, suggesting a timeline by which date the patient needed to report back, or the clinician would have to proceed with the notification as mandated by law. The clinician also set a time for calling the health department and patient to assure a smooth transition for the reporting and contact tracing.

REFERENCES

Campos-Outcalt, D., England, R., Porter, B., *et al.* (1991). Reporting of communicable diseases by university physicians. *Public Health Rep* **106**: 579–83.

Centers for Disease Control and Prevention (1999a). Ten great public health achievements: United States, 1900–1999. *MMWR Morb Mortal Wkly Rep* **48**: 241–3.

Centers for Disease Control and Prevention (1999b). Control of infectious diseases. *MMWR Morb Mortal Wkly Rep* **48**: 621–9.

Centers for Disease Control and Prevention (2006a). *Nationally Notifiable Infectious Diseases, United States.* Atlanta, GA: Centers for Disease Control and Prevention (http://www.cdc.gov/epo/dphsi/phs/infdis2006.htm) accessed 14 July 2006.

Centers for Disease Control and Prevention. (2006b). *Case definitions for Infectious Conditions under Public Health Surveillance.* Atlanta, GA: Centers for Disease Control and Prevention (http://www.cdc.gov/epo/dphsi/casedef/index.htm) accessed 14 July 2006.

Childress, J. F., Faden, R. R., Gaare, R., *et al.* (2002). Public health ethics: mapping the terrain. *J Law Med Ethics* **30**: 170–8.

Connecticut Department of Public Health (2006). Reportable diseases and laboratory findings, 2006. *Connecticut Epidemiol* **26**: 1–3.

Doyle, T. J., Glynn, M. K., Groseclose, S. L. (2002). Completeness of notifiable infectious disease reporting in the United States: an analytical literature review. *Am J Epidemiol* **155**: 866–74.

Epstein, R. M., Alper, B. S., Quill, T. E., (2004). Communicating evidence for participatory decision making. *JAMA* **291**: 2359–66.

Fox, D. M. (1986). From TB to AIDS: value conflicts in reporting disease. *Hastings Cent Rep* **16**(Suppl): 11–16.

Hagerty, R. G., Butow, P. N., Ellis, P., *et al.* (2005). Communicating prognosis in cancer care: a systematic review of the literature. *Ann Oncol* **16**: 1005–53.

Kass, N. E. (2001). An ethics framework for public health. *Am J Public Health* **91**: 1776–82.

Koo, D. and Wetterhall, S. F. (1996). History and current status of the National Notifiable Diseases Surveillance System. *J Public Health Manag Pract* **2**: 4–10.

Last, J. (ed.) (2001). *A Dictionary of Epidemiology*, 4th edn, Toronto: Oxford University Press.

Lo, B. and Katz, M. H. (2005). Clinical decision making during public health emergencies: ethical considerations. *Ann Intern Med* **143**: 493–8.

Menikoff, J. (2001). *Law and Bioethics.* Washington, DC: Georgetown University Press, p. 178.

National Advisory Committee on SARS and Public Health (2003). *Learning from SARS: Renewal of Public Health in Canada.* Ottawa: Public Health Agency of Canada.

Nixon, S., Upshur, R., Robertson, A., *et al.* (2005). Public health ethics. In *Public Health Ethics and Law*, ed. T. Bailey, T. Caulfield, and N. Ries. Toronto: LexisNexis Butterworths, Ch. 2.

Public Health Agency of Canada (2004). *Global Public Health Intelligence Network.* Ottawa: Public Health Agency of Canada (http://www.phac-aspc.gc.ca/media/nr-rp/2004/2004_gphin-rmispbk_e.html) accessed 14 July 2006.

Roberts, M. J. and Reich, M. R. (2002). Ethical analysis in public health. *Lancet* **359**: 1055–9.

Roush, S., Birkhead, G., Koo, D., Coob, A., and Fleming, D. (1999). Mandatory reporting of diseases and conditions by health care professionals and laboratories. *JAMA* **282**: 164–70.

St Lawrence, J. S., Montano, D. E., Kasprzyk, D., *et al.* (2002). STD screening, testing, case reporting, and clinical and partner notification practices: a national survey of US physicians. *Am J Public Health* **92**: 1784–8.

Sutherland, H. J., Lockwood, G. A., Tritchler, D. L., *et al.* (1991). Communicating probabilistic information to cancer patients: is there "noise" on the line? *Soc Sci Med* **32**: 725–31.

Taylor, Z., Nolan, C. M., and Bloomberg, H. M. (2005). Controlling tuberculosis in the United States. Recommendations from the American Thoracic Society, CDC, and the Infectious Diseases Society of America. *MMWR Recomm Rep* **54**(**RR-12**): 1–81.

Trepka, M. J., Beyer, T. O., Proctor, M. E., and Davis, J. P. (1999). An evaluation of the completeness of tuberculosis case reporting using hospital billing and laboratory data; Wisconsin, 1995. *Ann Epidemiol* **9**: 419–23.

University of Toronto Joint Centre for Bioethics. Pandemic Influenza Working Group (2005). *Stand on Guard for Thee: Ethical Considerations in Preparedness Planning for Pandemic Influenza*. Toronto: University of Toronto Press.

World Health Organization (1998). *Global Infectious Disease Surveillance*. Geneva: World Health Organization (http://www.who.int/mediacentre/factsheets/fs200/en/) accessed 14 July 2006.

World Health Organization (2003). *WHO Issues Emergency Travel Advisory*. Geneva: World Health Organization (http://www.who.int/mediacentre/news/releases/2003/pr23/en) accessed 14 July 2006.

37

Emergency and disaster scenarios

Harvey Kayman, Howard Radest, and Sally Webb

In October 2001, the USA was on edge following the discovery of several letters containing anthrax. People who worked in facilities that received letters containing anthrax were sometimes stigmatized within their communities. Some employees of American Media Inc., the site of the first anthrax case, were doubly victimized. Physically affected by their potential exposure to anthrax, they were also socially stigmatized by physicians who refused to care for them, schools that turned away their children, and employers of second jobs who refused to let them work: some American Media employees who moonlighted as housekeepers were not allowed into homes to clean (Malecki, 2001).

Suddenly, around 9:50, everything momentarily appears pale pink. There is an enormous bang. Some of my colleagues have looks of terror on their faces. We can see white smoke and debris raining down in the square. The fire alarms are sounding. Although staff members leave, the doctors stay ... After several minutes, we gingerly make our way to the front of the building and look down onto the stricken bus. ... I grab some surgical gloves and my ambulance service physician identity card ... On arrival downstairs, I meet the deputy chairman of the BMA Council ... Knowing of my prehospital emergency care experience, he asks me to take over the direction of clinical operations ... My assets are a building offering protection from all but a direct hit and 14 doctors, most of them experienced general practitioners with some training in emergency medicine. But we have no equipment, no communications, and no personal protective clothing. Armed with nothing, we set about maximizing the victims' chances of survival. I have trained for such a situation for 20 years – but on the assumption that I would be part of a rescue team, properly dressed, properly equipped, and moving with semimilitary precision. Instead, I am in shirtsleeves and a pinstripe suit, with no pen and no paper,

and I am technically an uninjured victim. All I have is my ID card, surgical gloves, and my colleagues' expectation that I will lead them though this crisis (Holden, 2005).

What are emergency and disaster scenarios?

In most situations, clinicians practice in an orderly milieu, often in coordination with other clinicians and with institutions that exist to cure disease, improve health, and/or prevent illness. Clinicians, like the rest of the population, may suddenly be faced with a chaotic world in the event of natural catastrophes, epidemics, or terror attacks: disasters that can cause terrible damage to peoples and societies. Standard ethical assumptions and medical practices may no longer be applicable. Both personal and professional equilibrium will be threatened. Ordinarily, clinicians do not face morally ambiguous situations and when they do, their own skill and experience is usually sufficient to deal with them. During a disaster, clinicians will ask themselves, "How will I resolve the dilemmas now facing me?" as they struggle with the disparate demands of their patients and the obligations of their profession (American Medical Association, 2004). In these settings, the needs of the individual patient will often conflict with the needs of the community and ethical conflicts will emerge in all phases of the disaster response (Gostin, 2003a; Institute for Bioethics Health Policy and Law, 2003). Advance disaster training and emergency medical preparedness must include planning and pre-paredness for sound ethical decision making in times of crisis.

National and international healthcare organizations have outlined recommendations for emergency preparedness plans. These plans often include mitigation, preparedness, response and recovery phases, and mandate frequent drills by responders. An effective response should be rapidly instituted; integrated between communities, law enforcement, public health officials, and healthcare facilities; and include the elements seen in Table 37.1, including our addition of attention to ethical issues.

Many critical problems exist in implementation of an effective disaster response. Mass casualties, especially in bioterrorism or radiation attack, will cause a sudden surge in demand for medical resources such as hospital beds, critical care equipment, medications, antidotes, staff, isolation rooms, and trained ancillary personnel, which may not be available (Church J for the Department of Defense, 2001; Hick *et al.*, 2004). Surge capacity, or the ability to handle an unexpected increase in patient volume, will be inadequate, since emergency departments remain overcrowded with patients, log-jammed awaiting admission to equally overcrowded hospitals. Critical nursing and other ancillary personnel shortages preclude increasing numbers of beds to alleviate overcrowding and improve access to care, even in ordinary times (American Hospital Association, 2007). In addition, communication systems may fail, leading to great uncertainty among medical personnel, who may be forced to grope about for the best strategies to minimize panic and restore order.

Responses to disasters and emergencies have enormous monetary costs to societies. Many medical facilities are now in tenuous financial health owing to falling reimbursements and increasing operating costs and will depend on state, federal, or international assistance to sustain their response efforts during the crisis and recovery phases of a catastrophe. Resource allocation and triage issues will challenge local leaders and clinicians in the acute phase, as hospitals usually have a limited supply of stored medications and equipment to utilize.

Table 37.1. Key elements of a response to a disaster or emergency

Mass casualty care challenges and procedures
Infrastructure preservation
Communication barriers/breakdowns
Incident command system and integration
Personal and scene safety issues
Contamination, containment, and security issues
Decontamination indications and sites
Maintenance of regular healthcare services
Personal protection and equipment issues
Personal behaviors and beliefs
Psychological impact
Secondary threats
Ethical issues

Adapted from Waeckerle *et al.* (2001).

Important ethical issues will surface during disasters including triage, access to care and other justice issues; privacy and confidentiality; the professional duty to treat; quarantine and its effect on patient autonomy, individual liberty and the right to refuse medical treatment; and transparency in public health planning (Pesik *et al.*, 2001; Singer *et al.*, 2003; Wynia and Gostin, 2004).

Why is preparation for emergency and disaster scenarios important?

Planning for a successful integrated, tiered, and flexible response team to ensure access to care for all citizens is necessary. Hospital staff and clinicians will have little experience with the wide array of partners with whom they will need to interact during a crisis. Law enforcement, the military, public health officials, emergency preparedness staff, community leaders, and politicians join the clinician under conditions of crisis (USDA Forest Service, 2004; Emergency Management Institute, 2005). These personnel may have little experience in dealing with jurisdictional disputes that will inevitably arise between federal, state, and local government officials, between law enforcement and firefighters, and between officials of various institutions in their communities.

Interaction with the community is essential to make sensible and equitable moral decisions, as well as to recruit practical logistical support (Glass and Schoch-Spana, 2002). Forums in which communities learn about clinical concerns (e.g., need for quarantine) and in which clinicians learn about community concerns (e.g., fear about loss of autonomous decision making) will be important in ensuring a transparent and reciprocal response to a catastrophic event. These advance programs should help clinicians and citizens to examine their own sense of vulnerability, understand impending threats, and recognize their own strengths and value (JCAHO, 2004). In crisis, it is usually impossible to provide the time and resources for identifying, reflecting, and dealing with these issues.

Resource allocation and access to care

In contrast with public health clinicians, practicing clinicians seldom have to deal with policy issues and community-based problems. They do not have to decide between patients or what resources will be committed to whom and for what outcomes. Indeed, ''rationing at the bedside'' is regarded as morally problematic in normal conditions, a probable violation of the physician's fiduciary duty to his or her patient (Council on Ethical and Judicial Affairs, 2004a). In the USA until very recently, it was not regarded as appropriate to think of the costs in time, money, and resources in deciding whether to treat or not to treat a given condition in a given patient. Clinicians will be forced to face tough resource-allocation decisions in catastrophic emergencies (Agency for Healthcare Research and Quality, 2002).

Most developed countries make universal healthcare available to their citizens. Where this is not the case, as in the USA, the commitment is nevertheless present to provide healthcare for everyone (Council on Ethical and Judicial Affairs, 2004b). Given the complexity of the US system, disparities in disease outcomes increasingly exist

between those who are reasonably well off and those who are not (Krieger and Birn, 1998). Ironically, as part of planning for health emergencies and disasters, health officials are committed to minimize death and illness in all populations. Paradoxically, crisis moves healthcare toward a fair distribution of benefits and burdens, although, as Hurricane Katrina revealed to Americans in 2005, the space between intention and reality can be very wide (Centers for Disease Control and Prevention, 2006). Whether effective or not, realistic or not, the restoration of the health of populations and communities and only secondarily of individuals is the primary concern in disaster response (Landesman, 2005).

Individuals who are poor or uninsured, however, may be reluctant to seek healthcare and are more vulnerable targets for bioterrorism attacks or mass casualties. Attempts to control contagious disease outbreaks will be unsuccessful if such affected populations fail to seek care or do so at late stages of infectivity.

Triage

Triage is commonly defined as the process of prioritizing sick or injured people for treatment according to seriousness of the injury. Clinicians will be expected to triage – to decide what groups must be left to survive on their own, what groups will get the limited resources that are available, and what groups will be judged capable of handling their own medical problems.

Urgent decisions are required in crisis situations where uncertainty prevails. These decisions will surely place lives at risk. Clinicians and their coworkers will need to be emotionally and morally prepared for doing and deciding what under normal conditions would be unthinkable (Glass and Schoch-Spana, 2002; American Medical Association, 2004).

Experts have made recommendations to help with this practice, which is unfamiliar to many primary care practitioners (Pesik et al., 2001). The Working Group on Emergency Mass Critical Care

(Rubinson *et al.*, 2005) have suggested using only interventions that are known to improve survival and without which death is likely, that are not very expensive, and that can be implemented without consuming extensive staff or hospital resources. These guidelines should also be used for patients already receiving care in an intensive care unit who are not casualties of an attack. Emergency workers and caregivers, even if asymptomatic, should probably be given priority for receiving medical care or prophylaxis to preserve the pool of available clinicians. However, every effort must be put forward to ensure non-discriminatory evaluation and treatment, as surveys have shown that the public believes that influence, wealth, and younger age impact the rapidity and degree of treatments given (Blendon *et al.*, 2003; Human Rights Center and East–West Center (Honolulu), 2005).

Clinicians will feel the need to protect themselves and their families. Ordinarily, they manage to balance conflicting obligations between their own needs, the needs of their families, the needs of their patients, and communities (Goldrich and Polk, 2004). Suddenly faced with serious risk to themselves or to their families, that ordinary balance is likely to be unavailable. It remains controversial whether it is ethically permissible to alter a triage algorithm to protect a clinician's family members if they are at less risk than others. However, those who then do not receive limited resources are likely to feel and express their outrage.

Quarantine

Clinicians may have to aid in placing entire populations into quarantine (Gostin, 2003a; Institute for Bioethics Health Policy and Law, 2003). To complicate matters further, some of these populations will be made up of people who have been wronged by their societies and who will be resentful and mistrustful of authority, including medical authority (Krieger and Birn, 1998; Covello and Sandman, 2001).

Transparent, understandable, and truthful communication about the potential for initiating quarantine during communicable disease outbreaks or acts of bioterrorism may alleviate some of the public's mistrust in advance. This becomes absolutely essential when crises strike (Kurland, 2002; Gostin, 2003b; Gostin *et al.*, 2003). Frightened and desperate people will not understand what is happening to them nor the reasons for the sacrifices of freedom, privacy, and comfort that they are asked to make. Quarantine may also cause significant economic harm to individuals who will lose their income by missing work. As epidemics or crises evolve, leaders may need to revise social distancing strategies, and these "course changes" may further alienate the public and lead to mistrust and confusion.

The first case outlined at the start of this chapter, hysteria and misunderstanding within the community led to the social stigmatization, discrimination, economic losses, and psychological injury seen not only in exposed victims but also in those with potential exposure to the deadly contagion. Similarly, linking severe acute respiratory syndrome (SARS) in North America to visitors from China caused widespread avoidance by the public of Asian businesses or communities, causing serious economic losses. Another example was seen in the Canadian SARS outbreak, where many people were denied access to healthcare during the quarantine process, and consequently some died from treatable diseases such as myocardial infarction or infections. During quarantine, such concerns about bodily integrity, right to privacy, a commitment to distributive and procedural justice, due process, and the right for people to control their own property and destiny will emerge (Kass, 2001; American Public Health Association, 2002).

Clinicians also need to prepare for the medical, emotional, and logistical challenges that they will face. Until social and political order can be restored, a shift in clinicians' commitments is necessary during both triage and quarantine from respecting the fiduciary relationship with a single patient to minimizing suffering for the largest possible number of patients in a fair and just manner. While some experts feel that only public health officers and not physicians should act in this broader "civic" role, many others stress that this shift in commitments to maximize the public's health is part of a physician's professional obligation (Wynia and Gostin, 2004).

Other ethical issues

As is evident from our description of what clinicians face in catastrophe, tools to help to deal with the deep moral concerns that will arise are as essential as the medical algorithms for treatment of mass casualties or toxic or infectious exposures. Ethics overlaps with legal issues (Gostin, 2002; The Turning Point Public Health Statute Modernization National Excellence Collaborative, 2003), law enforcement issues, psychological issues, spiritual issues, interpersonal issues, social issues, and communication issues (McKenna *et al.*, 2003). Yet ethics has its special role to play: to work out what clinicians ought and ought not to do in the situations in which they find themselves. Of course, clinicians do not come to crisis without a good deal of ethical experience and without their own moral values. Fortunately, ethical decision making is also facilitated by professional codes and practices. In other words, while some of the language of ethics may be esoteric, the essence of ethical deliberation is approachable if considered in advance and incorporated into preparedness plans.

How should I approach emergency and disaster scenarios in practice?

Preparing for ethical decision making in crisis must be part of training for catastrophe. Briefly, this should include how to identify ethical issues, how to deal with them, and not least of all, how to evaluate them in order to improve future moral performance (Singer *et al.*, 2003). Ethical decision making requires consideration of the medical, political, religious, social, and economic factors that taken together raise ethical issues. The values of the community in which they arise contribute as well to their complexity. So, insofar as possible,

ethical decision making needs an interdisciplinary approach. No single specialty or point of view can be adequate.

Many tools for approaching ethical dilemmas in public health are available (Public Health Leadership Society, 2002). One should be familiar with the foundational principles of bioethics decision making: autonomy, beneficence, non-maleficence, and justice (Beauchamp and Childress, 2001). Exploration of different moral perspectives like rights (Uzgalis, 2001), distributive justice (Rawls, 1971), consequences (Solomon, 2000), and universal ideals (Koterski, 2000) may enhance ethical deliberation in situations involving the tension between individual liberty and the common good. The "precautionary principle" provides an excellent framework for sound ethical decision making. It requires transparency of plans and actions, inclusiveness of the affected population in the decision-making process, a commitment to accountability, and an awareness that action, even coercive action, must be taken in the face of uncertainty when there is a serious threat to the public welfare (Tickner, 2002; Kayman, 2006).

In crisis, early recognition of the signs of ethical tension is important. For example, a growing sense of discomfort or an unwillingness to communicate openly about a situation suggests that there is likely an underlying ethical dilemma confounding the situation. When possible, consultation with a multidisciplinary team or bioethicist trained in ethical deliberation is recommended. Those in state, federal, and international public health leadership positions should begin a dialogue on how to best encourage the development of such deliberative bodies, even for ordinary times. A group including nurses, social workers, chaplains, administrators, and community members can provide moral perspective and support. In the midst of crisis, this may not be possible. But if it is – and it is advisable to make every effort to have such a group available – its members will understand that they must make decisions quickly with limited, perhaps incorrect, information.

One obvious tension in crisis situations is between individual rights and freedoms and the public's health and common good. It is likely that ethical problems will arise anytime that liberty, freedom of association, and freedom of movement are restricted. A landmark US Supreme Court ruling (1905) in *Jacobson* v. *Massachusetts* mandates that coercive public health action must be shown to be *effective, necessary, least restrictive possible, proportional*, and *impartial*. The Public Health Code of Ethics (Thomas *et al.*, 2002) can also provide guidance for public health officials and clinicians during catastrophes.

In the second case opening this chapter, another tension is highlighted: between a clinician's duty to treat and preserving one's own health and safety. As seen in this case and historically in the plague and the recent SARS epidemic, clinicians must weigh the considerable health risks to themselves and their families against their professional duty to care for others. The majority of health professionals rise to the challenge, even risking (and suffering) mortality. Although the original 1847 American Medical Association's Code of Ethics stated, "When pestilence prevails it is [physicians'] duty to face the danger ... even at the jeopardy of their own lives," some health professionals now place their own safety ahead of those patients who need their care. Because most professional codes emphasize duty over potential harm to self, healthcare institutions have an obligation during crises to promote the safety of and minimize risks to their healthcare workers. Individual clinicians are urged to consider in advance how their own moral decision making can help them to balance professional and personal obligations.

Retrospective analysis by bioethicists of ethical issues that emerge during crises, such as the SARS epidemic, can help to enable better preparation for future events and is strongly recommended (Singer *et al.*, 2003). The evaluation in the aftermath of a crisis might include outcomes indices in various population groups, including people from different socioeconomic situations, ethnicities, ages, and gender. Research efforts by interdisciplinary teams of policy makers, academicians, healthcare providers, and community groups should focus, not only on mortality, but on the incidence of displaced peoples, of social isolation or quarantine, of variable economic losses, and so on to help communities to improve future public health or management strategies. A recent report (Daniels, 2006) has emphasized utilizing five benchmarks to address dimensions of equity: exposure of people to public health risks, inequalities in the distribution of the social determinants of health; financial and non-financial barriers to access to care; inequalities in the benefits for different groups; and the burden of healthcare cost among those less able to pay.

The keys to minimizing ethical dilemmas in times of emergencies and disasters include a basic familiarity with ethical concepts and tools, and a recognition that although uncertainty and chaos can confound all situations, an equitable, transparent, and organized approach can foster trust and cooperation among large numbers of those affected. Interdisciplinary planning with clinicians, the community, law enforcement, public health officials, and politicians is of paramount importance. Clinicians will be faced with difficult moral choices favoring the health of the public over the health of the individual. A commitment should be made that the response system will be fair, and that people will have recourse to express their concerns to formulate improvement.

REFERENCES

Agency for Healthcare Research and Quality (2002). *Bioterrorism Preparedness and Response: Use of Information Technologies and Decision Support Systems*. Rockville, MD: Agency for Healthcare Research and Quality (http://www.ahrq.gov/clinic/epcsums/bioitsum.htm) accessed 27 August 2006.

American Hospital Association (2007). *The 2007 State of America's Hospitals: Taking the Pulse; Findings from the 2007 AHA Survey of Hospital Leaders (ppt)*. Washington, DC: American Hospital Association www.aha.org/aha/research-and-trends/.

American Medical Association (2004). *Core Disaster Life Support, Provider Manual*, version 2.0. Chicago, Il: American Medical Association.

American Public Health Association (2002). *Guiding Principles for a Public Health Response to Terrorism.* Washington, DC: American Public Health Association (http://www.apha.org/united/phresponseterrorism.htm) accessed 8 September 2006.

Beauchamp, T. and Childress, J. (2001). *Principles of Biomedical Ethics*, 5th edn. New York: Oxford University Press.

Blendon, R. J., DesRoches, C. M., Benson, J. M., *et al.* (2003). The public and the smallpox threat. *N Engl J Med* **348**: 426–32.

Centres for Disease Control and Prevention (2006). Public health response to Hurricanes Katrina and Rita: United States, 2005. *MMWR Morb Mortal Wkly Rep* **55**: 229–31.

Church, J. for the Department of Defense (2001). *Neighborhood Emergency Help Center: A Mass Casualty Care Strategy for Biological Terrorism Incidents.* Washington, DC: Government Printing Office (http://www.nnemmrs.org/documents/Neighborhood%20Emergency%20Help%20Center%20-%20A%20Mass%20Casualty%20Care%20Strategy%20for%20Biological%20Terrorism%20Incidents.pdf#search=%22neighborhood%20emergency%20help%20center%20mass%20casualty%20care%20strategy%22) accessed 27 August 2006.

Council on Ethical and Judicial Affairs (2004a). Opinion 2.03. Allocation of limited medical resources. In *Code of Medical Ethics: Current Opinions with Annotations*, 2004–2005 edn. Chicago, IL: AMA Press.

Council on Ethical and Judicial Affairs (2004b). Principle IX, principles of medical ethics. In *Code of Medical Ethics: Current Opinions with Annotations*, 2004–2005 edn. Chicago, IL: AMA Press.

Covello, V. and Sandman, P. (2001). Risk communication: evolution and revolution. In *Solutions to an Environment in Peril*, ed. A. Wolbarst. Baltimore, MD: Johns Hopkins University Press, pp. 164–78.

Daniels, N. (2006). Toward ethical review of health system transformations. *Am J Public Health* **96**: 447–51.

Emergency Management Institute (2005). *FEMA Independent Study Program: IS-l;195 Basic Incident Command System.* Washington, DC: Government Printing Office (http://www.training.fema.gov/EMIWeb/IS/is195.asp) accessed 27 August 2006.

Glass, T. A. and Schoch-Spana, M. (2002). Bioterrorism and the people: how to vaccinate a city against panic. *Clin Infect Dis* **34**: 217–23.

Goldrich, M. and Polk, S. (2004). Physicians' obligation to accept personal risk in the provision of medical care. In *Report 3-I-03 of the Council on Ethical and Judicial Affairs.* Chicago, IL: American Medical Association.

Gostin, L. O. (2002). *Public Health Law: Power, Duty, Restraint.* Berkeley, CA: University of California Press.

Gostin L. O. (2003a). *The Law and Bioethics Report*, Vol. 2, No. 4: *Public Health and Civil Liberties in an Era of Bioterrorism.* Louisville, KT: University of Louisville (http://www.louisville.edu/medschool/ibhpl/lab_report/index.html) accessed 27 August 2006.

Gostin, L. O. (2003b). When terrorism threatens health: how far are limitations on personal economic liberties justified? *Florida Law Rev* **55**: 1105.

Gostin, L. O., Bayer, R., and Fairchild, A. L. (2003). Ethical and legal challenges posed by severe acute respiratory syndrome: implications for the control of severe infectious disease threats. *JAMA* **290**: 3229–37.

Hick, J. L., Hanfling, D., Burstein, J. L., *et al.* (2004). Health care facility and community strategies for patient care surge capacity. *Ann Emerg Med* **44**: 253–61.

Holden, P. J. (2005). The London attacks – a chronicle: improvising in an emergency. *N Engl J Med* **353**: 541–3.

Human Rights Center and East–West Center (Honolulu) (2005). *After the Tsunami: Human Rights of Vulnerable Populations.* Berkeley, CA: University of California Press.

Institute for Bioethics Health Policy and Law (2003). *Quarantine and Isolation: Lessons Learned from SARS. A Report to the Centers for Disease Control and Prevention.* Louisville, KT: University of Louisville (http://www.louisville.edu/medschool/ibhpl/publications/SARS%20REPORT.pdf) accessed 27 August 2006.

Jacobson v *Massachusetts* (1905) 25 s. cf. 358.

JCAHO (2004). *Joint Commission International Newsletter. Standards link: Coordinating Community Efforts to Respond to Emergencies.* Oakbrook, Terrance, IL: Joint Commission on Accreditation of Healthcare Organizations (http://www.jcrinc.com/subscribers/intlnewsletter.asp?durki=7574&site=49&return=6757) accessed 27 August 2006.

Kass, N. E. (2001). An ethics framework for public health. *Am J Public Health* **91**: 1776–82.

Kayman H. (2006). From principles to public health programs through uncertainty. *J S Carolina Med Assoc*, in press.

Koterski, J. (2000). Natural law and human nature. In *The Great Courses.* Springfield, MA: The Teaching Company, course 4453.

Krieger, N. and Birn, A. E. (1998). A vision of social justice as the foundation of public health: commemorating 150 years of the spirit of 1848. *Am J Public Health* **88**: 1603–6.

Kurland, J. (2002). The heart of the precautionary principle in democracy. *Public Health Rep* **117**: 498–500.

Landesman, L. (2005). *Public Health Management of Disasters: The Practice Guide*, 2nd edn. Washington, DC: American Public Health Association.

Malecki, J. (2001). *Letters Laced with Anthrax*. Palm Beach, FL: Health Commission.

McKenna, V. B., Gunn, J. E., Auerbach, J., *et al.* (2003). Local collaborations: development and implementation of Boston's bioterrorism surveillance system. *J Public Health Manag Pract* **9**: 384–93.

Pesik, N., Keim, M. E., Iserson, K., *et al.* (2001). Terrorism and the ethics of emergency medical care. *Ann Emerg Med* **37**: 642–6.

Public Health Leadership Society (2002). *Principles of the Ethical Practice of Public Health*. New Orleans, LA: PHLS (http://www.phls.org/products.htm) accessed 27 August 2006.

Rawls, J. (1971). *A Theory of Justice*. Cambridge, MA: Belnap Press of Harvard University.

Rubinson, L., Nuzzo, J. B., Talmor, D. S., *et al.* (2005). Augmentation of hospital critical care capacity after bioterrorist attacks or epidemics: recommendations of the Working Group on Emergency Mass Critical Care. *Crit Care Med* **33**: 2393–403.

Singer, P. A., Benatar, S. R., Bernstein, A. S. *et al.* (2003). Ethics and SARS: lessons from Toronto. *BMJ* **327**: 1342–4.

Solomon, R. (2000). Mill's ultilitarianism. In *The Great Courses: The Great Minds of Western Intellectual Tradition*. Springfield, VA: The Teaching Company, course 470.

The Turning Point Public Health Statute Modernization National Excellence Collaborative (2003). *Model State Public Health Act: A Tool for Assessing Public Health Laws*. Seattle, WA: University of Washington (http://www.turningpointprogram.org/Pages/pdfs/statute_mod/MSPHAfinal.pdf) accessed 27 August 2006.

Thomas, J. C., Sage, M., Dillenberg, J., and Guillory, V. J. (2002). A code of ethics for public health. *Am J Public Health* **92**: 1057–9.

Tickner, J. A. (2002). Precautionary principle encourages policies that protect human health and the environment in the face of uncertain risks. *Public Health Rep* **117**: 493–7.

USDA Forest Service (2004). *Fire and Aviation Management*. Washington, DC: USDA Forest Service (http://www.fs.fed.us/fire/) accessed 27 August 2006.

Uzgalis, W. (2001). John Locke. In *The Stanford Encyclopedia of Philosophy*, ed. E. N. Zalta. Stanford, CA: University of Stanford (http://plato.stanford.edu/archives/fall2005/entries/locke/).

Waeckerle, J. F., Seamans, S., Whiteside, M., *et al.* (2001). Executive summary: developing objectives, content, and competencies for the training of emergency medical technicians, emergency physicians, and emergency nurses to care for casualties resulting from nuclear, biological, or chemical incidents. *Ann Emerg Med* **37**: 587–601.

Wynia, M. K. and Gostin, L. O. (2004). Ethical challenges in preparing for bioterrorism: barriers within the health care system. *Am J Public Health* **94**: 1096–102.

38

Rural healthcare ethics

William A. Nelson and Jared M. Schmidek

A primary care physician that works in a small, remote hospital diagnoses a patient with lung cancer and refers the patient to a distant large medical center for treatment. After several overnight trips to the medical center, the patient returns to the primary care provider to indicate that she is no longer willing to travel and wants to receive care at the small hospital.

A rural psychologist, also a member of the town's school board, discovers during a family counseling session that one of the patients, a schoolteacher, has missed many teaching days because of a significant alcohol problem.

A family physician treats a long-term patient for a minor work-related injury. The patient is very depressed and tearful but refuses to discuss it. The physician encourages the patient to see a mental health professional to be further assessed and, if needed, receive treatment. The patient acknowledges feeling depressed but does not want help. If people see his truck at the mental health provider's office, everyone will know that he has "that" type of problem. The patient also requests that the physician not make any reference to depression in his medical record, because his sister-in-law works at the doctor's office.

What is rural healthcare ethics?

In *A Fortunate Man*, Berger and Mohr (1967, pp. 13–15) provided a deeply compelling portrait of an English country doctor who lives and provides care in a remote, rural community: "Landscapes can be deceptive. Sometimes a landscape seems to be less a setting for the life of its inhabitants than a curtain behind which struggles, achievements and accidents take place. For those who are behind the curtain, landmarks are no longer only geographic but also biographical and personal." Rather than feeling discouraged by his professional isolation and stressful workload as a "one-man hospital" and its challenging situations, we are uplifted by the depth of his relationships and commitment to the people of a remote community. In this story of a country doctor, we are taken behind the curtain to a unique setting, unknown and rarely understood by many who live in metropolitan and urban settings.

Authors have reported from different countries that what makes the rural community unique is not just its small population density or distance to an urban setting but also the combination of its social, geographical, cultural, religious, and personal values as well as its residents' economic and health status (Flannery, 1982; Bushy, 1994; Ricketts *et al.*, 1998; Roberts *et al.*, 1999a; Ricketts, 2000; Gamm *et al.*, 2003; Kelly, 2003; Institute of Medicine, 2005). A rural community's health beliefs, overall health status, geographic isolation, access to healthcare, and limited ethics services play a influential role in the nature and frequency of ethical issues faced by healthcare professionals as well as in the manner in which they respond. Rural healthcare ethics focuses ethical reflection through the application of ethical concepts and ethical standards of healthcare practices to challenges that occur in rural settings. A need exists for the rural setting to be understood as culturally distinct from the urban setting, which has been the primary focus of healthcare ethics (Purtilo, 1987; Roberts *et al.*, 1999a; Cook and Hoas, 2001).

Why is rural healthcare ethics important?

There are four reasons for the importance of considering rural healthcare ethics. The first reason is the large number of people living, working, and receiving healthcare in rural communities. In 2001, 30.4% of Canada's population lived in rural communities (Canadian Rural Partnership Research and Analysis Unit, 2002). In the UK, 19% or 9.5 million people live in rural areas (Department for Environment, Food and Rural Affairs, 2004). In the USA, approximately 59 million people, roughly 21% of the population, live in rural, "non-metropolitian" communities according to the 2000 United States Census (Institute of Medicine, 2005); however, variations in the definition and methodologies used to define rural areas have resulted in several estimates (Institute of Medicine, 2005).

The second reason is the distinctive characteristics of residents of rural communities. In the USA, the rural population has a lower median income per household (US Department of Housing and Urban Development, 2000) and higher poverty rates than the urban population (Institute of Medicine, 2005). In 2000, 23% of US children in "completely rural, non-adjacent counties" lived in poverty (Economic Research Service, 2005). Rural residents are also more likely to be underinsured or uninsured (Ziller *et al.*, 2003), further increasing the financial hardship of interacting with the healthcare system (Ricketts, 2000). Compared with the urban population living in metropolitan counties, residents of the US rural population have a higher age-adjusted mortality rate (National Center for Health Statistics, 2005); a higher probability for a chronic or life-threatening disease (Braden and Beauregard, 1994); a higher proportion of vulnerable residents, specifically children and the elderly, who require more health services (National Center for Health Statistics, 2001a); higher rates of particular mental health issues including substance abuse (Institute of Medicine, 2005) and suicide (National Center for Health Statistics, 2001b); and encounter a greater prevalence of environmental and occupational related hazards (Ricketts, 2000).

A large study of US veterans concluded that, when compared with urban veterans, those living in a rural setting have worse health-related quality of life scores (Weeks *et al.*, 2004). Similar health inequalities between rural and urban populations have been reported in other countries, for instance, in Canada (Romanow, 2002).

The third reason is that there are fewer healthcare providers per capita for rural populations than for urban populations. About 9% of physicians practice in rural America although roughly 21% of the population lives in those areas (Rosenblatt and Hart, 1999; Institute of Medicine, 2005). These disparities encompass a wide range of healthcare professionals other than physicians, such as nurses, social workers, dentists, and, in particular, mental health professionals (Wagenfeld *et al.*, 1994; Goldsmith *et al.*, 1997; Holzer *et al.*, 1998; Rost *et al.*, 1998; Hartley *et al.*, 1999; Bird *et al.*, 2001; Baldwin *et al.*, 2006; Johnson *et al.*, 2006; Rosenblatt *et al.*, 2006).

In addition to these three factors shaping the frequency and nature of rural ethics issues, the fourth reason why rural healthcare ethics is important is because there are limited ethics resources focused on rural issues. In the USA, these limitations include the number of bioethicists (Nelson and Weeks, 2006), a rural-focused literature (Nelson *et al.*, 2006), ethics committees, adequately trained ethics consultants, and opportunities for rural ethics education (Niemira, 1988; Cook and Hoas, 2001; Cook *et al.*, 2002; Nelson, 2004). In addition, numerous barriers contribute to the lack of existing or effective ethics committees in rural communities, including the lack of ethics expertise, time and financial resources to support ethics training and education, an understanding of rural communities, and the use of a urban model for ethics committees in the rural healthcare facility (Niemira *et al.*, 1989a, b; Bushy and Rauh, 1991; Moss, 1999; Cook and Hoas, 2000, 2001; Cook *et al.*, 2000a; Nelson, 2006). As a consequence of the limited rural ethics-related resources, rural clinicians are hampered in their efforts to seek rural ethics training, and, when consulting the clinical ethics literature, find that the material has such an urban focus that it proves unhelpful (Roberts *et al.*, 1999b; Cook and Hoas, 2001; Cook *et al.*, 2000a). It has been noted that "bioethics is an urban phenomenon," because its focus emanates from large, university, tertiary care hospitals, and the "latest hot research topic," all intended for an urban audience (Hardwig, 2006, p. 53).

Ethics

With an understanding of rural healthcare comes an emerging awareness of the special ethical considerations inherent to clinical practice in closely knit, tightly interdependent small communities (Nelson and Pomerantz, 1992a; Bushy, 1994; Roberts *et al.*, 1999a; Cook and Hoas, 2001; Roberts and Dyer, 2004). Because of the distinct characteristics of the rural community, the identification and solutions that rural practitioners might employ to address ethical conflicts may differ from their urban counterparts (Roberts *et al.*, 1999a; Cook and Hoas, 2000, 2001; Nelson, 2004). In a rural setting, for example, it might be necessary to provide healthcare to a family member, friend, or neighbor; whereas, in a urban setting, it permits for greater role separation and clearer personal and professional boundaries since other healthcare clinicians, facilities, and more diverse health resources might exist in more the immediate area (Purtilo and Sorrell, 1986; Sobel, 1992; Schank, 1998; Roberts *et al.*, 1999a; Cook *et al.*, 2001; Roberts and Dyer, 2004).

Responses of healthcare professionals to all ethical conflicts are expected to be in accordance with generally accepted ethical principles or standards of practice, such as informed consent. However, community values inherent to rural settings influence healthcare decision making, including self-reliance and self-care; the use of informal supports, such as neighbors, family, and church members; a strong work ethic; and a different perception of illness, where, illness occurs when a person cannot work (Bushy, 1994). Roberts *et al.* (1999a, p. 33) commented that these "Cultural issues ... sometimes

exert a greater influence on rural than urban healthcare because local customs and practices may affect a greater proportion of a caregiver's practice." Since identification and solutions to ethical issues in rural areas may differ from urban areas (Roberts *et al.*, 1999a; Cook and Hoas, 2000, 2001; Nelson, 2004), rural clinicians may experience dissatisfaction with professional ethics codes and ethical standards of practice that are primarily urban focused (Niemira, 1988; Cook and Hoas, 2000; Roberts *et al.*, 1999b; Cook *et al.*, 2002) and, in general, provide inadequate insight into how the rural context might influence ethical decision making.

Several articles have suggested that the quality of care of rural residents might be adversely impacted because of the limited amount and variety of available healthcare services and the insufficient array of healthcare professionals (Moscovice and Rosenblatt, 2000; Cook *et al.*, 2002; Gallagher *et al.*, 2002; Weeks *et al.*, 2004). Isolation from specialists and specialized technological resources force the provider to make decisions based more on clinical impression rather than the most up-to-date specialty knowledge and technology. Some rural providers believe this compromises the quality of care they can deliver (Turner *et al.*, 1996; Cook and Hoas, 2000; Cook *et al.*, 2000b) and the ethical norms of the medical profession.

Geographic isolation of rural communities might also give rise to ethical issues. Distance to and between healthcare professionals and facilities in rural regions can be extensive, thereby limiting their accessibility to rural residents (Nelson and Pomerantz, 1992b; Bushy, 1994; Rosenthal *et al.*, 2005; Chan *et al.*, 2006). Distance to healthcare services can be additionally problematic because of the lack of public transportation, challenging roads, and weather-related barriers (Cook and Hoas, 2001).

Resistance or refusal to be transferred to urban and tertiary-care centers through fear of the unfamiliar urban setting is not uncommon among rural patients (Nelson and Pomerantz, 1992a). This resistance or refusal leaves many rural clinicians conflicted because a competent patient refuses care that the clinician believes is essential. Related ethical conflicts include how aggressively the clinician should attempt to persuade a patient to seek treatment in a distant, urban medical center. If the patient maintains their refusal, the clinician must address the burden by providing, presumably, less than an optimal level of care. This ethical issue is accentuated by legal concerns when professionals believe they are practicing outside their scope of competence (Roberts *et al.*, 1999b).

Overlapping or multiple relationships can influence and become the source of many ethical conflicts faced by rural healthcare professionals. Because healthcare clinicians might have multiple roles within the community, for example as a physician, as a school board member, and as a neighbor, relationships with patients in rural settings might foster boundary-related ethical conflicts (Purtilo and Sorrell, 1986; Miller, 1994; Roberts *et al.*, 1999a, b; Cook and Hoas, 2001; Cook *et al.*, 2001; Larson, 2001). However, disengagement of the provider from multiple relations may lead to a sense of rejection, a lack of trust, and produce a less productive clinical relationship (Cook and Hoas, 2001). Rural clinicians might experience ethical conflicts since they routinely try to balance competing needs, such as that of the individual patient versus the community.

Because of the familiarity and frequent contact among healthcare professionals with patients, their families, and other community members, rural healthcare providers might often face situations that make privacy and confidentiality difficult (Woods, 1977; Spiegel, 1990; Jennings, 1992; Sobel, 1992; Ullom-Minnoch and Kallail, 1993; Rourke and Rourke, 1998; Schank, 1998; Roberts *et al.*, 1999a, b; Simon and Williams, 1999; Glover, 2001; Cook *et al.*, 2002; Campbell and Gordon, 2003) resulting in ethical conflicts (Simon and Williams, 1999; Henderson, 2000). For example, healthcare facilities are one of the largest employers in some small towns, so it is not uncommon for a patient's relative or neighbor to be a member of the healthcare professional's staff or even the billing clerk who records diagnoses.

Disease stigma might lead to ethical conflicts because of the extent of knowledge rural residents have about one another (Roberts *et al.*, 1999a). Clinicians may be reluctant to record in a medical record a stigmatizing diagnosis, such as HIV, a mental illness, or a sexually transmitted disease. Rural residents may be uncomfortable with the prospect of disclosure of such information to the clinician or may not seek necessary care (Flannery, 1982; Purtilo, 1987; Nelson and Pomerantz, 1992a; Bushy, 1994; Ricketts *et al.*, 1998; Ricketts, 2000; Kelly, 2003).

Policy

Rural populations are a critical concern in discussions of the provision of an appropriate standard of care, health disparities, and the allocation of government healthcare resources in many countries, including the UK (Cox, 1997), Canada (Romanow, 2002; Maddalena and Sherwin, 2004), and the USA (Institute of Medicine, 2005). For instance, in the USA, the Institute of Medicine's report *Quality Through Collaboration: The Future of Rural Health Care* outlined a five-point strategy and made 11 recommendations regarding the quality of healthcare provided to or in rural populations (Institute of Medicine, 2005, pp. 1–18). The recruitment and education of physicians and other healthcare professionals to rural areas are recognized in many countries as particularly significant policy concerns. Strategies have been developed to address these needs of the vulnerable rural population (Cox, 1997; Boffa, 2002; Romanow, 2002; Institute of Medicine, 2005).

Since healthcare policy is regionalized in Canada, ethics committees to aid governing authorities exist to provide specialized reviews regarding research, clinical, or organizational ethics issues (Maddalena and Sherwin, 2004, p. 235). Ethics committees that help to supplement rural and remote health authorities face challenges and might even not exist owing to geographical isolation, the lack of adequate trained members, and insufficient financial support. Some authorities utilize the services of an urban ethics committee; however, such a committee is unable to take into account the rural perspective (Maddalena and Sherwin, 2004, pp. 235–7).

Empirical studies

Various studies have identified ethical issues encountered in rural settings in the USA (Purtilo and Sorrell, 1986; Robillard *et al.*, 1989; Ullom-Minnich and Kallail, 1993; Turner *et al.*, 1996; Roberts *et al.*, 1999a, b, 2005; Cook *et al.*, 2000a, b, 2002; Cook and Hoas, 2000, 2001; Warner *et al.*, 2005). The commonly noted ethical issues arising in rural communities included safeguarding confidentiality and privacy, boundary conflicts due to overlapping relations, access to healthcare services, allocation of healthcare resources, inability to pay for healthcare, disease stigma, clinician–patient relationship, informed consent, and community cultural value conflicts. In India, another study explored patient satisfaction with medical professionals' ability to communicate medical information among hospitalized patients between urban and rural settings (Sriram *et al.*, 1990). Although these studies provide an understanding of ethical issues occurring in rural settings, the generalizability of four studies (Purtilo and Sorrell, 1986; Robillard *et al.*, 1989; Turner *et al.*, 1996; Ullom-Minnich and Kallail, 1993) are limited since many had a small sample size, a low response rate, or were conducted in limited geographic locations (Roberts *et al.*, 1999a, p. 31). These limitations have continued in other studies.

Cook and others have noted differences between the availability, frequency, and competency of rural ethics committees (Cook *et al.*, 2000a). A survey of 117 rural hospitals, mainly of administrators, in six states in the USA found that only 41.2% of the hospitals had an ethics committee or similar mechanism. Data suggest a predictive relationship between the size of the hospital, the presence of an ethics committee, and accreditation from the Joint Commission on Accreditation of Healthcare Organizations.

In a literature review using an established methodology for conducting literature searches, Nelson and others found that despite initially identifying 57 000 articles broadly related to bioethics published between 1966 and 2004, only 86 publications specifically and substantively addressed rural healthcare ethics issues, with 55 of the publications related to the USA, including seven original research articles (Nelson *et al.*, 2006).

Using members of the American Society for Bioethics and Humanities (ASBH) as a representative cross-section of professional resources for healthcare ethics, Nelson and Weeks (2006) analyzed how ASBH members were distributed along the rural–urban continuum. The ratio of ASHB members to urban hospitals is about one in three, whereas in rural hospitals the ratio is one to one hundred. The ratio is even more dramatic when using hospital beds as the denominator. Using various comparisons, the authors consistently found that ASBH members are underrepresented in rural settings compared with urban settings, suggesting that the availability of professional bioethical resources may be inadequate in rural settings.

How should I approach rural healthcare ethics in practice?

Rural clinicians respond to ethical challenges based on their personal beliefs and experiences, community values, and/or their understanding of ethical guidelines. The quality of care a patient receives can be greatly influenced by the clinician's response to ethical challenges. Several strategies are suggested to support the efforts of rural clinicians in addressing ethical challenges.

- Rural clinicians can acquire an understanding of healthcare ethics, including an awareness of basic ethical standards of practice. Ethical standards are generally accepted guidelines to help to guide responses to common ethical conflicts. Even though these guidelines may lack a specific rural focus, they can provide an important foundation for how to respond to ethical challenges. Ethical standards can be found in a wide variety of sources, such as, the American Medical Association *Ethics Manual* (American College of Physicians, 1998), professional codes of ethics (American Psychiatric Association, 2006), and position papers. Articles covering ethics are regularly published in medical and/or ethics specialty journals.

- Rural clinicians can develop a network of colleagues who can be consulted to provide support or advice regarding ethical challenges (Cook *et al.*, 2000a). Another clinician's perspective, outside the immediate clinical situation, might provide insight, clarity, and supportive advice (Roberts *et al.*, 1999b).
- Rural clinicians can identify healthcare ethicists to provide consultation and training. Despite the general lack of trained ethicists that live or work in rural settings (Nelson and Weeks, 2006), many are available through the telephone, Internet, or tele-health programs. Most academic-based ethics centers have websites that can provide ethics resources. The development of networks with ethicists and clinicians can alleviate a sense of isolation (Roberts *et al.*, 1999b).
- Rural clinicians can identify those healthcare facilities with an ethics program or committee. Many committees do exist at small rural facilities, which could provide case consultation and education programs that might serve as a useful resource.
- Rural clinicians can collaborate with a network of clinicians, ethicists, and ethics committee members to proactively draft and disseminate ethics practice guidelines for recurring rural ethical conflicts. The process may seem time consuming, but the process can diminish future conflicts. Such an effort can also be facilitated through formal, established professional groups.
- Rural clinicians can develop and implement community-wide educational programs on healthcare issues, such as end of life decision making, privacy, and confidentiality, to foster community understanding of basic ethical concepts in healthcare. Educational events can be facilitated in collaboration with community leaders, such as clergy (Cook and Hoas, 2000, 2001). Clinicians can also develop pamphlets delineating their ethical standards of practice to complement discussions. Proactive initiatives can foster a community understanding by utilizing a "preventive ethics" approach (Forrow *et al.*, 1993).
- Rural clinicians can encourage healthcare education conference planners at regional or national professional meetings to include a focus on rural issues (Roberts *et al.*, 1999b). These meetings can provide an opportunity to engage with others concerning rural healthcare.
- Rural clinicians can actively participate on committees of national or international professional organizations that establish standards of care to ensure that a rural perspective is recognized.
- Rural clinicians can work with professional organizations, such as the National Rural Health Association, to advocate for adequate rural healthcare resources from government agencies.

The cases

All healthcare professionals must address ethical challenges. The clinician in each case must address ethical challenges that are inherent to the rural context and are familiar to all rural clinicians.

In the first case, limitations of resources generated healthcare access and quality of care concerns. The rural physician referred the patient to improve clinical care. However, the patient declined the specialized care because of the travel distance, possibly challenging roads, and the lack of her normal support system at the urban medical facility. After disclosing to the patient his clinical limitations as a non-specialist, the rural physician ought to provide the needed care. The physician, ethically, cannot refuse to provide care to the patient. To enhance quality of care of the patient, the physician should seek consultation with specialists for guidance, possibly by the usage of colleagues, professional organizations, or the Internet to create a consultation network. Proactively, physicians should educate their patients and the community about rural health issues, including the need of access to specialized care, and they should work with local social service agencies to diminish the barriers to receiving care in distant communities.

In the second case, competing professional obligations, as a physician and as a school board member, force the clinician to weigh whether or not to take administrative action against a teacher based upon privileged medical knowledge. There are no easy resolutions in this case; however, the patient did come to the psychologist to address family relationship issues. The psychologist should pursue a suitable treatment of the patient's alcohol problem and avoid using the information ascertained in the counseling session as a school board member. The situation could change if, the psychologist believed, students were harmed by the teacher's alcohol problem. Proactively, healthcare professionals should discuss over lapping relationships with all patients prior to providing healthcare. As in this case, there also needs to be a clear understanding with all school board members on ways to separate or diminish conflicting roles.

In the third case, the physician should encourage the patient to seek needed mental healthcare in the nearby community or in a more distant community where his truck may not be recognized. If the patient still continues to be unwilling to seek the needed specialized care, the family physician should attempt to address the mental health concerns using mental health colleagues to provide guidance on an adequate course of treatment. The concern of the patient regarding charting of the depression is reasonable because of the nature of a small, close-knit community. The physician may consider keeping personal notes out of the medical record. The physician should implement a privacy and confidentially protocol that includes discussions with patients only behind closed doors, keeping all records locked, and only sharing patient information and records with those that have a "need to know." The physician should proactively educate staff about the importance of privacy and the associated problems, including how breaches in confidentiality can be detrimental to care. Physicians can work collaboratively with mental health professionals using a single clinic to avoid stigma (Roberts *et al.*, 1999a; Roberts and Dyer, 2004).

REFERENCES

American College of Physicians (1998). Ethics manual: 4th edn, *Ann Intern Med* **128**: 576–94.

American Psychiatric Association (2006). *The Principles of Medical Ethics: With Annotations Especially Applicable to Psychiatry*, 2006 edn. Arlington, VA: American Psychiatric Association (http://www.psych.org/psych_pract/ethics/ppaethics.cfm) accessed 8 September 2006.

Baldwin, L. M., Patanian, M. M., Larson, E. H., *et al.* (2006). Modeling the mental health workforce in Washington State: using state licensing data to examine provider supply in rural and urban areas. *J Rural Health* **22**: 50–8.

Berger, J. and Mohr, J. (1967). *A Fortunate Man*. New York: Pantheon, pp. 13–5.

Bird D. C., Dempsey P., and Hartley D. (2001). *Addressing Mental Health Workforce Needs in Underserved Rural Areas: Accomplishments and Challenges*. [Working Paper No. 23.] Portland, ME: University of Southern Maine, Edmund S. Muskie School of Public Service, Institute for Health Policy, Maine Rural Health Research Center (http://www.muskie.usm.maine.edu/m_view_publication.jsp?id=954) accessed 8 September 2006.

Boffa, J. (2002). Is there a doctor in the house? *Aust N Z J Public Health* **26**: 301–4.

Braden, J. and Beauregard, K. (1994). *Health Status and Access to Care of Rural and Urban Populations. National Medicare Expenditure Survey Findings 18*. Rockville, MD: Agency for Health Care Policy and Research.

Bushy, A. (1994). When your client lives in a rural area. Part I: rural health care delivery issues. *Issues Ment Health Nurs* **15**: 253–66.

Bushy, A. and Rauh, J. R. (1991). Implementing an ethics committee in rural institutions. *J Nurs Admin* **21**: 18–25.

Campbell, C. D. and Gordon, M. C. (2003). Acknowledging the inevitable: understanding multiple relationships in rural practice. *Prof Psychol Res Pract* **34**: 430–4.

Canadian Rural Partnership Research and Analysis Unit (2002). *Rural Research Note: Canadian Rural Population Trends.* [Publication 2138/E.] Ottawa: Government of Canada, Agriculture and Agri-Food Canada (http://www.rural.gc.ca/research/note/note1_e.phtml) accessed 8 September 2006.

Chan, C., Hart, L. G., and Goodman, D. C. (2006). Geographic access to health care for rural Medicare beneficiaries. *J Rural Health* **22**: 140–6.

Cook, A. F. and Hoas, H. (2000). Where the rubber hits the road: implications for organizational and clinical ethics in rural health care settings. *HEC Forum* **12**: 331–40.

Cook, A. F. and Hoas, H. (2001). Voices from the margins: a context for developing bioethics-related resources. *Am J Bioethics* **1**: W12.

Cook, A. F., Hoas, H., and Guttmannova, K. (2000a). Bioethics activities in rural hospitals. *Camb Q Healthc Ethics* **9**: 230–8.

Cook, A. F., Hoas, H., and Joyner, J. C. (2000b). Ethics and the rural nurse: a research study of problems, values, and needs. *J Nurs Law* **7**: 41–53.

Cook, A. F., Hoas, H., and Joyner, J. C. (2001). No secrets on Main Street. *Am J Nurs* **101**: 67, 69–71.

Cook, A. F., Hoas, H., and Guttmannova, K. (2002). Ethical issues faced by rural physicians. *SDJ Med* **55**: 221–4.

Cox, J. (1997). Rural general practice: a personal view of current key issues. *Health Bull (Edinb.)* **55**: 309–15.

Department for Environment, Food and Rural Affairs. (2004). Appendix B – Summary of evidence base. In *The Rural Strategy 2004.* London: defra (http://www.defra.gov.uk/rural/strategy/annex_b.htm) accessed 8 September 2006.

Economic Research Service (2005). Child poverty declined between 1990 and 2000. In *Economic Information Bulletin Number 1: Rural Children at a Glance.* Washington, DC: US Department of Agriculture (http://www.ers.usda.gov/publications/EIB1/EIB1.htm) accessed 8 September 2006.

Flannery, M. A. (1982). Simple living and hard choices. *Hastings Cent Rep* **12**: 9–12.

Forrow, L., Arnold, R. M., and Parker, L. S. (1993). Preventive ethics: expanding the horizons of clinical ethics. *J Clin Ethics* **4**: 287–94.

Gallagher, E., Alcock, D., Diem, E., Angus, D., and Medves, J. (2002). Ethical dilemmas in home care case management. *J Healthc Manag* **47**: 85–96.

Gamm, L. D., Hutchinson, L. L, Dabney, B. J., and Dorsey, A. M. (eds.) (2003). *Rural Healthy People 2010: A Companion Document to Healthy People 2010.* College Station, TX: The Texas A&M University System Health Science Center, School of Rural Public Health, Southwest Rural Health Research Center.

Glover, J. J. (2001). Rural bioethical issues of the elderly: how do they differ from urban ones? *J Rural Health* **17**: 332–5.

Goldsmith, H. F., Wagenfeld, M.O., Manderscheid, R. W., and Stiles, D. (1997). Specialty mental health services in metropolitan and nonmetropolitan areas: 1983 and 1990. *Admin Policy Mental Health* **24**: 457–88.

Hardwig, J. (2006). Rural health care ethics: what assumptions and attitudes should drive the research? *Am J Bioethics* **6**: 53–4.

Hartley D., Bird D., and Dempsey P. (1999). Rural mental health and substance abuse. In *Rural Health in the United States*, ed. T.C. Ricketts. New York: Oxford University Press, pp. 159–78.

Henderson, C. B. (2000). Small-town psychiatry. *Psychiatr Serv* **51**: 253–4.

Holzer, C. E., Goldsmith, H. F., and Ciarlo, J. A. (1998). Effects of rural–urban county type on the available of health and mental health care providers. In *Mental Health, United States.* Washington, DC: US Government Printing Office [DHHS Pub. No. (SMA)99–3285], pp. 204–13.

Institute of Medicine (2005). *Quality Through Collaboration: The Future of Rural Health Care.* Washington, DC: National Academies Press.

Jennings, F. L. (1992). Ethics of rural practice. *Psychother Private Pract* **10**: 85–104.

Johnson, M. E., Brems, C., Warner, T. D., and Roberts, L. W. (2006). Rural–urban health care provider disparities in Alaska and New Mexico. *Adm Policy Ment Health* **33**: 504–7.

Kelly, S. E. (2003). Bioethics and rural health: theorizing place, space, and subjects. *Soc Sci Med* **56**: 2277–88.

Larson, L. (2001). How many hats are too many? *Trustee* **54**: 6–10.

Maddalena, V. and Sherwin, S. (2004). Vulnerable populations in rural areas: challenges for ethics committees. *HEC Forum* **16**: 234–46.

Miller, P. J. (1994). Dual relationships in rural practice: a dilemma of ethics and culture. *Hum Serv Rural Environ* **18**: 4–7.

Moscovice, I. and Rosenblatt, R. (2000). Quality-of-care challenges of rural health. *J Rural Health* **16**: 168–76.

Moss, A. H. (1999). The application of the Task Force report in rural and frontier settings. *J Clin Ethics* **10**: 42–8.

National Center for Health Statistics (2001a). Figure 3. Population by age, region, and urbanization level: United States, 1998. Data tables on urban and rural health. In *Health, United States, 2001 with Urban and Rural Health Chartbook*. Washington, DC: US Government Printing Office (DHHS Publ. No. (PHS) 01-1232), p. 93.

National Center for Health Statistics (2001b). Figure 19. Suicide rates among persons 15 years of age and over by sex, region, and urbanization level: United States, 1996–8. Data tables on urban and rural health. In *Health, United States, 2001 with Urban and Rural Health Chartbook*. Washington, DC: US Government Printing Office (DHHS Pub. No. (PHS) 01-1232), p. 109.

National Center for Health Statistics (2005). Table 33. Age-adjusted death rates, according to race, sex, region, and urbanization level: United States, average annual 1994–6, 1997–9, and 2000–2. In *Health, United States, 2005 with Chartbook on Trends in the Health of Americans*. Washington, DC: Government Printing Office (DHHS Pub. No. 2005-1232), p. 184.

Nelson, W. (2004). Addressing rural ethics issues. The characteristics of rural health care settings pose unique ethical challenges. *Healthc Exec* **19**: 36–7.

Nelson, W. (2006). Where's the evidence: a need to assess rural health ethics committee models. *J Rural Health* **22**: 193–5.

Nelson, W. A. and Pomerantz, A. S. (1992a). Ethics issues in rural health care. *Trustee* **45**: 14–15.

Nelson W. A. and Pomerantz A. S. (1992b). Ethics issues in rural health care. In *Choices and Conflict: Explorations in Health Care Ethics*, ed. E. Friedman. Chicago, IL: American Hospital Publishers, pp. 156–63.

Nelson, W. A. and Weeks, W. B. (2006). Rural/non-rural differences of American Society of Bioethics and Humanities membership. *J Med Ethics* **32**: 411–13.

Nelson, W., Lushkov, G., Pomerantz, A., and Weeks, W. B. (2006). Rural health care ethics: is there a literature? *Am J Bioethics* **6**: 44–50.

Niemira, D. A. (1988). Grassroots grappling: ethics committees at rural hospitals. *Ann Intern Med* **12**: 981–3.

Niemira, D. A., Meece, K. S., and Reiquam, C. W. (1989a). Multi-institutional ethics committees. *HEC Forum* **1**: 77–81.

Niemira, D. A., Orr, R. D., and Culver, C. M. (1989b). Ethics committees in small hospitals. *J Rural Health* **5**: 19–32.

Purtilo, R. (1987). Rural health care: the forgotten quarter of medical ethics. *Second Opin* **6**: 10–33.

Purtilo, R. and Sorrell, J. (1986). The ethical dilemmas of a rural physician. *Hastings Cent Rep* **16**: 24–8.

Ricketts, T. C. (2000). The changing nature of rural health care. *Annu Rev Public Health* **21**: 639–57.

Ricketts, T., Johnson-Webb, K., and Taylor, P. (1998). *Rural Definitions for Health Policy Makers*. Bethesda, MD: DHHS, Federal Office of Rural Health Policy.

Roberts L. W. and Dyer, A. R. (2004). Caring for people in small communities. In *Concise Guide to Ethics in Mental Health Care*, ed. L. W. Roberts and A. R. Dyer. Washington, DC: American Psychiatric Press, pp. 167–83.

Roberts, L. W., Battaglia, J., Smithpeter, M., and Epstein, R. S. (1999a). An office on main street: health care dilemmas in small communities. *Hastings Cent Rep* **29**: 28–37.

Roberts, L. W., Battaglia, J., and Epstein, R. S. (1999b). Frontier ethics: mental health care needs and ethical dilemmas in rural communities. *Psychiatr Serv* **50**: 497–503.

Roberts, L. W., Warner, T. D., and Hammond, K. G. (2005). Ethical challenges of mental health clinicians in rural and frontier areas. *Psychiatr Serv* **56**: 358–9.

Robillard, H. M., High, D. M., Sebastian, J. G., *et al.* (1989). Ethical issues in primary health care: a survey of practitioners' perceptions. *J Community Health* **14**: 9–17.

Romanow R. J. (2002). *Building on Values: The Future of Health Care in Canada, Ch. 7: Rural and Remote Communities*. Saskatoon: Commission on the Future of Health Care in Canada (http://www.hc–sc.gc.ca/english/care/romanow/hcc0023.html) accessed 19 September 2006.

Rosenblatt, R. A. and Hart, L. C. (1999). Physicians and rural America. In *Rural Health in the United States*, ed. T. C. Ricketts, III. New York: Oxford University Press, pp. 38–51.

Rosenthal, M. B., Zaslavsky, A., and Newhouse, J. P. (2005). The geographic distribution of physicians revisited. *Health Serv Res* **40**: 1931–52.

Rosenblatt, R. A., Andrilla, C. H. A., Curtin, T., and Hart, L. G. (2006). Shortages of medical personnel at community health centers: implications for planned expansion. *JAMA* **295**: 1042–9.

Rost, K., Owen, R. R., Smith, J., and Smith, G. R. (1998). Rural–urban differences in service use and course of illness in bipolar disorder. *J Rural Health* **14**: 36–43.

Rourke, L. L. and Rourke, J. T. (1998). Close friends as patients in rural practice. *Can Fam Physician* **44**: 1208–10, 1219–22.

Schank, J. A. (1998). Ethics issues in rural counseling practice. *Can J Counseling* **32**: 270–83.

Simon, R. I. and Williams, I. C. (1999). Maintaining treatment boundaries in small communities and rural areas. *Psychiatr Serv* **50**: 1440–6.

Sobel, S. B. (1992). Small town practice of psychotherapy: ethical and personal dilemmas. *Psychother Private Pract* **10**: 61–9.

Spiegel, P. B. (1990). Confidentiality endangered under some circumstances without special management. *Psychotherapy* **27**: 636–43.

Sriram, T. G., Radhika, M. R., Shanmugham, V., and Murthy, R. S. (1990). Comparison of urban and rural respondents' experience and opinion of ethical issues in medical care. *Int J Soc Psychiatry* **36**: 200–6.

Turner, L. N., Marquis, K., and Burman, M. E. (1996). Rural nurse practitioners: perceptions of ethical dilemmas. *J Am Acad Nurs Pract* **8**: 269–74.

Ullom-Minnich, P. D. and Kallail, K. J. (1993). Physicians' strategies for safeguarding confidentiality: the influence of community and practice characteristics. *J Fam Pract* **37**: 445–8.

US Department of Housing and Urban Development (2000). *Attachment 2: FY 2000 Median Family Income for States, Metropolitan and Nonmetropolitan Portions of States*. Washington, DC: Government Printing Office (http://www.huduser.org/DATASETS/IL/fmr00/medians2.html) accessed 18 September 2006.

Wagenfeld, M. O., Murray, J. D., Mohatt, D. F., and DeBruyn, J. C. (1994). *Mental Health and Rural America: 1980–1993. An Overview and Annotated Bibliography.* Washington, DC: HHSA, Office of Rural Health Policy.

Warner, T. D., Monaghan–Geernaert, P., Battaglia, J., *et al.* (2005). Ethical considerations in rural health care: a pilot study of clinicians in Alaska and New Mexico. *Community Ment Health J* **41**: 21–33.

Weeks, W. B., Kazis, L. E., Shen, Y., *et al.* (2004). Differences in health-related quality of life in rural and urban veterans. *Am J Public Health* **94**: 1762–7.

Woods, D. (1977). The rural doctor: among friends on the Canada–US border. *CMAJ* **117**: 809, 812–14.

Ziller, E. C., Coburn, A. F., Loux, S. L., Hoffman, C., and McBride, T. D. (eds.) (2003). *Health Insurance Coverage in Rural America: Chartbook.* [Publication 4093] Washington, DC: Kaiser Commission on Medicaid and the Uninsured.

39

Community healthcare ethics

Kyle W. Anstey and Frank Wagner

Staff in a community care agency provide service to an elderly, but capable, woman in her home. This woman is cared for by her son, who the staff believes is neglectful. The home care staff believes that the neglectful son is not providing adequate support to his mother while at the same time enjoying many financial benefits (e.g., rent and food) in this living arrangement. Further, the pair lives in a "rough" area of the city and staff has witnessed the son both purchasing from, and having loud arguments with, local drug dealers. The staff are concerned about their own and their client's safety and feel distress in relation to the situation each time after they visit the home; yet within their organization there exists no tools for them to discuss or work through the ethical issues faced in this situation.

What is community healthcare ethics?

Community healthcare ethics can be defined as an endeavor to promote the sector's philosophy of supporting clients' independence and ongoing integration (or reintegration) in their community. It does so by providing a unique view that is sensitive to how client's self-determination may be affected by the distinct supports offered by the sector, and the different settings they are provided in.

Such a definition is not unproblematic, as community healthcare ethics is ill defined: it lacks the rich literature, dedicated educational programs and professional roles, codes, and policies that treat ethical issues in institutional clinical practice. Thousands of articles have been published on the latter, which is also considered in many dedicated journals. In North America, clinical ethics education is frequently incorporated into the training of physicians and nurses, many of whom will later work hospitals with established ethics programs led by clinical ethicists. By comparison, our review of the literature shows that there is little scholarship available on ethical issues in community healthcare. There is no journal dedicated to this topic, and less than 100 peer-reviewed articles on this subject. Outside of the community care sector in the greater Toronto area (GTA) that we will focus on in this article, there are very few programs that include ethics training for community care staff such as personal support workers. Even fewer homecare organizations have established ethics policies, programs, or committees, and to our knowledge, none of these has its own ethicist.

One might question whether these differences demand a distinct analysis for community care and argue that institutional clinical ethics resources can continue to be applied as patients move from hospital or clinic to home. This position fails to give sufficient weight to the marked difference between these sectors with respect to philosophy of care, resulting range of supports, and, most importantly, setting of care provision. Institutional clinical care is focused on treatment, with a curative goal. As noted, the philosophy of community healthcare focuses on independence and ongoing integration (or reintegration) of clients in their community. We will not explore the ethical significance of the contrast between these "medical" and "social" models of care here, as this is well examined by theorists in areas of inquiry such as disability studies. However, it is important to acknowledge that these philosophies and the care provision that follows are not mutually exclusive: indeed, institutional clinical practices are essential to community healthcare. Clinical treatment may be necessary before a client can make use of community care supports, and may be essential to their bodily, person, and social-level functioning. Further, community care itself offers specialized care as found in acute clinical settings, such as dialysis, ventilator care and tube feeding, laboratory services, and physical and speech therapy. Additionally, however, community care also offers a myriad of distinct services that include personal care, homemaking and shopping assistance, repair and maintenance services, transportation, adult day care, and respite care. This complex combination of formal and informal care, and multiple non-health issues such as family dynamics, safety, and housing, creates ethical dilemmas that are not suitable for analysis or resolution using an ethical framework based on an institutional model.

Why is community healthcare ethics important?

The provision of services in the setting of the client's home (rather than the institution-based care described at the start of this chapter) itself creates ethical issues. The case illustrates a frequent scenario facing personal support workers: other people sharing the home setting (in this case, the son) may have a vested interest and benefit materially from the client continuing to be cared for at home. Further, the location of the client's home in the community is intimately related to the safety issues facing the workers who provide this assistance. Such examples of the significance of setting suggest that ethical approaches used in institutional clinical care cannot simply be transposed from hospital to community care.

There is clearly a need for a great deal of work on the significance of setting in community ethics.

Indeed, some of the small body of literature available on community care ethics treats this topic (Liaschenko, 1996; Aulisio *et al.*, 1998). Yet, beyond addressing the lack of community ethics literature, there is a pressing need for resources to aid community care staff in supporting their clients in the community. There has been an observed increase in the number and complexity of ethical dilemmas in the homecare sector (Committee to Advance Ethical Decision-Making in Community Health, 2001). Faced with an increasing number of complex cases and ethical dilemmas, there is evidence that staff in the homecare sector are experiencing considerable moral distress, which is commonly defined as an inability to translate moral choices into moral action (Elpern *et al.*, 2005: 523; Rushton, 2006, p. 161). Evidence suggests that the experience of moral distress in community care may be having an impact on the recruitment and retention of workers in the sector (Wojtak, 2002, p. 70).

The prevalence of these issues and the associate outcomes like moral distress are plausibly explained in part by a general increase in caseload and complexity. This results from a number of interrelated factors, including increased pressures from governments and payers worldwide to move from institutionally based healthcare to less-expensive community-based care. Increasing proportions of the population are aged, with chronic conditions, and continue to live at home dependent on in-home and community services. The impact of medical technology combined with a trend toward reduced length of stay (and subsequent earlier discharge of non-compliant and/or complex cases from hospital without effective communication with patient, family, or community support agencies) contribute to further distress. Furthermore, the related tendency toward ''silo-ing'' – the perception on the part of many decision makers in these institutions that their only responsibility is for care delivered in their own setting – leads to increased isolation for patient and caregivers after discharge.

How should I approach community healthcare ethics in practice?

To support their community-based staff in dealing with such complex issues as raised in the case above, the Toronto Community Care Access Centre and other community organizations in the GTA have formed innovative partnerships, and trialed an ethics toolkit for ethical decision making in community healthcare. We describe this toolkit, and the strategic community engagement process that informed it, in detail below. Our aim in doing so is to share with other community care sectors a common approach for their workers to identify, analyze, and address ethical issues arising in their service delivery, with the intention of improving client care and staff experience.

The main components in this community-based approach to ethics issues are: (i) a strategic community engagement process, (ii) a code of ethics, (iii) a decision-making worksheet, and (iv) ethics case documentation, review, and evaluation tools.

A strategic community engagement process

Since most bioethical decision-making resources are based on hospital cases and in hospital settings, the development of this approach began by letting those forming the community articulate their own experience with the unique community-based ethical dilemmas and decide what resources were important to support their work in this area. A strategic community engagement process was developed to identify specific issues facing workers in the sector and to address the need to build organizational ethics capacity to meet these challenges. In this way, the initiative was grassroots based, and the decision-making tool was grounded in the values of the community.

Most homecare organizations in the GTA community sector lack the resources necessary to mount their own ethics initiatives. However, many organizations in the sector indicated a real willingness

to cooperate in developing common tools and education for their staff. A joint research project to identify the major ethical issues facing their front-line staff was commissioned in 2001. The project included a literature review, as well as a questionnaire and oral interviews with over 200 staff and representatives from 45 agencies (over half of the interviewees were front-line workers). Analysis of responses revealed seven major categories of ethical issues faced by community health workers:
• making choices
• allocation of financial resources
• workplace demands
• environmental factors
• client safety
• worker safety
• consent.

These project results served as the catalyst for formalizing cooperation between the participating agencies and led to the establishment of the GTA Community Ethics Network in October 2005. This network has continued and developed a mission to provide the resources, coordination, and support necessary to advance the practice of ethics among its 30-member health service agencies. Regular meetings of agency representatives provide a supportive forum for members facing difficult ethical issues, as well as for coordinating and resourcing joint initiatives and tools for their staff. We are not aware of any other comparable collaboration between community agencies in Canada, or worldwide.

A code of ethics for community health

The Code of Ethics for Community Health resulted from a working group round-table discussion attended by approximately 200 people from 40 community-based provider agencies, and it was finalized in September 2003. The result was an agreed code that expresses in lay terms common values of the community sector members. A total of 10 principles are articulated in the code (Figure 39.1). These principles provide staff with

CODE OF ETHICS FOR THE COMMUNITY HEALTH AND SUPPORT SECTOR OF TORONTO

We, as employees of Community Health and Support Sector organizations, are committed to being an integral part of the communities we serve. We are responsible for: acting professionally and in a client-centred manner; upholding the dignity and honour of our clients; and practicing in accordance with ethical principles. This Code of Ethics is intended to provide us with specific ethical principles to address situations that we may encounter, and to guide us in our relationships with clients, family members and others in the support team, other health care practitioners, and the public. This code is intended to complement laws, codes and standards of professional practice.

Advocacy: We have the responsibility to help improve the awareness, the accessibility and the quality of our services by advocating on behalf of our clients. We will seek guidance both internally and externally from our organization for those situations that could place the organization and/or its clients at risk.

Client Confidentiality: Client information is confidential; we will ensure that clients and their legal substitute are informed of their right to consent to the sharing of necessary information with individuals and organizations directly involved in the client's care.

Commitment to Quality Services: We are committed to providing the highest quality services that will benefit our clients within available resources.

Conflict of Interest: We will not compromise services to our clients for our own personal benefit.

Dignity: In all our interactions we will demonstrate profound respect for human dignity. We will be responsive and sensitive to the diversity among our clients and staff groups.

Employee Safety: We recognize that the community work setting provides a unique working environment for all of us. We will take necessary measures to ensure our personal safety, and all safety concerns will be reported and addressed in a supportive and non-threatening way. After all options have been considered, we may withdraw service if our safety is compromised.

Fair and Equitable Access: We believe that each individual is entitled to an assessment. We will ensure that services are based on clients' needs, regardless of their income, age, gender, ethnicity or race, physical or mental ability, and any other factors such as diverse behaviors or lifestyle.

Health and Well Being: We will use a holistic approach to clients' health care needs by acknowledging all things important to them in their community.

Informed Choice and Empowerment: We believe that most individuals have the ability and the right to make decisions about their health. We will assist clients to make care plans and life choices in keeping with the client's values, beliefs and health care goals. We will ensure that clients are fully informed of their options and have all the information they need to make informed decisions about their health. If the client is mentally incapable of making these decisions, we will take directions from the client's legal substitute.

Relationships Among Community Agencies: We recognize there may be a competitive element in our working relationships, however we agree to respect one another's roles and to work together in the spirit of collaboration to maximize the effectiveness of client services.

Figure 39.1. The Code of Ethics of the Community Health and Support Sector of Toronto.

relevant concepts that help them to identify and articulate ethical issues and conflicts based on a common language within the community context.

A decision-making worksheet for community health

The third major component of the toolkit is a decision-making worksheet also designed, piloted, and modified with the input of over 200 frontline staff. The worksheet is a step-by-step field tool to be used by a staff member who is faced with an ethical dilemma out on a home visit or in another community setting. It is introduced to staff as part of a three-part training process that includes: (i) helping staff to discern true ethical dilemmas, (ii) providing tools and resources on how to deal with the dilemma, and (iii) confirming a commitment on behalf of the employer organization to provide supports and resources should the workers need help. The worksheet comprises four key sections or steps that are identified by the acronym "IDEA," to aid memory:

I   identify the facts
D   determine the ethical principles in conflict
E   explore the options
A   act on your decision and evaluate.

Ethics case documentation, review, and evaluation tools

Toolkits are ultimately only significant if they change the behavior of the staff and organizations that make use of them. A system of case documentation is now being trialed among members of the Community Ethics Network to provide the measurement necessary to evaluate whether this common approach will achieve its goal of enhancing practice around ethical decision making in the community health sector.

The Clinical and Community Ethics Database (CCED) allows ethics cases to be documented,

reviewed, and potentially evaluated in a secure environment. Data fields are grouped and may further structure and focus discussion, within the categories of the IDEA worksheet. Additionally, case reports can be generated in this format, and stripped of identifying fields to help to facilitate the sharing of case knowledge between organizations. Moreover, the database can report on trends across cases related to volume of consults, the time spent conducting them, as well as client demographic information. For example, an organization could query how many times it dealt with cases of family neglect and/or safety as described in the case above, the time spent conducting them, and what groups or individuals among its staff tended to refer them for consultation. All organizations within and outside the Community Ethics Network can freely use, modify, and distribute this open-source database.

The network has also initiated a follow-up case review process to facilitate and guide discussion about these documented cases, and to support staff decision-making processes by using these collected cases as a basis for new staff educational materials. There is considerable need for such material, as our literature reviews have produced mainly hospital-based case examples that do not reflect the unique variables of community care.

Cases and ethical consults documented via the CCED will provide a significant component for the development of materials for informal and formal education of community sector workers. Informally, they will serve as a reference point in debriefing affected staff through individual case reviews and for conducting discussions with wider staff groups likely to be affected by similar issues. In the education sector, documented cases will be incorporated into the formal education of nursing degrees and training for personal support workers as a result of a partnership between the Community Ethics Network and a local community college (George Brown College). This initiative will reinterpret and reformat the case-based materials developed by community workers to contribute to the development of formal educational material that is part of the Community Ethics Network strategic plan. Specifically, the material will focus on the inter-professional learning required to ensure appropriate ethical decision-making process by these and other workers in the community sector.

How should I approach community healthcare ethics in practice?

The cooperation of the GTA community sector has permitted the development of unique resources to support community healthcare staff as they face an increasing volume and complexity of moral issues. Beyond beginning to address the resulting moral distress staff may experience, the partnerships, tools, and processes of the GTA community sector are also important for addressing an altogether different type of pressure: namely, that brought by changing healthcare accreditation standards.

The Canadian Council for Health Services Accreditation (CCHSA) has expressed concern about the ability of small homecare organizations to build and maintain capacity in ethics (Murphy, 2006). The unique partnership of the Community Ethics Network addresses this concern by pooling resources so that all organizations have access to the same robust set of tools.

Furthermore, some of these tools are themselves relevant to accreditation, as the CCHSA is beginning to move beyond requiring mechanisms for conducting case consultations toward review of their results, and the impact of these outcomes for ethics services (Murphy, 2006). As noted above, the CCED collects the necessary information on service delivery for such evaluation research, which to date has never been conducted with community agencies, and very little among clinical ethics support services (Slowther *et al.*, 2001).

The CCED and other components of the toolkit will be of use in other regions. Indeed, some teaching hospitals in Toronto as well as in other parts of Ontario and Canada have used the toolkit

to assist in the education of their staff. These resources can be freely used with appropriate attribution, and downloaded from the Community Ethics Network website at: http://www.utoronto.ca/jcb/ethics/cen.htm

While the network's tools will be of use to individual homecare organizations, it is important to emphasize this partnership itself as a model for collaborative approaches to ethical issues facing other catchment areas. Again, this network provides a forum that enhances organizational capacity to review difficult cases that arise, and the resource pool required to further develop and teach new educational materials.

The case

The case illustrates the significant ethical issues arising from the delivery of community health services unique to the community healthcare setting. Using the ethics toolkit, the community care staff member first used the IDEA framework to collect the relevant facts, including the perspectives of the client on the situation. The client consistently maintained that she was quite happy with the quality of her life, and that she had absolutely no desire to be placed in a long-term care facility. While she acknowledged that her son was "not perfect," she did not feel neglected or abused, and found comfort in having a familiar face around the house.

Directed by the worksheet to reflect on her own emotions, feelings, and values about the situation, the staff member felt that the son's motives and the impact of his choices on client's quality of life was her primary concern. His criminal behavior was an issue for her more for this reason than for her own personal safety. Nevertheless, directed by the worksheet to examine the Code of Ethics in articulating the values in conflict (step 2), she felt reassured by the code's allowance for service being withdrawn where, after all options have been considered, employee safety remains compromised. Further, the code emphasized the need to respect choices that capable clients like this elderly woman make about their care plan, but to seek guidance in situation where clients like this elderly woman may be at risk. A district supervisor was involved, and together they determined that there was a conflict between their perception of the quality of the patient's life and her own. Given that the client was capable, and the staff member had informed her of the provider perspective on the potential consequences of her son's behavior and dependency (e.g., possibly not receiving service, danger in the home), the staff decided to respect the client's decision to live at home.

Next, the staff member took action (step 3 and step 4) and communicated her respect for the client's decision to her and her son. At this time, she also communicated to the son that he must offer the resources necessary to provide quality care to his mother, and that his capacity to do so would be evaluated. Further, he was informed that legal action would be taken if evidence of abuse was encountered in the future; that he could relinquish his role as caregiver if he wanted; or that staff would help to educate and support him in meeting his mother's medical and dietary needs. The son agreed to these conditions.

REFERENCES

Aulisio, M. P., May, T., and Aulisio M. S. (1998). Vulnerabilities of clients and caregivers in the homecare setting. *Generations* **22**: 58–63.

Committee to Advance Ethical Decision Making in Community Health (2001). *Final Report March 2001– December 2001*. Toronto: Community Access Care Centre Toronto.

Elpern, E. H., Covert, B., and Kleinpel, R. (2006). Moral distress of staff nurses in a medical intensive care unit. *Am J Crit Care* **14**: 523–30.

Liaschenko, J. (1996). A sense of place for patients: living and dying. *Home Care Provider* **1**: 270–2.

Murphy, T. (2006). *Ethics and CCHSA's Accreditation Program*. Toronto: Joint Centre for Bioethics.

Rushton, C. H. (2006). Defining and addressing moral distress: tools for critical care nursing leaders. *AACN Adv Crit Care* **17**: 161–8.

Slowther, A., Bunch, C., Woolnough, B., and Hope, T. (2001). Clinical ethics support services in the UK: an investigation of the current provision of ethics support to health professionals in the UK. *J Med Ethics* **27**: (Suppl. I): i2.

Wojtak, A. (2002). Practice based ethics as a foundation for human resources planning in community health care. *Healthc Manag Forum* **3**: 67–72.

Using clinical ethics to make an impact in healthcare

Introduction

Susan K. MacRae

A recent study was done in Canada to identify what clinical ethicists felt were the top 10 clinical ethical challenges facing Canadians in healthcare. (Breslin *et al.*, 2005; Table VII.1).

What is clear from this list is that many of these ethical issues are core to challenges of healthcare more broadly today. While this study was conducted in Canada, it is likely these same challenges may be similar in other healthcare systems, at least in the developed world.

Clinical ethics is a comparatively recent endeavor in healthcare, but despite its relative newness it provides an ideal model for initiatives that can impact healthcare because of its inherent interdisciplinary make-up and its unique capacity to impact care across the healthcare spectrum from "boardroom to bedside." While clinical ethics offers this unique perspective to address healthcare problems, it is often missing from the meetings where significant system-wide decisions are made. Many decision makers miss the key point that much of healthcare is grounded in values and many of the solutions may be found in the ethical field of inquiry. The most likely reason for this absence of clinical ethics at the decision tables in healthcare is related to the still developing nature of this work. What the chapters in this section show, however, is that perhaps clinical ethics is "coming of age" and is beginning to make serious arguments to the healthcare community about how its activities and frameworks can offer useful, real-world contributions to help to guide system decision makers, healthcare professionals, and the public.

In Ch. 40, the authors outline the importance of systems thinking in the practice of clinical ethics with the goal of impacting the overall professional and organization ethics culture and accountability of hospitals and other healthcare settings. The authors built their chapter around a challenge by Singer, Pelligrino and Siegler from their 2001 article "Clinical ethics revisited," who stated that the two significant challenges in the field of clinical ethics for this decade are (i) for clinical ethics practice (consultation and committees) to integrate clinical ethics work into the culture of health care organizations and (ii) to improve organizational accountability for clinical ethics. The authors take this challenge and offer systems thinking as an important response to these problems by arguing that clinical ethics must focus more on the underlying systems factors that give rise to many of the ethical concerns in healthcare rather than focusing only on cases and acute situations. The three authors provide leadership to major clinical ethics programs in Canada, the USA, and the UK and have each independently evolved to this systemic approach to clinical ethics. In this chapter, they describe their reasons for and experience with this approach. At the end of the chapter, the authors highlight their own top 10 leading practices in applying systems thinking to clinical ethics.

Chapter 41 reviews four innovative strategies that may improve clinical ethics effectiveness in healthcare organizations: (i) the hub and spokes model for clinical ethics service delivery, (ii) leadership and management skills training for clinical

Table VII.1. The top 10 ethical challenges facing Canadians in healthcare

Rank	Scenario	Score
1	Disagreement between patients/families and healthcare professionals about treatment decisions	113
2	Waiting lists	102
3	Access to needed healthcare resources for the aged, chronically ill, and mentally ill	89
4	Shortage of family physicians or primary care teams in both rural and urban settings	82
5	Medical error	76
6	Withholding/withdrawing life-sustaining treatment in the context of terminal or serious illness	56
7	Achieving informed consent	43
8	Ethical issues related to subject participation in research	40
9	Substitute decision making	38
10	The ethics of surgical innovation and incorporating new technologies for patient care	21

From Breslin *et al.*, 2005.

ethicists, (iii) ethics strategic planning and (iv) evaluation of clinical ethics services based on process indicators. These innovations were developed in the "laboratory" of the University of Toronto Joint Centre for Bioethics, where 15 healthcare organizations and 25 bioethicists collaborate across a broad spectrum of health care organizations (from acute care, home care, specialty hospitals, and a genomic institute) to model, pilot, test, and share innovations in clinical ethics service and practice. This chapter reviews these innovations in the context of clinical ethics effectiveness. In so doing, they give a brief history and outline some of the complexities involved in evaluating clinical ethics effectiveness. They make a further point that the unique patient populations, variability of ethics capacity in any given institution, and the different missions and values of different organizations will demand that "some component of evaluating clinical ethics effectiveness will necessarily [be] context-dependent." Nevertheless the authors challenge us to take this notion of effectiveness seriously, as ethics is increasingly recognized as an important component of high-quality clinical care and valued strongly by patients and their families.

In Ch. 42, the authors tackle the challenge of bioethics teaching in clinical practice and advocate for a clinician–teacher approach. The authors intend the chapter to encourage clinician–teachers

to accept the important responsibility of teaching bioethics and to provide them with some practical advice. While the focus in this chapter is on medical students and medical residents, the authors acknowledge that a similar clinical approach applies to teaching other clinicians, such as nurses. The authors organize their chapter around five questions for the clinical teacher. (i) Why should I teach? (ii) What should I teach? (iii) How should I teach? (iv) How should I evaluate? (v) How should I learn? The authors review the importance of a bedside or case-based approach as a way to capture the interest of the clinical audience. The authors quite extensively review various evaluation strategies for clinical training, including in-training evaluation reports, chart audits, objective structured clinical examination using standardized patients, multiple choice examinations, and short answer or essay examinations. Finally, the authors encourage clinicians to seek continued and further education for themselves if they are to teach bioethics as a specialized skill. The authors provide an extensive list of bioethics teaching resources in an appendix at the end of the chapter.

This section is a limited examination of only a few innovations in clinical ethics that strive to make an impact on the healthcare system. There are others in the field working toward the same goal. Perhaps it is now time for those individuals interested in clinical ethics as a vehicle for quality improvement and influence in healthcare to collaborate and share lessons and strategies. There are considerable opportunities to further research and gather evidence to demonstrate how changing the ethical culture in healthcare can make a significant impact to the current problems we face in healthcare.

REFERENCES

Breslin, J.M., MacRae, S.K., Bell, J., for the University of Toronto Joint Centre for Bioethics Clinical Ethics Group (2005). Top 10 health care ethics challenges facing the public: views of toronto bioethicists. *BMC Med Ethics* **6**: 5.

Singer, P.A., Pelligrino, E.D., and Siegler, M. (2001). Clinical ethics revisited. *BMC Med Ethics* **2**: 1.

40

Clinical ethics and systems thinking

Susan K. MacRae, Ellen Fox, and Anne Slowther

A health region, with multiple hospitals and community healthcare organizations, is faced with increased pressures to improve the ethical care of patients and improve staff experience across the system. Currently the patient satisfaction scores at many of the sites are quite low and recent Health Commission inspections in some hospitals have highlighted management of consent issues and patient-centered care as areas of major concern. The staff's morale is waning and moral distress seems to be increasing. The CEO of the Strategic Health Authority believes that clinical ethics could potentially make a significant difference to the overall culture of the system but feels that the existing mechanisms are not that effective. She begins to consult with experts in the field to discuss how clinical ethics can help her to improve her health system.

"ABC Health Care" has an established clinical ethics program that performs a variety of functions including case consultation, education, policy work, and scholarly writing. Although ABC has received positive accreditation ratings relating to clinical ethics, many within ABC – including both administrators and clinical staff – have a general sense that ABC's current clinical ethics program may not be fully addressing the organization's needs. For example, the program tends to focus on a narrow range of ethical concerns, mostly related to high-profile acute situations in the intensive care and emergency units. In contrast, staff experience a much broader range of ethical issues in their work day to day, and many issues and areas go unserved. Although the clinical ethics program devotes many hours to ethics consultation, similar ethical issues continue to recur again and again. At times, ethics program staff seems more concerned about philosophical questions and principles than about the practical realities

experienced by patients and healthcare staff. Overall, the clinical ethics program's impact on everyday behavior or on organizational culture is unclear, and no measures exist to evaluate the program's effectiveness. The CEO feels strongly that the clinical ethics program should be held accountable for its effects on the system (or lack thereof). He looks to other organizations for models of how clinical ethics programs can be used to make systems change.

What is systems thinking in clinical ethics?

According to Silverman (2000), systems thinking "is concerned with the key interrelationships, structures, and processes that control and monitor behaviour ... With systems thinking, the focus is not on individuals as objects of improvement, but rather, on examining interrelationships, communications, ongoing processes, and underlying causes of behaviour with an eye towards changing interactions or redesigning the system to produce different behaviours."

In the healthcare arena, systems thinking has been increasingly evident since the late 1980s (Berwick, 1989). Don Berwick, President of the Institute for Healthcare Improvement in the USA, has been instrumental in instilling the concept, now well recognized in healthcare, that "every system is perfectly designed to achieve the results it achieves" (Berwick, 1996). Also in the USA, the major organization that accredits healthcare organizations – the Joint Commission on Accreditation of Healthcare Organizations (JCAHO) – adopted a new set of *Principles of Organization and Management Effectiveness* in 1989 that strongly emphasized a systems approach to continuous quality improvement in patient care (JCAHO, 1991).

Unfortunately, clinical ethics has not caught on to this trend toward systems thinking in healthcare. To the contrary, clinical ethics has continued to focus more on the particulars than the general: more on, for example, reacting to acute situations on a case-by-case basis than on identifying and addressing the underlying systems factors that give rise to many of the ethical concerns in healthcare (Silva, 1998).

Why is it important to apply systems thinking to clinical ethics?

In 2001, three long-standing leaders in the field of clinical ethics wrote a paper that highlighted the history of clinical ethics, talked about key developments in the previous decade and outlined remaining challenges for the field in this decade (Singer *et al.*, 2001). The two top significant challenges they highlighted for clinical ethics practice (consultation and committees) was the need to integrate clinical ethics work into the culture of healthcare organizations and to improve organizational accountability for clinical ethics. What these authors were pointing to is a need to understand and impact the functioning of the larger context (the system) in which the ethical issues in healthcare exist.

A systems approach to clinical ethics offers a potential for significant impact across a broad scope of healthcare. Practically speaking, a systems approach focuses on the dynamic "assemblages of interactions within an organisation or between organisations" (Emanuel, 2000). As a result, this perspective can impact the broader healthcare culture and address the "silo" problem in clinical ethics consultation (where the consultation service

is perceived to operate in relative isolation from the rest of the organization) (Blake, 2000). A systems approach can improve ethics accountability by demonstrating a systemic commitment to ethics, by integrating ethics from "boardroom to bedside" (MacRae *et al.*, 2002), and by bridging the artificial gap between organizational and clinical domains (Foglia and Pearlman, 2004).

A systems approach can help clinicians, managers, and ethics facilitators to understand and address the components of the systems that drive ethical care and behavior. These components may relate to local dynamics and practice, or they may be broader in scope to include such things as financial models, information technology systems, philosophy of care issues, rewards and incentives, historical factors, or professional boundary issues. Systems thinking may also help to decrease moral distress and disempowerment among healthcare staff – a factor that has been shown to be a major cause of staff burn-out and turnover. Moral distress has been defined as "what happens when a staff person knows the right thing to do, but institutional constraints make it nearly impossible to pursue the right course of action" (Jameton, 1984) and is something that lends itself to a deeper inquiry using systems thinking. Systems thinking applied to the problem of staff moral distress inquires into the systemic challenges that create painful ethical challenges for healthcare professionals, moving the solution beyond the staffs' personal suffering to the possibility of changing institutional conditions that created this suffering in the first place. A similar approach can be used to move to a more patient-centered healthcare quality approach that addresses key patient and family concerns (Cleary and Edgman-Levitan, 1997).

A systems approach also helps to ensure that clinical ethics practice is collaborative with others in the healthcare organization or system. In the traditional models, clinical ethics programs and clinical ethics committees are poorly integrated across the organization and with other groups in the systems that have similar goals.

Finally, systems-based clinical ethics supports evidence-based practice and accountability to the end-users in healthcare. In this way the end-user provides the marker to the type of system that is in existence around a given situation and, therefore, lends insight into future opportunities for improvement. Such an approach requires serious study of the effects of various clinical ethics interventions on actual practice in order to drive innovation and change. This includes incorporating clinical ethics indicators into other system measurements such as patient satisfaction outcomes and accreditation scoring. The shift is one where a clinical ethics committee or consultant moves from asking questions such as, "Was this one consult or educational session successful?" to questions such as "How has clinical ethics impacted the overall healthcare culture in how it sets financial priorities, frames problems, addresses staff morale, etc?" – or even to such fundamental questions as, "Is this the system of healthcare we ought to have in order to achieve the goals we strive to achieve?"

There are no regulatory requirements for ethicists in Canada, the USA or the UK, and no formalized competency requirements or understanding of "effective" clinical ethics practice. This lack of standards in clinical ethics is strangely accompanied by drive to require clinical ethics services by oversight bodies (Canadian Counsel on Health Services Accreditation, 2004; Royal College of Physicians, 2005; JCAHO, 2007). It is only a matter of time before ethicists are going to need to define what counts as effective practice. One danger in this shift towards effective practice is that ethicists will respond to this challenge by being too inwardly focused and will spend time exclusively on their own professional issues such as their working conditions, core competencies, and codes of conduct for ethicists without, at the same time, looking outwardly for impact on the people that ethics is meant to serve. A field that is too inward looking may soon make itself irrelevant in the broader healthcare context and die under its own weight. It seems that a reasonable approach for those

in ethics may, therefore, be to look beyond the characteristics of individual consultants and consultations to an examination of how clinical ethics interventions are actually affecting patients, healthcare professionals, and organizations and healthcare more broadly (Fox and Tulsky, 1996; Leeman et al., 1997). In this way systems-based clinical ethics programs can offer leadership in the field as a standard bearer to which regulating bodies may turn.

How should I apply systems thinking to clinical ethics in practice?

Changing organizational behavior and/or culture is no small task. As leaders of three large clinical ethics networks in three different countries, we have each been working for a number of years to find innovative ways to meet this challenge. In the USA, EF leads the National Center for Ethics in Health Care of the Veterans Health Administration, which is the largest healthcare system in the USA, with roughly 8 million enrolled patients, 200 thousand employees, and 1300 sites of care delivery. In the UK, AS leads the support program for the national network of clinical ethics committees. This programme includes a website (http://www.ethics-network.org.uk) and educational resources for all clinical ethics committees in the UK, of which there are approximately 85. In Canada, SM is the Deputy Director of the Joint Centre for Bioethics, a partnership with the University of Toronto and 15 diverse healthcare organizations in the greater Toronto area and with the largest group of in-hospital full-time clinical bioethicists in Canada and perhaps in the world.

Despite the fact that the authors work in three different countries, with three different cultures, healthcare-funding structures, and settings, we have all evolved independently towards systems thinking in our clinical ethics practice. Below we have identified our top 10 leading practices that we agree are essential when applying systems thinking to clinical ethics.

The top 10 leading practices in applying systems thinking to clinical ethics

Have a clear organizational mandate

A clear organizational mandate means that clinical ethics programs must have a well-defined organizational role, clear responsibilities and expectations for that role, and the status, authority, and resources needed to carry out that role.

> EXAMPLE. The National Center for Ethics in Health Care (http://www.va.gov/ethics) is one of the major national program offices of the Veterans Health Administration. It is responsible for promoting ethical healthcare practices throughout the Veterans Health Care System and its roles and responsibilities are delineated in formal documents that are updated regularly. The Center's Director is a senior executive who reports to the organization's top leadership. The Center's budget supports 20 full- and part-time staff members.

Be and stay engaged with the "real world"

By engaging with the "real world," we mean that the clinical ethics program must be well attuned to the everyday reality of the healthcare organization and the "real world" it seeks to affect. From our experience, historically two streams of activity have struggled to claim the "ownership" of the field of clinical ethics: the highly academic field of applied ethics on the one hand and the grassroots movement of clinicians, clinical programs, and hospital ethics committees on the other. This has often resulted in a split in the field of clinical ethics between scholars studying bioethics in universities, who often have extensive theoretical training but relatively little experience with day-to-day healthcare conflicts and operations, and clinicians and members of clinical ethics teams in hospitals, who may have little formal ethics training but understand very well the practical realities of the modern healthcare organization and the ethical dilemmas therein. Systems thinking allows one to move beyond this ownership question to a question of impact and seeks to integrate theory and practice for the betterment of healthcare quality.

> EXAMPLE. The University of Toronto Joint Centre for Bioethics (http://www.utoronto.ca/jcb) seeks to bridge this theory-to-practice gap by involving scholars and practitioners alike in a common pursuit of "real world" bioethics solutions in an engaged way. These solutions range from ethics delivery models to evaluation studies of the field, as well as scholarship and models for practical problems faced by healthcare organizations and citizens. This approach involves engaging with the end-users of ethics knowledge in order to constantly redefine the models created in academia while at the same time presenting scholars with opportunities to apply their knowledge to actual dilemmas of the present reality of healthcare and its key stakeholders.

Take advantage of economies of scale

Application of a system-based clinical ethics program can benefit from creation of networks in a way that provides more impact and higher benefit and service to individuals belonging to the network than what they would be able to realize if a similar effort were made at the individual level.

> EXAMPLE. The UK Clinical Ethics Network includes all clinical ethics committees in the UK linked to a small support team at the Ethox Centre (http://www.ethox.org.uk). This model enables widespread dissemination of educational material and information to the individual committees, which, in turn, supports them in their efforts to improve ethical practices within their organization and avoids duplication of effort. The network provides a facility for sharing experience, best practice, and new ideas between committees, increasing the rate at which clinical ethics can develop in the individual organizations. For example, a committee dealing with a difficult case consultation around confidentiality in clinical genetics

can use the network email system to access expertise in other committees, who may be able to share examples of policies they have developed on this issue. The resulting discussion and exchange of information is open to all committees, so good practice is disseminated throughout several institutions.

Be practical and useful

A clinical ethics program should be practical and useful: that is, it should be focused on serving the practical needs of the organization of which it is part and helping to advance the organization's mission and goals. Some clinical ethics centers and programs have a strongly academic or theoretical bent, serving primarily as "think tanks." Some see it as their mission to enhance dialogue [http://wings.buffalo.edu/faculty/research/bioethics/news1], encourage debate [http://www.fom.sk.med.ic.ac.uk/medicine/about/divisions/ephpc/pcsm/research/meu/], or enrich the moral imagination [http://www.ethics.emory.edu/]. In contrast, centers like ours are service oriented and focus on results. Specifically, we aim to improve actual on-the-ground ethical behavior throughout the healthcare organizations we serve.

EXAMPLE. The mission of the National Center for Ethics in Health Care of the Veterans Health Administration is explicitly practical and behavior based. One of the Center's major national initiatives, called IntegratedEthics, is an organization-change initiative designed to help individual healthcare facilities improve "ethics quality" at three levels: decisions and actions, systems and processes, and environment and culture. "Ethics quality" is seen as essential to the core mission of the Veterans Health Administration: delivering high-quality healthcare.

Be proactive, not reactive

Systems thinking allows clinical ethics to be proactive and not just reactive. In the case of current ethics consultants, the practicing lone bioethicist often struggles with isolation and overwork, and lacks appropriate integration, sustainability, and accountability to move beyond a few priorities and reactive efforts (MacRae et al., 2002). Clinical ethics needs to function strategically if it is to do any more than react to crises. Clinical ethics that is geared at systems change is not as focused on the crisis situations as it is on the overall context of these situations, which may allow for more thoughtful, systematic, well-thought-out strategic directions for ethics interventions. As clinical ethics becomes more systems focused, interventions (e.g., consultation or educational sessions) are seen as opportunities to understand the "root cause" of a problem or behavior and to suggest changes or alternative systems models that will reduce rather than create ethical difficulties for clinicians and patients. The goal is wider than resolving the immediate ethical conflict involving an individual patient and his or her clinicians. In some cases, it can be to eliminate the underlying cause of the ethical conflict completely from the system. This "upstream approach," which looks at what causes the problems or what leads to certain behaviors, focuses not on the failures of individuals but instead on the opportunities in the system for improved outcomes. Ethicists may also choose to impact public policy, for example by choosing to collaborate with clinicians or scholars to conduct research to influence a thoughtful response to a larger trend they are noticing in the field. Or they may plan overall goals through a formal ethics strategic-planning process (Gibson et al., 2007) to help to highlight the institution's priorities with respect to ethics.

EXAMPLE. At the University of Toronto Joint Centre for Bioethics, an affiliated hospital was asked to create an ethics framework for allocation of scarce resources in the event of pandemic influenza. This framework was developed locally but was then adopted by the provincial health ministry as the ethical framework for the provincial plan. A white paper Stand On Guard for Thee (http://www.utoronto.ca/jcb/home/documents/pandemic.pdf) was also generated, which was subsequently adapted by healthcare organizations and health systems internationally, including the World Health Organization.

Build relationships

If the goal of clinical ethics is to effect change in the healthcare system then it requires that the ethics program/committee liaise and build relationships with others in the organization or region. These linkages may be with other departments, such as quality, patient relations, or risk management, or with key senior leaders and university scholars. One of the failures of traditional ethics committees has been that it often lacks the necessary relationships within the system to move the understanding of unique ethics problems to other parts of the system and thus effect more global change to systemic problems. A systems-based clinical ethics program builds networks of individuals from a variety of backgrounds. Programs that value the involvement of these different disciplines and that builds transdisciplinary communities enables the necessary critical approach that many ethics problems require. This diversity allows for a rich complexity of views and perspectives in the analyses, which can provide solutions that are well rounded, supportive, and inclusive.

> EXAMPLE. The UK Clinical Ethics Network acts as a link between the clinical ethics community "on the ground" and national organizations such as the General Medical Council and other professional bodies, facilitating ethical dialogue within the regulatory systems that guide professional practice. This provides local input into development of national policies governing professional behavior and improves the implementation of professional guidance at a local level.

> EXAMPLE. At the University of Toronto Joint Centre for Bioethics, the Clinical Ethics Group (made up of the 22 clinical bioethicists and the seven clinical ethics fellows) meets for three hours each week for ethics rounds,

case conference, and continuing education seminars. The group is also linked via an electronic listserv. Through this interdisciplinary group space, a sense of community is strengthened and harnessed to share material and resources, review cases, learn new material, conduct research and joint projects, and support each other emotionally and professionally. This community of support and practice has shown itself to be a key factor in the capacity of the bioethicists to do their work. Many bioethicists now consider community as a key factor in their effectiveness.

Maintain a constant improvement orientation

An improvement orientation focuses on achieving continuous improvement throughout the system: setting up an iterative process between individual committees, local programs and larger institutional bodies to develop and evaluate systems change. Providing a research or evidence base to clinical ethics system's approaches is a critical factor for achieving effectiveness in this field. The evidence may come from the use of case studies and the distillation of key themes and good practices.

> EXAMPLE. The National Center for Ethics in Health Care is spearheading a system-wide initiative to improve the quality of ethics consultation in Veterans Health Administration medical centers nationwide. A central part of that effort is the development, field testing, and deployment of ECWeb: a secure, web-based software program designed to standardize ethics consultation processes and to provide an electronic method of documenting, storing, and retrieving ethics consultation data. In addition, ECWeb can generate reports of service utilization, consultation processes, and participant satisfaction. Other features of ECWeb include secure access to authorized users through the Veterans Administration's own internet system, stratified access to information on a need-to-know basis, ability to

designate certain consultation records as quality-improvement reviews with special legal confidentiality protections, automated (email) reminders of planned consultation activities, automated (email) notification of consultation referrals, ability to attach electronic documents to records (e.g., Word documents, PDF files), ability to search records by key word, and categorization of consultations into standardized content domains and topics for quality improvement and reporting purposes.

Understand key stakeholders

Understanding the individuals or groups that can affect or be affected by an ethics program is also essential. To be effective, an ethics program must be able to reach its stakeholders and earn their trust. This requires insight into stakeholder characteristics, including their preexisting knowledge, how they like to receive information, plus their needs, interests, and values. Effective ethics programs appreciate the importance of understanding their stakeholders and actively seek out information to inform their approach.

> **EXAMPLE**. The recent Project Examining Effectiveness (PEECE) research study conducted at the University of Toronto's Joint Centre for Bioethics (Godkin *et al.*, 2005) asked key stakeholders, including patients/families, healthcare staff and physicians, bioethicists, ethics committee members, and senior healthcare administrators and funders, to define clinical ethics and what they consider to be effective clinical ethics practice. This grassroots case-study approach to examining clinical ethics effectiveness allowed for a more nuanced snapshot description of what the end-users of healthcare think, rather than prescribing a model created by bioethicists. A similar model is currently being applied to case studies in organizational ethics as a method to elucidate current practices and lessons in this area.

Ensure accountability for the ethics program

Accountability requires that ethics committees, consultants, and programs work to an appropriate standard, have clear lines of reporting, and are situated in such a way to impact change at the level required at the institution.

> **EXAMPLE**. Clinical ethics committees in the UK are situated within the clinical governance structure of each institution. This ensures that the work of the committee feeds into clinical management by raising awareness at an executive level of the issues facing clinicians on the ground. It also provides an opportunity for the committee to play an active role in policy and guideline development within the institution. The UK Clinical Ethics Network is currently developing guidance for all committees on core competencies, and on procedures for assessing the acquisition and maintenance of competencies by committees. This includes an ability to identify and engage with ethical issues at a systems level as well as responding to individual conflicts within the system.

Target root cause organizational factors that influence behavior

Many ethics programs make the mistake of focusing exclusively on specific decisions and actions on a case-by-case basis. But to have a real and lasting impact on ethical behavior, ethics programs must target not just individual behaviors but also the underlying root cause organizational factors that influence them. In particular, individual behaviors are powerfully influenced by an organization's systems, processes, environment, and culture (http://www.va.gov/integratedethics/primer.cfm).

If an ethics program focuses only on specific decisions and actions, without addressing broader organizational influences that may facilitate or impede ethical practices, employees are more likely to experience moral distress or a feeling that they know the right thing to do but are unable to do it (http://www.cna-nurses.ca/cna/documents/

pdf/publications/Ethics_Pract_Ethical_Distress_ Oct_2003_e.pdf#search=%22moral%20distress%22). In contrast, when ethics is integrated throughout an organization's systems, processes, environment, and culture, employees recognize ethical concerns and discuss them openly. They feel empowered to behave ethically and know they will be supported when they "do the right thing."

> EXAMPLE. The IntegratedEthics initiative of the National Center for Ethics in Health Care is a multilevel organizational change project that is being rolled out to all Veteran Health Administration facilities nationwide. The initiative seeks to improve "ethics quality" by explicitly targeting not only individual decisions and actions but also the underlying factors that influence behavior. It includes specific mechanisms for dealing with ethics quality gaps on a systems level, as well as specific interventions for fostering a positive ethics environment. The initiative's evaluation tools assess not only specific ethical practices but also ethics-related structures, processes, environment, and culture (http://www.va.gov/ integratedethics/index.cfm).

The cases

Both of the cases at the beginning of this chapter represent scenarios that could benefit from systems thinking. In the first case, the situation is based in a health region that spans many healthcare delivery sites, while the second scenario is based in an organization. In both cases, a systems approach to clinical ethics requires an explicit recognition by clinical ethicists and other ethics facilitators of the different interrelational systems of values within and outside the organization as well as a focus on culture-wide ethical integrity.

More specifically, a systems approach to clinical ethics in these cases requires using the original functions associated with clinical ethics – consultation, education, policy development, and scholarly work – for the purpose of improving the overall culture and system of care delivery, including, but moving beyond, care of the individual patient. It means seeking an impact at all levels of the organization from "boardroom to bedside," making ethics as available and visible at senior executive meetings for example, as it is in clinical rounds. It means working with senior leaders to effect change throughout the organization, sitting at the senior tables and clinical tables and offering useful and effective tools and resources to help them to manage the real problems they face. It requires that the ethicist understands the context of healthcare and its business model and structure in order to identify how change can occur within that particular setting, while still appreciating the considerable variation in cultures that occurs from one healthcare organization to another. It may also mean building liaisons with other departments and with professionals focused on organizational change, such as quality departments, patient relations, and risk management, while maintaining the unique viewpoint that ethics offers to the discussions that usually surface in these arenas. It means acknowledging the many different ethical codes (professional, financial, personal) and clashes that exist in the complex systems of healthcare (Thurber, 1999). It also means integrating ethics into the key "thrust" areas in the network, organization or region (such as patient safety, pandemic influenza planning) as an important contribution from ethics that may affect the overall system of care.

References

Berwick, D. M. (1989). Continuous improvement as an ideal in health care. *N Engl J Med* **320**: 53–6.

Berwick, D. M. (1996). A primer on leading the improvement of systems. *BMJ* **312**: 619–22.

Blake, D. C. (2000). Reinventing the health care ethics committee. *HEC Forum* **12**: 8–32.

Canadian Council for Health Services Accreditation (2004). The Canadian Health Accreditation Report 2004. Ottawa: Canadian Council for Health Services Accreditation. (http://www.cchsa.ca/pdf/2004report. PDF), accessed 5 June 2006.

Cleary, P. D. and Edgman-Levitan, S. (1997). Health care quality, incorporating consumer perspectives. *JAMA* **278**: 1608–12.

Emanuel, L. (2000). Ethics and the structures of healthcare. *Camb Q Healthc Ethics* **9**: 151–68.

Foglia, M. B. and Pearlman, R. A. (2004). Integrating clinical and organizational ethics. A systems perspective can provide an antidote to the "silo" problem in clinical ethics consultation. *Chest* **125**: 2367–8.

Fox, E. and Tulsky, J. (1996). Evaluation research and the future of ethics consultation. *J Clin Ethics* **7**: 146–9.

Gibson, J., Godkin, M. D., Tracy, C. S., and MacRae, S. K. (2007). *Innovative Strategies to Improve Effectiveness in Clinical Ethics. Bioethics for Clinicians.* Cambridge, UK: Cambridge University Press.

Godkin, M. D., Faith, K., Upshur, R. E. G., for the PEECE Group Investigators (2005). Project Examining Effectiveness in Clinical Ethics (PEECE): phase 1 – descriptive analysis of nine clinical ethics services. *J Med Ethics* **31**: 505–12.

Jameton, A. (1984). *Nursing Practice: The Ethical Issues.* Englewood Cliffs, NJ: Prentice-Hall.

JCAHO (Joint Commission on Accreditation of Healthcare Organizations) (1991). Principles of organization effectiveness in healthcare organizations and management. *J Qual Assur* **13**: 26–9.

JCAHO (2007). Overview of 2007 Leadership Standards. Oakbrook Terrace, IL: Joint Commission on Accreditation of Healthcare Organizations (http://www.jointcommission.org/NR/rdonlyres/A55ACEC4-E027-4FE0-8532-C023E8817A30/0/07_bhc_ld_stds.pdf, p. 20).

Leeman, C. P., Fletcher, J. C., Spencer, E. M., and Fry-Revere, S. (1997). Quality control for hospitals' clinical ethics services: proposed standards. *Camb Q Health Ethics* **6**: 257–68.

MacRae, S., Chidwick, P., Berry, S., *et al.* (2002). Clinical bioethics integration, sustainability, and accountability: the hub and spokes strategy. *J Med Ethics* **31**: 256–61.

Royal College of Physicians (2005). *Ethics in Practice: Background and Recommendations for Advanced Support.* London: Royal College of Physicians.

Silva, M. (1998). Organizational and administrative ethics in health care: an ethics gap. *Online J Issues Nurs* **3**: 1–13 (http://www.nursingworld.org/ojin/topic8/topic8_l.htm.) accessed 5 June 2006.

Silverman, H. J. (2000). Organizational ethics in healthcare organizations: proactively managing the ethical climate to ensure organizational integrity. *HEC Forum* **12**: 202–15.

Singer, P. A., Pelligrino, E. D., and Siegler, M. (2001). Clinical ethics revisited. *BMC Med Ethics* **2**: 1.

Thurber, C. F. (1999). Assessing quality in HCOs: a paradigm for organizational ethics. *HEC Forum* **11**: 358–63.

Innovative strategies to improve effectiveness in clinical ethics

Jennifer L. Gibson, M. Dianne Godkin, C. Shawn Tracy, and Susan K. MacRae

A large tertiary healthcare organization has a full-time clinical ethicist who is responsible for ethics consultation, education, policy development, and research. A recent accreditation survey identified a number of gaps in clinical ethics services across the organization. The clinical ethicist is already over-extended and is at risk of burning out. The Vice-President responsible for overseeing the ethics portfolio wonders what can be done to enhance support for the clinical ethicist, strengthen ethics capacity across the organization, and improve the overall effectiveness of clinical ethics services.

What is clinical ethics effectiveness?

The ultimate goal of any clinical ethics delivery model is improved patient care. As more healthcare resources are invested in clinical ethics services, questions are increasingly raised about whether these services are effective in improving the quality of patient care and whether they justify investments of limited healthcare resources. In this chapter, we identify some key challenges to existing clinical ethics delivery models and suggest four innovative strategies to improve effectiveness in clinical ethics services in healthcare organizations.

Since 1995, when James Tulsky and Ellen Fox convened the *Conference on Evaluation of Case Consultation in Clinical Ethics* (AHCPR, 1995), there has been a marked increase in scholarly attention to the study and evaluation of clinical ethics, particularly related to the ethics consultation component of clinical ethics (e.g., McClung *et al.*, 1996; Orr *et al.*, 1996; Schneiderman *et al.*, 2000). This has

been described as a new phase in the clinical ethics movement (Aulisio, 1999). As the field of clinical ethics continues to develop, it will not be sufficient for clinical ethicists "merely to mean well"; they must also be able to demonstrate effectiveness (Aulisio, 1999). While the goals of clinical ethics are generally clear – namely, the identification, analysis, and resolution of ethical concerns arising in the delivery of patient care (Siegler and Singer, 1988) – it remains unclear how clinical ethics effectiveness should be defined and evaluated.

Defining and evaluating clinical ethics effectiveness is complex for several reasons: (i) the different perspectives of multiple stakeholders on effectiveness (e.g., healthcare managers, patients, clinicians, society), (ii) the different levels at which evaluation can take place (i.e., individual ethicist, clinical ethics service, organization), and (iii) the diverse activities within the clinical ethics portfolio that must be evaluated (i.e., consultation, education policy development and research) (Griener and Storch, 1992; Aulisio *et al.*, 2000). To date, most evaluative efforts have focused on identifying core competencies for clinical ethics practice (ASBH, 1998) and benchmarks of clinical ethics effectiveness from the perspective of those who deliver the services (Godkin *et al.*, 2005). The perspectives of other stakeholders, such as patients, family members, and healthcare managers, have not been adequately explored (Cleary and Edgman-Levitan, 1997). For healthcare organizations, the most relevant concern is whether clinical ethics services are effective in improving *local* delivery of patient care.

Consequently, the unique patient populations served by an organization, existing clinical ethics capacity within the organization, and the mission and values of the organization would be key considerations in evaluating the effectiveness of clinical ethics service in improving patient care. So while it is important that there be a continued emphasis on identifying evidence-based practices in clinical ethics and developing general benchmarks of clinical ethics effectiveness to use across clinical ethics programs, some component of evaluating clinical ethics effectiveness will necessarily be context dependent.

Why is clinical ethics effectiveness important?

Ethics is increasingly recognized as an important component of high-quality clinical care (Woolf, 1994; Cleary and Edgman-Levitan, 1997; Wynia, 1999, 2006; CCHSA, 2004; JCAHO, 2007). Indeed some commentators, such as Wynia (2006), have suggested that ethics "just might be the realm of quality that many patients care about most of all." Demonstrating clinical ethics effectiveness is important in healthcare institutions for the purposes of assessing quality and identifying areas for improvement, increasing efficiency and impact, justifying allocation of resources, influencing policy, and disseminating knowledge (Silva, 1998; Wynia, 2006). Additionally, in Canada and the USA, accreditation standards now require healthcare organizations to have formal mechanisms in place to help staff to deal with ethical issues related to client care and business practices (CCHSA, 2004) and to demonstrate "ethical behavior in care, treatment, and services and business practices" (JCAHO, 2007).

The dominant model for clinical ethics service delivery in healthcare institutions has been the lone ethics consultant model – also referred to in the literature as the "lone ranger" (Fox *et al.*, 1998) or "beeper ethicist" model (McGee, 1995) – operating with or without the support of an ethics committee. The role of the clinical ethicist (or ethics committee) generally includes ethics consultation (including

research ethics), policy development, education, and research (Storch and Griener, 1992; McNeill, 2001; Slowther *et al.*, 2001). The lone ethics consultant model faces three challenges: integration, sustainability, and accountability (Silva, 1998; Berchelmann and Blechner, 2002; MacRae *et al.*, 2005). When accountability for clinical ethics is delegated to the clinical ethicist alone, it is difficult to achieve integration of ethics across the organization and to meet demand for clinical ethics support in a sustainable way. Accessibility of clinical ethics services among patients and family members is often particularly limited within this model.

How should I approach clinical ethics effectiveness in practice?

In this section, we describe four innovative strategies to improve the effectiveness of clinical ethics services in healthcare organizations. These practical strategies were developed and piloted by the University of Toronto Joint Centre for Bioethics (JCB) in response to the challenges identified above: integration, sustainability, and accountability. The JCB is a partnership network among the University of Toronto and 15 health organizations (13 academic and/or community hospitals, one community care access center, and one science organization), each of which has at least one full-time clinical ethicist. The strategies include (i) the "hub and spokes" model for clinical ethics service delivery, (ii) leadership and management skills training for clinical ethicists, (iii) ethics strategic planning, and (iv) evaluation of clinical ethics services.

Strategy 1: the "hub and spokes" model for clinical ethics service delivery

The hub and spokes model is an innovative model of clinical ethics delivery. In contrast to the traditional lone ethics consultant model, the hub and spokes model envisages an integrated institution-wide ethics network comprising the clinical ethicist ("hub"), who provides core ethics leadership, and

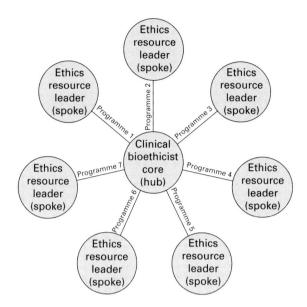

Figure 41.1 The hub and spokes model. (From MacRae *et al.*, 2005.)

ethics resource leaders with training in ethics ("spokes," e.g., clinical staff), who help to build local ethics awareness, knowledge, and skills in clinical settings across the organization (Figure 41.1).

One of the strengths of this model is its adaptability to different organizational contexts, as well as its flexibility in operational design. For example, within the JCB partnership network, the spokes at one acute care hospital are physicians in three core clinical areas (critical care, oncology, family medicine), a portion of whose salary is paid by the organization for the purpose of providing local ethics support. By contrast, one rehabilitation hospital has professional practice staff (e.g., social workers, physiotherapists) as spokes, whose local ethics roles are written into their job descriptions as protected time. Some organizations within the JCB network augment the model with a "clinical ethics forum," made up of the hub and spokes, a senior management representative, and other key stakeholders (e.g., patient/family representatives, board members, quality and risk managers, chaplains). In addition to providing an important community of support for the hub and spokes, the forum is a mechanism for developing strategies to

improve and monitor clinical ethics effectiveness and for reinforcing ethics accountability in the organization (MacRae *et al.*, 2005).

The hub and spokes model contributes to improved clinical ethics effectiveness in three ways. Firstly, it improves ethics *integration*. By positioning spokes locally, ethics support is more readily accessible to staff, patients, and family members and can be more immediately incorporated into patient care decision making. Secondly, it improves *sustainability*. The integrated structure offers a more sustainable clinical ethics service because it does not depend exclusively on the efforts of any single individual, thereby lessening the risk of isolation and burnout characteristic of the lone clinical ethicist model. Finally, it improves *accountability*. Although it has generally been recognized that healthcare institutions are accountable for ethics in clinical care, this model takes an important step toward formalizing this accountability and recognizing clinical ethics "not just as the clinical ethicist's role, but as an integrated part of everyone's role" (MacRae *et al.*, 2005).

The hub and spokes model can also be implemented *across* organizations. For example, the

JCB's Clinical Ethics Group, which is made up of all of the clinical ethicists and clinical ethics fellows who work in JCB partner organizations along with members of the JCB's leadership team, meets on a weekly basis for case review, professional development, and collaboration on creating and testing innovative clinical ethics practices. The group places significant emphasis on peer support and quality assurance, which group members describe as an invaluable component of their local clinical ethics effectiveness (Chidwick *et al.*, 2004).

Strategy 2: leadership and management skills training for clinical ethicists

Leadership can be defined as "the process through which an individual attempts to intentionally influence another individual or a group in order to accomplish a goal" (Pointer and Sanchez, 2005). The hub and spokes model involves a significant shift in the clinical ethicist's role. As the hub, the clinical ethicist's responsibilities include providing core leadership to the integrated ethics network, mentoring and coordinating the spokes, strategic planning, and evaluating and monitoring clinical ethics effectiveness (MacRae *et al.*, 2005). In some institutions, it may also involve budgeting, managing staff, and reporting to senior management or the board of directors. As healthcare organizations face budget constraints, many clinical ethicists face the challenge of justifying the "value-for-money" of their activities. Sustainability may depend in part on the clinical ethicist's ability to influence the decision-making process, whether through a senior management champion or their own persuasiveness. Senior managers in JCB partner organizations are increasingly calling for clinical ethicists to play a greater ethics leadership role, including participation in broader organizational initiatives that have significant ethical implications for patient care (e.g., pandemic influenza planning, resource allocation). Consequently, clinical ethics effectiveness requires a certain amount of institutional intelligence (i.e., practical knowledge about how

the organization works functionally and politically), as well as leadership skills.

Clinical ethics training does not typically involve professional development in leadership or management skills. What leadership training clinical ethicists do receive tends to be informal (i.e., learning from experience) or a combination of formal mentorship by a senior manager, executive coaching, or continuing education seminars in management for clinicians. To our knowledge, there is no leadership program developed with clinical ethicists in mind. To fill this gap, the JCB developed and piloted a six-month leadership program for its affiliated clinical ethicists and clinical ethics fellows in 2005/2006. With the academic support of faculty from a local management school, the program was designed to link the classroom experience with the practical realities of ethical leadership in healthcare organizations. Classroom learning focused on three key themes: effective leadership, change management, and interpersonal skills related to networking and dealing with interpersonal conflict. Over the course of the program, each clinical ethicist conducted a leadership project in their organization under the preceptorship of his/her senior manager and with the peer advice of two or three other clinical ethicists. On the last day of the program, each clinical ethicist had the opportunity to present his or her leadership project and to receive constructive feedback from a panel of senior managers from JCB partner organizations.

Strategy 3: ethics strategic planning

The demand for ethics service is often so great and so varied that ethicists feel they must be all things to all people, which is an unsustainable objective. The JCB has developed an ethics strategic-planning process and has piloted it across eight partner organizations. The objectives of the ethics strategic-planning process are (i) to develop a vision for the clinical ethics portfolio aligned to the organization's strategic directions (mission/vision/values), (ii) to reach agreement on focused priorities related to the vision, and (iii) to develop an action plan that includes clear mechanisms and indicators of effectiveness. The strategic planning process is conducted in three steps.

Step 1 is an institutional scan. The purpose of the institutional scan is to gather information about the organization's ethics needs, the perceived effectiveness of existing clinical ethics services, and possible future directions for clinical ethics in the organization. Focus groups and interviews are conducted with a broad range of internal stakeholders "from boardroom to bedside," including patients and family members whenever possible. Scan findings are collated, validated by a member check with participants, and benchmarked against leading practices in other healthcare organizations. The final institutional scan report is the key input for the ethics strategic planning retreat (in step 2).

Step 2 is an ethics strategic planning retreat. The purpose of the retreat is to draft a strategic plan, including a vision statement, three to five year priorities, and performance indicators for clinical ethics in the organization. Retreat participants include a broad range of internal and relevant external stakeholders. The final ethics strategic plan document provides a guide to yearly action planning for the clinical ethics portfolio (in step 3).

Step 3 is a yearly action plan. The purpose of the action plan is to specify key action steps, timelines, performance indicators, and accountabilities to operationalize the priorities in any given year. The clinical ethicist is accountable for developing the action plan and monitoring its implementation in consultation with the reporting senior manager and in coordination with other ethics resource leaders (e.g., "spokes") in the organization. The action plan provides an accountability framework for evaluating clinical ethics effectiveness on a yearly basis.

A key strength of the ethics strategic planning process is its broad engagement of institutional stakeholders. This strengthens the *integration* of clinical ethics by aligning clinical ethics services with stakeholders' needs, building a sense of shared responsibility for ethics across the organization, and

creating a network of support for the hub and spokes. Moreover, by linking the clinical ethics service to the organization's mission, vision, and values, the ethics strategic plan advances the organization's strategic directions. Finally, it provides an explicit *accountability* framework for monitoring, improving, and evaluating organizational performance in relation to clinical ethics and, ultimately, for justifying a *sustainable* resource base.

Strategy 4: evaluation of clinical ethics services

All clinical ethics services should have explicit performance standards and a formal evaluation strategy to monitor progress, facilitate ongoing quality improvement, ensure alignment with current organizational needs and goals, and hence, enhance *accountability* for the organizational resources invested in the service. Clinical ethics services can be evaluated against a number of benchmarks and quality indicators, including strategic plan priorities, locally developed indicators (e.g., action plan), and/or accreditation standards. This suggests the need for a multimodal evaluation strategy, including both qualitative and quantitative data related to short- and long-term goals of the clinical ethics service as well as to the overall goal of improving patient care.

To address some gaps in knowledge around clinical ethics effectiveness, the JCB initiated the Project Examining Effectiveness in Clinical Ethics (PEECE). The study objectives were three-fold: (i) to examine the services, structures, and activities of nine clinical ethics services in JCB partner hospitals (see Godkin *et al.* [2005] for a detailed review of findings related to this objective); (ii) to identify specific policies, processes, and practices stakeholders defined as effective; and (iii) to investigate stakeholders' views on clinical ethics effectiveness. To address objectives two and three, individual interviews and focus groups were conducted with a broad range of stakeholders including senior managers, clinical ethicists, ethics committee members, clinicians, patients, and family members. Stakeholders defined clinical ethics effectiveness primarily in terms of process indicators

Table 41.1. Key parameters for evaluating clinical ethics effectiveness

Internal parameters	External parameters
• Strategic alignment (i.e., compliance with organization's mission, vision, values, and goals) • Strategic focus (i.e., achievement of priorities in ethics strategic plan) • Clinical performance (e.g., patient/family satisfaction, staff satisfaction) • Professional performance (e.g., all-round evaluation, peer evaluation)	• Accreditation standards (e.g., CCHSA, JCAHO) • Professional competencies (e.g., ASBH core competencies) • Leading practices from the field (e.g., institution-wide focus, peer support) • Resource benchmarks (e.g., one ethicist for every 48 intensive care beds; Godkin *et al.*, 2005)

related to quality issues (e.g., patient-centered care, communication, inclusiveness) rather than more clinically oriented indicators such as number of hospital admissions or length of stay (Tracy *et al.*, 2005). In addition, they saw clinical ethics effectiveness as a bedside-to-boardroom phenomenon, which should be evaluated at both the clinical and the organizational level and should include patients' and family members' views. A number of potential quantitative and qualitative evaluation strategies were suggested by stakeholders including, for example, global assessments of organizational culture, performance measurement tools (e.g., patient/staff satisfaction surveys, staff and board performance evaluations), and formal debriefings with affected stakeholders following clinical ethics interventions (e.g., consultation, education sessions). Based on the PEECE data and our experience with JCB partner organizations, Table 41.1 identifies key parameters, for which specific local indicators could be derived, to evaluate clinical ethics effectiveness in practice.

A key lesson learned in the clinical ethics services of JCB-affiliated institutions is the importance of incorporating a formal evaluation strategy into daily clinical ethics practice. This type of daily management of clinical ethics effectiveness can be likened to a sailor embarking on a sea journey with a clear destination in mind, a map to guide the way, and the necessary skills to steer the ship – but who must adjust course according to the wind and the sea conditions in order to reach the destination successfully. Experience shows that clinical ethics services are more likely to be effective if the clinical ethicist has clear goals linked to the needs, values, and goals of the organization, gathers real-time information and feedback from key stakeholders related to these goals, and uses this information to make mid-course corrections in clinical ethics services.

The case

The Vice-President and the clinical ethicist should consider taking the following steps. Firstly, they should explore developing a broader network of ethics support throughout the organization (e.g., the hub and spokes model). Secondly, depending on the previous experience of the clinical ethicist, it may be advisable to augment the clinical ethicist's expertise with leadership and management skill training. Thirdly, an ethics strategic-planning process should be conducted to create an institution-wide vision for clinical ethics and ensure that the clinical ethics service's priorities are aligned with the organization's mission/vision/values and ethics needs, and to build on the organization's existing ethics capacity. Finally, an evaluation strategy should be developed to monitor, improve, and evaluate the performance of the clinical ethics service in relation to its action plan and other indicators of clinical ethics effectiveness. Following these steps will help to ensure that the organization's clinical ethics service is integrated, sustainable, accountable, and ultimately more effective.

REFERENCES

AHCPR (1995). *Conference on Evaluation of Case Consultation in Clinical Ethics*. Chicago, IL: University of Illinois press for the Agency for Health Care Policy and Research.

ASBH (1998). Core competencies for health care ethics consultation. Washington, DC: American Society for Bioethics and Humanities (http://www.asbh.org/publications/core.html).

Aulisio, M. P. (1999). Ethics consultation: is it enough to mean well? *HEC Forum* **11**: 208–17.

Aulisio, M. P., Arnold, R. M., and Youngner, S. J. (2000). Health care ethics consultation: nature, goals, and competencies. *Ann Int Med* **133**: 59–9.

Berchelmann, K. and Blechner, B. (2002). Searching for effectiveness: the functioning of Connecticut clinical bioethics committees. *J Clin Bioethics* **13**: 131–45.

CCHSA (2004). *The Canadian Health Accreditation Report 2004*. Ottawa: Canadian Council for Health Services Accreditation (http://www.cchsa.ca/pdf/2004report.PDF) accessed 5 June 2006.

Chidwick, P., Faith, K., Godkin, D., and Hardingham, L. (2004). Clinical education of ethicists: the role of a clinical ethics fellowship. *BMC Med Ethics* **8**: 5.

Cleary, P. D. and Edgman-Levitan, S. (1997). Health care quality: incorporating consumer perspectives. *JAMA* **278**: 1608–12.

Fox, M. D., McGee, G., and Caplan, A. (1998). Paradigms for clinical ethics consultation practice. *Camb Q Healthc Ethics* **7**: 308–14.

Godkin, M. D., Faith, K., Upshur, R. E. G., MacRae, S. K., and Tracy, C. S. (2005). Project Examining Effectiveness in Clinical Ethics (PEECE): phase 1 – descriptive analysis of nine clinical ethics services. *J Med Ethics* **31**: 505–12.

Griener, G. G. and Storch, J. L. (1992). Hospital ethics committees: problems in evaluation. *HEC Forum* **4**: 5–18.

JCAHO (2007). *Overview of 2007 Leadership Standards*. Oakbrook Terrace, IL: Joint Commission on Accreditation of Healthcare Organizations, p. 20 (http://www.jointcommission.org/NR/rdonlyres/A55ACEC4-E027-4FE0-8532-C023E8817A30/0/07_bhc_ld_stds.pdf).

MacRae, S., Chidwick, P., Berry, S., *et al.* (2005). Clinical bioethics integration, sustainability, and accountability: the hub and spokes strategy. *J Med Ethics* **31**: 256–61.

McClung, J. A., Kaner, R. S., DeLuca, M., and Barger, H. J. (1996). Evaluation of a medical ethics consultation service: opinions of patients and health care providers. *Am J Med* **100**: 456–60.

McGee, G. (1995). Therapeutic ethics. *Uni Pennsylvania Cent Bioethics Newslet* **1**: 3–4.

McNeill, P. M. (2001). A critical analysis of Australian clinical ethics committees and the functions they serve. *Bioethics* **15**: 443–60.

Orr, R. D., Morton, K. R., deLeon, D. M., and Fals, J. C. (1996). Evaluation of an ethics consultation service: patient and family perspectives. *Am J Med* **101**: 135–41.

Pointer, D. and Sanchez, J. (2005). Leadership: a framework for thinking and acting. In *Healthcare Management: Organizational Behaviour and Design*, 5th edn, ed. S. Shortell and A. Kaluzny. Albany: Delmar, pp. 106–29.

Schneiderman, L. J., Gilmer, T., and Teetzel, H. D. (2000). Impact of ethics consultations in the intensive care setting: a randomized, controlled trial. *Crit Care Med* **28**: 3920–4.

Siegler, M. and Singer, P. A. (1988). Clinical ethics consultation: godsend or "god squad"? *Am J Med* **85**: 759–60.

Silva, M. (1998). Organisational and administrative ethics in health care: an ethics gap. *Online J Issues Nurs* **3**: 1–13 (http://www.nursingworld.org/ojin/topic8/topic8_1.htm) accessed 5 June 2006.

Slowther, A., Bunch, C., Woolnough, B., and Hope, T. (2001). Clinical ethics support services in the UK: an investigation of the current provision of ethic support to health professionals in the UK. *J Med Ethics* **27**: 2–8.

Storch, J. L. and Griener, G. G. (1992). Ethics committees in Canadian hospitals: report of the 1990 pilot study. *Healthc Manag Forum* **5**: 19–26.

Tracy C. S., MacRae S. K., Upshur, R. E.G., for the Clinical Ethics Group (2005). Project Examining Effectiveness in Clinical Ethics (PEECE): findings of a case study comparison of nine clinical ethics services. In *Proceedings of the 2nd International Clinical Ethics Conference*, Basel, Switzerland.

Woolf, S. M. (1994). Quality assessment of ethics in health care: the accountability revolution. *Am J Law Med* **20**: 105–28.

Wynia, M. (1999). Performance measures for ethics quality. *Effect Clin Pract* **2**: 294–9 (http://www.acponline.org/journals/acp/novdev99/wynia.htm) accessed 3 June 2006.

Wynia, M. (2006). Who is measuring the ethical quality of care in American medicine? No one, yet. *Med Gen Med* **8**: 49 (http://www.medscape.com/viewarticle/531920) accessed 31 May 2006.

42

Teaching bioethics to medical students and postgraduate trainees in the clinical setting

Martin F. McKneally and Peter A. Singer

As he reviews the curriculum for his surgical residency training program, Dr. A is concerned about how to prepare his residents to gain understanding of biomedical ethics as it relates to the specialty and to use their understanding to improve patient care (Royal College of Physicians and Surgeons of Canada, 2001). Last year, he invited a moral philosopher to give a guest lecture, which focused on theoretical issues with no reference to how these concepts relate to clinical experience. The residents' evaluations were unfavorable: "a waste of our time," "not relevant to the problems we face." Recently, the residents and nurses were troubled by a difficult situation on the ward: Mr. B, a 46-year-old patient, was found to have unresectable pancreatic cancer, but his wife insisted that the staff withhold the diagnosis from him because he is prone to depression. Dr. A wonders whether this situation could serve as a learning opportunity for the residents and staff and whether he should try to lead a seminar about this problem. He pages the chief resident.

What is bioethics teaching and why is it important?

Bioethics is now taught in most medical schools as part of the standard curriculum. Many accrediting bodies require residency training programs to teach bioethics as a condition of approval, and there is increasing interest in bioethics in continuing medical education. We need teachers who can help clinicians to learn bioethics, an inherent aspect of

good clinical medicine (Jonsen *et al.*, 1998). The purpose of this chapter is to encourage clinician–teachers to accept this important responsibility and to provide them with practical advice. Teaching bioethics to clinicians such as nurses, physiotherapists, physicians, residents, and medical students is facilitated by using a clinical approach.

How should I approach bioethics teaching in practice?

Working with physicians in training with their clinician–teachers, we have developed a practical approach that we outline by answering five questions: Why should I teach? What should I teach? How should I teach? How should I evaluate? How should I learn?

Why should I teach?

The primary goal of teaching bioethics to clinicians is to enhance their ability to care for patients and families at the bedside and in other clinical settings. Dealing effectively with a bioethical problem depends on recognizing the ethical issue, applying relevant knowledge, analyzing the problem, deciding on a course of action, and implementing the necessary steps to improve the situation (Jonsen *et al.*, 1998). Clinicians confront

An earlier version of this chapter has appeared: McKneally, M. F. and Singer, P. A. (2001). Teaching bioethics in the clinical setting. *CMAJ* **164**: 1163–7.

ethical problems in a charged public setting, where their values and beliefs, and those of their patients, may not be congruent (Engelhardt, 1996). Enhancing clinicians' knowledge and skills in resolving ethical quandaries can increase their ability to deal with issues that cause moral distress and thus enable better team and institutional performance in caring for patients.

We favor enlisting interested and respected clinicians as primary teachers of bioethics and encouraging them to pursue additional training in ethics or bioethics. Their expressed values and approach to ethical problems will penetrate widely as part of the informal but powerful cultural network that has been described as the hidden (Hafferty and Franks, 1994) or informal (Hundert *et al.*, 1996) curriculum. Bioethicists, moral philosophers, chaplains, and other non-clinicians are valuable collaborators in presenting the clinical ethics curriculum and can enrich and illuminate the educational experience; however, in our view, they should not displace the clinician–teacher (Siegler, 1981; Shalit, 1997). Unlike other students of ethics, clinician learners are grounded in experiential work with patients; in our experience, they respond better to clinician role models as teachers than to those whose understanding of ethical issues is based on more abstract knowledge. Clinician–teachers' credibility in the biomedical aspects of care and their unchallenged passport into the clinical domain make them ideal communicators of the ethics curriculum.

What should I teach?

Clinicians in most specialties regularly deal with a common set of ethical issues, such as truth telling, consent, capacity, substitute decision making, confidentiality, conflict of interest, end of life issues, resource allocation, and research ethics. These topics are well suited to an introductory bioethics teaching program. Curricular modules, including teaching cases, discussion questions, suggested answers, summaries, and references, such as those prepared for the Royal College of Physicians and

Surgeons of Canada Bioethics Education Project (Royal College of Physicians and Surgeons of Canada, 2004), are useful for introductory teaching of bioethics in the first and second years of residency training. Cases that focus on the management of problems that are specific to a particular clinical area are effective in specialty conferences. For example, physiatrists will be attracted to an analysis of the issue of justice in the treatment of disabled people. Urologists may find more salience in the case in which a family demands postmortem sperm aspiration and in vitro fertilization of a surviving partner as a condition for organ donation (Murphy, 1995). Discussion of these topics offers an opportunity to deepen the discourse with clinicians about the humanistic and holistic aspects of medicine that are an important part of a well-rounded medical education.

What *not* to teach? Resist the temptation to teach theory unrelated to cases, particularly at the start. Clinicians want to learn the right thing to do and how to do it; they will learn the theoretical background that guides the ethical decision-making process when they see its applicability to making good decisions.

How should I teach?

Because it is most closely linked to patient care, bioethics should ideally be taught at the bedside or in the clinic. We are unaware of models for bedside teaching of bioethics or systematic evaluation of its effectiveness, and the uneven and hectic pattern of clinical medicine limits the predictability of bedside and clinic teaching. Nevertheless, we encourage clinician–teachers to innovate and expand on this potent pedagogical experience.

Case-based conferences provide an alternative method that is also closely linked to clinical care. Clinicians learn well when they are actively involved in case discussions (Davis *et al.*, 1999). We recommend taking advantage of this in teaching both the practical and theoretical aspects of bioethics. A problem case captures the interest of the clinical audience. The discussion that follows the case presentation provides a broader exposition of pertinent theory and empirical evidence. It closes with a return to the case. Resolution is achieved by using the definitions, principles, and reasoning introduced during the discussion to clarify the best options for management. When presenting clinical cases, whether on paper or in video format, clinician–teachers can use interactive techniques by asking participants to describe how they would manage the case, explain the reasoning that led them to their position, and outline their approach to mediating the conflicts inherent in the case. Standardized patients or role playing intensifies the experience for medical students and junior residents; more experienced clinician learners are less engaged by this approach. Cases that have caused some measure of moral anguish to the clinicians are especially effective. The strong feelings revived at morbidity and mortality conferences make this a powerful, formative learning experience that is vividly remembered by residents and other clinicians exposed to this tradition (Bosk, 1979). Interactive discussion with peers is a potent catalyst to learning to articulate and analyze ethical issues.

Many clinical medical ethicists recommend the presentation of clinical cases using four main headings: medical factors, patient preferences, quality of life issues and contextual features (Table 42.1; Jonsen *et al.*, 1998). This analytic framework is helpful for identifying issues that require ethical analysis and resolution. Like the ''review of systems'' in an Oslerian clinical history, it provides structure and reminds students of important but less bioscientific aspects of the case that should be considered in the ethical analysis. One of us (MM) uses a modified form of this analytic tool for case-based teaching.

If Dr. A chooses to use this approach in a facilitated discussion of the case of Mr. B outlined at the beginning of this chapter, he might first ask the residents to provide information on the following.

1. **Medical factors**. How do we make the diagnosis of pancreatic cancer preoperatively? What intraoperative findings preclude resection? What are

Table 42.1. An approach used for case-based teaching of clinical and ethical decision making

Areas of consideration	Characteristics
Medical factors	Diagnosis, treatment, prognosis
Quality of life	Before, during, after
Preferences	Patient, family, team
Context	Support system, cost, availability, special circumstances

Based on information in Jonsen *et al.* (1998).

the treatment alternatives? What is the survival rate and prognosis?

2. **Preferences**. Do patients really want detailed scientific explanations of the extent of their disease? Do family members feel that they can protect the patient from despair or disappointment by dissembling? Why do science-based medical team members insist on disclosure?

3. **Quality of life**. Discussion might focus on the quality of residual life, the psychological harm from deception, loss of confidence in physicians who misled, and deprivation of the patient's opportunity to settle emotional as well as financial accounts, or to realize deferred personal goals.

4. **Contextual features**. What are the unique psychological or social factors particular to the patient that might justify an exception to the general recommendation that truth telling is the best policy? Cultural beliefs about the harm from disclosure of a diagnosis of terminal illness might be elicited from the residents.

In contrast to the ''review of systems'' approach in the model by Jonsen *et al.* (1998), experienced clinician–teachers often use problem-specific frameworks to organize their thinking. Experienced clinicians have a specific approach to common clinical problems; for example, rather than a single framework (i.e., a type of Starling curve) to diagnose and treat all cardiology problems, they use individual frameworks for common paradigm cases such as heart failure, coronary artery disease, and arrhythmias. Similarly, experienced bioethics teachers can use paradigmatic frameworks for analyzing truth telling, consent, end of life issues, priority setting, and other common ethical problems. In the scenario faced by Dr. A, the paradigm would be truth telling (Hébert *et al.*, 1997). There are specific arguments to use in conversations with patients and families about telling the truth, such as: Mr. B needs time to prepare for death; he may know anyway; when he finds out, he will lose faith in his care team; and he has the right to know. If these arguments fail to convince Mr. B's wife, an intermediate strategy between withholding the truth and burdening the patient with the truth is to "offer truth" (Freedman, 1993): that is, explicitly ask him if he would like his wife to handle all the medical information or to learn of the medical findings himself directly from his physician.

Small group conferences allow clinicians to develop their skills through active participation in discussion. The large group lecture is a less effective venue, although gifted teachers can be effective, even in this format, if they can evoke the emotional responses associated with important prior clinical experiences of the audience. Debates can introduce humor, tension, and active learning; they may increase the intensity of vicarious participation in the larger group format if they focus on "what should we do?" The learning experience is most intense for the debaters, but requiring members of the audience to take a stand, vote, and defend their position increases their participation and active learning. Well-informed individuals in the audience who have completed assigned reading can help to enliven the debate and stimulate other members of the larger group to become better informed. Residents respond well to this form of peer learning pressure.

How should I evaluate?

In-training evaluation reports (ITERs), a well-established method of evaluation in residency training programs, record the discussion of performance between teachers and their clinician trainees. Such reports are a valuable source of feedback to residents about their clinical performance, and a reminder to program directors of the domains of performance that should be evaluated. Adding a bioethics domain to the ITER emphasizes to both the teacher and the learner that it is important. Turnbull and colleagues (1998) have provided helpful advice on how to use the ITER process effectively; their recommendations may be applied to bioethics. To our knowledge, the ITER has not been evaluated in relation to bioethics. Innovative methods to get feedback from patients and other members of the healthcare team may be particularly applicable to bioethics.

Chart audits can measure clinical performance. Many aspects of performance with respect to ethical issues may not be recorded in the chart because of the customary telegraphic recording of bioscientific aspects of patient care in hospital records. Despite this limitation, Sulmasy and colleagues (1994) used chart audits as a method of evaluating the impact of bioethics teaching on residents' performance. Their study demonstrated that bioethics education improved clinician learners' performance in writing and clarifying do-not-resuscitate orders.

Objective structured clinical examinations (OSCEs), using standardized patients, are also used to evaluate clinical performance. We have conducted studies using OSCEs with standardized patients for evaluating bioethics performance (Singer *et al.*, 1993, 1994). This method is feasible and has adequate inter-rater reliability, content validity, and construct validity. However, as with OSCEs for other specific topics, it shares the problem of low internal consistency; a reliable estimate of bioethics performance would require more OSCE stations than is feasible in most settings.

Multiple-choice written examinations, although limited in value, are accepted as reliable methods of evaluating clinical knowledge and judgement. However, they may be better suited to evaluating bioscientific aspects of medicine than the value-based judgements and reasoning processes that characterize ethical discourse. Other evaluative formats such as short-answer or essay questions are commonly used in undergraduate and graduate bioethics teaching. A reasonable strategy would be to combine the reliability of these methods with the validity of some of the methods described above.

In addition to measuring learners' performance, process measures evaluating a bioethics teaching program also describe the number of teaching sessions, the topics, the teaching materials distributed, the number of participating clinicians, the clinicians' critique of the content and method, and the learners' evaluations of the session. This record will be helpful when accreditors ask, "How are you teaching bioethics?"

How should I learn?

Teaching bioethics to clinicians is a specialized skill, but one that is not difficult to learn for clinicians who are already effective teachers. The content material for learning bioethics is available to teachers and students on the World Wide Web and in journals, books, conferences, and educational programs adapted to their needs. Graduate programs specifically geared at clinicians are now available, as are summer intensive programs. A partial list of resources that may be helpful to clinicians who are interested in bioethics is included in the Appendix at the end of the chapter.

The case

Dr. A discusses his intentions for an education session with the chief resident. He decides against a lecture and helps the chief resident organize a case-based clinical conference about the issue of truth telling, using a debate or discussion format. All of the residents are asked to read about cultural variations in the practice of truth telling about the diagnosis and extent of cancer spread (Thomsen et al., 1993) before attending the conference. Two opinion leaders among them are asked to read additional information about legal and ethical views on truth telling (Hébert et al., 1997). Enlisting opinion leaders is an effective strategy for implementing change (Stross, 1996). One of the two residents is advised to consult with the psychiatry service, the other with the moral philosopher, inviting both to participate in the discussion of whether withholding the diagnosis is appropriate to forestall depression. Dr. A decides to use the truth-telling module of the Royal College of Physicians and Surgeons of Canada curriculum for his basic teaching plan and references. He prepares copies of the "Bioethics Bottom Line" component of the truth-telling module to distribute at the end of the session as a record of the main points of the discussion. To strengthen his effectiveness in teaching bioethics, Dr. A plans to explore available intensive courses, conferences and workshops. Participants in these programs have described the experience as intellectually engaging and personally rewarding.

REFERENCES

Bosk, C. L. (1979). *Forgive and Remember*. Chicago: University of Chicago Press.

Davis, D., O'Brien, M. A., Freemantle, N., et al. (1999). Impact of formal continuing medical education: do conferences, workshops, rounds, and other traditional continuing education activities change physician behavior or health care outcomes? *JAMA* **282**: 867–74.

Engelhardt, H. T., Jr. (1996). *The Foundations of Bioethics*, 2nd edn, New York: Oxford University Press, pp. 74–84.

Freedman, B. (1993). Offering truth: one ethical approach to the uninformed cancer patient. *Arch Int Med* **153**: 572–6.

Hafferty, F. W. and Franks, R. (1994). The hidden curriculum, ethics teaching, and the structure of medical education. *Acad Med* **69**: 861–71.

Hébert, P. C., Hoffmaster, B., Glass, K. C., and Singer, P. A. (1997). Bioethics for clinicians: 7. Truth telling. *CMAJ* **156**: 225–8.

Hundert, E. M., Douglas-Steele, D., and Bickel, J. (1996). Context in medical education: the informal ethics curriculum. *Med Educ* **30**: 353–64.

Jonsen, A. R., Siegler, M., and Winslade, W. J. (1998).
Introduction. In *Clinical Ethics*, 4th edn, ed. A. R. Jonsen,
M. Siegler, and W. J. Winslade. New York: McGraw-Hill,
pp. 1–12.

Murphy, T. F. (1995). Sperm harvesting and post-mortem
fatherhood. *Bioethics* **9**: 380–98.

Royal College of Physicians and Surgeons of Canada
(2001). *General Standards of Accreditation*. Ottawa:
Royal College of Physicians and Surgeons of Canada
(http://rcpsc.medical.org/residency/accreditation/gen
standards_e.html) accessed 14 June 2006.

Royal College of Physicians and Surgeons of Canada (2004).
Bioethics Education Project. Ottawa: Royal College of
Physicians and Surgeons of Canada (http://rcpsc.
medical.org/ethics/index.php) accessed 14 June 2006.

Shalit, R. (1997). When we were philosopher kings. *The
New Republic* **28**: 24.

Siegler, M. (1981). Cautionary advice for humanists.
Hastings Cent Rep **11**: 19–20.

Singer, P. A., Cohen, R., Robb, A., and Rothman, A. (1993).
The ethics objective structured clinical examination.
J Gen Intern Med **8**: 23–8.

Singer, P. A., Robb, A., Cohen, R., Norman, G., and
Turnbull, J. (1994). Evaluation of a multicenter ethics
objective structured clinical examination. *J Gen Intern
Med* **9**: 690–2.

Stross, J. K. (1996). The educationally influential physician. *J Cont Educ Health Prof* **16**: 167–72.

Sulmasy, D. P., Terry, P. B., Faden, R. R., and Levine, D. M.
(1994). Long-term effects of ethics education on the
quality of care for patients who have do-not-resuscitate
orders. *J Gen Intern Med* **9**: 622–6.

Thomsen, O. O., Wulff, H. R., Martin, A., and Singer, P. A.
(1993). What do gastroenterologists in Europe tell
cancer patients? *Lancet* **341**: 473–6.

Turnbull, J., Gray, J., and MacFadyen, J. (1998). Improving
in-training evaluation programs. *J Gen Intern Med* **13**:
317–23.

Appendix: bioethics teaching resources

The Royal College of Physicians and Surgeons
Bioethics Education Project (http://rcpsc.
medical.org/ethics/index.php) provides curricular modules for teaching bioethics to
residents in medicine, surgery, obstetrics and
gynecology, psychiatry, and pediatrics.

The College of Family Physicians of Canada has
prepared a bioethics curriculum that is available on its website (www.cfpc.ca/English/cfpc/
communications/health%20policy/Bioethics%
20Curriculum/default.asp?s-1).

The Canadian Bioethics Society website (www.
bioethics.ca/) provides links to university bioethics centers and bioethics organizations
throughout Canada.

Useful websites for US organizations include the
US National Institutes of Health Bioethics
Resources on the Web (www.nih.gov/sigs/
bioethics); the Georgetown University Kennedy
Institute of Ethics (www.georgetown.edu/
research/kie/) and the Georgetown University
National Reference Center for Bioethics Literature (www.georgetown.edu/research/nrcbl),
which holds the center's database of bioethics
organizations and provides assistance for
using BIOETHICSLINE, an online medical
ethics database available through Internet
Grateful Med (http://www.frame-uk.demon.co.
uk/guide/grateful_med.htm). The American
Society for Bioethics and Humanities offers
multiple resource links on its website (www.
asbh.org); The Center for Law and the Public's
Health at Georgetown and Johns Hopkins
website (http://www.who.int/ethics/en/) links
to national and international ethics resources.

The International Research Ethics Network for
Southern Africa (http://www.irensa.org/cgi/
about.cgi) provides educational resources,
regional contacts and news on current
research.

UNESCO Bangkok website (http://www.
unescobkk.org/index.php?id=41) provides a
downloadable textbook and accompanying
teacher's guide. The site also links to multiple
regional bioethics resources and organizations.

The Bioethics and Society Research Registry,
Oxford University website (http://www.
bioethicsandsociety.org/) provides links to
bioethics courses offered in the UK.

The Council of Europe Bioethics Division
website (http://www.coe.int/T/E/Legal_affairs/

Legal_co-operation/Bioethics/) provides news and links to bioethics events in Europe.

The International Association of Bioethics website (http://www.bioethics-international. org/iab-2.0/index.php?show=index) is a good venue for communicating with colleagues from around the world.

More extensive educational programs that are accessible to clinicians while they continue their professional work include the Alberta Provincial Health Ethics Network Distance Education Course: Introduction to Bioethics (www.phen. ab.ca/disted/); the MHSc Bioethics Program at the University of Toronto Joint Centre for Bioethics (www.utoronto.ca/jcb/Education/ mhsc.htm); the Medical College of Wisconsin Center for the Study of Bioethics distance learning programs (http://www.mcw.edu/ bioethics/depage.html); and the Alden March Bioethics Institute at Albany Medical College (http://www.bioethics.org/), which provides formal graduate training to clinician–teachers.

Global health ethics

Introduction

Solomon R. Benatar

In an increasingly interdependent world we are all threatened by widening disparities in wealth and health, and by failure to achieve the goal of more widespread respect for basic human rights. In such a world, further complicated by significantly different cultural perspectives on the good life, it is necessary to consider how relationships between individuals, institutions, and nations should be structured in order to reduce injustice and improve prospects of human well-being, peace, and security.

In Ch. 43, Solly Benatar outlines global disparities, defines global bioethics, argues that global bioethics is important, and examines how cross-cultural differences could be considered and reconciled in theory and in medical practice without resorting to moral relativism.

In Ch. 44, Jerome Singh examines the legal and ethical responsibilities of health professionals in relation to care of those who are victims of torture and degrading treatment. After defining dual loyalty and describing how dual loyalty dilemmas arise, he refracts the rights of detainees through the "lens" of the principles of biomedical ethics, and shows how international human rights law, several United Nations Resolutions and international medical ethics guidelines provide a framework for protecting such vulnerable persons. His chapter, inclusive of a description of how it is possible for those in authority to become complicit in abusing detainees, is of special topical interest given the recent treatment of detainees in Guantanamo Bay and Abu Ghraib prisons.

The HIV/AIDS era has focused world attention on lack of access to essential life-extending drugs for millions of people. Moving from concerns about individuals to concerns for whole groups of people, Jillian Clare Cohen and Patricia Illingworth address in Ch. 45 the question of how access to medicines for all could be improved. They attribute the imbalance in access at a global level to government and market failures and then describe how changes to Trade-Related Aspects of Intellectual Property (TRIPS) coupled to enhanced corporate social responsibility could facilitate improved access to necessary drugs globally.

Moving to what ought to be done to narrow injustice at a global level, Gopal Sreenivasan concludes the section by arguing in Ch. 46 that, in the absence of a theory of international distributive justice to which all could agree, it would be possible to reduce disparities in wealth and health significantly through the application of ideas emanating from a theory of non-ideal justice.

A clinician might ask, "Why should clinicians care about global health ethics? I am already faced with a multitude of local ethical dilemmas and issues, why should I think global bioethics affects my clinical practice?" Firstly, because this book is aimed at clinicians in both industrialized and developing nations, it illustrates that, to varying degrees, there are problems in many healthcare settings with access to and distribution of medical services and in respecting human rights. Secondly, clinicians practicing in the industrialized world should have some sense of solidarity with their colleagues in the developing world, especially regarding some of the more pressing issues they face. Thirdly, it highlights to clinicians the importance of recognizing the existence of reasonable ethical pluralism in bioethics and how different cultural and political conditions affect our conception of bioethics in industrialized nations.

The chapters in this section do not attempt to deal comprehensively with all aspects of global bioethics and global health ethics. However, we hope that they provide readers both with a sensitizing introduction to a broad set of ethical considerations on issues that impact profoundly on the health of whole populations and with references through which to pursue further study.

43

Global health ethics and cross-cultural considerations in bioethics

Solomon R. Benatar

The AIDS Clinical Trials Group Study 076 (ACTG 076) made an important contribution to prevention of HIV infection when it established that mother-to-child transmission of HIV (MTCT) in the USA and France could be significantly reduced by giving antiretroviral drugs to pregnant women orally for 8 weeks or more prior to childbirth (median 14 weeks) and intravenously during labor, as well as to the newborn child for 6 weeks in the absence of breast feeding (Connor et al., 1994). A major controversy developed when in subsequent studies of MTCT in developing countries shorter courses of treatment were compared with placebo. Although there is no reason to believe that the ACTG 076 regimen would not work in developing countries if it could be applied, placebo studies were undertaken instead. The rationale was that use of the ACTG 076 regimen was precluded in developing countries, not only by its extremely high cost but, more relevantly, because women do not present early enough in pregnancy to receive this prolonged and intensive regimen. In addition they are anemic and malnourished, unable to stop breast feeding, and have difficulty providing treatment to a child for a six-week period (Varmus and Satcher, 1997). Consequently, cheaper and more easily applied preventive methods needed to be studied to enable rapid application of this preventive method to save many lives in developing countries.

What is global health ethics?

Global health ethics is a suggested means through which to promote widely values that include meaningful respect for human life, human rights, equity, freedom, democracy, environmental sustainability, and solidarity (Benatar *et al.*, 2003). It is contended that failure to pursue adequately such values that play an essential role in improving population health is the underlying basis for new threats to health, life, and security within nations and across the world. Global health ethics could promote this set of values – which combines genuine respect for the dignity of all people and a conception of human development that goes beyond that conceived within the narrow, individualistic "economic" model of human flourishing (Doyal and Gough, 1991; Bensimon and Benatar, 2006). Foremost among the values to promote is solidarity, without which we ignore distant indignities, violations of human rights, inequities, deprivation of freedom, undemocratic regimes, and damage to the environment.

A framework that combines an understanding of global interdependence with enlightened long-term self-interest has the potential to promote a broad spectrum of beneficial outcomes, especially in the area of global health. Health and ethics provide a framework within which such an agenda could be developed and promoted across borders and cultures. An extended public debate through a multidisciplinary approach to global health ethics could promote the new mindset needed to improve health and to deal with threats to health at a global level.

This chapter utilizes material from the following previously published articles with permission from the publishers: Benatar, S. R., Daar, A. S., and Singer, P. A. (2003). Global health ethics: the rationale for mutual care. *Int Affairs* **79**: 107–38; Benatar, S. R. (2004). Towards progress in resolving dilemmas in international research ethics. *J Law Med Ethics* **32**: 574–82; Benatar, S. R. (2004). Rationally defensible standards for research in developing countries. *Health Human Rights* **8**: 197–202.

That mindset requires recognition that health, human rights, economic opportunities, good governance, peace, and development are all intimately linked within a complex, interdependent world. The challenge of the twenty-first century is to explore these links, to understand their implications, and to develop processes that could harness economic growth to human development, narrow global disparities in health, and promote peaceful coexistence. This process requires that interest in health and ethics be extended beyond the micro level of interpersonal relationships and individual health to include ethical considerations in relation to public and population health at the levels of institutions, nations, and international relations (Benatar *et al.*, 2003).

A global agenda must, therefore, extend beyond interpersonal ethics and mere rhetoric on universal human rights to include greater attention to individual and institutional duties, social justice, and interdependence. The relatively new interdisciplinary field of bioethics, when expanded in scope to embrace widely shared foundational values, could make a valuable contribution to the improvement of global health. A vision, discussed in detail elsewhere, offers a way forward for global health reform through five transformational approaches (Benatar *et al.*, 2003):

- developing a global state of mind
- promoting long-term self-interest and not merely short-term interests
- striking a balance between optimism and pessimism about globalization
- developing capacity in disadvantaged groups
- achieving widespread access to public goods such as education, basic subsistence needs, and work; this requires collective action, including financing (to make sure they are produced), and good governance (to ensure their optimum distribution and use).

Why is global health ethics important?

Global health: disparities and implications

Since the birth of modern bioethics in the 1960s, the world has changed profoundly. Major expansion of the world economy has been associated with spectacular progress in science, technology, knowledge, healthcare, and in speed of travel and communication, which have been beneficial for many. The dark side of progress includes widening disparities in wealth and health, rapid population growth, the emergence of new infectious diseases, escalating ecological degradation, numerous local and regional wars, a stockpile of nuclear weapons, and dislocation of millions of people (Benatar, 1998). The gap between the income of the richest and poorest 20% of people in the world increased from a nine-fold difference at the beginning of the twentieth century to 30-fold by 1960 – and since then to almost 80-fold by 2000. The gap in health status across the world has also widened (Benatar, 2001). This is illustrated by the fact that although life expectancy improved dramatically worldwide during the second half of the twentieth century this trend has been reversed in the poorest countries in recent years (Kaiser Network, 2006). The emergence and spread of new infectious diseases pose déjà vu dilemmas and, together with new terrorist threats, demonstrate how interconnected we all are (Singer, 2002). The recent epidemic of severe acute respiratory distress syndrome (SARS) (Booth *et al.*, 2003; Lee *et al.*, 2003) is a small-scale example of the new, acute, rapidly fatal infectious diseases that may, like the 1918–19 influenza epidemic, sweep through the world with high mortality rates in all countries and accompanying profound social and economic implications. This recrudescence of a public health threat also provided ethical insights into the implications of the interconnectedness of individuals and society and the need to reconsider the ethics of overriding individual rights (Singer, *et al.*, 2003). Consequently, in the first decade of the new millennium we face the grim reality of human life, health, and security being under severe threat.

Growing global instability and threats to human security and well-being from the widening gulf between the world's "haves" and the "have-nots" call for new ways of thinking and acting. Distinctions between domestic and foreign policy have become blurred, and the need for coherence between local and international policies is increasingly being acknowledged. Public health, even in the most privileged nations, is arguably now more closely linked than ever to health and disease in impoverished countries. Under such circumstances, linkage of local action to an expanded global health agenda based on shared values and the application of new concepts in public health ethics (Nixon *et al.*, 2005) could facilitate significant improvements in global health.

Cross-cultural considerations in bioethics

In a world characterized by many different value systems and cultures, wide disparities in wealth and health, and common threats (for example new pandemics and environmental degradation), it is of special importance to give consideration to whether there are universal ethical principles that potentially bind us all more closely than we appreciate. If there are, how could these be applied rationally in specific social contexts? This is important both in relation to clinical care of patients (Berger, 1998; Bowman, 2004) and in international collaborative research (Benatar, 2004a).

Rather that attempting to review the extensive debate on ethical universalism and moral relativism (Horton, 1995; Macklin, 1999; Beauchamp, 2003; DeGrazia, 2003; Turner, 2003; Hinman, 2006), I explore here whether areas of disagreement in making ethical decisions may be explicable by failure to understand others and by differing perceptions of social relations. I shall suggest that universal ethical principles applied through moral reasoning, with appropriate consideration of morally relevant local factors, could allow us to find a rational middle ground between the seemingly polarized perspectives of ethical universalism and ethical relativism.

There are two requirements for finding such middle ground. Firstly, it is necessary for scholars to acquire deeper insights into their own value systems and the value systems of others. Secondly, and of equal importance, is the need to avoid either uncritically accepting the moral perspectives of all cultures as equally valid or rejecting them all as invalid. Instead, and despite the shortcomings perceived by some of such an approach, moral reasoning should be used to evaluate when and how local considerations can be morally relevant in the application of universal principles in local contexts.

Understanding others

Understanding others is essential in a globalizing world. Understanding ourselves and others requires what Ninian Smart (1995) has called "structured empathy" and "cross-disciplinary study of world views/belief systems." Belief systems provide ways of "seeing" the world that, "through symbols, actions, and mobilization of feelings and wills to act ... serve as engines of social and moral continuity and change" (Smart, 1995). As world views represent powerful and different starting points from which people think and argue (and generate conflict), it is necessary to understand how they are constructed, used, and abused. While Smart describes several dimensions of world views with special emphasis on these dimensions within religions, his analysis is also relevant for secular world views (Smart, 1995).

Understanding others also requires mutually respectful dialogue. Martha Nussbaum (1997) eloquently argued that three capacities are essential for intelligent dialogue and cooperation between people from different backgrounds in today's interdependent world: (i) the capacity for critical examination of oneself and one's traditions, (ii) the capacity to see oneself as bound to all other human beings, and (iii) the capacity to imagine what it might be like to be in the shoes of a person very different from oneself. Jonathan Glover (2001), in his descriptions of numerous genocides across the world during the twentieth century and his quest for understanding why these are perpetrated, concluded that it is only our moral imagination that could enable us to significantly alter our outlook and actions.

Bioethics in the context of a more nuanced understanding of social relations

Anthropologists and social scientists have been critical of modern bioethics on the grounds that it is based on Western moral philosophy and western biomedical perspectives. An additional criticism is that bioethics is located within a theoretical framework that emphasizes the application of scientifically rigorous medical care to people who are sufficiently autonomous to make self-interested decisions about themselves in a context of minimal social connectedness. It is claimed that such a highly reductionist and individualistic approach takes insufficient consideration of the social and cultural contexts of illness or associated ethical dilemmas. In addition, it isolates bioethical issues from spiritual perspectives on health and neglects the dynamic nature of relationships between individuals, their families, and their communities (Fox and Swazey, 1985, 2005; Hoffmeister, 1990; Lieban, 1990; Weisz, 1990; Christakis, 1992; Marshall, 1992).

Some critics of modern bioethics favor a more embracing communitarian conception of the individual that acknowledges and values closer links with other people. As an example, the African notion of a person values links with the past (ancestors), the present (family and community), and with other animate beings (and even inanimate objects such as earth) within a "web of relations" that has been labeled as an "eco-bio-communitarian perspective" (Tangwa, 2000). Within this more embracing context of the African perspective, and similarly within many other traditional cultures, illness represents more than mechanical dysfunction. Here understanding and dealing with illness requires an explanatory model that includes attention to the influence of external social interactions, luck, fate, and magico-religious considerations. These arguments also apply in clinical practice, where ethical decision making could be facilitated in cross-cultural contexts by considering differences in how people in various cultures understand the meaning of personhood, what they view as harms and benefits, how the human body and illness are to be interpreted, and

the role of religion and belief systems in health and alleviation of suffering (Helman, 1990). It is necessary to understand that such differences may give rise to abhorrence in some cultures of issues that are taken for granted in others – for example truth telling about fatal diseases, the use of advance directives, removal of life support, and donation of organs (Berger, 1998; Bowman, 2004).

These two views of people, within social relationships defined in a polarized manner either as individualistic or communitarian along a single dimension, have generated much debate in relation to ethical considerations in cross-cultural research (Loue et al., 1996; Nairn, 1998; Tangwa, 2002). Some scholars insist that the individualistic approach is the best universal model and that it must be rigorously applied (Macklin, 1999). Others argue that this is a "particular rationality" about human life; one that is attractive in its abstract form but lacks resemblance to the real world in which people live (Fox and Swazey, 1985).

Mary Douglas and colleagues have offered a more complex framework for understanding social relations and interactions. This framework hopes to bridge the gap between a conception of all humans as fundamentally the same in being rational and self-interested and another conception that views people as differing greatly in what they consider to be rational and what is indeed in their own self-interest (Douglas et al., 2003). These scholars posit that both polar views rest on shaky foundations because cultures and societies vary across time, such that social differences cannot be explained so simply. They also make the case that if we are indeed all totally different it would be hard to understand history and to cooperate across cultures and that it is not necessary to have to choose between these extremes.

They propose a cultural theory in which four basic ways of life can be derived from two dimensions (Figure 43.1), and from which a large variety of ultimate forms of social and cultural life can be derived. Each of the four ways of life identified in this analysis, "consists of a specific way of structuring social relations and a supporting cast of particular

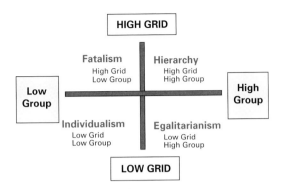

Figure 43.1. Four forms of social solidarity. (Adapted from Douglas *et al.*, 2003.)

beliefs, values, emotions, perception and interests" (Douglas *et al.*, 2003). This analysis illustrates the wider spectrum of middle ground that lies between the usually described extremes of individualism and community, and the inadequacy of always focusing on the polar extremes of dichotomous options.

Cultures are also dynamic and undergoing continuous change. Some traditional hierarchical societies are moving towards greater democracy and placing more emphasis on individualism, for example in the new South Africa with its liberal constitution and Bill of Rights. In addition, multicultural modern societies are acknowledging the need for more emphasis on community, and the need for solidarity is increasingly appreciated in a globalizing and interdependent world. However, it is important to note that in such pluralistic societies respect for democracy should take precedence over the preservation of cultural traditions that undermine democracy and human rights. Under these circumstances, egalitarianism (see Figure 43.1) is becoming an attractive and challenging common ground on which diverse cultures could hopefully meet.

How should I approach global health ethics in practice?

In a multicultural, pluralistic world, it is proposed that healthcare professionals and researchers

should have a deeper understanding of the global forces that profoundly influence health. They should also be educated about the social, economic, and political milieu that frames the context in which the clinical practice of medicine and the conduct of international collaborative research take place and be sensitive to the differing perceptions of research and healthcare that prevail in such contexts (Benatar, 2002; Marshall and Koenig, 2004; Fox and Swazey, 2005).

The example of international collaborative research illustrates the need to understand others and for finding a middle ground between ethical universalism and ethical relativism, because it is in this field more than in any other that serious efforts have been made to understand what it means to do research on vulnerable people in developing countries (Benatar, 2004a; Fogarty International Center, 2005). In addition, given the high profile of, and interest in, research, the example of standards set in the research context and linkage of research to improvements in healthcare could provide the stimulus towards achieving greater commitment to improving global health.

I have proposed a two-dimensional framework, along the lines of the analysis offered by Douglas and colleagues, to facilitate understanding disagreements about some of the ethical dilemmas that arise in cross-cultural collaborative research (Figure 43.2; Benatar, 2004a). One dimension of this framework stretches from a pole representing the abstract philosophical construction of universal ethical concepts and principles to a contrasting pole where the local ethos (defined as the "mores" that are influenced by time, geographical location, culture, and other social forces) defines the different worlds that have been studied and described by anthropologists and social scientists. A second intersecting dimension stretches from the ability to use moral reasoning to negotiate the application of universal principles within local contexts to positions of moral dogmatism and "instruction manual" approaches to ethics.

This is a more nuanced analysis than one that pits ethical universalism against moral relativism

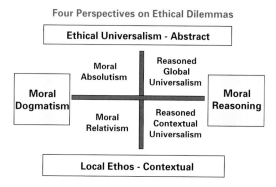

Figure 43.2. Four perspectives on ethical dilemmas. (From Benatar, 2004a.)

along a single dimension. It enables distinctions to be drawn between four broad positions: moral absolutism, moral relativism, reasoned global universalism, and reasoned contextual universalism. *Moral absolutism* describes the position taken by those who believe in ethics as prescribed and immutable. *Moral relativism* contends that morality is entirely relative to time, place, and culture. The position of *reasoned global universalism* is reached through the application of a set of abstract ethical principles that have been developed and justified through a reasoned process. The position of *reasoned contextual universalism* is reached by taking morally relevant local factors into consideration in applying reasoned global universalism.

Seeking morally justified practical applications within the position of reasoned contextual universalism acknowledges the relevance of history, geography, culture, economics, and other factors to the interpretation of universal principles so that they can be utilized effectively and progressively in differing contexts (Benatar, 2002). The influence of such factors on shaping values, belief systems, and the real world is evident in the evolution of bioethics and its methodology in the western world since the early 1960s (Sugarman and Sulmasy, 2001).

Many continue to seek research ethics guidelines that can be uniformly adopted to resolve controversial ethical dilemmas. However, it should be more widely acknowledged that just as it is not possible to spell out precisely in any particular jurisdiction what is constitutional or unconstitutional in all situations and at all times without judicial interpretation so it is a fruitless exercise to attempt to write detailed "instruction manual" type directions spelling out precisely what is ethical or unethical in all situations at all times. The place of ethical universalism is at the abstract and conceptual levels, and then there is the need to seek reasoned ways of specifying how abstract principles are to be applied at the local level.

As with considerations of social solidarity, the position of reasoned contextual universalism allows for the rational application of universal approaches within local contexts. Achieving such middle ground avoids the abstraction that is blind to context while also avoiding the perils of moral relativism (London, 2000, 2001). An essential requirement here is to have deeper insights (a difficult task) into when and how it is morally appropriate to take local contexts (ethos/mores) into consideration in applying universal ethical principles. Considerations of major importance will include whether local cultural values inflict harms that could and should be avoided (or are harmless) and whether (or not) they infringe on human rights or abrogate respect for human dignity – in the full acknowledgement that these concepts too are not easily defined in acceptable ways to all (Benatar, 2004a; Ashcroft, 2005).

The case

The HIV/AIDS pandemic has had a powerful influence on expanding the discourse about global health and human interconnectedness across the globe. It has also sensitized researchers to the complexities of applying universal principles in medical research. The case study selected here is used to illustrate the need for a broader, more global approach to health and to bioethics and the need to find rational means of applying universal ethical principles in different contexts without resorting to moral relativism.

The ideas outlined above have been applied to facilitate resolution of persisting ethical dilemmas in international collaborative research and to assist in determining when a placebo control is justified in clinical research (Benatar, 2004b). I have suggested that under the very different circumstances in which pregnant mothers present for delivery in developing countries the research question that needs to be asked about preventing MTCT of HIV infection differs somewhat from the question asked about how to reduce MTCT in wealthy countries. So, the question to study becomes, "to what extent can MTCT of HIV be prevented in resource-poor settings where pregnant mothers only present to clinics a few weeks or hours before labor, are often anemic and malnourished, and where breast-feeding cannot be avoided?"

The balance of benefits and harms associated with a research project pursuing this question, and the feasibility of then introducing into everyday clinical practice an affordable preventive regimen, differ very significantly from the original studies. When few women present early enough to be treated with the full ACTG 076 regimen, the legitimacy of a different study design, which may include a placebo, is based on this significantly different research question being asked in a totally different social context with very different implications for the local society. Important relevant differences include inability to enroll enough women presenting early enough to receive the ACTG 076 regimen (those few who do present early could receive it), inability to prevent breast-feeding, and the great public health value of obtaining an answer to the research question as rapidly and efficiently as possible in the face of a major pandemic where many threatened lives in developing countries could be saved.

So, if we agree that (i) double standards should be avoided, (ii) that different standards may be acceptable when there are relevant contextual differences, and (iii) that consideration of relevant differences is part of the moral reasoning process, then we can agree that different standards may not be double standards. Such arguments can lead to the conclusion that the use of a placebo in the comparative arm of a study of short-course antiretroviral treatment in MTCT could be ethical (Benatar, 2004b).

This argument can also be taken one step further in the quest to link research to improvements in medical care in developing countries. For example, in the ACTG 076 study in wealthy countries, the researchers were not faced with needing to treat their research subjects for malaria, tuberculosis, or other concomitant diseases that may afflict them during the study, as treatment for these would be available to them through locally available health services. In developing countries, however, it would surely be unethical of researchers not to treat their research subjects for such conditions if treatment were not otherwise available to them. So we have provided a reasoned account of why and how researchers should be required to provide a broader and *different* standard of overall care in these two research situations (Shapiro and Benatar, 2005), and that this is not an example of double standards, but rather of morally legitimate *different* standards (Benatar, 2004a).

Making progress in global health will require new paradigms of thinking. Progress could be made through an extended notion of global bioethics and by coupling research to improvements in health through a broader conception of the standard of care that links research to sustainable development through partnerships and strategic alliances.

REFERENCES

Ashcroft, R. E. (2005). Making sense of dignity. *J Med Ethics* **31**: 679–82.

Beauchamp, T. L. (2003). A defense of the common morality. *Kennedy Inst Ethics J* **13**: 259–74.

Benatar, S. R. (1998). Global disparities in health and human rights. *Am J Public Health* **88**: 295–300.

Benatar, S. R. (2001). Health in developing countries. In *International Encyclopedia of the Social and Behavioral Sciences*, ed. N. J. Smelser and P. B. Baltes. Amsterdam: Elsevier, pp. 6566–70.

Benatar, S. R. (2002). Some reflections and recommendations on research ethics in developing countries. *Soc Sci Med* **54**: 1131–41.

Benatar, S. R. (2004a). Towards progress in resolving dilemmas in international research ethics. *J Law Med Ethics* **32**: 574–82.

Benatar, S. R. (2004b). Rationally defensible standards for research in developing countries. Review of "Double Standards in Medical Research in Developing Countries" by Ruth Macklin, Cambridge University Press. *Health Human Rights* **8**: 197–202.

Benatar, S. R., Daar, A. S., and Singer, P. A. (2003). Global health ethics: the rationale for mutual caring. *Int Affairs* **79**: 101–38.

Bensimon, C. A. and Benatar, S. R. (2006). Developing sustainability: a new metaphor for progress. *Theor Med Bioethics* **27**: 59–79.

Berger, J. T. (1998). Culture and ethnicity in clinical care. *Arch Intern Med* **158**: 2085–90.

Booth, C. M., Matukas, L. M., Tomlinson, G. A., *et al.* (2003). Clinical features and short-term outcomes of 144 patients with SARS in the greater Toronto area. *JAMA* **289**: 1–9.

Bowman, K. (2004). What are the limits of bioethics in a culturally pluralistic society? *J Law Med Ethics* **32**: 664–9.

Christakis, N. A. (1992). Ethics are local: engaging cross-cultural variations in the ethics for clinical research. *Soc Sci Med* **35**: 1079–91.

Connor, E., Sperling, R., Gelber, R., *et al.* (1994). Reduction of maternal–infant transmission of human immuno-deficiency virus type 1 with zidovudine treatment. *N Engl J Med* **331**: 1173–80.

DeGrazia, D. (2003). Common morality, coherence, and the principles of biomedical ethics. *Kennedy Inst Ethics J* **13**: 219–30.

Douglas, M., Thompson, M., and Verweij, M. (2003). Is time running out? The case of global warming. *Daedalus* **Spring**: 98–107.

Doyal, L. and Gough, I. (1991). *A Theory of Human Need*. London: MacMillan.

Fogarty International Center (2005). *International Research Ethics Education and Curriculum Development Award*. http://www.fic.nih.gov/programs/training_grants/ bioethics/index.htm. Accessed June 2007.

Fox, R. C. and Swazey, J. (1985). Medical morality is not bioethics: medical ethics in China and the United States. *Perspect Biol Med* **27**: 337–60.

Fox, R. C. and Swazey, J. P. (2005). Examining American bioethics: its problems and perspectives. *Camb Q Healthc Ethics* **14**: 361–73.

Glover, J. (2001). *Humanity: a Moral History of the 20th Century*. New Haven, CT: Yale University Press.

Helman, C. G. (1990). *Culture, Health and Illness*, 2nd edn. London: Butterworth–Heinemann.

Hinman, L. M. (2006). Internet philosophical sources on moral relativism. *Ethics Updates* (http://ethics.sandiego. edu/theories/Relativism) accessed 26 July 2006.

Hoffmeister, B. (1990). Morality and the social sciences. In *Social Science Perspectives on Medical Ethics*, ed. G. W. Weisz. Dordrecht, the Netherlands: Kluwer, pp. 241–60.

Horton, R. (1995). African traditional thought and Western science. In *African Philosophy*, ed. A. Mosely. Englewood Cliff, NJ: Prentice Hall, pp. 310–38.

Kaiser Network (2006). *Global Challenges: Life Expectancy in Sub-Saharan Africa Decreases*. http://www. kaisernetwork.org/daily_reports-rep_index.cfm?DR_ID= 38068. Accessed 26 July 2006.

Lee, N., Hui, D., Wu, A., *et al.* (2003). A major outbreak of severe respiratory distress syndrome in Hong Kong. *N Engl J Med* **348**: 1986–94.

Lieban, R. W. (1990). Medical anthropology and the comparative study of medical ethics. In *Social Science Perspectives on Medical Ethics*, ed. G. W. Weisz. Dordrecht the Nehtherlands: Kluwer, pp. 221–39.

London, A. J. (2000). The ambiguity and the exigency: clarifying 'standard of care' arguments in international research. *J Med Philos* **25**: 379–97.

London, A. J. (2001). Equipoise and international human-subjects research. *Bioethics* **15**: 312–32.

Loue, S., Okello, D., and Kawama, M. (1996). Research bioethics in the Ugandan context. *J Law Med Ethics* **24**: 47–53.

Macklin, R. (1999). *Against Relativism: Cultural Diversity and the Search for Ethical Universals in Medicine*. New York: Oxford University Press.

Marshall, P. A. (1992). Anthropology and bioethics. *Med Anthropol Q* **6**: 49–73.

Marshall, P. and Koenig, B. (2004). Accounting for culture in a globalized bioethics. *J Law Med Ethics* **32**: 252–66.

Nairn, T. (1998). The use of Zairian children in HIV vaccine experimentation: a cross-cultural study in medical ethics. In *On Moral Medicine*, 2nd edn, ed. S. Lammers and A. Verhey. Grand Rapids MI: Eerdmans, pp. 919–31.

Nixon, S., Upshur, R., Robertson, A., *et al.* (2005). Public health ethics. In *Public Health and Law Policy in Canada*, ed. N. Ries, T. Caulfield, T. Bailey. Toronto: Lexis Nexis, pp. 39–58.

Nussbaum, M. C. (1997). *Cultivating Humanity: A Classical Defense of Reform in Liberal Education.* Cambridge, MA: Harvard University Press.

Shapiro, K. and Benatar, S. R. (2005). HIV prevention research and global inequality: towards improved standards of care. *J Med Ethics* **31**: 39–47.

Singer, P. (2002). *One World: The Ethics of Globalization.* New Haven: Yale University Press.

Singer, P. A., Benatar, S. R., Bernstein, P., *et al.* (2003). Ethics and SARS: lessons from Toronto. *BMJ* **327**: 1342–4.

Smart, N. (1995). *Worldviews: Cross-cultural Explorations of Human Beliefs*, 2nd edn. Englewood Cliffs, NJ: Prentice Hall.

Sugarman, J. and Sulmasy, D. P. (eds.) (2001). *Methods in Medical Ethics.* Washington, DC: Georgetown University Press.

Tangwa, G. (2000). The traditional African perception of a person: some implications for bioethics. *Hastings Cent Rep* **30**: 39–43.

Tangwa, G. (2002). International regulations and medical research in developing countries: double standards or differing standards?. *Notizie di Politeia* **XVIII**: 46–50.

Turner, L. (2003). Zones of consensus and zones of conflict: questioning the "common morality" presumption in bioethics. *Kennedy Inst Ethics J* **13**: 193–218.

Varmus, H. and Satcher, D. (1997). Ethical complexities of conducting research in developing countries. *N Engl J Med* **337**: 1003–5.

Weisz, G. W. (ed.) (1990). *Social Science Perspectives on Medical Ethics.* Dordrecht, the Netherlands: Kluwer, pp. 221–39.

44

Physician participation in torture

Jerome Amir Singh

Hours after a bomb kills 23 people in a busy marketplace, state armed forces arrest a suspect. Dr. A, a state physician, is summoned to the city's detention facilities. When he arrives, he finds the suspect unconscious and covered in blood from severe beatings inflicting by the security forces. He is asked to resuscitate the patient for further interrogation. Angered at the bombing, Dr. A complies. Shortly thereafter, in an attempt by detaining authorities to extract information from the detainee, Dr. A is asked to administer sodium pentothal (also known as "truth serum") to the detainee. Before doing so, the suspect dies from his injuries sustained from the beatings. The detaining authorities instruct Dr. A to record the death as a suicide, which he does. Later, Dr. A wonders whether his actions and silence in the matter makes him complicit in the torture and subsequent cover-up of the incident. He is also uncertain whether he is obliged to act in the best interests of his employer (the state), himself, or his patient in such instances.

Dr. B, a psychiatrist in a detention center, is informed by one of her patients that he has not been charged or tried for any crime since his detention months earlier. In addition, he is regularly shackled and held in solitary confinement for prolonged periods, made to stand in awkward positions for hours on end, and deprived of sleep by the detaining authorities. Dr. B is unsure what to do with this information.

C, a prison nurse, overhears correctional services officials at her prison boast about their interrogation and humiliation of detainees who were recently transferred there as a result of extrajudicial renditions, a practice whereby detainees

are deported by countries without going through proper court channels. Their accounts include, amongst others, stripping detainees naked and photographing them, and scaring them with prison dogs while they are blindfolded. C, who has not personally witnessed any of these acts, nor knowingly treated such patients, confronts her colleagues, who inform her that such detainees have no recognition or protection under international law. C is unsure of her moral and legal duties towards the detainees.

What is torture?

In the World Medical Association's (WMA) Declaration of Tokyo of 1975 (hereafter the *Tokyo Declaration*) torture is defined as: "the deliberate, systematic or wanton infliction of physical or mental suffering by one or more persons acting alone or on the orders of any authority, to force another person to yield information, to make a confession or for any other purpose." "Any other purpose" could include simply punishing and terrorizing persons (McQuoid-Mason and Dada, 1999). In 1984, the United Nations (UN) adopted the *Convention Against Torture and other Cruel, Inhumane or Degrading Treatment or Punishment* (hereafter *Convention Against Torture*). In Article 1 of this convention, torture is defined as "any act by which severe pain or suffering, whether physical or mental, is intentionally inflicted in order to obtain

This chapter is based on: Singh, J. A. (2003). American physicians and dual loyalty obligations in the "war on terrorism." *BMC Med Ethics* **4**: 1–10 (http://www.biomedcentral.com/1472-6939/4/4).

a confession, to punish or to intimidate in cases where such suffering is inflicted with the connivance of a public official'' (UN General Assembly, 1984).

Why are ethical and legal issues surrounding torture important?

Dual loyalty conflict defined

In 2003 the International Dual Loyalty Working Group proposed a comprehensive set of guidelines on dual loyalty conflicts, entitled *Dual Loyalty and Human Rights in Health Professional Practice* (DLHR) (Physicians for Human Rights and University of Cape Town Health Sciences Faculty, 2003). This defined a dual loyalty as a ''clinical role conflict between professional duties to a patient and obligations, express or implied, real or perceived, to the interests of a third party such as an employer, insurer or the state.'' This paper addressed these issues in the context of a health professional's clinical role conflict between serving his or her detainee patient and serving his or her country or employer.

How dual loyalty dilemmas can arise

History and recent events have demonstrated that health professionals of a detaining power are not above being complicit in detainee abuse (British Medical Association, 2001; Lifton, 2004; Marks, 2005). If a detainee is being subjected to poor detention conditions, or abusive or humiliating interrogation by a detaining power, health professionals could experience a conflict of interest between (i) their duty to care for, and protect, that patient (which would ideally require the professional to actively protest against, or report, abusive treatment to the appropriate authorities), and (ii) their patriotic duty to protect and serve the interests of their employer or country (which might arguably require the professional to remain silent about such treatment). Conversely, a government's openly negative views towards detainees could induce health professionals not to *want* to provide reasonable care

to, or protect the interests of, such detainees. This could conceivably occur where health professionals come to believe (rightly or wrongly) in the detainee's complicity or guilt in actual, incomplete, or prospective crimes against the professional's country. This mindset could conflict with the professional's ethical duty to care for the detainee.

International human rights law

The *Universal Declaration of Human Rights* adopted by the UN General Assembly in 1948 states that ''no one shall be subjected to torture or to cruel, inhumane or degrading treatment or punishment.'' Although this declaration is not binding on countries, it carries considerable moral weight. Article 7 of the *Covenant on Civil and Political Rights* of 1966 (which is an instrument that is binding on states that ratify it) replicates this right word-for-word (UN General Assembly, 1966). In its General Comments on this clause, the UN's Human Rights Committee stressed that this prohibition relates not only to ''acts which cause physical pain but also to acts that cause mental suffering to victims'' (Kellberg, 1998). Indefinite solitary confinement, a measure practiced by some countries, can be seen as a form of mental suffering. The Committee has also stated that no justification or extenuating circumstances excuses a violation of Article 7, including an order from a superior officer or a public authority.

In 1978, the European Court of Human Rights ruled that the use by British forces in Northern Ireland of tactics such as hooding, forced standing, sleep deprivation, subjection to noise, and deprivation of food and drink was not torture. However, the Court did find that such methods were ''inhuman and degrading'' and, therefore, unlawful under various treaties (*Ireland* v. *UK*, 1978). Moreover, in 1999, the Israeli Supreme Court unanimously ruled that certain Israeli interrogation methods (including forced uncomfortable postures and sleep deprivation) were unlawful (*Public Committee against Torture in Israel et al.* v. *Government of Israel et al.*, 1999).

The Israeli Supreme Court also ruled that the State (of Israel) could not use the defense of "necessity" to justify such treatment. These cases illustrate that the techniques outlined above are clearly considered repugnant internationally. Health professionals of countries practicing such techniques should not be party to such treatment. Professionals who witness such treatment have an ethical duty to speak out against it. This resonates with the benevolent advocacy role for health professionals postulated above.

International humanitarian law

The international treaties governing armed conflicts are known as international humanitarian law or the "law of war." Disregard of these treaties can easily lead to degrading and/or abusive treatment of detainees, which, in turn, could impact negatively on their mental and physical health. In the international conflict context, "prisoner of war" (POW) status entitles detainees to basic rights under several international treaties, including the Third Geneva Convention. The four Geneva Conventions established rules for the conduct of international armed conflict (UN, 1949). The Geneva Convention applies "to all cases of declared war or of any other armed conflict which may arise between two or more of the High Contracting Parties, even if the state of war is not recognized by one of them." "Common Article 3," as it has become known, is found identically in all four conventions and is taken to define a "hard core" of obligations that must be respected in *all* armed conflicts. This is generally taken to mean that no matter what the nature of the war or conflict certain basic rules cannot be abrogated. Common Article 3 states (UN, 1949):

> The following acts are and shall remain prohibited at any time and in any place whatsoever: violence to life and person, in particular murder of all kinds, mutilation, cruel treatment and torture; outrages upon personal dignity, in particular humiliating and degrading treatment

Under the Geneva Conventions, POW status also bestows upon detainees a plethora of rights, many of which directly or indirectly involve military physicians. These include Articles 3, 13, 15, 17, 19, 21, 22, 31, and 46. Article 17 is of particular relevance. It states that no physical or mental torture, nor any other form of coercion, may be inflicted on POWs to secure from them information of any kind whatsoever. It also states that prisoners who refuse to answer questions may not be threatened, insulted, or exposed to any unpleasant or disadvantageous treatment of any kind. This would clearly rule out the application of any robust interrogation methods on detainees by a detaining power.

Non-binding United Nations resolutions

Although UN General Assembly resolutions are generally not binding on member states (unless they agree to be bound), like the *Universal Declaration of Human Rights*, they carry considerable moral weight as they reflect the moral conscience and general consensus of the collective international community. According to the 1982 UN General Assembly resolution entitled *Principles of Medical Ethics relevant to the Role of Health Personnel, particularly Physicians, in the Protection of Prisoners and Detainees against Torture and Other Cruel, Inhuman or Degrading Treatment or Punishment* (hereafter the *Principles of Medical Ethics*), it is a contravention of medical ethics for health personnel to apply their knowledge and skills in order to assist in the interrogation of prisoners and detainees in a manner that may adversely affect their physical or mental health and which is not in accordance with the relevant international instruments, and to certify, or to participate in the certification of, the fitness of prisoners or detainees for any form of treatment or punishment that may adversely affect their physical or mental health (Principle 4). Further, it is a gross contravention of medical ethics, as well as an offence under applicable international instruments, for health personnel to engage, actively or passively, in acts which constitute participation in, complicity in, incitement to, or attempts to commit torture or other cruel, inhuman, or degrading treatment or punishment (Principle 2). It also explicitly stipulated that there may be no derogation from the foregoing principles on any ground whatsoever, including public emergency (Principle 6).

According to the 1988 UN General Assembly resolution entitled *Body of Principles for the Protection of All Persons under Any Form of Detention or Imprisonment* (hereafter *BOP*) *all* persons under *any form* of detention or imprisonment shall be treated in a humane manner and with respect for the inherent dignity of the human person (Principle 1). Nor may that individual be subjected to torture or to "cruel, inhuman or degrading treatment or punishment" (Principle 6). This is to be interpreted so as to "extend the widest possible protection against abuses, whether physical or mental, including the holding of a detained or imprisoned person in conditions which deprive him, temporarily or permanently of the use of any of his natural senses, such as sight or hearing, or of his awareness of place and the passing of time" (Principle 6). Under this provision, *no circumstance whatsoever* may be invoked as a justification for torture or other cruel, inhuman or degrading treatment or punishment. Significantly, the *BOP* explicitly stipulates that officials who "have reason to believe that a violation of this Body of Principles has occurred or is about to occur" must report the matter to their superior authorities and, where necessary, to "other appropriate authorities or organs vested with reviewing or remedial powers" (Principle 7(2)). Thus, health professionals need to be mindful that even detainees who are assigned unilateral classifications such as "unlawful combatant" are protected against undue advantage being taken against them during interrogations (Principle 21).

The UN *Standard Minimum Rules for the Treatment of Prisoners* made it clear that its provisions cover the general management of institutions and are applicable to all categories of prisoners, criminal or civil, untried or convicted, including prisoners subject to "security measures" (UN Congress, 1955; Articles 4(1), 84(1), 84(2), 95). Countries that disregard the rights of detainees could also be violating a UN resolution pertaining to the protection of human rights and fundamental freedoms while countering terrorism (UN General Assembly, 2002). This resolution affirms, among others, that states must ensure that any measure taken to combat terrorism complies with obligations under international law, in particular international human rights, refugee, and humanitarian law.

International medical ethics guidelines

According to the *Tokyo Declaration* (WMA, 1975), a physician should not "countenance, condone or participate in the practice of torture or other forms of cruel, inhuman or degrading procedures, whatever the offence of which the victim of such procedures is suspected, accused or guilty, and whatever the victim's beliefs or motives, and in all situations, including armed conflict and civil strife" (Article 1). It stated that the physician "shall not provide any premises, instruments, substances or knowledge to facilitate the practice of torture or other forms of cruel, inhuman or degrading treatment or to diminish the ability of the victim to resist such treatment" (Article 2). Physicians who participate in interrogation sessions, either directly or by resuscitating unconscious detainees for the purposes of further interrogation by the detaining power, could be deemed as having diminished the ability of detainees to resist such treatment. The mere presence of any physician during any inhumane treatment of detainees is also a violation of the *Tokyo Declaration* (Article 3). Physicians cannot justify their involvement in such interrogations on the basis of any political ideology (such as a country's "national security" interest) as the *Tokyo Declaration* states that the physician's fundamental role is to alleviate the distress of his or her fellow men, and no motive whether personal, collective, or political shall prevail against this higher purpose (Article 4). According to *DLHR*, the health professional should not perform medical duties or engage in medical interventions for "security purposes" (Guideline 14).

According to Article 1 of the *Regulations in time of Armed Conflict* (also known as the *Havana Declaration*) (WMA, 1956), medical ethics in time of armed conflict is identical to medical ethics in times of peace. Article 2 of this document makes clear that as the primary task of the physician is to preserve health and save life, it is unethical for physicians to (a) give advice or perform prophylactic, diagnostic or therapeutic procedures that are not justifiable in the patient's interests, (b) weaken the physical or mental strength of a human being without therapeutic justification, and (c) employ scientific knowledge to imperil health or destroy life.

Provisions (a) and (c) prohibit physicians treating or resuscitating detainees in furtherance of further invasive interrogations. Provision (b) could be interpreted as forbidding physicians from declaring detainees mentally competent for indefinite solitary confinement or administering a truth serum to detainees for interrogation purposes.

The *Manual on Effective Investigation and Documentation of Torture and Other Cruel, Inhumane or Degrading Treatment* (the *Istanbul Protocol*) is the first set of international guidelines intended to serve for the assessment of persons who allege torture and ill-treatment, for investigating cases of alleged torture, and for reporting such findings to the judiciary and any other investigative body (Action for Torture Survivors, and Amnesty International, and Association for the Prevention of Torture *et al.*, 1999). If physicians witness or suspect the abuse of detainees, they should consider it their ethical duty to use the *Istanbul Protocol* to document and report such abuse. This approach is endorsed by the *DLHR* guidelines on prison, detention, and other custodial settings, although it cautions (Guideline 6): "The health professional must, however, weigh this action against any reprisal or further punishment to the prisoner that may result. When appropriate, the health professional should gain the consent of the prisoner before making such a report."

But how should clinicians handle risks of reprisals against themselves? Those few documented accounts that do exist of brave clinicians laudably acting in the interests of their tortured detainee patients despite the threat of serious repercussions if they did so reveal that many were themselves subsequently abused or tortured (CPT [European Committee for the Prevention of Torture and Inhumane or Degrading Treatment or Punishment], 2001). Physicians in Iraq during the Hussein era, for example, participated in state-inflicted torture because they feared for their lives if they failed to comply with army directives (Reis *et al.*, 2004), while physicians in Turkey routinely also do not report torture for fear of reprisal (Physicians for Human Rights, 1996). But does the failure to report actual or suspected abuses against detainees constitute a transgression of law or ethics? From a legal perspective, health professionals in many countries are deemed to have a "special duty" relationship with their patients that obliges them to act in their patient's best interests. A failure to do so usually constitutes an "omission" in law, which is actionable in criminal and civil law. However, the health professional is not obliged to act if doing so could reasonably compromise his or her life. Accordingly, if a health professional reasonably believes that his or her life or safety would be endangered by any torture-related disclosure to outside parties, his or her special duty obligation to act in the patient's interests would arguably not immediately apply. The health professional's duty in this regard, though, would be triggered as soon as the threat ended and/or the opportunity to disclose to relevant third parties arose, if applicable. In this regard, the CPT stated (2001; Principle 5; italics added for emphasis):

Doctors have a duty to monitor and speak out when services in which they are involved are unethical, abusive, and inadequate or pose a potential threat to patients' health. In such cases, they have an ethical duty to take prompt action as failure to take an immediate stand makes protest at a later stage more difficult. They should report the matter to appropriate authorities or international agencies who can investigate but *without exposing patients, their families or themselves to foreseeable serious risk of harm.*

Moral disengagement, ideological totalism, and victim blame

The participation of health professionals in torture (e.g., advising torturers on methods, evaluating individuals to determine whether they can survive additional torture, and using medical skills in the process of torture) is well documented (Stover and Nightingale, 1985; Reis *et al.*, 2004). Health professionals, like others who witness or are aware of incidents of torture in their settings, fail to denounce torture for a variety of reasons, including fear, self-interest, and self-promotion. Such individuals may not wish to acknowledge that torture is perpetuated by their government, and/or their ignorance may mean that they are unaware that torture is *never* justifiable (British Medical Association, 1999).

There may be social circumstances and particular factors that precipitate a loss of moral perspective (Weinstein, 1988). These may have colonial and imperial roots. The negative labeling or devaluing of a group by influential forces can breed a culture of fundamentalism or extremist ideology (also known as "ideological totalism"). "Moral disengagement" occurs when subordinates of a labeling group regard the interests of the labeled group as less relevant because of the political culture under which they live (British Medical Association, 2001). Health professionals must avoid morally disengaging from their patients regardless of the political culture patients emerge from. "Victim-blame" is a tendency to hold victims responsible for their own fate. If professionals knowingly or unknowingly adopt this mentality, their ethical obligations towards patients may become compromised. They should note that ideological totalism, moral disengagement, and victim blame were factors that facilitated the abuse of detainees in apartheid South Africa. Health professionals must ensure that they do not make the same mistakes when carrying out their duties.

Extrajudicial renditions

The transfer of terror suspects (primarily from countries in the developed world) for interrogation to (primarily developing) countries known for practicing torture is a growing practice. The deportation has been labeled "extrajudicial rendition" and occurs without due process through proper legal channels;usually a court has to approve a deportation before it can occur (Garcia, 2006). To ensure that detainees have access to the outside world and as a safeguard against human rights violations such as "disappearance" and torture, all detained people have the right to be held only in an officially recognized place of detention, located if possible near their place of residence, and under a valid order committing them to detention (UN General Assembly, 1977 [Rule 7(2)], 1988 [Principles 11(2) and 20], 1992 [Article 10]; Council of Europe Committee of Ministers, 1987 [Rule 7(1)]; Organization of American States, 1994 [Article XI]). Physicians who certify detainees fit for travel for the purposes of extrajudicial rendition, treat them for illnesses and injuries in furtherance of being declared fit for such travel (if fitness for travel is even an issue in such instances), or who treat them on their arrival in preparation for interrogation should be mindful that their actions amount to complicity in torture. The relevant principles of ethics and international law in regard to complicity in torture apply equally to them in these instances. Such physicians have a duty to speak out against such practices and to expose them.

In November 2002, the *Optional Protocol to the Convention against Torture* was adopted by the UN Economic and Security Council. This instrument seeks, *inter alia*, to establish a system of unannounced inspections of prisons and detention centers. Because of its binding nature, some countries are refusing to ratify it. The duty of beneficence sometimes necessitates the health professional adopting an advocacy role. Given that the optional protocol seeks to enhance detainee patients' rights, members of the international health professions community (in conjunction with respective domestic professional associations) should regard it as their ethical duty to pressure relevant government to accede to it. These measures will resonate with the health provider's beneficent duties to promote good and prevent harm. Health professionals should press their government to realize that if their country fails to respect the laws of war and detainee health rights it cannot expect its enemies to do any better if its own troops are captured.

How should I act when encountering torture in practice?

By acting as whistleblowers, health professionals can play an important role in reducing gross human rights violations (British Medical Association, 2001). When professionals stationed in military detention camps observe that detention conditions of detainees fall short of the standards required under international humanitarian law, or are of the professional opinion that such conditions are compromising, or could compromise, the health interests of detainees, the health professional's duty to protect the well-being of detainees must be regarded as paramount.

Detainees who have incommunicado status are especially vulnerable and powerless to resist abuse. Health professionals should strive to change this situation by reporting suspected violations of detainee rights to the UN Special Rapporteur on Torture. Alternatively, they can approach organizations such as the International Committee of the Red Cross, Medécins Sans Frontiéres, Amnesty International, Physicians for Human Rights, or Human Rights Watch. These organizations could at least use their profile to publicize the incidents and apply pressure on relevant governments to investigate such allegations. To discourage victimization of whistleblowers, domestic health professional associations should press their governments to explicitly endorse their code of ethics. They should also offer express support to professionals who experience, or who are likely to experience, dual loyalty conflicts.

While the post 9–11 torture and abuse of detainees by US forces has been comprehensively documented and rightfully evoked outrage (Physicians for Human Rights, 2005), it is the participation and complicity of US physicians in these acts that is of particular concern (Singh, 2003; Gregg Bloche, 2004; Lifton, 2004; Marks, 2005; Miles, 2004; Rubenstein, 2004a; Slevin and Stephens, 2004). Proponents of such deeds argue that in times of war: "A patient's rights to life and self-determination contract; human dignity strains under the barrage of military necessity; and the interests of the state and political community may outweigh considerations of patients' welfare". Moreover, that "medical ethics in war are not identical to medical ethics in times of peace" (Gross, 2004: 22). Such arguments are weak as they are seemingly engineered to defend misguided national self-interests and simplistically side step fundamental multilateral principles of law and medical ethics. They too, have justifiably been condemned (Rubenstein, 2004b).

If a health professional experiences a conflict of interest between his/her duty to care for, and protect, a detainee from abusive treatment and the patriotic duty to protect and serve the interests of his/her country, he or she should consider it their legal and ethical obligation to report or actively protest against such treatment to appropriate authorities. Detainees have rights by virtue of several international legal conventions and ethical declarations, which are not elastic in nature. A unilateralist and isolationist mentality based on military might, self-interest, and a sense of impunity can lead to a disregard of international law, medical ethics, and, consequently, detainee rights. This mindset must be avoided by health providers.

If faced with a conflict between following national policies and universally embraced multilateral principles of international law and ethics, health professional should consider themselves morally bound to follow the latter. Conversely, even in situations where they come to believe (rightly or wrongly) in the detainee's complicity or guilt in actual, incomplete, or prospective crimes against the health professional's country, and where the professional finds him or herself not *wanting* to protect the interests of a detainee because of his/her government's policies, the health professional's core duty to care for the detainee patient must still prevail.

Health professionals should always remember that the duty of care supersedes any blanket notion of loyalty, obligation, allegiance, or patriotism they may feel is owed to their station. Health professionals involved in treating detainees, particularly victims of torture, must always strive to practice ethics-based care. History will judge their failure to do so.

The cases

Dr. A's role in the torture of the terror suspect and the subsequent cover-up of the suspect's true cause of death constitutes complicity in torture according to international law and guidelines on medical ethics. Dr. A ought to have acted in the best interests of the detainee by refusing to participate in the interrogation session and reporting the true cause of death to the relevant authorities.

Dr. B is legally and ethically obliged to report the detainee's allegation to her superiors (and if possible, keep his identity confidential, or if requested to do so by the detainee). Failing any relief, she should consider reporting the matter to higher authorities or outside bodies.

C is legally and ethically obliged to report her colleagues' conduct to her superiors. Moreover, she should note that extrajudicial renditions are unlawful according to international law. Failing any action from her immediate superiors, she should consider reporting the matter to higher national authorities or outside bodies.

REFERENCES

Action for Torture Survivors, Amnesty International, Association for the Prevention of Torture, *et al.* (1999). *Manual on the Effective Investigation and Documentation of Torture and Other Cruel, Inhuman or Degrading Treatment or Punishment (The Istanbul Protocol).* Submitted to the United Nations High Commissioner for Human Rights (http://www.phrusa.org/research/istanbul_protocol/ist_prot.pdf).

British Medical Association (1999). *Withholding and Withdrawing Life-Prolonging Medical Treatment: Guidance for Decision Making.* London: BMJ Books, pp. 81–2.

British Medical Association (2001). *The Medical Profession and Human Rights: Handbook for a Changing Agenda.* London: Zed Books.

Council of Europe Committee of Ministers (1987). *European Prison Rules Recommendation No. R(87)3.* Brussels: Coucil of Europe (http://www.iuscrim.mpg.de/info/aktuell/lehre/docs/EUPrisonRules.pdf).

CPT (2001). *Physicians Acting at the Authorities' Request for Non-medical Purposes.* Brussels: European Committee for the Prevention of Torture and Inhumane or Degrading Treatment or Punishment (http://www.cpt.coe.int/EN/working-documents/cpt-2001-65-eng.pdf).

Garcia, J. G. (2006). *Renditions: Constraints Imposed by Laws on Torture.* Washington, DC: Congressional Research Service Report for the US Congress (http://www.fas.org/sgp/crs/natsec/RL32890.pdf).

Gregg Bloche M. (2004). After Abu Ghraib; physician, turn thyself in. *New York Times* June, A27.

Gross, M. L. (2004). Bioethics and armed conflict: mapping moral dimensions of medicine and war. *Hastings Cent Rep* **34**: 22–30.

Ireland v. *UK* (1978) 2 EHRR 25, paragraph 168 (http://www.law.qub.ac.uk/humanrts/ehris/ni/icase/intcaseA.htm).

Kellberg, L. (1998). Torture: international rules and procedures. In: *An End to Torture: Strategies for its Eradication*, ed. B. Duner. London: Zed Books.

Lifton, R. J. (2004). Doctors and torture. *N Engl J Med* **351**: 415–16.

Marks, J. H. (2005). Doctors of interrogation. *Hastings Cent Rep* **35**: 17–22.

McQuoid-Mason, D. J. and Dada, M. A. (1999). *Guide to Forensic Medicine and Medical Law.* Durban: Independent Medico-Legal Unit.

Miles, S. (2004). A troubling silence from prison medics. *Minneapolis Star Tribune* 18 May (http://www.commondreams.org/views04/0518-09.htm).

Organization of American States (1994). *Inter-American Convention on Forced Disappearance of Persons* Belém do Pará, 1994 (http://www.oas.org/juridico/English/Treaties/a-60.html).

Physicians for Human Rights (1996). *Torture in Turkey and its Unwilling Accomplices*. Boston, MA: Physicians for Human Rights.

Physicians for Human Rights (2005). *Break Them Down: the Systematic Use of Psychological Torture by US Forces*. Boston, MA: Physicians for Human Rights (http://www.phrusa.org/research/torture/pdf/psych_torture.pdf).

Physicians for Human Rights and University of Cape Town Health Sciences Faculty (2003). *Dual Loyalty and Human Rights in Health Professional Practice: Proposed Guidelines and Institutional Standards*. Boston, MA Physicians for Human Rights (http://www.phrusa.org/healthrights/dual_loyalty.html).

Public Committee against Torture in Israel et al. v. *Government of Israel et al.* (1999). Piskei Din 3 (4) 817 (HCJ 5100/94) (http://www.stoptorture.org.il//eng/images/uploaded/publications/18.pdf).

Reis, C., Ahmed, A. T., Amowitz, L. L., *et al.* (2004). Physician participation in human rights abuses in southern Iraq. *JAMA* **291**: 1480–6.

Rubenstein L (2004a). *Statement of Leonard Rubenstein, Executive Director, Physicians for Human Rights*. Boston, MA: Physicians for Human Rights (http://www.aclu.org/news/NewsPrint.cfm?id=13965&c=36).

Rubenstein, L. (2004b). Medicine and war. *Hastings Cent Rep* **34**: 3.

Scheer R. (2004). Tout torture, get promoted. *Los Angeles Times* 15 June (http://www.alternet.org/columnists/story/18950/).

Singh, J. A. (2003). American physicians and dual loyalty obligations in the ''war on terrorism.'' *BMC Med Ethics* **4**: 1–10.

Slevin, P. and Stephens, J. (2004). Detainees' medical files shared: Guantanamo interrogators' access criticized. *Washington Post* 10 June A1.

Stover, E. and Nightingale, E. O. (1985). *The Breaking of Bodies and Minds*. New York: Freeman.

UN (1949). *Geneva Convention of 27 July 1929 Relative to the Treatment of Prisoners of War, As Amended in 1949*. New York: United Nations (http://www.icrc.org/IHL.nsf/52d68d14de6160e0c12563da005fdb1b/eb1571b00daec90ec125641e00402aa6?OpenDocument).

UN Congress (1955). *First Congress on the Prevention of Crime and the Treatment of Offenders*, Geneva. New York: United Nations (http://193.194.138.190/html/menu3/b/h_comp34.htm).

UN Economic and Security Council (2002). *Resolution 2002/27: Optional Protocol to the Convention Against Torture and Other Cruel, Inhuman or Degrading Treatment or Punishment*. New York: United Nations (http://www1.umn.edu/humanrts/instree/optprotort.html).

UN General Assembly (1948). *Resolution 217 A (III): Universal Declaration of Human Rights*. New York: United Nations (http://www.un.org/Overview/rights.html).

UN General Assembly (1966). *Resolution 2200A (XXI): International Covenant on Civil and Political Rights*. New York: United Nations (http://www.iidh.ed.cr/docweb/instrumentos/ing/pacto%20internacional%20de%20devechos%20civiles%20y%20politics.htm).

UN General Assembly (1977). Resolution 663C(XXJV): *Standard Minimum Rules for the Treatment of Prisoners*.

UN General Assembly (1982). *Resolution 37/194: Principles of Medical Ethics*. New York: United Nations (http://www.un.org/documents/ga/res/37/a37r194.htm).

UN General Assembly (1984). *Resolution 39/46: Convention Against Torture and Other Cruel, Inhuman or Degrading Treatment or Punishment*. New York: United Nations (http://www.unhchr.ch/html/menu3/b/h_cat39.htm).

UN General Assembly (1988). *Resolution 43/173: Body of Principles for the Protection of All Persons under any Form of Detention or Imprisonment*. New York: United Nations (http://www.nchre.org/readingroom/undocuments/bpi1.shtml).

UN General Assembly (1992). *Resolution 47/133: Declaration on the Protection of all Persons from Enforced Disappearance*. New York: United Nations (http://www.unhchr.ch/huridocda/huridoca.nsf/(Symbol)/A.RES.47.133.En?OpenDocument).

UN General Assembly (2002). *Resolution A/RES/57/219: The Protection of Human Rights and Fundamental Freedoms While Countering Terrorism*. New York: United Nations (http://www.hri.ca/fortherecord2002/documentation/genassembly/a-res-57–219.htm).

Weinstein, H. (1988). *Psychiatry and the CIA: Victims of Mind Control*. Washington, DC: American Psychiatric Press.

WMA (1956). *Tenth World Medical Assembly: The Havana Declaration*. Washington, DC: World Medical Associations (http://www1.umn.edu/humanrts/instree/armedconflict.html).

WMA (1975). *29th World Medical Assembly, General Assembly: The Tokyo Declaration*. Washington, DC: World Medical Associations (http://www.wma.net/e/policy/a20.htm).

45

Access to medicines and the role of corporate social responsibility: the need to craft a global pharmaceutical system with integrity

Jillian Clare Cohen-Kohler and Patricia Illingworth

Dr. D is a primary healthcare worker in a large city in an East European country. He struggles to make ends meet for his family given his paltry income. Recently, Dr. D was approached by a multinational pharmaceutical company at his practice. He was told that for every prescription of the company's product for high blood pressure, he will receive an additional 5 dollars. Dr. D believes it is a pretty good medication but knows there are other equally effective, though much less expensive medications. He does not want to engage in unethical prescribing, but the monetary incentives offered to him make this a difficult choice.

Company E has a new drug that could considerably help to cure inflicted populations in Africa and elsewhere. However, this new product is priced well beyond the purchasing power of most persons in developing countries and would significantly drain already limited health budgets of developing country governments. The company argues that it needs to price the drug at a rate that will enable it to recoup its significant research and development costs. But people will die without access to it.

What is access to medicines and corporate social responsibility?

The phrase "access to medicines" as used in this context refers to the social problem of providing medicines to those who need them both domestically and globally. The problem exists primarily because of the high cost of these medicines. In addition, the phrase "access to medicines" has also been used to refer to the need to create medicines for disease that primarily afflict those in the developing world for which there is no market.

The term "corporate social responsibility" refers to the moral duty of corporations to provide these medicines even if it entails sacrificing profit.

Why is access to medicines and corporate social responsibility important?

Access to medicines is important both to us as individuals and collectively. From an individual point of view, pharmaceuticals make us feel better when we are sick by either treating existing health conditions to help us live or to heal us. When we are well, pharmaceuticals can prevent adverse health conditions from developing. Pharmaceuticals, if used appropriately, have the power to improve and prolong our lives. As pharmaceuticals have curative and therapeutic qualities, they cannot be considered as simply ordinary goods. Moreover, access to essential and good-quality medicines has been argued by many to be a basic human right. This is understood from the *Universal Declaration of Human Rights* and consequent covenants, although not universally accepted on the basis of philosophical reasoning.

The collective problem relates to the practical issue of ensuring access to medicines. Should we pay for individual drug treatment no matter what the price? If we assume as our premise that access to medicines is a basic human right, then what implications does this have for pharmaceutical organizations and their shareholders? Access to essential medicines has become a central topic within international policy making. It is increasingly viewed as a fundamental human right, with international human rights law placing attendant obligations on states to ensure access (Cullet, 2003). Specifically, Article 12 of the United Nations (UN) *International Covenant on Economic, Social and Cultural Rights* outlines the "right to the highest attainable standard of health," which includes the right to the availability of essential medicines as defined by the World Health Organization (WHO) (UN Committee on Economic, Social and Cultural Rights, 2000). Through the legal obligations to "respect," "protect" and "fulfill" the right to health, governments have implicit duties to ensure that pharmaceutical systems are institutionally sound, transparent, and have appropriate mechanisms to reduce the likelihood of corruption or undue influence. This includes sufficient regulation of the pharmaceutical industry to ensure that the "appropriate" corporate behavior is being practiced. Regulation of the pharmaceutical system is a core government responsibility. Unfortunately, in most developing countries, weak regulatory agencies result in lax standards.

As the required duties are not being followed, the global pharmaceutical system is unsatisfactory on several moral grounds, the most compelling of which is that access to pharmaceuticals is often a life and death issue. Until the global population has equitable and regular access to essential medicines, this morally reprehensible situation will persist. In this chapter, we argue for the need to develop global pharmaceutical systems that are commensurate with the right to essential medicines and the moral importance of access to those medicines.

To begin with, we need to address market and governmental failures and start authentically caring for others, particularly those who live beyond our borders. This perspective requires a rethinking of the primacy of market principles, particularly the primacy of shareholder interest in profit maximization over individual health needs – in this case, the right to access to affordable medicines. Access here implicitly refers to public health policies that promote affordable, appropriate, good-quality medicines as needed.

In Ghana, as an example, despite availability of pharmaceuticals in many health facilities across the country, access to drugs is largely limited by financial barriers for the majority of the population, particularly the poorest of the poor. As Management Sciences for Health (MSH) has reported, recent data indicate that 40% of Ghana's population earns less than the minimum wage and that this proportion is even higher in rural areas (MSH, 2003). As a result, the poverty level makes it difficult for patients to purchase drugs. The cost of a recommended adult treatment course for pneumonia for a minimum wage earner will be two days of wages from a private pharmacy, one and three-quarters days from a private healthcare facility, and one and a half days from a public healthcare facility (MSH, 2003).

Explaining the global drug imbalance

Global inequities in access to pharmaceuticals are stark between developed and developing countries because of market and government failures and income differences (Reich, 2000). People in developing countries make up about 80% of the population but only represent about 20% of global pharmaceutical sales (MSF [Médecins Sans Frontiéres], 2001). More specifically, high drug costs, weak or corrupt purchasing patterns and distribution systems, and the potential consequences of the Trade Related Aspects of Intellectual Property (TRIPS) agreement further constrain drug access (Henry and Lexchin, 2002). Inadequate access to essential drugs is not only a concern in less-developed countries. In the USA, for example, many seniors and uninsured people cannot afford the drugs they need (Henry and Lexchin, 2002). Even in Canada, many patients with needs for particular drug therapies (e.g., for cancer) are denied treatment because of the exorbitant drug costs.

While spending on pharmaceuticals represents less than 20% of total public and private health spending in most countries belonging to the Organisation for Economic Co-operation and Development, it represents 15–30% of health spending in transitional economies and 25–66% in developing states. In most low-income states, pharmaceuticals are the largest public expenditure on health after personnel costs and the largest household health expenditure. Family illness, including drugs, is a major cause of household poverty in developing states (Velasquez *et al.*, 1998). One of the major differences between developing countries and advanced economies is that in developing countries the majority of pharmaceutical expenditure represents out-of-pocket payments: anywhere from 50% to 90% (Velasquez *et al.*, 1998). Consider that, along with the fact that about 1.3 billion persons survive on a dollar a day, and we understand plainly why there is a drug gap. If provision of pharmaceuticals is not being covered within the public sector and patients must rely on out-of-pocket payments for their drug needs, many will simply not be able to afford them.

How should I approach access to medicines and corporate social responsibility in practice?

Government failures

Many of the problems with access to essential medicines are best corrected by governments and international organizations. The inequities in the pharmaceutical system do not result from one single factor but rather from a complex interweaving of many. One of these is government deficiencies. More government spending on health generally and pharmaceuticals (including infrastructure) in particular is a necessary condition for improving access to pharmaceuticals. The WHO's Commission on Macroeconomics and Health found that basic healthcare spending in the poorest countries would require $57 billion in 2007. This would be the necessary annual health outlay for both health infrastructures and the care against infectious diseases and nutritional deficiencies (WHO, 2001). In many of these developing countries, the overall health expenditure may be as little as US$10–12 per person per year (WHO, 2003). Furthermore, in 1999, 39 of 94 reporting countries (41%) had a public drug expenditure of less than US$2 per person per year despite having large numbers of people living with the human immunodeficiency virus (HIV) and the acquired immunodeficiency syndrome (AIDS) (WHO, 2000). On top of this inadequate percentage of spending on health and drug expenditure, inefficiencies and/or corruption in the prescription, storage, and use of drugs in developing countries are such that some countries do not gain enough from allocated budgets. (See Cohen [2006] for more on this issue.) The failures of developing country governments are both internal – through poor governance – and external – through external forces such as structural adjustment programs that enforce reduced expenditure on healthcare systems. In addition, the arms trade and the mechanisms through which debts are created by developed nations further impoverish poor countries.

Market failures

Markets work effectively and efficiently when there is real price competition, comprehensive and accurate information, an adequate supply of drugs, consumers are able to make informed and beneficial choices between competing products, and there are few barriers for entry to the market. However, there is significant evidence that allowing markets to reign supreme in relation to pharmaceuticals does not lead to desirable outcomes because pharmaceutical markets are not typical for a myriad of reasons. Firstly, consumers do not typically make choices about their pharmaceutical needs. Their healthcare provider prescribes a medicine for them and may not always act in the best interest of the patients but rather on the basis of self-interest. This is the classic principal-agent dilemma. Secondly, there are information asymmetries between consumers and healthcare providers, between healthcare providers and manufacturers, as well as between manufacturers and governments. Patent protection means that there are market monopolies for products, which prevents price competition and essentially distorts the market.

We are compelled to think about access of the poorest to essential medicines because as the numbers point out the inequities are glaring. There is an 80/20 distortion in the global pharmaceutical market. Even though developing countries represent about 80% of the global population, they represent a relatively small proportion of the global pharmaceutical market, about 20% of the global value, thus providing limited market incentives for the development of new drugs specific to diseases of those countries (including many tropical diseases). Since 1973, more than 25 new infectious diseases have emerged, all requiring treatment with pharmaceuticals. Some infectious diseases, such as HIV/AIDS, are global in their scope and are particularly devastating. Other diseases like cholera, tuberculosis, and malaria are mainly disease burdens of developing states. New infectious diseases such as the severe acute respiratory syndrome (SARS) continue to evolve and require drug treatments.

One of the arguments industry raises for the application of robust intellectual property law is that it could conceivably promote research and development of products in those markets that formerly did not adhere to strict intellectual property standards. But this is unlikely to happen anytime in the near future given that we see limited spending on diseases of the poor despite increased global expenditure on health research and development. In 2001, an estimated US$70 billion was invested globally in health research and development, with the private sector in the USA alone accounting for just under half of the spending (MSF, 2001). An analysis of drug development outcomes since 1975 shows that only 15 new drugs were indicated for tropical diseases and tuberculosis (MSF, 2001). These diseases primarily affect poor populations and account for 12% of the global disease burden. In comparison, 179 new drugs were developed for cardiovascular diseases that represent 11% of the global burden of disease. Finally,

out of the 1393 new drugs approved between 1975 and 1999, only 16 (or just over 1%) were specifically developed for tropical diseases and tuberculosis, diseases that account for 11.4% of the global disease burden. The WHO's Commission on Intellectual Property Rights, Innovation, and Public Health (CIPIH, 2006, p. 13) identified an interdependence between poverty, disease burden, and research capacity: "poverty affects purchasing power, and the inability of poor people to pay reduces effective demand, which in turn affects the degree of interest of for-profit companies."

How commensurate are pharmaceutical prices with the costs of research and development? And, should profit maximization supersede life-saving medicines for those most in need? If market principles encourage profit maximization, surely we need to rethink its incentive structures and use regulatory methods to infuse a criterion of compassion, along with equity, fairness, and interdependence, in the quest for profit maximization. The view that corporations can make profits and do "good" should not be an empty slogan but a real practice. The issue of fair profits also tends to creep into pharmaceutical policy dialogue. This is raised primarily because of the corporate success of the research-based pharmaceutical industry. Critics of the pharmaceutical industry also focus on issues beyond the ethical problems associated with drug access. Drs. Arnold Relman and Marcia Angell (former editors of the *New England Journal of Medicine*) wrote a highly controversial article in which they criticized drug companies for lack of innovation and noted that most of the new drugs are simply copies of those which are already in the market (Relman and Angell, 2002). These types of drug are known by the industry as "me too" pharmaceuticals; many new innovative drug are based on government research. They are not alone in citing this point. The National Institute for Health Care Management (2002) reported that the majority of drug application approvals by the US Food and Drug Administration from 1989 to 2000 were for drugs that contained active ingredients already in the market.

Relman and Angell (2002) were also critical of drug company efforts to extend their patent rights through patent extensions, known as "evergreening", in an effort to block competition from the production of less-costly generic drugs.

The moral dilemmas of intellectual property law for pharmaceuticals

The TRIPS Agreement extended patent protection to a lengthy period of 20 years (prior to TRIPS, even the USA, which has had a robust patent regime for pharmaceuticals, had a shorter period for the patent life: 17 years). The TRIPS Agreement included and surpassed most of the past provisions of the international agreements on the protection of intellectual property rights (Schott, 2000). It required each member state to maintain sufficient procedures and remedies within its body of domestic law to ensure protection of intellectual property. These procedures and remedies must also be made available to foreign right holders.

We argue that the TRIPS Agreement is morally unsatisfactory because it does not help to improve global drug access even with the inclusion of its "safety valves." For example, the Doha *Declaration on the TRIPS Agreement and Public Health* by the World Trade Organization (2001) and the implementation of paragraph 6 in August 2003 suggested a means for selective disengagement by permitting those countries that do not have the capacity to manufacture medicines to still use compulsory licensing by contracting-out agreements with firms in other countries. This unleashes the potential for more competition in the pharmaceutical market, more drug supply for those in need. For now, this is particularly relevant for antiretroviral therapy. Despite the positive outcome, the accord is limited by a number of administrative procedures, such as requiring both the importing and exporting countries to issue compulsory licenses, ensuring that the World Trade Organization is involved in the overseeing of the procedures, plus other stipulations; these effectively limit its application in countries.

Access to medicines and corporate social responsibility

There are a number of ways that the obligation to provide essential medicines to the developing world might be met (Cohen and Illingworth, 2003) by the private sector and also the healthcare professional. Those obligations fall on many different parties and are grounded in a variety of moral concerns. There are, in other words, enough moral obligations and responsibilities to go around. Similarly, there are a number of different ways that help can be rendered, such as through greater investment in infrastructure and the training and development of sufficient personnel to administer medicines to those who need it. Our obligations to the "distant needy" have been defended and are based on many different considerations, including, and perhaps most persuasively, that which states that those of us in the developed world have both *inflicted* harms on people living in the developing world and *benefited* from the corruption and inhumanity that exist there (Pogge, 2004).

We thus begin with the assumption that everyone in the developed world has obligations to those in the developing world (Pogge, 2004; Singer, 2004). The question is, then, whether or not pharmaceutical companies are for some reason exempt from these obligations. Arguably, pharmaceutical companies have a competing obligation to their shareholders that overrides the standing obligation all people have to those in the developing world (Friedman, 2004). We argue that while pharmaceutical companies do indeed have an obligation of loyalty to shareholders that obligation does not override the obligations they have to fulfill the right to essential medicines of people in the developing world. We reason that not only are pharmaceutical companies not exempt from the obligation shared by all in the developed world but, if anything, they have a special duty to provide medical aid, in the way of essential medicines, by virtue of the fact that the medical sphere is morally special. This imperative applies to both international and local pharmaceutical producers, the latter being major producers in many low- and middle-income countries, such as Brazil, India, and South Africa.

Corporate social responsibility and the right to essential medicines

Corporate social responsibility is the obligation of corporations to do good and to confer benefits on the community: to give back to the community (Freeman, 2004). It implies a duty on the part of corporations to give, even when satisfying the duty may be inconsistent with the making of excessive profits. Corporate social responsibility can be justi-fied on a number of different moral bases. It can, for example, be justified on the grounds of beneficence, the duty to do good and to avoid or prevent harm (Frankena, 1973). It could also be justified on a utilitarian basis, that corporate social responsibility will maximize good consequences, and has been justified on the basis of stakeholder obligations (Freeman, 2004). At present, few pharmaceutical corporations would quarrel with the need to engage in some kind of corporate social responsibility and, specifically, to contribute to world health (Mills *et al.*, 2006). Indeed, many pharmaceutical companies already donate some essential medicines to those who need them in the developing world and include a statement about such giving in their corporate mission statements. Although we applaud these charitable acts of pharmaceutical companies, we do not think they go far enough, since premature and unnecessary death continues in such countries. Consequently, it may be that the mere act of giving, as a matter of corporate social responsibility, is not adequate to meet the *rights* to essential medicines of those in the developing world. By asking that pharmaceutical companies fulfill the duty to do good, we also argue that they need to modify their marketing practices particularly in developing countries so that healthcare workers are not unduly influenced to prescribe a particular drug.

There is certainly a moral right on the part of the world's poor and sick, often children, to essential medicines, and that right is based on the dire urgency of the need. Many of the diseases that afflict those in the developing world are indirectly associated with poverty, some of which is historic-ally linked to the adverse activities of the developed world (Pogge, 2004). In addition, as Thomas Pogge has argued, assisting the world's poor is at least partially a negative duty to stop inflicting harms (e.g., sustaining corrupt powers).

When rights are at issue, considerations of justice demand enforcement of the rights (Ashford, 2007). Rights cannot be left to the whimsy of the supererogatory duties implicit in corporate social responsibility. Rights would seem to require that pharmaceutical companies set aside some of their property rights (e.g., patents) for the sake of those in the developing world who may not have a strict legal claim in that property. Patents are not the only problem for those in the developing world. Rights may require that pharmaceutical companies undertake research and development in order to identify treatment for neglected diseases.

There have been important approaches to creat-ing ways to meet the right to essential medicines. Thomas Pogge (2004) has identified an interesting revision to the pharmaceutical incentive system that might overcome some of these incentive problems, and public–private partnerships suggest another way of meeting this problem (Light, 2006). Both these approaches, however, try to meet pharmaceutical companies on their own terms; that is, they try to appeal to the profit motive of pharmaceutical companies and their shareholders. This, of course, has the distinct advantage of pro-viding an attractive, realistic, and potentially long-term solution to the problem. Although we applaud both of these approaches, we believe that it is important, nonetheless, to keep uppermost in our minds the deeply held moral conviction that people have a *right* to essential medicines. As a result, failure to provide them is a human rights violation. The language of human rights *is* important not only because it establishes the standard of justice to be invoked but also because it carries with it an important narrative meaning about our moral and perhaps legal obligations to the developing world.

The duty to help the developing world falls on many, including pharmaceutical companies (Scientific Organising Committee for the Montréal Statement, 2005). There are many reasons why pharmaceutical companies are obligated to meet these rights, many of which have been stated elsewhere (Cohen *et al.*, 2006). Pharmaceutical companies not only share the same duty to help with all members of the global community but they also have an even higher responsibility. We argue that pharmaceutical companies as medical entities committed to human health have the duty to render aid to the sick. Healthcare needs, as well as the people and organizations that meet them, have heightened responsibilities. Medical needs are special and they have been uniformly recognized as special (UN Department of Public Information, 2005; WHO, 2006). In part, they are special because of the role they play in sustaining the lives of humans (Scientific Organising Committee for the Montréal Statement, 2005) and in maintaining the security, value, and integrity of those lives. Arguably, individuals and entities involved in the medical field incur certain special responsibilities because of the moral importance of medical needs. Physicians are expected to meet medical needs, such as providing emergency care, even when it is inconvenient, or they may be required to put themselves at risk in order to help others, as with contagions or bioterrorism.

Healthcare providers, unlike the common bystander, are presumed to be in a position to render reasonable aid. This important duty of medical providers also suggests that people's physical well-being is valued morally, and because providers are well positioned to render medical aid, they have a duty to do so. (There is not, for example, and regrettably, such a duty to render IT services in the event of an emergency computer crash.) Arguably, the moral intuitions that underlie this duty should also hold true for pharmaceutical companies – unless they have a conflicting obligation that overrides this duty. Just as healthcare providers are required to render aid in an emergency, so, we believe, are pharmaceutical companies. Pharmaceutical companies, like

physicians, have the knowledge and skills needed to meet important healthcare needs and rights. Both have a duty to ensure that pharmaceutical prescribing represents the right drug for the right person at the right time.

The dire need alone of the afflicted and dying in a global community should be a sufficiently compelling reason to have pharmaceutical companies act for the benefit of them. Of course, this reasoning could also be applied to other organizations with the unique wherewithal and skill set to render aid. Farmers, grocery stores, and other food purveyors, for example, are likely to have a duty to provide food to the global hungry. Indeed, such a duty was enacted in the USA at the national level with the Federal Bill Emerson Good Samaritan Food Donation Act (US Congress, 1996).

Just as physicians are asked, and expected, to put themselves at risk, to help the sick, it is reasonable to expect pharmaceutical companies to risk some profits in order to provide essential medicines to those in the developing world who will die without them. We believe that a moral paradigm shift is required to complement the needed revisions of the patent system, proposed by Pogge (2006) and others. That shift must include the conviction that rights trump profits. Such a right would, of course, extend beyond the case of pharmaceutical companies. It would also apply to healthcare plans such as managed care organizations. If, and especially in the healthcare arena, the best way to ensure that rights are not sacrificed to profits is through nationalized healthcare systems, such an approach would be morally required.

It would indeed be difficult to make the case that money is more important than saving lives. This is especially so if it were also the case that most of those profits were to fall on those who live in wealthy western countries and who have, in some sense and even if indirectly, caused the poverty and associated disease (Pogge, 2004; Ashford, 2007). There are no compelling arguments to justify putting money before lives.

One might argue in defense of pharmaceutical companies that they and their shareholders are entitled to these profits, and the actions that are necessary to yield these profits, because of an implicit or explicit agreement between shareholders and pharmaceutical companies. But are there not many reasons to think that, if this agreement unnecessarily entails that some people die while others line their pockets with corporate dividends, it is unconscionable. Although agreements are in general respected, in the case of necessities the courts have been more flexible, as they should be, and have set aside signed contracts that impair the ''right'' to necessities (*Hennigsen* v. *Bloomfield Motors, Inc.*, 1960). Shareholders who benefit from the patent system, while part of an unjust system, may have an even greater moral responsibility for the harm that indirectly results from this system. In any case, as Elizabeth Ashford (2007) has so eloquently argued, there is good reason to think that many in the West are indirectly causally responsible for the denial of basic human rights.

The cases

It is important to keep in mind that physicians are professionals, and that they must at all times meet the high ethical standards of their profession. These standards can guide clinicians through the moral dilemmas posed by access issues, including those presented in the cases with which we began. Dr. D's primary duty is to his patients' welfare including cultivating and maintaining the trust between doctor and patient. Prescribing medicines on the basis of personal gain would jeopardize trust between patient and physician and is, therefore, unethical (Illingworth, 2006). Professionalism also includes a commitment to advocate on behalf of medical service, to patient welfare in general, and social justice worldwide. Given this, physicians and other providers can engage in activism directed at ensuring essential medicines worldwide.

We have argued that pharmaceutical companies, such as company E, have an obligation to *aid* the sick and dying in the developing world in much the same way that physicians have such a duty. We argued for this obligation on the basis that pharmaceutical companies have indirectly caused harm to those in the developing world; the conflicting duties that pharmaceutical companies have to shareholders are easily defeated by showing that the human right to basic necessities overrides shareholders' rights to unlimited profits, and pharmaceutical companies (and their investors) have special duties in virtue of the medical mission. This also demands that pharmaceutical companies do not price products out of reach for those in need and also do not resort to unethical marketing practices such as through material incentives to those healthcare workers who are most susceptible. In addition, healthcare workers who prescribe medicines need to ensure that they are prescribing with the patient's health as a priority and are not prescribing a product because of the influence of a particular pharmaceutical company. This involves ensuring that any interaction with the pharmaceutical industry does not represent personal gain.

REFERENCES

Ashford, E. (2007). The duties imposed by the human right to basic necessities. In *Freedom From Poverty as a Human Right: Who Owes What to the Very Poor?* ed. T. Pogge. Oxford: Oxford University Press, p. 210.

CIPIH (2006). *Public Health, Innovation and Intellectual Property Rights*. Geneva: World Health Organization Commission on Intellectual Property Rights, Innovation and Public Health.

Cohen, J. (2006). Pharmaceuticals and corruption: a risk assessment. In *Transparency International, Global Corruption Report 2006*. London: Pluto Press for Transparency International, p. 77.

Cohen, J. and Illingworth, P. (2003). The dilemma of international property rights for pharmaceuticals: the tension between securing access of the poor to medicines and committing to international agreements. *Devel World Bioethics* **3**: 27–48.

Cohen, J., Illingworth, P., and Schuklenk, U. (eds.) (2006). *The Power of Pills: Social, Ethical, and Legal Issues in Drug Development, Marketing, and Pricing*. London: Pluto Press.

Cullet, P. (2003). Patents and medicines: the relationship between TRIPS and the human right to health. *Int Affairs* **79**: 139–60.

Frankena, W. (1973). *Ethics*. Englewood Cliffs, NJ: Prentice Hall.

Freeman, R. (2004). A stakeholder theory of the modern corporation. In *Ethical Theory and Business*, ed. T. L. Beauchamp and N. E. Bowie. Upper Saddle River, NJ: Pearson Prentice Hall, pp. 55–64.

Friedman, M. (2004). The social responsibility of business is to increase its profits. In *Ethical Theory and Business*, ed. T. L. Beauchamp and N. E. Bowie. Upper Saddle River, NJ: Pearson Prentice Hall, pp. 50–5.

Hennigsen v. *Bloomfield Motors, Inc.* (1960). 32 N.J. 358, 161 A.2d 69.

Henry, D. and Lexchin, J. (2002). The pharmaceutical industry as a medicines provider. *Lancet* **360**: 1590–5.

Illingworth, P. (2006). *Trusting Medicine*. London: Routledge.

Light, D. (2006). Advance purchase commitments: moral and practical problems. In *The Power of Pills: Social, Ethical and Legal Issues in Drug Development, Marketing and Pricing*, ed. J. Cohen, P. Illingworth, and U. Schuklenk. London: Pluto Press, pp. 230–43.

Mills, A., Werhane P., and Gorman M. (2006). The pharmaceutical industry and its obligations in the developing world. In *The Power of Pills: Social, Ethical and Legal Issues in Drug Development, Marketing and Pricing*, ed. J. Cohen, P. Illingworth, and U. Schuklenk. London: Pluto Press, pp. 57–74.

MSF (2001). *Fatal Imbalance: The Crisis in Research and Development for Drugs for Neglected Diseases*. Geneva: Medécins Sans Frontiéres Access to Essential Medicines Campaign and the Drugs for Neglected Diseases Working Group (http://www.msf.org/source/access/2001/fatal/fatalshort.pdf) accessed 9 October 2001.

MSH (2003). *Strategies for Enhancing Access to Medicines (SEAM), Ghana: Key Findings*. Management Sciences for Health Cambridge, MA (www.msh.org) accessed 5 November 2003.

National Institute for Health Care Management (2002). *Changing Patterns of Pharmaceutical Innovation*. Washington, DC: National Institute for Health Care Management (www.nihcm.org).

Pogge, T. (2004). "Assisting" the global poor. In *The Ethics of Assistance*, ed. D. K. Chatterjee. Cambridge, UK: Cambridge University Press, pp. 260–88.

Pogge, T. (2006). The Montréal Statement on the Human Right to Essential Medicines. *Camb Q Healthc Ethics*. **16**: 97–108.

Reich, M. (2000). The global drug gap. *Science* **287**: 1979–81.

Relman, A. S. and Angell, M. (2002). America's other drug problem. *The New Republic* **16**: 27–41.

Schott, J. (ed.) (2000). *The WTO after Seattle*. Washington, DC: Institute for International Economics, p. 115.

Scientific Organising Committee for the Montréal Statement (2005). *The Montréal Statement on the Human Right to Essential Medicines*. International Workshop on Human Rights and Access to Essential Medicines. Montréal: University of Montréal.

Singer, P. (2004). *One World: The Ethics of Globalization*. New Haven, CT: Yale University Press.

UN Committee on Economic, Social and Cultural Rights (2000). *General Comment No. 14: Substantive Issues Arising in the Implementation of the International Covenant on Economic, Social and Cultural Rights, E/C.12/2000/4*. New York: United Nations (http://www.unhchr.ch/tbs/doc.nsf/(symbol)/E.C.12.2000.4.En?OpenDocument) accessed 24 March 2005.

UN Department of Public Information (2005). *The Universal Declaration of Human Rights*. Geneva: United Nations (http://www.unhchr.ch/udhr/index.htm) accessed 2 June 2006.

United States Congress (1996). The Federal Bill Emerson Good Samaritan Food Donation Act of 1996, Pub. L. No. 104–210.

Velasquez, G., Madrid, Y., and Quick, J. (1998). *Health Reform and Drug Financing, Selected Topics. Health Economics and Drugs*. DAP series [No. 6; WHO/DAP/98.3] Geneva: World Health Organization (http://whqlibdoc.who.int/hq/1998/WHO_DAP_98.3.pdf).

WHO (2000). *WHO Medicines Strategy: 2000–2003. Framework for Action in Essential Drugs and Medicines Policy*. Geneva: World Health Organization Department of Essential Drugs and Medicines Policy, Health Technology and Pharmaceuticals Cluster (http://www.who.int/medicines/strategy/strategy.pdf).

WHO (2001). *Macroeconomics and Health: Investing in Health for Economic Development.* Geneva: World Health Organization Commission on Macroeconomics and Health (www3.who.int/whosis/cmh/cmh_report/e/pdf/cmh_english).

WHO (2003). Access to essential medicines: a global necessity. *Essential Drugs Monitor* **32**: 13 (http://www.who.int/medicines/mon/32_6.pdf).

WHO (2006). *The Declaration of Alma-Ata.* Geneva: World Health Organization (http://www.who.int/chronic_conditions/primary_health_care/en/almaata_declaration.pdf) accessed 2 June 2006.

World Trade Organization (2001). *Declaration on the TRIPS Agreement and Public Health.* Geneva: World Trade Organization.

46

Global health and non-ideal justice

Gopal Sreenivasan

The United Nations Development Program (2005) gave the following statistics for 2003.

Japan has a population of 127.7 million people and a per capita income of $27 967. Average life expectancy is 82 years, highest in the world.
Earth has a population of 6.3 billion people and a per capita income of $8229. Average life expectancy is 67.1 years.
Yemen has a population of 19.7 million people and a per capita income of $889. Average life expectancy is 60.6 years.
Zambia has a population of 11.3 million people and a per capita income of $877. Average life expectancy is 37.5, fifth lowest in the world.

International inequalities in life expectancy are simply staggering. Ten countries, all in sub-Saharan Africa, have average life expectancies at birth that are, like Zambia's, 25 years or more below the global *average* (and 40 years or more below that for Japan). In 33 countries, all but two in sub-Saharan Africa, life expectancy at birth is 15 years or more below the global average. Intuitively, these inequalities in basic life prospects seem plainly unjust. But can this intuitive conviction be vindicated by an argument? If present international inequalities in life expectancy *are* unjust, what obligations do rich nations – or their individual citizens – have to remedy the injustice? This chapter offers answers to both questions.

What are the obligations of international distributive justice?

For simplicity, we can divide competing views of the obligations owed to the global poor into three categories: the global rich owe them a lot, a little, or nothing. The traditional utilitarian answer is that the global rich owe them *a lot*. In particular, they (i.e., we) are obligated to give as much of our personal income to the global poor as is required to bring them up to our level of well-being. Peter Singer (1972), the Australian philosopher, famously argued for this answer on the basis of what is, in effect, a Good Samaritan principle: if one can prevent a very grave harm from befalling another person, at no more than a trivial cost to oneself, then one is obligated to prevent the harm, that is, to help the other person. However, many people reject the utilitarian answer because the obligation it imposes is "too demanding," and Singer's argument for it is controversial, not least because it depends on a rather controversial interpretation of which costs are properly discounted as "trivial."

Despite these controversies, the Good Samaritan principle itself remains eminently plausible. This suggests a simple argument for the second kind of view, on which the global rich at least owe the global poor *a little*. Let us consider a more specific version of this answer: the richest nations minimally have an obligation to transfer 1% of their gross domestic product (GDP) to the poorest nations. For added concreteness, imagine this as an obligation incumbent on the "major seven" (G7) countries of the Organisation for Economic Co-operation and Development (OECD). In that case, for 2004, we are considering an obligation to transfer some $241.5 billion (OECD, 2005, p. 13). By contrast, in 2004, official development assistance (ODA) from the G7 was a mere 0.22% of GDP or $56.686 billion (OECD, 2005, p. 65). So even a 1% transfer would represent a clear improvement over the status quo.

From the standpoint of a rich nation (or individual), 1% of annual income is a trivial cost. I take it that this holds true on a completely straightforward and uncontroversial interpretation of "trivial cost." Hence, according to the Good Samaritan principle, if transferring 1% of GDP can prevent very grave harms from befalling the inhabitants of poor countries, the G7 has an obligation to make the transfer. Unlike the utilitarian obligation, a 1% obligation cannot be rejected as "too demanding." If that is right, then it seems there is little to be said – at least, not at the level of principle – in favor of the third view, on which the global poor are owed *nothing*.

Why is it important to act on the 1% obligation?

But is 1% *enough* to prevent very grave harms from befalling (very many of) the global poor? To invoke the Good Samaritan principle, we must be able to supply an affirmative answer on this point. Perhaps any obligation that imposes only a trivial burden on the rich would likewise produce only a trivial benefit for the poor. Fortunately, this is decidedly not the case. To see how much good 1% of G7 GDP might do, as well as to bring out the connection between global health and global justice, let us examine what might reasonably be expected from spending the 1% on improving the *health* of the globally worst off.

Global health

We should begin by reviewing the fundamental *determinants* of health in developing countries, which is what efforts to improve the health of the globally worst off would need to target.

1. **Basic health care**. Public health and primary healthcare systems are important determinants of health, especially in developing countries. Preston (1980) estimated that at least 50% of the improvements in mortality rates by developing countries between 1940 and 1970 were the result of factors *other than* income, literacy, and nutrition. While this remainder includes unknown factors, he attributed a significant part of it to public health measures. Immunization, vector control, clean water, and sanitation all play a significant role in reducing mortality in developing countries (Caldwell, 1986).

2. **Individual income**. There is general agreement that, at least in developing countries, an individual's absolute income (i.e., its *non*-comparative level) makes a significant contribution to his or her life expectancy. Certain conditions of absolute material deprivation – notably inadequate nutrition, but also lack of clean water and sanitation, and poor housing – constitute well-recognized risks for ill-health and death. A very plausible causal pathway runs from low levels of individual income through these material risk factors to lower individual life expectancy (Preston, 1980; Caldwell, 1986).

3. **Education**. A final fundamental determinant of health is education. In developing countries, *female* education in particular correlates very highly with infant and child (under five) life expectancy, even after controlling for income and other factors (Hobcraft, 1993; Subbarao and Raney, 1995). Mothers with primary schooling have child mortality rates 26% lower than mothers with no schooling, while mothers with secondary schooling have rates 36% lower again than mothers with only primary schooling (Filmer and Pritchett, 1999). Subbarao and Raney (1995) estimated that doubling female secondary school enrollments in 1975 (to 38%, from the actual 19%) would have lowered annual infant deaths in 1985 by 64%.

As this brief review suggests, to improve the health of the globally worst off, resource transfers should be targeted at (i) primary health care and public health, (ii) basic nutrition and income support, and (iii) education (especially for girls and women). If we allocated 0.25% of G7 GDP to each of these fundamental determinants, that would still leave

0.25% to cover existing development commitments (presently, recall, at 0.22%). A transfer of 0.75% of GDP from the G7 would fund a per capita package of $144 for 1.26 billion people, which covers the world's poorest quintile.

Suppose, then, that $144 were spent annually per capita on the three fundamental determinants of health in jurisdictions where life expectancy is 15 years or more below the global average: this includes not only many countries of sub-Saharan Africa but also the worst-off Indian states and Chinese provinces (Gwatkin *et al.*, 1999). What kind of improvement in life expectancy might one reasonably expect? To judge by the historical record, the answer is "a very significant improvement." I have in mind the experience of those developing countries that have achieved exceptional life expectancy despite a very low GDP. Among "open societies," they include Sri Lanka (life expectancy, 71 years), Kerala (71 years; an Indian state, but with a population of 30 million), and Costa Rica (77 years). Among "closed" societies, they include China (71 years), Cuba (77 years), and Vietnam (71 years). In all of these societies, life expectancy is notably *higher* than the global average (67.1), and this was achieved precisely by following the path of concerted investment in (i) primary healthcare and public health; (ii) the provision of a nutritional floor; and (iii) basic education, including for girls (and, thus, a high degree of literacy among women) (Caldwell, 1986; Mehrotra and Jolly, 1997). As Caldwell concluded (1986, p. 209): "These findings ... show that low mortality is indeed within the reach of all countries."

Equally important for our purposes is the fact that the absolute cost of following this path to higher life expectancy is quite low. In fact, 0.75% of G7 GDP is enough to fund the described per capita package for the world's poorest quintile at levels comparable to those actually employed by the high-achieving developing countries. That is partly because $144 per capita is a real dollar figure, whereas cross-national comparisons should be made in purchasing power parity (PPP) equivalents. Since the relevant PPP multiplier can be conservatively set at three,

$144 (PPP) can be spent per capita on *each* of the three fundamental determinants. By way of comparison, in Sri Lanka for example, total health expenditure in 2002 was $131 (PPP) per capita (UN Development Program, 2005) and public educational expenditure in 1995–7 was $100 (PPP) per capita (UN Development Program, 2001) (recently, it has been less).

Now this is not to claim that any developing country that manages to spend $432 (PPP) annually per capita on the fundamental determinants of health will succeed in lifting the life expectancy of its inhabitants above (or even, to) the global average. However, the evidence does make it reasonable to expect substantial progress in that direction. To fix ideas, let us say that life expectancy in the worst-off jurisdictions could thereby be raised 10 years. Since a 10 year *loss* in life expectancy certainly qualifies as a "very grave harm," the opportunity to avert this outcome at a trivial cost, therefore, satisfies the terms of a Good Samaritan obligation. On this basis, we may conclude that the G7 are obligated to transfer 1% of their GDP to the world's worst-off jurisdictions.

Non-ideal theory

If the global rich owe the global poor at least a little, it follows that they do not owe them nothing. But it does not follow that the global rich do not owe *more* than just a little. It may still be, for example, that they owe 5 or 10% of GDP, rather than simply 1%. On what basis can we say that the global rich do not owe more than 1%? As far as the ideal theory of justice is concerned, we cannot say it – how much more, if anything, the rich owe remains an open question.

Yet if we adopt the perspective of non-ideal theory, things are different. In non-ideal theory, the aim is not to settle the ideal requirements of justice, finally and completely. Rather, it is (among other things) to define *interim* targets for practical action, toward which progress can be made before a complete ideal has been settled in theory. Non-ideal theory proceeds here by anticipating the minimum requirements that any plausible and complete ideal theory of justice will include, and it does so by identifying a common core of requirements on which plausible contending ideal theories agree. Hence, for practical purposes, non-ideal theory simply sets the question of what *else* justice may require aside. Theoretical disagreements about whether the G7 owe more than 1% of GDP need not, and should not, obstruct efforts to act on the 1% obligation in the here and now.

In fact, for similar reasons, we need not regard the Good Samaritan argument as *the* decisive basis of the obligation either. Agreement on the 1% obligation can be secured among a significant coalition of rival moral theories. Each can endorse the obligation for its own reasons. Arguably, this coalition includes utilitarians, global egalitarians and prioritarians of various kinds, decent humanitarians, as well as many decent ordinary people. More specifically, potential members include such diverse theorists as Singer himself (2002, p. 192) and Thomas Pogge (2002, Ch. 8), both of whom explicitly endorse a 1% minimum, and, outside of philosophy, (economist) Jeffrey Sachs (2005, Ch. 15) and (musician–activist) Bono, who endorse the UN's Pearson target of 0.7% of GDP.

Moreover, this coalition can be made broader still. For example, Rawls (1999, pp. 114–18) rejected the idea of *permanent* obligations of international distributive justice. Nevertheless, he did acknowledge certain obligations of transitional justice, which aim to assist "burdened societies" to become "well-ordered," in part through meeting the basic needs of their inhabitants. Transitional obligations are distinguished from permanent ones by their built-in "cut-off point." To bring Rawls and his followers on board, then, it suffices to add a suitable cut-off point to the 1% obligation. Let us say that the obligation cuts off when no country – better still, *or* Indian state or Chinese province – has an average life expectancy of 10 years or more below the global average. When that point has been reached, the question of whether the G7's obligation to transfer 1% of GDP annually to the worst-off jurisdictions

is a permanent obligation or not will acquire practical purchase. But until then, non-ideal theory can safely ignore it.

Likewise, libertarians may reject the idea that the 1% transfer is an obligation of *justice*, or perhaps even that it is in any way *obligatory*, preferring instead to regard it as a humanitarian act of *charity*. Often this stance is driven as much by the conviction that humanitarian relief is always discretionary and supererogatory as it is by opposition to claims of (international) distributive justice. Now, as a philosophical matter, it is actually a mistake to think that charity is never strictly obligatory or morally mandatory (Buchanan, 1987). Again, in non-ideal theory, this does not matter so much. The crucial qualification for membership in our coalition is *willingness* – willingness to transfer 1% of income to improve the well-being of the globally worst off – including, if need be, willingness accompanied by insistence on the description "discretionary transfer." Consequently, libertarian scruples need be no impediment, either to a G7 nation's transferring 1% of its GDP to the worst-off jurisdictions or to a moral theory's endorsing the transfer.

How might the 1% obligation work in practice?

Since clinicians are professionally committed to improving the health of those in need, and likely sensitive to the urgent claims of the worst off, many may feel that the most pressing concerns about the 1% obligation are practical, rather than theoretical. While there is a whole level of important detail that we do not have space to address here – concerning the issue of aid effectiveness, for example, or subdivisions of responsibility between global and local actors – I do want briefly to address a pair of strategic practical objections. I thereby hope to allow the proposal at least to keep its foot in the doorway to action.

In the real world, of course, not everyone discharges his or her obligations adequately. When some actors shirk their obligations within a given distributive scheme, and so do less than their fair share, what does justice require of the remaining actors – the compliant ones, who have already done their (original) fair share? Does justice consequently require the compliant to do yet more, and to pick up the slack created by the non-compliant? Certainly not, as this would be extremely unfair (Murphy, 2000).

Accommodating this concern belongs to a different branch of non-ideal theory, which functions to calibrate the requirements of justice under conditions of *partial* compliance. In the present instance, we should regard the 1% obligation assigned to each G7 nation as *invariant* under non-compliance by other G7 nations. That is to say, if one of the G7 were to transfer 1% of its GDP annually to developing nations (at present, none does), then the non-ideal theory of justice would require nothing further of it. Its fair share is limited to 1% – even if no other G7 nation complies at all with *its* obligation, with the result that life expectancy remains 15 years or more below the global average in many more jurisdictions than would reasonably be expected under full compliance by the G7.

A slight twist on this point also helps to answer a second practical objection to the 1% proposal, which has to do with the prevalence of corruption and waste. Even someone who accepts, in principle, an obligation to improve the well-being of the globally worst off, and who is also prepared to act on it, may reasonably baulk if it turns out that, in fact, this 1% will simply disappear down a black hole of corruption. There is no obligation to line the pockets of the corrupt, no matter how many destitute there may be, unreached, in the background.

The objection is well-taken up to a point, but it still does not defeat the proposal. Invariance under non-compliance cuts both ways: while each G7 nation is only responsible for its fair share, it remains responsible for its fair share *even if* none of the others comply. Let me illustrate and then explain. I shall take Italy as my example, since in 2004 Italian ODA (0.15%) was actually the furthest from 1% in the G7 (OECD, 2005, p. 64). But in 2004, 0.85% of Italian GDP (1% minus existing ODA) was $13.687 billion (OECD, 2005, p. 12). Under full compliance (by the G7), Italy would be responsible for transferring that $13.687 billion at a rate of $144 per capita. In other words, Italy's fair share of improvements in the fundamental determinants of health among the world's poorest quintile would cover a population of 95.05 million people.

Non-compliance by the rest of the G7 does not relieve Italy of *its* obligation to transfer 1% of GDP. Moreover, 1% is also small enough that no G7 nation can – and hence, Italy cannot – plausibly claim that solitary compliance will put it at any serious relative disadvantage within its peer group (i.e., the G7). If need be, then, Italy should simply go it alone and transfer $13.687 billion annually to the globally worst off at the full compliance rate of $144 per capita. To do so, Italy would have to choose a mix of jurisdictions where life expectancy is 10 years or more below the global average (our cut-off point, recall), up to a total population of 95.05 million people (e.g., roughly a seventh of the population of sub-Saharan Africa).

Transferring its 1% on this basis would enable Italy to cover the same fair share of the globally worst off as it would cover under full compliance by the G7 – neither more nor less. But in that case, corruption and waste are only relevant to Italy's action if they are so prevalent that insufficient non-corrupt (and badly off) jurisdictions exist for Italy to reach its fair share of 95.05 million people effectively. To put it the other way round, if there are enough non-corrupt (and badly off) jurisdictions – as I believe there are – that Italy *can still* reach its fair share effectively, by simply avoiding corrupt jurisdictions altogether, then, corruption and waste are no impediment to *Italy's* action on its 1% obligation. At worst, they are an impediment to later full compliers, which is not Italy's problem.

Of course, Italy only serves here as an example. The analysis could be repeated, with somewhat different numbers, for whichever of the G7 cared to increase its ODA to 1% first. Since each of the G7 is in the same boat as Italy, the corruption and waste objection at least begins by being irrelevant.

The cases

According to the non-ideal theory of justice we have discussed, which of our opening cases represent examples of global distributive injustice? What are rich nations obligated to do about it?

In Yemen, life expectancy (60.6 years) is *less* than 10 years below the global average (67.1 years). It, therefore, exceeds the cut-off point we added to the 1% obligation, in order to bring Rawls (1999) and his followers into our coalition of the willing. This means that, in non-ideal theory, Yemen is not a case of global distributive injustice. It also means that worse-off jurisdictions (those below the cut-off point) have *priority* over Yemen for receiving transfers from the G7.

In Zambia, life expectancy (37.5 years) is almost 30 years below the global average (67.1), well below the cut-off point. Zambia *is*, therefore, a case of global distributive injustice. Any nation in the G7 that has not already expended its 1% elsewhere – that is, *every* G7 nation (including Japan), since none has reached 1% – can make progress in discharging its obligations by transferring $1.627 billion annually to Zambia (i.e., $144 per capita) to improve the fundamental determinants of its population's health. Zambia is one of the countries with priority over Yemen.

This chapter condenses and simplifies material from Sreenivasan (2002 and 2007), which interested readers may wish to consult. For more on current debates about international distributive justice, see Caney (2005, Ch. 4). For more on the social determinants of health, see Marmot and Wilkinson (1999). For more on global health and development, see Mehrotra and Jolly (1997) and Leon and Walt (2001). Life expectancy figures given are for 2003 and have been taken from the 2005 *Human Development Report* (UN Development Program, 2005), except in the case of Kerala, where they are for 1988–91 (Krishnan, 1997).

REFERENCES

Buchanan, A. (1987). Justice and charity. *Ethics* **97**: 558–75.

Caldwell, J. (1986). Routes to low mortality in poor countries. *Pop Devel Rev* **12**: 171–220.

Caney, S. (2005). *Justice Beyond Borders*. Oxford: Oxford University Press.

Filmer, D. and Pritchett, L. (1999). The impact of public spending on health: does money matter? *Soc Sci Med* **49**: 1309–23.

Gwatkin, D., Guillot, M., and Heuveline, P. (1999). The burden of disease among the global poor. *Lancet* **354**: 586–9.

Hobcraft, J. (1993). Women's education, child welfare, and child survival: a review of the evidence. *Health Transit Rev* **3**: 159–75.

Krishnan, T. N. (1997). The route to social development in Kerala: social intermediation and public action. In *Development with a Human Face*, ed. S. Mehrotra and R. Jolly. Oxford: Clarendon Press, pp. 204–34.

Leon, D. A. and Walt, G. (eds.) (2001). *Poverty, Inequality, and Health: An International Perspective*. Oxford: Oxford University Press.

Marmot, M. and Wilkinson, R. (eds.) (1999). *Social Determinants of Health*. Oxford: Oxford University Press.

Mehrotra, S. and Jolly, R. (eds.) (1997). *Development with a Human Face*. Oxford: Clarendon Press.

Murphy, L. (2000). *Moral Demands in Nonideal Theory*. New York: Oxford University Press.

OECD (2005). *OECD in Figures*. Paris: Organisation for Economic Co-operation and Development.

Pogge, T. (2002). *World Poverty and Human Rights*. Oxford: Blackwell.

Preston, S. H. (1980). Causes and consequences of mortality declines in less developed countries during the twentieth century. In *Population and Economic Change in Developing Countries*, ed. R. Easterlin. Chicago, IL: University of Chicago Press, pp. 289–360.

Rawls, J. (1999). *The Law of Peoples*. Cambridge, MA.: Harvard University Press.

Sachs, J. (2005). *The End of Poverty*. New York: Penguin Press.

Singer, P. (1972). Famine, affluence, and morality. *Philos Public Affairs* **1**: 229–43.

Singer, P. (2002). *One World*. New Haven, CT: Yale University Press.

Sreenivasan, G. (2002). International justice and health: a proposal. *Ethics Int Affairs* **16**: 81–90.

Sreenivasan, G. (2007). Health and justice in our non-ideal world. *Pol Philos Econ* **6**: 218–36.

Subbarao, K. and Raney, L. (1995). Social gains from female education: a cross-national study. *Econ Devel Cult Change* **44**: 105–28.

United Nations Development Program (2001). *Human Development Report* 2001. New York: Oxford University Press.

United Nations Development Program (2005). *Human Development Report* 2005. New York: Oxford University Press.

Religious and cultural perspectives in bioethics

Introduction

Joseph M. Boyle, Jr. and David Novak

There is no doubt that modern clinical medicine in the West is practiced in a pluralistic and multicultural context. Yet nowadays, there is frequently a divide between the moral values of clinicians and those of their patients. Whereas many clinicians, whatever their own personal beliefs, ascribe to a basically secular morality that emphasizes such values as individual autonomy and social utility, many of their patients ascribe to cultural and religious traditions that emphasize such values as obedience to God and the responsibility of families and communities to care for their own. In addition, whereas it is usually quite easy to negotiate respect for the strictly ritual requirements of such patients in such areas as prayer and diet, it is more difficult to negotiate great differences in moral perspectives between clinicians and their patients when it comes to practical questions involved in medical treatment in general and the treatment of the patient at hand in particular. Sometimes these differences need to be more generally negotiated in the public policy discussions that take place in hospital ethics committees or even in legislative and judicial settings. Other times, these differences need to be more particularly negotiated on a case-by-case basis between clinicians and their patients and the patients' immediate families, plus those from their traditional communities authorized by patients and their families, such as priests, rabbis, pastors, or imams, to provide them with moral guidance or even moral governance.

This section aims to acquaint clinicians with such potential differences between their moral values and the moral values of their patients and their families and communities. It does not suggest, much less propose, ways that these moral differences can be negotiated in a clinical setting. This section is, therefore, descriptive and not prescriptive. Nevertheless, such information will surely be useful in making informed moral judgements when dealing with patients who come from the religious and cultural traditions discussed in this chapter.

Here the distinctive views on basic issues in biomedical ethics from a significant number of the world's major religions and cultures are represented. The authors of these distinct contributions to this section of the book are all experts in the ethics of their respective religious and cultural traditions, especially in the way their traditions deal with biomedical questions. Despite their intellectual expertise in both the theoretical and applied ethics of their own traditions, the contributions of all the authors in this section will be easily understood by those having little or no familiarity with these traditions. Also, accessible references in English for further reading and inquiry are provided.

In terms of the relation of religion and culture at work in all of these contributions in one way or another, one can see that if "culture" is the way of life of a particular community having historical continuity from a premodern time into the present and intending to persevere into the future, then one can see that "religion" lies at the core of all these cultures. But what is "religion"? Clearly, there is no one overriding general definition of a class called "religion" in which all the "religions" discussed here (or anywhere else) are simply its specific manifestations. Instead, one can only see certain overlappings between the various traditions themselves. That is, there are some things that some social phenomena usually called "religions" have in common with some other "religions," and other things they have in common with some other "religions." Nevertheless, perhaps one can say that what all of the religions dealt with in this section have in common is that moral decisions in all of them are made by reference to some transcendent reality; that is to something or someone beyond human making and human control. As such, ethics in all of them is in one way or another part of worship. Other than that, though, almost all the other commonalities are between specific cultural traditions rather than among all of them, let alone encompassing them all in some larger structure.

The force of various forms of what might be called *traditional* moral beliefs and sentiments varies from patient to patient. Some patients are quite articulate and coherent in expressing their moral beliefs and sentiments, or they are quite clear about whom they themselves designate to articulate these beliefs and sentiments for them. Other patients are less articulate, less coherent, and frequently less than wholehearted in affirming any traditional moral view for themselves. Then, there are patients who affirm no traditional moral view or who have rejected the traditions in which they were once participants, whether actively or only passively (as in the case of a tradition into which one was only born, yet recognized by others as being a member of it). Therefore, it is extremely important that the clinician should not only be aware of the tradition from which his or her patient comes but also should evoke from the patient just what his or her relation is to that tradition: wholehearted, halfhearted, rejecting, or non-existent. Frequently, especially in situations of long-term treatment, such information about the patient's religious position is as important, or almost as important, as information about the patient's physical condition. Minimally, such information should be sought when the psychological state of the patient is being examined and assessed.

The recognition that the patient's moral perceptions require attention in the clinical setting does not, of course, imply that those perceptions are correct or valuable for the whole process of clinical treatment. There are patients who are often very much misinformed about what their own tradition teaches about a particular moral issue. In fact, there are even times when a so-called "religious" position masks psychological pathology. Therefore, this section of the book, with its brief but accurate accounts of the moral positions on basic biomedical issues of the various traditions considered, can be helpful to a clinician when trying to ascertain whether a patient is accurately representing his or her own tradition on the moral question at hand, or whether the patient is expressing his or her private confusion or pathology. (Of course, such knowledge will be of no use to a clinician who considers all religion to be pathological per se, which is also an issue that needs to be examined when treating a religious patient.) Yet, even when a patient is correct about the position of his or her tradition on the moral question at hand in his or her own treatment and no psychological pathology is evident, such religious points of view cannot be allowed to dominate the ethical aspects of clinical decision making. These traditions should have a voice but not a veto. Clinicians and other healthcare professionals are bound by their own moral convictions, professional ethics, often by mission statements of the healthcare institutions where they work, and by the law. For example, the dominant role of the family in many traditionally based moralities can run counter to modern secular notions that only the autonomy of the individual patient is to be taken into consideration. This is especially important to note when a child is the patient and who cannot be expected to make his or her own moral decisions, but also in the case of many adults who would say that they freely accept the authority of their family and their traditional community (often seen as an extension of the family) to make major decisions affecting their lives and their health.

The attention of clinicians to the religious views of their patients can also enrich their own personal process of developing a cogent moral point of view. When this happens, there is genuine dialogue between clinicians and patients and the communities in which they all live – both with each other and apart from each other. This section seeks to contribute to that ongoing dialogue.

47

Aboriginal bioethics

Jonathan H. Ellerby

Mr. A, a 70-year-old Aboriginal elder who speaks only Ojibway, is admitted to a tertiary care hospital for diagnostic investigation of possible prostate cancer. Initially, only a female interpreter is available, and she has difficulty translating the physician's references to the penis while obtaining consent for cystoscopy. When asked to tell Mr. A that the procedure would aid in cancer diagnosis, she refuses to translate the concept of cancer directly and, instead, uses the word for "growth." The patient responds that he does not fully understand the diagnostic test but trusts the interpreter and the urologist and agrees to sign the consent form. During cystoscopy, both his son and a male interpreter, are present to translate. Following the biopsy and other diagnostic tests, Mr. A, his son, the male interpreter, and the urologist meet. Addressing the son and the interpreter, the urologist explains that Mr. A has advanced cancer spreading to bone. When asked by the son about treatment, the urologist replies that any attempted curative treatment would probably cause more risk and discomfort than would pain relief and other palliative measures. The interpreter begins to translate the urologist's summary, but his explanation of the diagnosis is interrupted by the son, who says that he will communicate directly with his father. He states that the interpreter should not have used the Ojibway word "manitoc," which denotes cancer through the cultural metaphor of "being eaten from within," and that direct reference to cancer and his father's terminal prognosis will promote fear and pain. He adds that his father has given him responsibility to interpret and to act as his proxy decision maker. The son further opposes the physician's attempt to communicate the prognosis directly to Mr. A, stating that direct references to death and dying
may "bring death closer." The urologist argues that Mr. A needs to understand his diagnosis and give informed consent for possible treatment or the more likely palliative measures. The son replies that he will not lie to his father but that he needs time to communicate with his father through a more gradual and indirect process. The physician and son finally agree that the son will involve other family members over the next 48 hours. The physician and family arrange to meet again in two days and, in the meantime, to hold a "sharing circle" (Table 47.1, below) in which patient, family members, and caregivers will discuss palliative care and answer Mr. A.'s questions.

What is Aboriginal bioethics?

The literal translation of Aborigine is "the people who were here from the beginning," which is not synonymous with "indigenous," and referred to the Australian Aborigines. There are groups all over the rest of the word who are referred to as Aboriginal peoples and who have distinct cultures. This chapter is based on those in North America. Although philosophies and practices analogous to bioethics do exist in Aboriginal cultures, the concept of bioethics is not generally differentiated from the ethical values and frameworks for decision making that are applied in all dimensions of living. Accordingly, ethical values that may be held by Aboriginal people will be addressed rather than a formal, codified

An earlier version of this chapter has appeared: Ellerby, J. H., McKenzie, J., McKay, S. *et al.* (2000). Aboriginal cultures. *CMAJ* **163**: 845–50.

Table 47.1. North American Aboriginal people and their culltures[a]

Term	Description
Aboriginal peoples	Groups or nations who were originally living in North America before European exploration
Elder	Spiritual and community leader recognized by the Aboriginal community; elders are cultural experts with special knowledge of community ethical values and some are also counselors and healers
First Nations	Aboriginal societies that existed in North America before Europeans arrived; some Aboriginal people, including Inuit, do not see themselves as members of First Nations
Inuit	A circumpolar Aboriginal people living in Canada, Greenland, Alaska, and Siberia
Métis	A distinct and independent people whose ancestors were both of Aboriginal and European heritage and who currently do not have defined status within federal legislation
Registered Indians	Aboriginal people who are registered under the Indian Act of Canada
Sharing circle	An Aboriginal process in which each person has an opportunity to speak in turn; it is used for seeking consensus in decision making, resolving conflicts between participants, and building community trust
Smudging	A cleansing ceremony using the smoke from plant medicine
Treaty Indians	Aboriginal people who are registered under the Indian Act of Canada and can prove descent from a band that signed a treaty

[a] Aboriginal categories based on definitions proposed by Pohl (2000, pp. 28–32) and on the Statistics Canada website (1996).

system of Aboriginal bioethics. Table 47.1 defines a number of Aboriginal terms that are used in this chapter.

A review of the literature revealed that little has been published on the subject of Aboriginal health ethics (Gariépy, 1999). In the scope of cultural bioethics, Aboriginal systems are unique in their respect for the visions and beliefs of the individual and concomitant respect for the community (Hultkrantz, 1987). Aboriginal values are frequently discounted by Western colonial culture. Primarily rooted in the context of oral history and culture, Aboriginal ethics are best understood as a process and not as the correct interpretation of a unified code (Gariépy 1999; Ong, 1982, pp. 57, 86, 145). In their approach to ethical decision making, Aboriginal cultures differ from religious and cultural groups that draw on scripture and textual foundations for their ethical beliefs and practices. Despite these challenges, common themes and the diversity within Aboriginal ethics may be highlighted. Research conducted with Aboriginal elders provides the basis for identifying widely held values in Aboriginal frameworks for decision making (Ellerby, 2005).

Themes in approaches to communication and caregiving

Some essential qualities of ethical approaches to communication and caregiving involving Aboriginal peoples are summarized in Table 47.2. Although these ethical values are important to understand and apply, examining specific applications of ethical care in detail is not as useful as developing a more generalized understanding of how to approach ethical decision making with Aboriginal people in actual clinical settings. Aboriginal ethical decisions are often situational and highly dependent on individual values and on the context of the family and community. In general, Aboriginal ethical values include the concepts of holism, pluralism, autonomy, community- or family-based decision making, and the maintenance of

Table 47.2. Essential qualities of ethical approaches to communication and caregiving involving Aboriginal patients

Qualities	Characteristics
Respect the individual	Individual experience and beliefs are viewed to be as valid and important as tradition or cultural norms (Gariépy, 1999). Although closely bound to family and community in identity, individuals are recognized as having authority over their own health and "healing journey." When communicating with an Aboriginal person, it is important to show respect, especially for the aged and those with high status such as elders
Practice conscious communication	Try to listen well and note responses, not only in speech but also, if possible, in body language. Emotional control is common among Aboriginal people and it may be difficult for non-Aboriginal people to "read" intonation and body language
Use interpreters	Use an interpreter if there is any doubt as to fluency and understanding in English or French. Interpreters often assist in explaining and advocating for the patient (Kaufert and Koolage, 1984)
Involve the family	Often Aboriginal families will wish to be present during decision making. Family members can be helpful in understanding the patient's beliefs and wishes. Patients may not strongly differentiate their own best interest from that of their family. Because of the individuality of values, however, family members may not always be suitable as interpreters. "Immediate family" can include many extended relations and may be very large and thus should be affirmed (Preston and Preston, 1991)
Recognize alternative approaches to truth telling	Aboriginal people may believe that speaking of a future illness or consequence will bring it to pass. Family members may not wish "bad news" to be communicated directly (Carrese and Rhodes, 1995; Kaufert et al., 1999). Mystery is an acceptable frame of reference for many Aboriginal people, and uncertainty in prognosis or disease progression is often easily accepted by Aboriginal people in contrast to non-Aboriginal people. Beneficence must be weighed carefully against the expressed wishes of Aboriginal patients and their families
Practice non-interference	A patient's decisions should be based on a comprehensive reporting of options and be respected except for reasons of misunderstanding. Some decisions will be based on cultural knowledge or personal identity, and it will not be possible to reconcile these with medical knowledge. Also, many Aboriginal people accept medical advice without question as a sign of trust and respect for people in the role of "healer." It is important not to abuse this non-challenging trust when presented. Rational persuasion may be experienced as coercion by Aboriginal people (Brant, 1990)
Allow for Aboriginal medicine	Aboriginal patients may desire the involvement of Aboriginal elders, healers, medicine people, or priests in their treatment. These practitioners are understood to be vital to the overall integrated health of a person and should be respected and honored whenever possible. Sharing circles, smudging (using herbal-based incense) and traditional herbal remedies may be aspects of cultural medical treatments (Table 47.1)

quality of life rather than the exclusive pursuit of a cure. Most Aboriginal belief systems also emphasize achieving balance and wellness within all domains of human life (e.g., mental, physical, emotional, and spiritual). Aboriginal North American cultures share some ethical practices, such as the need to respect the integrity of the human body after death (Hultkrantz, 1987; Gariépy, 1999). Spirituality and cultural understandings of death, loss and the existence of Spirit Beings often play a role in the bioethical decisions of Aboriginal patients and families (Gariépy, 1999). Acceptance is a common, deeply rooted aspect of Aboriginal relationships to death and the passage of time during illness (Hultkrantz, 1981 [pp. 11–28], 1989, 1992 [pp. 15–16, 164–8]; Deloria, 1993 [pp. 62–77, 165–84]). Maintaining quality of life is commonly seen as paramount to extending life. Simultaneously, life is to be preserved and should be pursued whenever meaningful quality can be maintained. Affirming the dignity of life is essential (Brant, 1990).

Some Aboriginal people have a problem with advanced technology, and it is important to acknowledge this in treatment. Problems arise when a cultural heritage of nature-based medicine encounters biomedical treatment emphasizing technological interventions. Healthcare institutions such as urban teaching hospitals may be associated with a "culture of colonization," emphasizing technological solutions. There are diverse perspectives in Aboriginal communities regarding the use of technologically advanced and aggressive treatments such as transplantation, dialysis, and mechanical ventilation. However, many Aboriginal people, particularly the young, may be open to and desirous of using the full range of medical technologies available.

Barriers

Ethical care of Aboriginal peoples may include the current emphasis in bioethics on the moral context of individual relationships in clinical interactions. However, this approach does not fully engage the broader structural context of barriers that impede access to care or interfere with healing processes. Barriers include language problems, lack of cultural competence among healthcare providers, problems of transportation and communication in service delivery to remote communities, and institutional discrimination.

Applications of the bioethical principles of autonomy, beneficence, and justice in contemporary relationships must recognize the historical context of power relationships between Aboriginal people and providers of health and social services. The dominant emphasis on respect for individual autonomy in bioethics may need to incorporate Aboriginal values emphasizing non-interference. The Aboriginal psychiatrist Clare Brant (1990) observed, "the ethic of non-interference is a behavioural norm of North America Native tribes that promotes positive interpersonal relations by discouraging coercion of any kind, be it physical, verbal or psychological."

Approaches to guaranteeing autonomy in communication involving consent and truth telling must accommodate this value of avoiding coercion. Direct, unmediated communication of bad news involving terminal prognosis or risks of impending death may violate the values of some individuals and communities. Cultural and spiritual traditions, including those of Navajo people in the USA and Dene people in Canada, assert that speaking explicitly about terminal illness and death may hasten death (Carrese and Rhodes, 1995; Kaufert et al., 1999). Some families may, therefore, ask to be present to mediate communication of bad news and support the family. One potential way of recognizing alternative approaches to truth telling in consent may resemble Freedman's (1993) concept of "offering truth." This framework avoids "imposing truth" by allowing the person to define the level and explicitness of the information they require to interpret care options.

Emphasis on guaranteeing informed consent and minimizing risks to individuals in the decision-making process may be unduly influenced by historical relationships that discount Aboriginal values, which emphasize protection of the family and the community. In making consent decisions, Aboriginal patients and their families may balance the risks and benefits to the individual with the interests of the family and community. For example, a patient may defer to the wisdom of an elder or healer or elect to use a proxy decision maker from the family in signing consent agreements or advance directives (Kaufert *et al.*, 1999).

In ethical decision making, power differences may be accentuated by language barriers among patients who are monolingual speakers of Aboriginal languages or who have limited fluency in English or French. In these situations, ethical communication should involve the use of trained Aboriginal health interpreters, who have competence in both biomedical terminology and Aboriginal concepts of health and healing.

Diversity and pluralism

Diversity and pluralism are essential dimensions of Aboriginal ethics. Aboriginal ethics emphasize a pluralistic perspective that accepts that a wide spectrum of values and perspectives may be held by family members. In allowing for the expression of a plural spectrum of values, autonomy among individual family members is emphasized and respected. Aboriginal cultures and communities are diverse, and therefore it is difficult to develop generalizations about values or decision-making practices. Across North America, for instance, and within individual states, provinces, and territories, there is a wide spectrum of cultural and language groups, and variations between individual Aboriginal communities and regional organizations. For example, Manitoba is home to Cree, Ojibway (Annishinabe), Métis, Inuit, Dene, and Dakota people. Despite some shared beliefs, each cultural group must be treated with respect and an understanding of inherent diversity.

In considering the diversity of beliefs among Aboriginal people, one needs to recognize the impact of Christianity on Aboriginal communities. In many communities and families, the introduction of Christianity increased the diversity of values

influencing ethical decision making. In some cases, the result has been division and animosity between family and community members who hold traditional Aboriginal values and those who assert Christian values.

Why is Aboriginal bioethics important?

Population

The population of Aboriginal people who may benefit from culturally appropriate ethical decision making is growing. There are alternative ways to define the Aboriginal population. For instance, data from the 1996 Canadian census indicated that about 800 000 people identified themselves with one or more Aboriginal groups: North American Indian, Métis, or Inuit (Statistics Canada, 1996). The population includes about 41 000 who identified themselves as Inuit and about 210 000 as Métis. Approximately 44% of Aboriginal people live in urban areas (Royal Commission on Aboriginal Peoples, 1996). Of the more than 550 000 respondents who identified themselves as "North American Indian," approximately 60% indicated that they were a member of a First Nation or Band or had treaty status as defined by the Indian Act of Canada (Statistics Canada, 1996; see Table 47.1). The ongoing transfer of control over health services to individual First Nations or Bands will mean that mandates to apply Aboriginal values in ethical decision making will be emphasized in primary and tertiary health programs.

Access to care

The importance of understanding Aboriginal perspectives on health ethics is often linked with differences in health status and utilization of health services. Lower health status and barriers to medical care access are engaged within the ethical context of distributive justice and equality. Research documenting the disproportionate burden of morbidity and mortality and high levels of health service utilization among Aboriginal people is often cited in medical literature. However, some Aboriginal health policy makers have recently emphasized that epidemiological comparisons do not express the importance of individual and community historical relationships or contemporary experiences of racism in residential schools, social welfare program, or the healthcare system (O'Neil *et al.*, 1998). In addition, there are many culturally distinct practices among Aboriginal people that necessitate a unique ethic of care.

Equitable access to high-quality health services is a central focus for both rural and urban Aboriginal people. Because of the centrality of family in Aboriginal people's experience of illness and treatment, and restrictions in the access of friends and family members, Aboriginal patients often feel isolated when in hospital. Aboriginal approaches to decision making commonly involve members of the extended family, and offering opportunities for family involvement should be considered a prerequisite of providing ethical and culturally appropriate services (Kaufert *et al.*, 1999).

How should I approach Aboriginal bioethics in practice?

To understand Aboriginal health ethics in clinical practice, several fundamental dimensions need to be recognized. Healthcare providers must recognize the risks of applying stereotyped values and spiritual beliefs, as well as the futility of attempting to develop generalized ethical formulas for communicating with Aboriginal patients. Plural belief systems and variation among individuals preclude the direct application of knowledge in reconciling Aboriginal beliefs with biomedical and bioethical criteria.

Aboriginal bioethics can best be viewed as an interpersonal process. Immediate and clearly defined approaches should not be expected. Aboriginal bioethical positions are largely situational; adopting a case-specific approach is, therefore, important. Healthcare providers working with Aboriginal people must first try to acknowledge the importance of autonomy, the centrality of family to health and

identity, the diversity in beliefs and practices among Aboriginal people, and the value of developing and maintaining personal and emotionally sincere relationships with patients. Provider ethics emphasizing the maintenance of professional distance may contravene the Aboriginal affirmation of the power of human relationships in the healing process. Trust is paramount.

Healthcare providers might consider adopting the role of learner, allowing Aboriginal elders and each patient to lead in the articulation of the ethical principles guiding care. Not only is the process of family consultation critical in making decisions about acute and emergency care, but it is also an important dimension of day-to-day primary care. Healthcare providers should recognize that biomedical values may not always be reconcilable with Aboriginal values, despite improved communication methods or increased cross-cultural awareness.

If healthcare providers ignore differences related to Aboriginal culture, they will not be able to understand the wide spectrum of beliefs and attitudes that Aboriginal people draw on in making ethical decisions. For example, although certain values such as respect for dignity, non-interference, sharing and the importance of family and community are widespread, other beliefs such as those about truth telling may differ, even among members of the same family. Healthcare providers cannot take Aboriginal beliefs for granted and need to explore these carefully with each person. As well as respecting beliefs, healthcare providers need to respect the decisions of patients and families who request involvement of Aboriginal healers, elders, and medicine people in their care (see Table 47.2).

The future of ethics and Aboriginal people

Aboriginal cultures can be identified as premodern in the sense that there is no separation between the self and the universe; between self, family, and community; or between mind, body, and spirit. Therefore, healing is not possible without spirituality, nor without relationships to family and community, and to the cosmos. Restoring these values and beliefs can balance biomedical treatments and lead to healing of the person as well as cure of disease.

Recent Western history has emphasized scientific and technological advances at the expense of, and exclusion of, spirituality. The consequences of this have been traumatic for many traditional Aboriginal people. When in need of healthcare, many Aboriginal people view healthcare institutions as dehumanizing: they experience mind–body separation and separation from family and community, and they are asked to participate in ethical decision making guided by biomedical values.

The postmodern paradigm, which questions the existence of universal norms, scientific truth, and "superior" cultures, presents an interesting challenge to modern medicine and its claims of exclusive efficacy in achieving cure. The current popularity of alternative healing methods, such as Aboriginal medicine, and the thirst for spiritual values are but two indications of a postmodern culture that is more inclusive and holistic and thus more akin to traditional Aboriginal culture.

Aboriginal ethics is an important area of study because of its potential to make exceptional contributions to more generalized understandings of bioethical practice in increasingly diverse clinical and sociocultural environments. The emphasis in Aboriginal ethics on pluralism, diversity, and the maintenance of a high level of respect for individuality challenges Western biomedical paradigms to adjust to become more responsive and dynamic in their approach to ethical decision making. By incorporating a model of ethics that acknowledges pluralism and cultural context, medicine has the opportunity to develop models of ethics and care that are relevant to the cross-cultural treatment of the whole person (Dacher, 1996).

The case

The young female interpreter, out of respect for Mr. A's age, sex, and status, cannot discuss the urological procedure with him directly. However, by adhering to Ojibway beliefs, she does use a genera-lized term to refer to cancer and thus avoids contravening the belief that "speaking the future may bring it to pass." Although the male interpreter is able to use anatomic language without disrespect, Mr. A's son feels that explicit truth telling about cancer is against traditional practice. In giving his son permission to be his interpreter and to be a proxy decision maker, Mr. A is not undermining his own personal autonomy and instead is demonstrating shared family and communal responsibility in decision making. This is in contrast to the usual Western view of autonomy as conceding supremacy to the individual rather than to anyone else in making decisions. Only recently has the importance of relationships, especially as propounded in feminist ethics, been given a place in bioethics. Though it is worrisome for some that a cognitively competent individual is not being involved in making decisions about his future, Mr. A has chosen to delegate responsibility to his son. Given the principle of non-interference among Aboriginal people, the father's values and beliefs may differ considerably from those of his family. An important task of the interpreter and caregivers is to determine whether such differences are present. Aboriginal language interpreters are, therefore, necessary not just for translation but also to bring cultural awareness and sensitivity to interactions between patients, family members, and healthcare providers. If differences in values are present, the physician may need to "offer truth" to ensure that Mr. A's views are respected. For example, Mr. A might be asked, "Are you the sort of person who likes to know all available information, or are you happy for your son to make decisions for you?" In this case, it is reasonable that the father is not immediately told about his prognosis, since curative treatment is not being recommended. By being given extra time and a cultural medical treatment (i.e., a sharing circle in which caregivers, family, and the patient participate), Mr. A achieves balance between his diagnosis, the biomedical view, and his spiritual beliefs in a culturally appropriate manner. Following the sharing circle and a family meeting, the son, the urologist, and the interpreter meet with Mr. A, his wife, and two of his other children. After this process of family consultation and gradual and prolonged truth telling by the family, Mr. A understands his diagnosis and the implications of metastatic cancer. Together with his family, he consents to palliative care, including pain control and palliative radiation.

REFERENCES

Brant, C. C. (1990). Native ethics and rules of behavior. *Can J Psychiatry* **35**: 534–9.

Carrese, J. A. and Rhodes, L. A. (1995). Western bioethics on the Navajo reservation: Benefit or harm? *JAMA* **274**: 826–9.

Dacher, E. (1996). Towards a post-modern medicine. *J Altern Complement Med* **2**: 531–7.

Deloria, V. (1993). Thinking in time and space. In *God is Red: A Native View of Religion*, ed. V. Deloria. Golden CO: Fulcrum, pp. 62–7.

Ellerby, J. H. (2005). *Working with Aboriginal Elders: Understanding Aboriginal Elders and Healers and the Cultural Conflicts Involved in Their Work in Health Care Agencies and Institutions*. Winnipeg: Aboriginal Issues Press, University of Winnipeg.

Freedman, B. (1993). Offering truth: one ethical approach to the uninformed cancer patient. *Arch Intern Med* **153**: 572–6.

Gariépy, G. J. (1999). *End of Life Issues in Aboriginal North America*. Winnipeg: University of Manitoba.

Hultkrantz, A. (1981). North American Indian religion in a circumpolar perspective. In *North American Indian Studies: European Contributions*, ed. P. Houins. Gottingen the Netherlands: Hovens, pp. 11–28.

Hultkrantz, A. (1987). *Native Religions of North America: The Power of Visions and Fertility*. San Francisco, CA: HarperCollins.

Hultkrantz, A. (1989). Health, religion and medicine in Native North American traditions. In *Healing and Restoring: Health and Medicine in the World's Religious Traditions*, ed. L. E. Sullivan. London: Macmillan, pp. 327–58.

Hultkrantz, A. (1992). *Shamanic Healing and Ritual Drama: Health and Medicine in Native North American Religious Traditions*. New York: Crossroad.

Kaufert, J. and Koolage, W. (1984). Role conflict among culture brokers: the experience of Native Canadian medical interpreters. *Soc Sci Med* **18**: 383–6.

Kaufert, J. M., Putsch, R. W., and Lavallée, M. (1999). End-of-life decision making among Aboriginal Canadians: interpretation, mediation, and discord in the communication of "bad news." *J Palliat Care* **15**: 31–8.

O'Neil, J., Reading, J., and Leader, A. (1998). Changing the relations of surveillance: the development of a discourse of resistance in Aboriginal epidemiology. *Hum Organ* **57**: 230–7.

Ong, W. J. (1982). *Orality and Literacy*. New York: Methuen.

Pohl, A. (2000). *Building International Awareness on Aboriginal Issues*. Toronto: Citizens for Public Justice.

Preston, R. J. and Preston, S. (1991). Death and grieving among northern forest hunters: an East Cree example. In *Coping with the Final Tragedy: Cultural Variations in Dying and Grieving*, ed. D. R. Counts and D. Ayers Counts. Amityville, NY: Baywood, pp. 135–56.

Royal Commission on Aboriginal Peoples (1996). *Gathering Strength*. Ottawa: The Commission.

Statistics Canada (1996). *Census 1996: Population by Aboriginal Group*. Ottawa: Statistics Canada.

Related websites

- Aboriginal healing and wellness links (Turtle Island Native Network): www.turtleisland.org
- Association of American Indian Physicians: www.aaip.com
- Health Canada First Nations and Inuit Health Programs: www.hc-sc.gc.ca/msb/fnihp
- Indian Health Service, US Department of Health and Human Services: www.ihs.gov

48

Buddhist bioethics

Damien Keown

Mrs. B is aged 35 and lives in a remote part of the Chiang Mai region of northern Thailand. She is an agricultural worker with only a basic education. She does not use contraception because there is no local family planning facilities. She is married with three children, and has just found out she is eight weeks' pregnant. She and her husband barely earn enough to support their existing children, and a fourth child would place an unbearable economic strain on family resources.

The Venerable C, a Burmese monk resident in the USA, suffered a severe stroke at the age of 59. He had a history of diabetes, poorly controlled high blood pressure, atrial fibrillation, congestive heart failure, and chronic obstructive pulmonary disease. He had undergone a cardiac bypass operation several years earlier. The prognosis was guarded at best, even with surgery. The attending neurosurgeon asked whether Venerable C would want emergency surgery or if he would prefer to forgo aggressive measures. The monk had not discussed his wishes previously with his fellow monks or students, had made no advance directives, and remained unconscious throughout (Hood, 2005).

What is Buddhist bioethics?

Buddhism is a body of religious teachings attributed to an historical individual called Siddhartha Gautama, who lived in northeast India in the fifth century BCE. Following a profound spiritual transformation at the age of 35, he became known by the honorific title of "Buddha" ("enlightened one"). In common with other Asian traditions, Buddhism believes in reincarnation and teaches that individuals undergo a potentially infinite series of rebirths. However, Buddhism is distinctive in lacking a belief in a supreme being, as well as denying the existence of a personal soul. Buddhists follow the Buddha's teachings (or *Dharma*) in the hope of putting an end to rebirth by attaining the transcendent state of nirvana. Buddhism has no head or central authority, and in resolving moral dilemmas Buddhists are encouraged to reflect on the teachings preserved in scripture, to seek the guidance of advanced practitioners such as monks, and to meditate on all aspects of a situation in order to ensure that any decision they reach is in harmony both with the spirit of the teachings and their conscience. There are no international organizations or colleges of Buddhist physicians that serve to formulate policy for the guidance of healthcare professionals. Despite this lack of central authority, there are fundamental moral values and principles that virtually all schools of Buddhism accept. Chief among these are compassion (*karuna*) and "non-harming" or respect for life (*ahimsa*), which between them underpin Buddhism's approach to bioethics.

The most widespread set of precepts in Buddhism are the Five Precepts, and the first of these prohibits causing harm or injury to living creatures (human and otherwise). This is interpreted quite strictly and has an important bearing on bioethics, especially in relation to questions such as abortion and euthanasia. At a theoretical level, recent studies have suggested that Buddhism can best be understood as a form of virtue ethics (Whitehill, 2000; Keown, 2001a, 2005a; Cooper and

James, 2005), and if so this offers an opportunity for dialogue with similar approaches to bioethics being developed in the West. The literature on Buddhist bioethics itself, however, remains limited at this time (e.g., Ratanakul, 1986; Harvey, 2000; Keown, 2001b; Tsomo, 2006).

Buddhism is a world religion with a large following both in Asia and the West. However, Buddhists are influenced not just by the formal teachings of their religion but also by the beliefs and practices of their indigenous cultures. In some cases, the influence of the latter may be so strong that it overrides the former, leading to the impression that there is little agreement or uniformity among Buddhists as a whole. For example, there is general agreement among Buddhists in Asia that abortion is contrary to the First Precept, but wide variation among countries where Buddhism is practiced as to what is legally permitted. There is also a diversity of views on this question among Buddhist converts in the West. In traditional Buddhist countries, the nucleus of social concern – as in many Asian cultures – is the extended family rather than the individual, and ethical questions, therefore, tend to be analyzed primarily in terms of duties rather than rights.

Since Buddhism is a transcultural phenomenon, it is impractical to discuss questions of law and policy here at any length. By way of example, some reference will be made to particular Buddhist countries, but readers should bear in mind that there is considerable legal and cultural diversity in the regions of Asia where Buddhism is practiced. More detailed information on local conditions may be found in the references.

Why is Buddhist ethics important?

Buddhism has had a major influence on Asian culture, spreading to every part of Asia and is now growing rapidly in the West. There are approximately five million Buddhists in the USA and around one million in Europe. The total number of Buddhists worldwide is put at 500 million. Given its

global distribution, many individuals now look to Buddhist teachings for ethical guidance when facing problematic decisions on medical treatment. It is, therefore, important for physicians and other care providers to understand the underlying values that may influence Buddhist patients in taking treatment decisions. Furthermore, as an Asian culture, Buddhism can provide a complementary perspective on ethics and may have much to contribute to Western discussions.

How should I approach Buddhist ethics in practice?

Buddhism imposes few special requirements on either patients or physicians in connection with medical treatment, and there is no reason why the care of Buddhist patients should pose any special problems. The only exception would be that it would not be appropriate for a monk or nun to be on a mixed ward, and it would be preferable for them to be treated by a physician of the same sex. Unlike Western clergy, Buddhist monks do not function as chaplains, nor do they visit hospitals in a pastoral role or to perform religious services for the sick.

Buddhism is a flexible and moderate religion in which concepts of taboo and religious purity have little, if any, part to play. Religious law imposes no special requirements or limitations on medical treatment, nor are there any special hygiene, purificatory, or dietary requirements (while many Buddhists are vegetarians, others are not). Cremation is the most common means of disposing of the dead.

In practice, local custom tends to have a greater bearing on the physician–patient relationship than Buddhist doctrine. It is difficult to generalize about local customs, but provided the conventions of normal medical etiquette are respected there is no reason why difficulties should arise. This is particularly so in the case of the many Westerners who have converted to Buddhism and who are unlikely to have any problems with the conventions of

Western medical practice. As with all societies there is diversity among Buddhist populations arising from socioeconomic factors and level of education, which makes it difficult to generalize how any individual Buddhist is likely to react. At the village level in Asia, for instance, Buddhism coexists with animism, and belief in the power of local gods and spirits to cure illness is widespread. Allowance, therefore, needs to be made for such variation, and the temptation to generalize should be avoided.

Notable differences are found across Asia, particularly between the countries of East Asia, such as China, Japan, and Korea, and those of South Asia, such as Burma, Thailand, and Sri Lanka. The former group follow the Mahayana form of Buddhism, while in the latter the more conservative Theravada form predominates. To highlight just one example, in Japan, the criterion of brain death is deeply unpopular because of its association with cadaver transplants. Being a party to what is seen as the desecration of the corpse of a close relative, particularly a parent, causes deep unease (LaFleur, 2001). There is also skepticism about the validity of the brain death criterion itself as a reliable test for human death, a skepticism increasingly voiced by dissidents in the West (Youngner *et al.*, 1999; Potts *et al.*, 2000).

Another distinctive feature of the Buddhist perspective is the emphasis it places on mindfulness and mental clarity, as seen in the practice of meditation. Buddhism emphasizes the importance of an unclouded mind, particularly when a patient is close to death, as it is believed this can lead to a better rebirth. Some Buddhists may, therefore, be unwilling to take pain-relieving drugs or strong sedatives, and even those who are not in a terminal condition may prefer to remain as alert as possible rather than take analgesics that will impair their mental or sensory capacities.

Abortion

Most Buddhists regard fertilization as the point at which individual human life commences and

believe that the embryo is entitled to moral respect from that time onwards. Abortion is, therefore, seen as morally in the same category as the intentional killing of an adult. The only exception is likely to be when the procedure is necessary to save the life of the mother.

The contemporary legal position varies from country to country. The more conservative Buddhist countries of southeast Asia, such as Thailand and Sri Lanka, have laws prohibiting abortion, except when necessary to save the life of the mother. Nevertheless, illegal abortions are common. Somewhat surprising for a country in which Buddhism is the state religion, abortions in Thailand are running at some 50% higher than the number in the USA for the equivalent number of citizens. Married women, who appear to use it as a means of birth control, account for 85% or more of abortions. Recent studies refer to an estimated 300 000 abortions per year, the vast majority of which are illegal. The Thai Penal Code of 1956 allows abortion in only two circumstances: first, "if it is necessary for the sake of the woman's health" and, second, in cases of rape. Official figures from the 1960s record as few as five legal abortions in some years. Opinion polls in Thailand also reveal an intriguing paradox: while most Thais regard abortion as immoral, a majority also believes the legal grounds for obtaining it should be relaxed (Florida, 1991, p. 22).

In east Asian countries, attitudes are more liberal. The rate of abortion in Japan has been very high in recent years, perhaps peaking at over a million (some would put the figure much higher) before decreasing in the last few years as the contraceptive pill has become more easily available. Central to the contemporary Japanese experience is the phenomenon of *mizuko kuyo*, a memorial service held for aborted children. This service involves erecting a small statue to commemorate the lost child and includes an apology to the spirit of the aborted fetus. William LaFleur (1992) has explored the complex symbolism and cultural history of the practice, and a feminist perspective has been provided by Hardacre (1997).

Korea provides an interesting comparison with Japan. Both countries have a very high rate of abortion, but in Japan it is legal (since 1948) whereas in Korea, it is not. Annual figures of between one and two million are quoted for Korea, a country with a population of around 46 million. Over a quarter of the population are Buddhists, which makes them the main religious group. Statistics quoted by Tedesco (1999) reveal that Buddhists are slightly more likely to have abortions than other segments of the population. In 1985, an anti-abortion movement began to gain ground following the publication of a book by the Venerable Sok Myogak (1985), a Buddhist monk of the Chogye order. His book, entitled *My Dear Baby, Please Forgive Me!* became popular, and readers began to demand rites and services for aborted children similar to the Japanese *mizuko kuyo* service, although distinctively Korean in form.

Some Western Buddhists take a more liberal stance on the abortion question. James Hughes (1999) suggested that "clear and defensible distinctions can be made between fetuses and other human life," and found the moral logic of utilitarianism persuasive in the context of abortion, although tempered by the requirements of a virtue ethic, which takes into account the mindset of the actors. Abortion may, therefore, be allowable where the intention is compassionate and the act achieves the best outcome for all concerned. One American Zen Buddhist group, the Diamond Sangha, has produced a liturgy that can be performed following an abortion or miscarriage.

Euthanasia

By euthanasia is meant intentionally causing the death of a patient by act or omission in the context of medical care. We are concerned here only with voluntary euthanasia, that is, when a mentally competent patient freely requests medical help in ending his life.

As a case of intentionally taking life, euthanasia is generally regarded as prohibited by the First Precept. As noted above, however, compassion is also an important Buddhist moral value, particularly when linked to the concept of the Bodhisattva, a Buddhist saint distinguished by self-sacrificing compassion for others. Some sources reveal an increasing awareness of how a commitment to the alleviation of suffering can create a conflict with the principle of the inviolability of life. Opinion on these questions divides between conservative and liberal positions, although the great majority of traditional Buddhists would see euthanasia as prohibited by the First Precept.

Despite opposition to euthanasia, however, it does not follow that Buddhism teaches that there is a moral obligation to preserve life at all costs. Recognizing the inevitability of death is a central element in Buddhist teachings. Death cannot be postponed forever, and Buddhists are encouraged to be mindful and prepared for the evil hour when it comes. To seek to prolong life beyond its natural span by recourse to ever more elaborate technology when no cure or recovery is in sight is a denial of the reality of human mortality and would be seen by Buddhism as arising from delusion (*moha*) and excessive attachment (*tanha*).

In terminal care, and in cases where a permanent vegetative state has been conclusively diagnosed, there is no need to go to extreme lengths to provide treatment where there is little or no prospect of recovery. There would, therefore, be no requirement to treat subsequent complications, for example pneumonia or other infections, by administering antibiotics. While it might be foreseen that an untreated infection would lead to the patient's death, it would also be recognized that any course of treatment that is contemplated must be assessed against the background of the prognosis for overall recovery. Rather than embarking on a series of piecemeal treatments, none of which would produce a net improvement in the patient's overall condition, it would often be appropriate to reach the conclusion that the patient was beyond medical help and allow events to take their course. In such cases it is justifiable to refuse or withdraw treatment that is either futile or too burdensome in the light of the overall prognosis for recovery.

Table 48.1. Essential considerations of ethical approaches to communication and caregiving involving Buddhist patients

In view of Buddhism's diversity, caution must be exercised when generalizing about what Buddhists believe
There is a danger of superimposing inappropriate Western assumptions about religious belief on Buddhism
In Buddhism there is no religious law imposing special dietary requirements or restrictions on medical treatment
Hospitals should have a strategy in place for dealing with patients from non-Western religious backgrounds
Buddhist monks and nuns should prepare advance directives or make provision for a surrogate in the event they become incapacitated, especially when resident abroad
Buddhist monks and nuns do not generally visit hospitals or work as chaplains
Key Buddhist values are non-harming (*ahimsa*) and compassion (*karuna*)
There is a strong presumption against the taking of life enshrined in the First Precept, which generates conservative positions on issues such as abortion and euthanasia
As yet little work has been done in the field of Buddhist bioethics however, it appears to resemble Western systems of virtue ethics in key respects

For further discussion of end of life issues see Keown (2001b, 2005b). Table 48.1 details the essential considerations discussed in this chapter.

The cases

Mrs. T attended one of the many illegal abortion clinics in Thailand and had a termination at 14 weeks. In Thailand, abortion is used as a method of birth control by married women because of the lack of family planning clinics and contraceptive advice, particularly in rural areas. As is usual, Mrs. T did not discuss her plans with any member of the Buddhist clergy, since intimate family matters are not seen as appropriate matters of concern for celibate monks who have renounced worldly concerns. In having the abortion, Mrs. T felt she had done wrong and would incur bad karma as a result. However, she believed she had no alternative, and hoped to mitigate any negative karmic effects by performing good works and making offerings at the local temple.

Since he did not fit the mould of the standard American patient, there was confusion as to who had authority to make treatment decisions on behalf of Venerable C. Staff had little understanding

of Buddhism, and so the hospital ethics committee sought a court-appointed guardian to manage the case. In the end, the surgery went ahead. This was not because Buddhist teachings required it, and a decision not to operate would equally have been in accordance with Buddhist ethics. Deciding against intervention, even with the expectation that this would shorten the patient's life, would not have been regarded as an instance of passive euthanasia since at no time was the death of the patient the outcome sought.

REFERENCES

Cooper, D. E. and James, S. P. (2005). *Buddhism, Virtue and Environment*. Aldershot: Ashgate.
Florida, R. (1991). Buddhist approaches to abortion. *Asian Philos* **1**: 39–50.
Hardacre, H. (1997). *Marketing the Menacing Fetus in Japan*. Berkeley, CA: University of California Press.
Harvey, P. (2000). *An Introduction to Buddhist Ethics: Foundations, Values and Issues*. Cambridge, UK: Cambridge University Press.
Hood, R. (2005). Buddhism and the practice of bioethics in the United States. In *Buddhist Studies from India to America. Essays in Honor of Charles S. Prebish*, ed. D. Keown. London: Routledge Curzon, pp. 32–44.

Hughes, J. J. (1999). Buddhism and abortion: a western approach. In *Buddhism and Abortion*, ed. D. Keown. London: Macmillan, pp. 183–98.

Keown, D. (2001a). *The Nature of Buddhist Ethics*. Basingstoke, UK: Palgrave.

Keown, D. (2001b). *Buddhism and Bioethics*. London: Palgrave.

Keown, D. (2005a). *Buddhist Ethics: A Very Short Introduction*. Oxford, Oxford University Press.

Keown, D. (2005b). End of Life: the Buddhist View. *Lancet* **366**: 952–5.

LaFleur, W. A. (1992). *Liquid Life: Abortion and Buddhism in Japan*. Princeton, NJ: Princeton University Press.

LaFleur, W. A. (2001). From agape to organs: religious difference between Japan and America in judging the ethics of the transplant. In *Ethics in the World Religions*, ed. J. Runzo and N. M. Martin. Oxford: Oneworld, pp. 271–90.

Myogak, S. (1985). *Aga ya, yongs'o haedao*. [*My Dear Baby, Please Forgive Me*.] Seoul: Changusa.

Potts, M., Byre, P. A., and Nilges, R. G. (2000). *Beyond Brain Death: The Case Against Brain Based Criteria for Human Death*. Dordrecht: Kluwer Academic.

Ratanakul, P. (1986). *Bioethics, An Introduction to the Ethics of Medicine and Life Sciences*. Bangkok: Mahidol University.

Tedesco, F. (1999). Abortion in Korea. In *Buddhism and Abortion*, ed. D. Keown. London: Macmillan, pp. 121–55.

Tsomo, K. L. (2006). *Into the Jaws of Yama, Lord of Death. Buddhism, Bioethics and Death*. Albany, NY: SUNY Press.

Whitehill, J. (2000). Buddhism and the virtues. In *Contemporary Buddhist Ethics*, ed. D. Keown. Richmond, UK: Curzon Press, pp. 17–36.

Youngner, S. J., Arnold, R. M., and Schapiro, M. P. H. (1999). *The Definition of Death. Contemporary Controversies*. Baltimore, MD: Johns Hopkins Press.

49

Chinese bioethics

Kerry W. Bowman and Edwin C. Hui

Mr. D is a 75-year-old Chinese Canadian who has been admitted to the intensive care unit because of respiratory failure. He has a long history of respiratory problems. Mechanical ventilation is started. Mr. D is oriented to time, person, and place. He spends much of his time reading and enjoys his family's visits. Attempts to wean him from the ventilator have failed; consequently, he is facing a situation of permanent dependence on the breathing machine. It is unclear as to what Mr. D's wishes related to this would be. The physician in charge wishes to inform Mr. D that he is unable to get him to a point where he can be taken off the ventilator and wants to introduce the option of gradually weaning him off the ventilator and keeping him comfortable so that nature may take its course and he may die in peace. The patient's eldest son is described to the healthcare team as "the decision maker." He approaches the physician and asks emphatically that his father not be told that he is permanently dependent on the ventilator as it would take away his hope, terrify him and, in turn, make him sicker. The son feels that telling his father would be cruel and is, therefore, unjustifiable.

What is Chinese bioethics?

Bioethics as a discipline does not formally exist within traditional Chinese culture. For many Chinese who have grown up or spent much of their lives in a culture characterized by strong communal values and an emphasis on social harmony, the process of explicit bioethical deliberation will be unfamiliar. Much of conventional Western bioethical analysis is based on such dichotomies as autonomy versus paternalism and duties versus rights. "Either/or" distinctions contrast sharply with the conception of moral order in Chinese culture, which treats apparent opposites, such as the individual and the group, as complementary rather than mutually exclusive. Thus the "person," "family," "clan," and "community" exist in a dynamic state of reciprocal definition (Fox and Swazey, 1984).

The concept of autonomy best highlights the contrast between Western and Chinese cultures. In the West, the principle of autonomy implies that every person has the right to self-determination. In the context of healthcare, this means that the patient is the best person to make healthcare decisions. Within Chinese culture, however, the person is viewed as a "relational self" – a self for whom social relationships, rather than rationality and individualism, provide the basis for moral judgement. From this perspective, an insistence on self-determination erodes the value placed on personal interconnectedness and the social and moral meaning of such relationships.

In traditional Chinese society, the influences of which still endure, the family is based on an extended or clan structure and plays a central role in an individual's life. The family is a semi-autonomous unit consisting of an elaborate hierarchy of kin and is held responsible for the

An earlier version of this chapter has appeared: Bowman, K. W. and Hui, E. C. (2000). Chinese bioethics. *Canadian Medical Association Journal* **163**: 1481–5.

care of its aged, sick, unemployed, and disabled members. The traditional family structure is patriarchal, with communication and authority flowing downward (Unschuld, 1985). All major decisions made by the family are thus informed by these hierarchical structures. This pattern of familial collectivity has deep roots. In the second century BC, a Confucianist social order that was focused on the quality of selflessness began to evolve. This notion emphasized allegiance – first to the family, second to the clan, and finally to the community. In Chinese culture, the family functions as collective decision maker and also as a powerful conduit for moral, religious, and social norms (Kleinman *et al.*, 1978; Siven, 1987). The family's role in self-determination is, therefore, integral to any notion of Chinese bioethics.

Conceptions of illness

All cultures generate explanatory models that attempt, either explicitly or implicitly, to account for the phenomenon of illness and its place in human existence. Such models undertake to define what a disease is, how it occurs, why it exists, what measures can prevent or control it, and why some people and not others are affected. Identifying and reconciling differences between cultural models is crucial to the successful treatment of illness (Kleinman, 1980, p. 35). In Western medicine, the primary explanatory model of illness focuses on abnormalities in the structure and function of bodily organs and systems. Traditional Chinese medicine, by comparison, views the body, soul, and spirit as an integrated whole. Furthermore, because human beings are considered products of nature, humankind and the natural environment are seen to be inseparably and interdependently related; protecting the integrity of the human–nature dyad is consequently fundamental to health.

The Chinese understanding of nature and the cosmos is expressed in three important theoretical concepts: *ch'i* (material or vital force), *yin* and *yang* (complementary, interdependent opposites), and *wu-hsing* (the five elements).

Ch'i. Traditional Chinese medicine identifies 12 main channels in the human body through which the ch'i moves. Health implies that the ch'i is flowing normally between the organs, which is detected by the pulse. Accordingly, one of the main causes of disease is an obstruction of ch'i in the body. For example, the symptoms of a stroke may be attributed to the obstruction of ch'i at a point of vital energy flow in the body.

Yin and yang. This is a dialectical concept that attempts to explain phenomena that appear to be simultaneously dependent on and in opposition to each other. All bodily functions are the result of the harmony of yin and yang; a mild imbalance implies a diseased state, and a total disruption of the harmony leads to death. Many foods and food groups are divided into yin–yang categories. For example, if an illness is believed to be caused by too much yang, one way to compensate would be to eat foods that are considered yin.

Wu-hsing. The five elements are fundamental categories of matter. Because the human body is part of nature, the five elements are distributed to the five most important organs in the body, which determine the functions of all the other parts of the body, including emotions. Thus, the liver is associated with wood, the heart with fire, the spleen with earth, the lungs with metal, and the kidneys with water. Through this system, traditional Chinese medicine explains not only the various interactions between the body organs but also the influence of environmental factors (e.g., seasons and weather) on the human body and emotions (Veith, 1967, p. 23).

From the perspective of traditional Chinese medicine, a person enjoys perfect health when she or he has a strong and unobstructed flow of ch'i, is under the influence of well-balanced yin–yang forces, and is in harmony with the five elements. The focus is thus primarily on maintaining and promoting the flow of ch'i (building up body resistance) and only secondarily on pathogenic factors. Thus, traditional Chinese medicine emphasizes preventive medicine and health maintenance; therapeutic intervention to dispel pathogenic factors is reserved for acute conditions. Even for acute conditions, health maintenance procedures (measures to strengthen resistance) are usually implemented simultaneously with therapeutic interventions.

Another significant consideration in assessing Chinese patients' attitudes toward health and illness is the degree to which they have acquired Western beliefs through acculturation or the recent effort in Mainland China to combine both Chinese and Western medicine.

Why is Chinese bioethics important?

General issues

The roots of both traditional and modern Chinese culture and philosophy are simultaneously diverse and tightly intertwined. This legacy has produced a people, a culture, and a moral perspective that are neither homogeneous nor in any sense monolithic. Furthermore, for Chinese patients, the process of acculturating to Western life adds yet another layer of complexity. Attitudes toward bioethical questions are, therefore, likely to be variable, complex, and difficult to predict.

Demographics

Since the 1980s, for example, at least a million ethnic Chinese from the Far East have settled in North America. In the 1980s, Cantonese-speaking Chinese, primarily from Hong Kong, made up the majority of the immigrants. In the last decade, Mandarin-speaking Chinese from Taiwan and Mainland China have rapidly grown in number. As people from this population enter the healthcare systems in the West, it is crucial that healthcare professionals understand their cultural perspectives. Although Chinese immigrants from these three geographical areas have much in common, subcultural differences between and among these groups add to the need for healthcare providers to recognize the diversity within Chinese culture and to avoid broad-based assumptions.

How should I approach Chinese bioethics in practice?

The moral perspective of traditional China is influenced primarily by Confucianism, but also by Taoism and Buddhism (see Ch. 48). Some areas that highlight the differences between Western bioethics and Chinese tradition include beginning of life issues, death and dying, informed consent, and communication.

Beginning of life issues

The Chinese conception of the relational self has significant ethical implications for beginning of life issues. For example, one of the most important ways to show filial piety (a responsibility or sense of duty to one's parents) is to provide offspring, especially male offspring. This explains why births in general – and male births in particular – are welcome events in Chinese society. Hence, the Chinese attitude toward abortion is generally negative, especially for male fetuses if the sex of the fetus is known. Life is always viewed as precious, and the taking of a life is something to be done only with careful consideration and the utmost caution.

Death and dying

In Confucian teaching, death is evaluated in terms of accomplishment in this world (i.e., the fulfillment of *jen*). *Jen* denotes the cultivation of positive human attributes such as humaneness, charity, and beneficence. A death is a "good" one – worthy and acceptable – only when most, if not all, of one's moral duties in life have been fulfilled. Resistance to acknowledging a terminal illness or to forgoing futile medical treatments may reflect a patient's perception of unfinished business and his or her desire to extend life in order to complete unfinished tasks or fulfill moral duties.

But even when an elderly Chinese patient is resigned to a "good death," his or her children may be reluctant to grant this wish for reasons related to filial piety. Because filial piety can be expressed only when a parent is alive, to extend an ailing parent's life is to extend the opportunity to show filial piety. For this reason, children may not consent to a physician's judgement that further intervention is futile and insist that heroic measures be taken for their dying parent.

Another significant reason to resist inevitable death is the beliefs of religious Taoism, which teaches the postmortem survival of the whole bodily person and an afterlife of torture and suffering in endless Hell. To avoid this, Taoism focuses on maintaining youth and attaining longevity and immortality. Patients with a strong Taoist religious background may, therefore, consider death an obstacle to be overcome and desperately cling to any means of extending life.

Philosophical Taoism, however, has a radically different perspective, which is reflected in the phrase, "Man comes into life and goes out to death." For this reason, one should view death with equanimity. In the face of death, acceptance is the only appropriate response. Any artificial or heroic measures contradict the course of natural events and should not be undertaken.

Informed consent

The notion of respect for an individual's right to self-determination is not prominent in traditional Chinese culture. In fact, the Confucian concept of relational personhood challenges the assumption that the patient should be given the diagnosis and prognosis and the opportunity to make his or her own medical decisions. Social and moral meaning rests in *interdependence*, which overrides self-determination. Consequently, many Chinese patients may give the family or community the right to receive and disclose information, to make decisions, and to coordinate patient care, even

when they themselves are competent. If not acknowledged, these differences in perspective can lead to a complete breakdown in communication.

Communication

It is important to remember that Western and Chinese cultures may hold sharply divergent views about autonomy and the nature and meaning of illness. The most effective way to address such cultural differences is through open and balanced communication. When healthcare workers are uncertain about how a Chinese patient or family perceives a situation, it is best simply to ask. Frequently, differences are easily negotiated. Many Chinese patients already hold blended cultural perspectives and views of health. The mere acknowledgement of such differences will usually lead to improved communication. Although the notion of Chinese bioethics does not exist in any traditional sense, healthcare workers should consider the essential qualities of ethical approaches to communication and care giving involving Chinese patients that are outlined in Table 49.1.

The case

In the Confucian social hierarchy, the elderly sick person can expect to be cared for by his or her family. The patient is relieved of a large share of personal responsibility, including decision making, even though he or she may be rational and competent. Furthermore, from a Confucian point of view, which is governed by the rule of filial piety and protection, a parent should not be given the news of a terminal illness; it is considered morally inexcusable to disclose any news that may cause further harm to one's parent (Veith, 1967; Feldman *et al.*, 1999; Pang Mei-che, 1999).

In the face of serious illness, Mr. D's family, much like many people of non-Western cultures (Kaufert and O'Neil, 1990; Dalla-Vorgia *et al.*, 1992; Caralis, 1993; Thomsen *et al.*, 1993; Orona *et al.*, 1994; Asai *et al.*, 1995; Murphy *et al.*, 1996; Ip *et al.*,

Table 49.1. Essential qualities of ethical approaches to communication and caregiving involving Chinese patients

Qualities	Characteristics
Assume diverse opinions	There is no monolithic Chinese culture; when dealing with Chinese patients, a broad range of beliefs should be anticipated. Furthermore, culture is not static, particularly in the case of immigration. Many Chinese immigrants hold beliefs and attitudes that are both blended and in transition. When uncertain of beliefs and perspectives, avoid assumptions and ask the patient or family directly
Acknowledge potential differences in emotional expression	Chinese patients may not be comfortable with frank, direct styles of communication. Emotional containment does not mean indifference. Be cautious in assessing a person's emotional reaction. Anticipate different views on informed consent: many of the values common to traditional Chinese culture differ from the concept of autonomy that underpins Western bioethics. The Chinese patient may not strongly distinguish his or her wishes from those of the family. For many Chinese patients, withholding a diagnosis or controlling negative information may be seen as a way of fostering and maintaining hope in a patient. Identifying and negotiating these differences is, therefore, crucial to effective healthcare
Use interpreters	Use an interpreter if there is any doubt about fluency in or understanding of English. It is always best to avoid using family members or close family friends as interpreters because they may not be comfortable with the direct nature of informed consent. Involve the family: Chinese patients may believe that consent is a family – rather than an individual patient – decision. Making decisions based solely on a patient's wishes or perspectives on quality of life may be foreign to many Chinese patients. Moreover, "immediate family" may include multiple generations. Allow for large or multiple-generation family conferences. Applying the notion of autonomy cross-culturally may, therefore, warrant accepting each person's terms of reference for his or her definition of self. We respect patients' and families' autonomy by bringing their cultural values and beliefs into the decision-making process
Anticipate differences in the understanding and meaning of illness	Because of radically different cultural and historical roots, some Chinese patients may hold perspectives on the nature and meaning of illness that differ substantially from a Western biomedical view. Again, it is best to ask about and negotiate these differences when building a treatment plan

1998), believe that focusing on the negative may be a way of creating negative outcomes. His family has made it clear that hope was central to their concern for their father. All societies seem to recognize "the need for hope," yet each differs in understanding the conditions for hope. In contemporary North American healthcare, the doctor is often perceived to be someone who works in partnership with the terminally ill patient to maintain the patient's dignity, quality of life, personal choice over treatments, and hope. In Western terms, therefore, hope appears to be upheld through autonomy and active participation in treatment choices and regimens.

However, Mr. D's family believes that hope is best maintained through the family's absorption of the impact of the illness and diagnosis, and through the family's control of medical information transmitted to Mr. D. Their wishes reflect a belief in the shared responsibility of the illness with other family members, and an awareness of the potential physical or emotional harm that truth telling might bring.

By inquiring about Mr. D's and his family's perspective on this illness, the patient and family, in turn, felt both respected and understood, leading to improved communication and a negotiated treatment plan.

REFERENCES

Asai, A., Fukuhara, S., and Lo, B. (1995). Attitudes of Japanese and Japanese–American physicians towards life-sustaining treatment. *Lancet* **346**: 356–9.

Caralis, P. V., Davis, B., Wright, K., and Marcial, E. (1993). The influence of ethnicity and race on attitudes toward advance directives, life-prolonging treatments, and euthanasia. *J Clin Ethics* **4**: 155–65.

Dalla-Vorgia, P., Katsouyanni, K., Garanis, T. N., *et al.* (1992). Attitudes of a Mediterranean population to the truth-telling issue. *J Med Ethics* **18**: 67–74.

Feldman, M. D., Zhang, J., and Cummings, S. R. (1999). Chinese and US internists adhere to different ethical standards. *J Gen Intern Med* **14**: 469–73.

Fox, S. and Swazey, J. P. (1984). Medical morality is not bioethics: medical ethics in China and the United States. *Perspect Biol Med* **27**: 336–60.

Ip, M., Gilligan, T., Koenig, B., and Raffin, T. A. (1998). Ethical decision-making in critical care in Hong Kong. *Crit Care Med* **26**: 447–51.

Kaufert, J. M. and O'Neil, J. D. (1990). Biomedical rituals and informed consent: native Canadians and the negotiation of clinical trust. In *Social Science Perspectives on Medical Ethics*, ed. G. Weisz. Philadelphia, PA: University of Pennsylvania Press, pp. 41–63.

Kleinman, A. (1980). *Patient and Healers in the Context of Culture: An Exploration of the Borderland Between Anthropology, Medicine, and Psychiatry*. Berkeley, CA: University of California Press.

Kleinman, A., Eisenberg, L., and Good, B. (1978). Clinical lessons from anthropologic and cross-cultural research. *Ann Intern Med* **88**: 251–8.

Murphy, S. T., Palmer, J. M., Azen, S., *et al.* (1996). Ethnicity and advance directives. *J Law Med Ethics* **24**: 108–17.

Orona, C. J., Koenig, B. A., and Davis, A. J. (1994). Cultural aspects of nondisclosure. *Camb Q Healthc Ethics* **3**: 338–46.

Pang Mei-che, S. (1999). Protective truthfulness: the Chinese way of safeguarding patients in informed treatment decisions. *J Med Ethics* **25**: 247–53.

Siven, N. (1987). Traditional medicine. In *Contemporary China*. Ann Arbor, MI: Center for Chinese Studies, University of Michigan, pp. 94–112.

Thomsen, O. Ø., Wulff, H. R., Martin, A., and Singer, P. A. (1993). What do gastroenterologists in Europe tell cancer patients? *Lancet* **341**: 473–6.

Unschuld, P. U. (1985). *Medicine in China*. Berkeley, CA: University of California Press.

Veith, I. (1967). *The Yellow Emperor's Classic of Internal Medicine*. Berkeley, CA: University of California Press.

50

Hindu and Sikh bioethics

Harold Coward and Tejinder Sidhu

Mrs. E is a married 35-year-old Hindu woman expecting her fourth child. She has three daughters and on several occasions has expressed her desire to have a son. Because of her age, she is referred for amniocentesis to rule out genetic anomalies. A healthy female fetus is reported, whereupon Mrs. E requests a termination of pregnancy. The pregnancy is now at 20 weeks. Mr. and Mrs. E are referred for counseling.

Mr. and Mrs. F, an orthodox Sikh couple, are happily anticipating the birth of their first child. The pregnancy is uneventful until 32 weeks, when gestational hypertension is diagnosed. Over the next two weeks, Mrs. F's condition continues to deteriorate despite bed rest, hospital care, and intensive medical management. Mr. and Mrs. F consent to cesarean section to save the lives of mother and child. At 34 weeks, a female infant is delivered by cesarean section under general anesthetic. The baby is grossly edematous, looks dysmorphic, and has an Apgar score of 1 at one minute. Her birth weight is 1000 g, and the placenta is small and calcified. Mrs. F is still under general anesthetic, and Mr. F is not in the operating room. The physicians need to decide on the degree of intervention. Fortunately, the infant responds to basic stimulation from toweling and drying under a prewarmed radiant heater and to resuscitation with oxygen by facemask. Her Apgar score is 6 at five minutes and 8 at ten minutes. The baby is transferred to the neonatal intensive care unit, and a buccal smear is sent for karyotyping to rule out chromosomal abnormality. Following the surgery, the physicians meet with Mr. F to discuss the baby's condition. The neonatal specialist, considering the baby's condition to be grave and irremediable, advises against intensive intervention.

What are Hindu and Sikh bioethics?

Hinduism is the most ancient religion of India, dating from about 2500 BC. Sikhism, which has influences from Hinduism, arose as a separate religion some 500 years ago. The majority of Sikhs live in the Punjab, whereas Hindus are found throughout India. The first wave of Sikh immigration into North America occurred between 1905 and 1915; however, the majority of Sikhs entered North America between 1960 and 1985. Hindus began immigrating into North America in the 1960s.

In the Hindu and Sikh traditions, there is no great distinction between religion and culture, and ethical decisions are grounded in both religious beliefs and cultural values. In contrast to the contemporary secular approach to bioethics, which is predominantly rights based, Hindu and Sikh bioethics is primarily duty based. Indeed, there is no word for rights in traditional Hindu and Sikh languages. (Although most Sikhs speak Punjabi, Hindus speak a variety of languages, including Hindi, Bengali, Marathi, Tamil, and Malayalam.) Traditional teachings deal with the duties of individuals and families to maintain a lifestyle conducive to physical and mental health. Although there are profound differences between the Hindu and Sikh religions and considerable diversity within them, these traditions share a culture and worldview that includes ideas of karma and rebirth, collective

An earlier version of this chapter has appeared: Coward, H. and Sidhu, T. (2000). Hinduism and Sikhism. *Canadian Medical Association Journal* **163**: 1167–70.

versus individual identity, a strong emphasis on purity, and a preference for sons.

The notion of karma and a belief in rebirth will be important for many Hindu and Sikh patients as they make ethical decisions surrounding birth and death. Unlike the linear view of life taken in Judaism, Christianity, and Islam, for Hindus and Sikhs, life, birth, and death are repeated, for each person, in a continuous cycle. The fundamental idea is that each person is repeatedly reborn so that his or her soul may be purified and ultimately join the divine cosmic consciousness (Radhakrishnan, 1968). What a person does in each life influences the circumstances and predispositions experienced in future lives. In essence, every action or thought, whether good or evil, leaves a trace in the unconscious that is carried forward into the next life. When a similar situation is encountered, that memory trace arises in the consciousness as an impulse to perform an action or think a thought similar to the earlier one. This impulse does not necessarily compel the person to repeat the act or thought. He or she can still exercise free will by either nurturing or uprooting what has been laid down in the unconscious. Karma theory rejects any absolute beginning and assumes that life has always been going on. Consequently, each person is thought to have a huge store of memory traces from previous lives that are transferred at birth and that, with the additions and deletions made through free choice in the current life, will influence rebirth in the next life (based on the *Yoga Sutras of Patanjali*, written around 2000 years ago; Woods, 1966). From this perspective, the moment of conception is the rebirth of a fully developed person who has lived many previous lives. Termination by abortion sends the soul back into the karmic cycle of rebirth.

Another major difference between Hindu and Sikh cultures and Western cultures concerns the question of identity. Who is the ethical agent in decision making: the patient or the family? In Western secular society, the individual person is viewed as having autonomy in ethical decision making. In Ayurveda (traditional south Asian medicine) the person is viewed as a combination of mind, soul, and body in the context of family, culture, and nature (Kakar, 1982). Thus, the person is seen not as autonomous but rather as intimately integrated with his or her extended family, caste, and environment. This necessitates a holistic approach to ethical matters such as informed consent, one that includes the patient's societal context as well as the religious or spiritual dimension of his or her experience.

Purity is an important value in Hindu and Sikh culture (Madan, 1985). In the classical Indian tradition, there are two terms for purity. *Suddha* (or *shudh* in Punjabi) evokes the image of the human body or elements of nature (e.g., the Ganges river) in their most pure, perfect, and desired state of being. *Sauca* (*sucha* in Punjabi) also means ''pure'' but relates more specifically to personal cleanliness. The most impure (*asauca*, or *jutha* in Punjabi) substances are the discharges of one's body. Women, since they have more discharges than men, are seen as being more impure. Only before puberty or after menopause does a female approach the standard of purity of a male. The matter is even more complex because the purity–impurity axis in daily life is bisected by the auspicious–inauspicious axis (*subha–asubha*). For example, childbirth is auspicious if it occurs under the right circumstances. However, even if the circumstances are favorable, the act of childbirth itself, involving the discharge of bodily fluids, renders the mother impure. The baby is also impure, but this impurity becomes insignificant in view of the auspiciousness of birth, particularly the birth of a son, which is duly celebrated through ritual performance and social ceremonies during the following 11–13 days, culminating in the ritual of purification (Coward *et al.*, 1989).

There is a general bias in favor of males over females in Hindu and Sikh culture. The roots of this bias are two-fold. In Hinduism, for example, the eldest son is required to light his father's funeral pyre and to perform yearly rituals for the wellbeing of the father in the next life. The eldest son is also the head of the extended family and has the responsibility to protect and provide for the women in the family; this includes a moral obligation to ensure that sexual mores are preserved. Sons at marriage receive a dowry with their wife, which adds to the family wealth. Daughters, in taking a dowry with them at marriage, do the reverse. The responsibility of eldest sons to provide for and protect the women in their extended families means that there is often a strong male dominance in matters of consent.

Why are Hindu and Sikh bioethics important?

The ethical theories employed in healthcare today tend to apply a Western philosophical framework to issues such as abortion, euthanasia, and informed consent. Yet the diversity of cultural and religious assumptions with respect to human nature, health and illness, life and death, and the status of the individual demands that physicians be sensitive to and respectful of the varied perspectives patients bring to ethical decision making (Coward and Ratanakul, 1999). Hindus and Sikhs are important minority groups in North America. For instance, in Canada, recent census figures show that about 500 000 South Asians, of whom Hindus and Sikhs make up the majority, are living in Canada. There are more than 1 billion South Asians in the world population. Many Hindus and Sikhs, especially those who are second and third generation in western countries, have acculturated to the dominant rights-based approach of Western bioethics, but recent immigrants, particularly older people, may apply the duty-based approach of their own tradition when considering treatment options.

How should I approach Hindu and Sikh bioethics in practice?

To avoid miscommunication, physicians need to understand and respect the religious and cultural traditions of their Hindu and Sikh patients. They also need to recognize the diversity of beliefs and practices within these populations. Individual patients' reactions to a particular clinical situation will be influenced by a number of factors, including how recently they or their families arrived in Canada, their level of education, whether their roots are rural or urban, their socioeconomic status, and their religious stance (e.g., fundamentalist versus moderate). Table 50.1 summarizes essential points to keep in mind when providing care to Hindu and Sikh patients. Extended families are common and provide family members with social support and financial security. Tradition favors frequent visits to an ill person by friends and members of the extended family to offer support. Therefore, the physician may encounter more visitors at the patient's bedside than he or she is accustomed to. Elderly members of the extended family provide advice, help with childcare, and are accorded respect. The family spokesperson, with whom issues of consent will usually have to be negotiated, is usually the most financially established senior person in the family; however, if there is a language barrier, a younger member of the family may fulfill the communication role for the family.

If the patient and physician do not speak the same language, every effort should be made to find a trained and impartial interpreter who is familiar with the patient's traditions and culture. It is particularly important in issues of consent to ensure that information given to or received from the patient is not being censored or altered by the interpreter. Because of their deep sense of modesty and of purity, Hindu and Sikh women may not feel comfortable with male physicians or interpreters. Family members such as a teenaged daughter may function well as an interpreter for minor problems; however, an older, trained Hindu or Sikh woman who understands medical terminology and is not a family member will make the best interpreter, especially in urological and gynecological matters. In some circumstances a female relative or the patient's husband may have to serve as an

Table 50.1. Essential qualities of ethical approaches to communication and caregiving involving Hindu and Sikh patients

Quality	Characteristics
Recognize the concept of karma and rebirth	Ideas of karma and rebirth are important when ethical issues surrounding birth and death are considered. The fetus is not developing into a person but, rather, is already a person from the moment of conception. Therefore, abortion is unacceptable except to save the mother's life. Every effort to save premature babies will likely be desired by devout parents
Involve the family	Regarding matters of diagnosis, treatment, and consent, the extended family, with the senior elder as spokesperson, will probably expect to be involved. The ethical agent in Hindu and Sikh traditions is usually understood to be the collective (extended) family rather than the autonomous individual. However, there is still a sense of individuality that must be respected. Thus, involve the extended family but ensure that the wishes of the individual are respected
Respect modesty and purity concepts	Because of their deep sense of modesty, Hindu and Sikh women may not feel comfortable with male physicians or interpreters, especially if urological and gynecological matters are involved. In particular, newly arrived immigrants and elders will be reluctant to uncover their bodies, especially in front of the opposite sex. Women will generally avert their gaze as a sign of respect, or when embarrassed. In traditional thinking, mucous secretions are seen as very impure
Use interpreters	If there are language barriers, use a trained and impartial interpreter who is familiar with Hindu or Sikh religious and cultural traditions. Female patients will need a female interpreter; if necessary, a female relative or the patient's husband could act as interpreter, although this is not preferred, especially in view of the importance of preserving the confidentiality of the physician–patient relationship
Allow for Ayurvedic medicine	Many South Asian people, especially Hindus, may wish to use Ayurveda, the traditional Indian medicine, alongside Western medicine. Ayurvedic medications are largely herbal and are used along with changes in diet, habits, and thoughts to overcome an imbalance in the three bodily humors: vata (wind), pitta (bile), and kapha (phlegm). (Klostermaier, 1998)

interpreter, but, in view of the importance of pre-serving the confidentiality of the physician–patient relationship, using an interpreter who knows the patient personally is not the preferred approach.

The physician may need to alter his or her usual communication style in caring for Hindu and Sikh patients. By planning for a longer interview and adopting an indirect conversational approach, the physician is likely to learn more. It also helps to be alert to untranslatable Hindi or Punjabi words commonly used to express psychosomatic symptoms; for example, the phrase *dil* (heart) *kirda* (fragmenting) *dubda* (sinking), which an interpreter or the patient may express in English as "a sinking heart," implies tremendous anxiety that may result from a headache, nausea, stomach pain (especially epigastric), or generalized malaise. The physician should rule out organic disease before adopting a psychosomatic interpretation. He or she should also be alert for the term *nazar* ("evil eye") accompanied by a black mark behind the ear or a black thread around the wrist to protect the patient against the malevolent wishes of another. In many Hindu and Sikh households, there is an attachment to traditional medicines (e.g., Ayurveda and Siddha), which may be used together with modern medicine

(Azariah *et al.*, 1998). Cultural beliefs about health, disease and treatment often differ significantly from standard Western medical practice, and there are likely to be differing dietary practices as well, ranging from veganism (no meat, fish, eggs, or dairy products) to a rejection of beef but acceptance of chicken or fish.

The cases

Contrary to the physician's expectation, Mr. and Mrs. E do not wait for the counseling appointment but travel to the USA to have the pregnancy terminated. For Hindus and Sikhs, the single most important ethical consideration surrounding the start of life is their belief in karma: that the fetus is not developing into a person but, rather, is already a person from the moment of conception. Abortion at any stage of fetal development is thus judged to be murder. However, abortion is accepted by Hindus and Sikhs if essential to preserve the life of the mother (Coward 1993). Furthermore, the religious prohibition of abortion is sometimes at odds with the cultural preference for sons. For Mr. and Mrs. E, the desire for a son outweighs the stance of their religion against abortion.

Mr. F affirms his religious belief in the sanctity of life and insists on maximum medical intervention. Baby F's edema resolves by 50% over the next 24 hours and resolves completely by 72 hours. She requires minimal medical intervention and leaves the hospital at 10 days. Karyotyping results are normal. In this example, it might have been easy to allow the cultural bias against female babies to prevail. However, unlike in the first case, the parents' religious beliefs overruled their cultural biases – and the clinical and ethical judgement of the physician involved.

REFERENCES

Azariah, J., Azariah, H., and Macer, D. R. J. (eds.) (1998). *Bioethics in India. Proceedings of the International Bioethics Workshop in Madras: Biomanagement of Biogeo-resources*, Jan 1997, University of Madras. Christchurch, NZ: Eubios Ethics Institute.

Coward, H. G. (1993). World religions and reproductive technologies. In *Social Values and Attitudes Surrounding New Reproductive Technologies*, Vol. 2. Ottawa: Royal Commission of New Reproductive Technologies, Research Studies, pp. 454–63.

Coward, H. G., Lipner, J. J., and Young, K. K. (1989). *Hindu Ethics: Purity, Abortion and Euthanasia*. Albany, NY: State University of New York Press.

Coward, H. and Ratanakul, P. (eds.) (1999). Introduction. In *A Cross-cultural Dialogue on Health Care Ethics*, ed. H. Coward and P. Ratanakul. Waterloo, ON: Wilfrid Laurier University Press, pp. 1–11.

Kakar, S. (1982). Indian medicine and psychiatry: cultural and theoretical perspectives on ayurveda. In *Shamans, Mystics and Scholar*, Ch. 8. Boston, MA: Beacon Press.

Klostermaier, K. K. (1998). *A Concise Encyclopedia of Hinduism*. Oxford: Oneworld.

Madan, T. N. (1985). Concerning the categories of subha and suddha in Hindu culture. In *Purity and Auspiciousness in Indian Society*, ed. J. B. Caorman and F. A. Marglin. Leiden: EJ Brill, pp. 11–29.

Radhakrishnan, S. (1968). *The Principal Upanisads*. London: Allen and Unwin.

Woods, J. H. (trans) (1966). *Yoga Sutras of Patanjali* II: 12–14 and IV:7–9, Vol. 17. Varanasi: Motial Banarsidass, Harvard Oriental Series.

51

Islamic bioethics

Abdallah S. Daar, Tarif Bakdash, and Ahmed B. Khitamy

An 18-year-old Muslim man sustains severe head injures in a traffic accident while riding his motorcycle. He is declared brain dead. The transplant coordinator approaches the grieving mother to obtain consent for organ donation. At first, the patient's mother is shocked at this approach. She then politely says that she would like to wait for her family to arrive before making a decision.

A 38-year-old Muslim woman is found to have a rapidly growing carcinoma of the breast. She requires surgery and postoperative chemotherapy. She is five weeks into her first pregnancy and is advised to terminate the pregnancy before the chemotherapy.

What is Islamic bioethics?

In Islam, human beings are the crown of creation and are God's vicegerents on earth. (Qur'an, 2:30) They are endowed with reason, choice, and responsibilities, including stewardship of other creatures, the environment, and their own health. Muslims are expected to be moderate and balanced in all matters (al Khayat, 1995) including health. Illness may be seen as a trial or even as a cleansing ordeal, but it is not viewed as a curse or punishment or an expression of Allah's (God's) wrath. Hence, the patient is obliged to seek treatment and to avoid being fatalistic.

Islamic bioethics is intimately linked to the broad ethical teachings of the Qur'an and the tradition of the Prophet Muhammad, and thus to the interpretation of Islamic law. Bioethical deliberation is inseparable from the religion itself, which emphasizes continuities between body and mind, the material and spiritual realms, and between ethics and jurisprudence (al Faruqi, 1982) The Qur'an and the traditions of the Prophet have laid down detailed and specific ethical guidelines regarding various medical issues. The Qur'an itself has a surprising amount of accurate detail regarding human embryological development, which informs discourse on the ethical and legal status of the embryo and fetus before birth (Bucaille, 1979; Albar, 1996).

Islamic bioethics emphasizes the importance of preventing illness, but when prevention fails, it provides guidance not only to the practicing physician but also to the patient (Ebrahim, 1989). It teaches that the patient must be treated with respect and compassion and that the physical, mental, and spiritual dimensions of the illness experience be taken into account. The Muslim physician understands the duty to strive to heal, acknowledging God as the ultimate healer.

The main principles of the Hippocratic oath are reflected in Islamic bioethics, although the invocation of multiple gods in the original version, and the exclusion of any god in later versions, have led Muslims to adopt the Oath of the Muslim Doctor, which invokes the name of Allah. It appears in the

An earlier version of this chapter has appeared: Daar, A. S. and Khitamy, A. (2001). Islamic bioethics. *CMAJ* **164**: 60–3.

2003 *Islamic Code of Medical Ethics*, which deals with issues such as organ transplantation and assisted reproduction. In Islam, life is sacred: every moment of life has great value, even if it is of poor quality. The saving of life is a duty, and the unwarranted taking of life a grave sin. The Qur'an affirms the reverence for human life in reference to a similar commandment given to other monotheistic peoples: "On that account We decreed for the Children of Israel that whosoever killeth a human being ... it shall be as if he had killed all humankind, and whosoever saveth the life of one, it shall be as if he saved the life of all humankind" (Qur'an, 5:32). This passage legitimizes medical advances in saving human lives (Sachedina, 1995) and justifies the prohibition against both suicide and euthanasia.

The Oath of the Muslim Doctor includes an undertaking "to protect human life in all stages and under all circumstances, doing [one's] utmost to rescue it from death, malady, pain and anxiety. To be, all the way, an instrument of God's mercy, extending ... medical care to near and far, virtuous and sinner and friend and enemy."

Islamic bioethics is an extension of Shariah (Islamic law), which is itself based on two foundations: the Qur'an (the holy book of all Muslims, whose basic impulse is to release the greatest amount possible of the creative moral impulse [Rahman, 1979] and is itself "a healing and a mercy to those who believe" [Qur'an, 41:44]); and the Sunna (the aspects of Islamic law based on the Prophet Muhammad's words or acts). Development of Shariah in the Sunni branch of Islam over the ages has also required *ijmaa* (consensus) and *qiyas* (analogy), resulting in four major Sunni schools of jurisprudence. Where appropriate, consideration is also given to *maslaha* (public interest) and *urf* (local customary precedent) (Kamali, 1991). The Shia branch of Islam has in some cases developed its own interpretations, methodology, and authority systems, but on the whole its bioethical rulings do not differ fundamentally from the Sunni positions. In the absence of an organized "church" and ordained "clergy" in Islam, the determination of valid religious practice, and hence the resolution of bioethical issues, is left to qualified scholars of religious law, who are called upon to provide rulings on whether a proposed action is forbidden, discouraged, neutral, recommended, or obligatory.

Islamic scholars have been writing about bioethical issues for a very long time. For example, the four bioethics principles of beneficence, non-malevolence, autonomy, and justice popularized by Beauchamp and Childress (2001) were discussed by Muslim scholars as early as the thirteenth century (Aksoy and Tenik, 2002; Aksoy and Elmai, 2002; Ajlouni, 2003).

To respond to new medical technology, Islamic jurists, informed by technical experts, have regular conferences at which emerging issues are explored and consensus is sought. Over the past few years, these conferences have dealt with such issues as organ transplantation, brain death, assisted conception, technology in the intensive care unit, and even futuristic issues such as testicular and ovarian grafts. The broader Islamic bioethics discourse has included work on human embryonic stem cell research (Serour and Dickens, 2001; Walters, 2004; Aksoy, 2005), organ transplantation (Daar, 2000; Goolam, 2002; Khalil, 2002; Shaheen *et al.*, 2004; Todorova and Kolev, 2004; Golmakani *et al.*, 2005), triage (Elcioglu and Unluoglu, 2004), informed consent (Moazam, 2001; Rashad *et al.*, 2004), end of life decision making (Hedayat and Pirzadeh, 2001; Clarfield *et al.*, 2003; Lundqvist *et al.*, 2003; Rodríguez Del Pozo and Fins, 2005), abortion (Daar and al Khitamy, 2001; Moosa, 2002; Al-Kassimi, 2003; Mohammed, 2003; Asman, 2004; Wong *et al.*, 2004; Schenker, 2005), assisted reproduction and genetic testing (El Dawla, 2000; Schenker, 2000, 2002, 2005; Fadel, 2001, 2002; Serour and Dickens, 2001; Albar, 2002; Arbach, 2002; Tsianakas and Liamputtong, 2002; Ahmed, 2003; Raz and Atar, 2003; Raz, *et al.*, 2003; Sher *et al.*, 2004), nursing (Rassool, 2000; Lundqvist *et al.*, 2003; Ott *et al.*, 2003; Rashad *et al.*, 2004), and pharmacy (Chipman, 2002). Many medical schools in countries with Muslim majorities have bioethics curricula. There are established mechanisms for addressing emerging biomedical and bioethics issues, and curricula are updated accordingly.

The Islamic Organization for Medical Sciences, (www.islamset.com) also holds conferences and publishes the *Bulletin of Islamic Medicine*. Most Islamic communities, however, would defer to the opinion of their own recognized religious scholars.

Islam is not monolithic, and a diversity of views in bioethical matters does exist. This diversity derives from the various schools of jurisprudence, the different sects within Islam, differences in cultural background, and different levels of religious observance.

There is little that is strange or foreign in Islamic bioethics for Western physicians, who are often surprised at the similarities of approach to major bioethical issues in the three monotheistic religions, particularly between Islam and Judaism (Daar, 1994, 1997).

If secular Western bioethics can be described as rights based, with a strong emphasis on individual rights, Islamic bioethics is based on duties and obligations (e.g., to preserve life, seek treatment), although rights (Shad, 1981) (of God, the community, and the individual) do feature in bioethics, as does a call to virtue (Ihsan).

Why is Islamic bioethics important?

The number of Muslims worldwide is estimated to be over 1.2 billion and their numbers are projected to increase. Even in Western countries, the number of Muslims is increasing; for example in Canada the number of Muslims had reached 550 000 by 1999 (Hamdani, 1999).

Many Muslims incorporate their religion into almost every aspect of their lives. They invoke the name of God in daily conversation and live a closely examined life in relation to what is right or wrong behavior, drawing often from the Qur'an, the traditions of the Prophet, and subsequent determinations by Muslim jurists and scholars, believing that

their actions are very much accountable (Qur'an, 52:21, 4:85) and subject to ultimate judgement.

Although individuals are given certain concessions on assuming the status of a patient, some try to live their lives in a Muslim way as patients, even when admitted to hospital. Greater understanding of Islamic bioethics would enhance the medical care of Muslims living in Western societies.

How should I approach Islamic bioethics in practice?

In the West, information about Islamic bioethics can be obtained most easily on the Internet (see related websites below). Another source is Muslim patients themselves. However, many Muslim patients may not be aware of contemporary discourse on bioethical issues. If the community has religious leaders or its own social workers, these can be useful sources. Hospitals should keep their contact numbers close at hand, especially in emergency departments.

There are varying degrees of observance of traditional Muslim beliefs and practices. Physicians need to be sensitive to this diversity and avoid a stereotyped approach to all Muslim patients.

At the practical level, physicians who are aware of Islamic bioethics will understand that the provision of simple measures can make big differences for their Muslim patients. In addition to understanding the religion and culture, there are a few practical considerations that may apply, particularly for the more devout Muslim (Table 5.1).

The cases

The first case raises the issue of organ transplantation. Organ transplantation is practiced in most countries with Muslim majorities. This generally involves kidney donations from living relatives, but cadaveric donation is increasing (Daar, 1997, 2000; Goolam, 2002; Khalil, 2002; Shaheen *et al.*, 2004; Todorova and Kolev, 2004; Golmakani *et al.*, 2005).

Table 51.1. Essential qualities of ethical approaches to communication and caregiving involving Muslim patients

Qualities	Characteristics
Diet	Muslims have fairly strict dietary rules. Pork is forbidden, as is alcohol (although it can be used externally). Meat must be processed in special ways (halal), but if halal meat is unavailable, kosher meat (and kosher food in general) may be acceptable
Privacy	Women tend to be reluctant to uncover their bodies. If possible, physicians should ask female patients to uncover one area of their body at a time; they should be particularly careful and gentle when examining breasts or genitalia, and explain in advance what they are about to do. A chaperone should be present, particularly if the physician is male. Although not absolutely necessary, many Muslim families will prefer to have a female physician for the female family members, especially for gynecological examinations, and a male physician for the male members, if circumstances permit
Communication	Muslims who have arrived in the West in the recent past may have language barriers. It is advisable, therefore, to have an interpreter present who is preferably, but not necessarily, of the same sex as the patient
Religious observance	In general, health concerns override all religious observances. However, the more devout Muslims and those who are physically able, along with their companions, may wish to continue some religious observances in hospital. They would need running water for ablutions and a small quiet area to place a prayer mat facing Mecca (*qibla*). Staff should avoid disturbing them during the 10 minutes or so that it takes to pray, usually up to five times a day. Some patients will also frequently recite silently from the Qur'an or appear to be in meditation. During the month of Ramadhan, Muslim patients may ask about fasting, even though they are not required to fast when ill. Muslims regard both fasting and praying as being therapeutic.
Consent	Essentially, the principles and components of consent that are generally acceptable in Western countries are also applicable to Muslims, although Muslims (depending on their level of education, background, and culture) will often want to consult with family members before consenting to major procedures. Particular care should be exercised when the consent involves abortion, end of life issues, or sexual and gynecological issues.
Hygiene	Muslims are on the whole very conscious of matters pertaining to bodily functions and hygiene. Bodily discharges such as urine and feces are considered ritually unclean and must, therefore, be cleaned in certain ways. Ablutions are especially important before prayers, and so it is crucial to provide running water close to the patient, with sandals to wear in the toilet. Muslim patients will resist having a colostomy because it makes ritual cleanliness for prayers difficult to achieve. The surgeon, therefore, needs to spend more time than usual explaining the medical need and the steps that can be taken to minimize soiling

Many Muslim scholars have permitted cadaveric organ donation (Albar, 1995a; Yaseen, 1995; Daar, 1997, 2000; Daar *et al.*, 1997; Habgood *et al.*, 1997; Goolam, 2002; Khalil, 2002; Shaheen *et al.*, 2004; Todorova and Kolev, 2004; Golmakani *et al.*, 2005). The Qur'anic affirmation of bodily resurrection has determined many religious and moral decisions regarding cadavers (Sachedina, 1995). Mutilation,

and thus cremation, is strictly prohibited in Islam. However, carrying out autopsies, although currently uncommon in Muslim countries, is permitted under certain circumstances, for example when there is suspicion of foul play (Sachedina, 1995).

Death is considered to have occurred when the soul has left the body, but this exact moment cannot be known with certainty. Death is, therefore, diagnosed by its physical signs. The concept of brain death was accepted by a majority of scholars and jurists at the *Third International Conference of Islamic Jurists* in 1986 (Albar, 1995a; Moosa, 1999). Most, but not all, countries with Muslim majorities now accept brain death criteria. In Saudi Arabia, for example, about half of all kidneys for transplantation are derived from cadavers, with application of brain death criteria (Shaheen and Ramprasad, 1996).

The mother of the recently deceased boy in the intensive care unit was initially shocked because she did not expect an approach so soon after her son's death. The coordinator, however, has been specifically trained and is very experienced and culturally sensitive. She allows the mother time to reflect and wait for her family to arrive. The mother's faith has taught her that God decides when a life is to end, and although she is grieving she knows that nothing could have saved her son when the moment of death arrived. A friend of the family, a professor of Islamic studies at a local university, arrives and confirms that it is acceptable in Islam to donate organs under such circumstances. The family jointly agrees to the donation. The surgical team is made aware of the Muslim requirement to bury the body on the same day and arranges for the organs to be removed that afternoon.

The second case raises issues of the commencement of life. The general Islamic view is that, although there is some form of life after conception, full human life, with its attendant rights, begins only after the ensoulment of the fetus. On the basis of interpretations of passages in the Qur'an and of sayings of the Prophet, some Muslim scholars agree that ensoulment occurs at about 120 days after conception (Albar, 1995b, 1996), while other scholars hold that it occurs at about 40 days after conception (Albar, 1995b).

Islamic law scholars do have some differing opinions about abortion. Abortion has been allowed after implantation and before ensoulment in cases in which there were adequate juridical or medical reasons. Accepted reasons have included rape. However, many Shias and some Sunnis have generally not permitted abortion at any stage after implantation, even before ensoulment, unless the mother's life is in danger. Abortion after ensoulment is strictly forbidden by all Islamic authorities, but the vast majority do make an exception to preserve the mother's life. If a choice has to be made to save either the fetus or the mother, then the mother's life would take precedence. She is seen as the root, the fetus as an offshoot.

In the case presented here, the chemotherapy is necessary for the mother's health, although it might cause a miscarriage or severe developmental abnormalities in the fetus. The pregnancy itself may worsen her prognosis. These are medical indications for termination. Although not generally accepted, some modern Islamic opinions (Ghanem, 1984) and rulings (Muslim World League Conference of Jurists, 1990) have also accepted prenatal diagnosis and accept severe congenital anomalies and malformations per se as a reason for termination before ensoulment.

Two physicians certify that the chemotherapy and abortion are necessary, and the pregnancy is terminated with the consent of the patient and her husband. The couple says that they would dearly love to have a child in the future and inform the physician that Islam permits in vitro fertilization (Serour, 1992; Albar, 1995c; Fadel, 2001, 2002; Serour and Dickens, 2001; Al-Qasem, 2003). They ask if it is possible before chemotherapy to retrieve and freeze her ova, to be fertilized later. This would be permissible provided the sperm, with certainty, came from her husband, and that at the time of fertilization they are still married and the husband is alive. The option of surrogacy is broached by the physicians as an alternative. On checking with their local religious scholar, the couple is informed that, under Islamic law, the birth mother, not the ovum donor, would be the legal mother (Ebrahim, 1989; Al-Qasem, 2003). The couple decides not to pursue surrogacy.

REFERENCES

Ahmed, H. K. (2003). Adapting biotechnology to culture and values. [In *International Conference on Ethics: How to Adapt Biotechnology to Culture and Values*, Beirut, Lebanon, March 2003.] *Bull Med Ethics* **188**: 23–4.

Ajlouni, K. M. (2003). Values, qualifications, ethics and legal standards in Arabic (Islamic) medicine. *Saudi Med J* **24**: 820–6.

Aksoy, S. (2005). Making regulations and drawing up legislation in Islamic countries under conditions of uncertainty, with special reference to embryonic stem cell research. *J Med Ethics* **31**: 399–403.

Aksoy, S. and Elmai, A. (2002). The core concepts of the "four principles" of bioethics as found in Islamic tradition. *Med Law* **21**: 211–24.

Aksoy, S. and Tenik, A. (2002). The "four principles of bioethics" as found in 13th century Muslim scholar Mawlana's teachings. *BMC Med Ethics* **3**: e4.

al Faruqi, I. R. (1982). Tawhid its implications for thought and life. Kuala Lumpur: International Institute for Islamic Thought.

al Khayat, M. H. (1995). Health and Islamic behaviour. In *Health Policy, Ethics and Human Values: Islamic Perspective*, ed. A. R. El-Gindy. Kuwait: Islamic Organization of Medical Sciences, pp. 447–50.

Albar, M. A. (1995a). Organ transplantation: an Islamic perspective, *Contemporary Topics in Islamic Medicine*, Ch. 1. Jeddah: Saudi Arabia Publishing and Distributing House, pp. 3–11.

Albar, M. A. (1995b). When is the soul inspired? *Contemporary Topics in Islamic Medicine*, Ch. 15. Jeddah: Saudi Arabia Publishing and Distributing House, pp. 131–6.

Albar, M. A. (1995c). Contraception and abortion: an Islamic view. *Contemporary Topics in Islamic Medicine*, Ch. 14. Jeddah: Saudi Arabia Publishing and Distributing House, pp. 147–53.

Albar, M. A. (1996). *Human Development as Revealed in the Holy Qur'an and Hadith*. Jeddah: Saudi Arabia Publishing and Distributing House.

Albar, M. A. (2002). Ethical considerations in the prevention and management of genetic disorders with special emphasis on religious considerations. *Saudi Med J* **23**: 627–32.

Al-Kassimi, M. (2003). Cultural differences: practising medicine in an Islamic country. *Clin Med* **3**: 52–3.

Al-Qasem, L. (2003). Islamic ethical views on in vitro fertilization and human reproductive cloning.

M.Sc. Thesis, McGill University [*Masters Abst Int* **42–05**: 669].

Arbach, O. (2002). Ethical considerations in Syria regarding reproduction techniques. *Med Law* **21**: 395–401.

Asman, O. (2004). Abortion in Islamic countries: legal and religious aspects. *Med Law* **23**: 73–89.

Beauchamp, T. L. and Childress, J. F. (2001). *The Principles of Biomedical Ethics*, 5th edn. Oxford: Oxford University Press.

Bucaille, M. (1979). Human reproduction. *The Bible, the Qur'an and Science*. Indianapolis, IN: North American Trust Publications, pp. 198–210.

Chipman, L. N. B. (2002). The professional ethics of medieval pharmacists in the Islamic world. *Med Law* **21**: 321–38.

Clarfield, A. M., Gordon, M., Markwell, H., and Alibhai, S. M. H. (2003). Ethical issues in end-of-life geriatric care: the approach of three monotheistic religions: Judaism, Catholicism, and Islam. *J Ame Geriatr Soc* **51**: 1149–54.

Daar, A. S. (1994). Xenotransplantation and the major monotheistic religions. *Xeno* **2**: 61–4.

Daar, A. S. (1997). A survey of religious attitudes towards donation and transplantation. In *Procurement and Preservation and Allocation of Vascularized Organs*, ed. G. M. Collins, J. M. Dubernard, W. Land, and G. G. Persijn. Dordecht: Kluwer Academic, pp. 333–8.

Daar, A. S. (2000). Cultural and societal issues in organ transplantation: examples from different cultures. *Transplant Proc* **32**: 1480–1.

Daar, A. S. and al Khitamy, A. B. (2001). Bioethics for clinicians: 21. Islamic bioethics. *CMAJ* **164**: 60–3.

Daar, A. S., Shaheen, F. M., Albar, M., and al Khader, A. (1997). Transplantation in developing countries: issues bearing upon ethics. *Pakistan J Med Ethics* **2**: 4–7.

Ebrahim, A. M. (1989). *Abortion, Birth Control and Surrogate Parenting. An Islamic Perspective*. Indianapolis, IN: American Trust Publications.

El Dawla, A. S. (2000). Reproductive rights of Egyptian women: issues for debate. *Reprod Health Matt* **8**: 45–54.

Elcioglu, O. and Unluoglu, I. (2004). Triage in terms of medicine and ethics. *Saudi Med J* **25**: 1815–9.

Fadel, H. E. (2002). The Islamic viewpoint on new assisted reproductive technologies. *Fordham Urban Law J* **30**: 147–57.

Fadel, M. (2001). Islam and the new genetics. *St Thomas Law Rev* **13**: 901–11.

Ghanem, I. (1984). [Abortion as a necessity.] *Al Faisal Med J* **9**: 61–5.

Golmakani, M. M., Niknam, M. H., and Hedayat, K. M. (2005). Transplantation ethics from the Islamic point of view. *Int Med J Exp Clin Res* **11**: RA105–9.

Goolam, N. M. I. (2002). Human organ transplantation: multicultural ethical perspectives. *Med Law* **21**: 541–8.

Habgood, J., Spagnolo, A. G., Sgreccia, E., and Daar, A. S. (1997). Religious views on organ and tissue donation. In *Organ and Tissue Donation for Transplantation*, ed. J. R. Chapman, M. Deirhoi, and C. Wight. London: Arnold, pp. 23–33.

Hamdani, D. H. (1999). Canadian Muslims on the eve of the twenty-first century. *J Muslim Minority Affairs* **19**: 197–209.

Hedayat, K. M. and Pirzadeh, R. (2001). Issues in Islamic biomedical ethics: a primer for the pediatrician. *Pediatrics* **108**: 965–71.

Islamic Code of Medical Ethics (2003). (www.islamset. com).

Kamali, M. H. (1991). Urf (custom). *Principles of Islamic Jurisprudence*. Cambridge: Islamic Texts Society, pp. 283–96.

Khalil, K. J. (2002). A sight of relief: invalidating cadaveric corneal donation laws via the free exercise clause. *DePaul J Health Care Law* **6**: 159–78.

Lundqvist, A., Nilstun, T., and Dykes, A. K. (2003). Neonatal end-of-life care in Sweden: the views of Muslim women. *J Perinat Neonatal Nurs* **17**: 77–86.

Moazam, F. (2001). Reconciling patients' rights and God's wisdom: medical decision making in Pakistan. *Responsive Community* **11**: 43–51.

Mohammed, I. (2003). Issues relating to abortions are complicated in Nigeria. *BMJ* **326**: 225.

Moosa, E. (1999). *Occasional Paper 35: Languages of Change in Islamic Law: Redefining Death in Modernity*. Islamabad: Islamic Research Institute.

Moosa, N. (2002). A descriptive analysis of South African and Islamic abortion legislation and local Muslim community responses. *Med Law* **21**: 257–79.

Muslim World League Conference of Jurists (1990). *Twelfth Session: Regarding Termination of Pregnancy for Congenital Abnormalities*, February Mecca.

Ott, B. B., Al-Khadhuri, J., and Al-Junaibi, S. (2003). Preventing ethical dilemmas: understanding Islamic health care practices. *Pediatr Nurs* **29**: 227–30.

Rahman, F. (1979). Legacy and Prospects. Islam. 2nd edn. Chicago, IL: University of Chicago Press, pp. 235–54.

Rashad, A. M., MacVane Phipps, F., and Haith-Cooper, M. (2004). Obtaining informed consent in an Egyptian research study. *Nurs Ethics* **11**: 394–9.

Rassool, G. H. (2000). The crescent and Islam: healing, nursing and the spiritual dimension. Some considerations towards an understanding of the Islamic perspectives on caring. *J Adv Nurs* **32**: 1476–84.

Raz, A. E. and Atar, M. (2003). Nondirectiveness and its lay interpretations: the effect of counseling style, ethnicity and culture on attitudes towards genetic counseling among Jewish and Bedouin respondents in Israel. *J Genet Couns* **12**: 313–32.

Raz, A. E., Atar, M., Rodnay, M., Shoham-Vardi, I., and Carmi, R. (2003). Between acculturation and ambivalence: knowledge of genetics and attitudes towards genetic testing in a consanguineous bedouin community. *Commun Genet* **6**: 88–95.

Rodríguez Del Pozo, P. and Fins, J. J. (2005). Death, dying and informatics: misrepresenting religion on MedLine. *BMC Med Ethics* **6**: E6.

Sachedina, A. (1995). Islam. In *Encyclopedia of Bioethics*, revised edn, ed. W. T. Reich. New York: Simon and Schuster/Prentice Hall International, pp. 1289–97.

Schenker, J. G. (2000). Women's reproductive health: monotheistic religious perspectives. *Int J Gynaecol Obstet* **70**: 77–86.

Schenker, J. G. (2002). Gender selection: cultural and religious perspectives. *J Assist Reprod Genet* **19**: 400–10.

Schenker, J. G. (2005). Assisted reproductive practice: religious perspectives. *Reprod Biomed* **10**: 310–19.

Serour, G. I. (ed.) (1992). Islamic views. In *Proceedings of the First International Conference on Bioethics in Human Reproduction Research in the Muslim World*, December 1991, Cairo. Cairo: International Islamic Center for Population Studies and Research, Al Azhar University, pp. 234–42.

Serour, G. I. and Dickens, B. M. (2001). Assisted reproduction developments in the Islamic world. *Int J Gynecol Obstet* **74**: 187–93.

Shad, A. R. (1981). *The Rights of Allah and Human Rights*. Lahore: Kazi.

Shaheen, F. A. M. and Ramprasad, K. S. (1996). Current status of organ transplantation in Saudi Arabia. *Transpl Proc* **28**: 1200–1.

Shaheen, F. A. M., Al-Jondeby, M., Kurpad, R., and Al-Khader, A. A. (2004). Social and cultural issues in organ transplantation in Islamic countries. *Ann Transpl* **9**: 11–3.

Sher, C., Romano-Zelekha, O., Green, M. S., and Shohat, T. (2004). Utilization of prenatal genetic testing by Israeli Moslem women: a national survey. *Clin Genet* **65**: 278–83.

Todorova, B. and Kolev, V. (2004). Theological and moral aspects of cadaverous donation-heart transplantation from the point of view of Islam. *Formos J Med Human* **5**: 29–36.

Tsianakas, V. and Liamputtong, P. (2002). Prenatal testing: the perceptions and experiences of Muslim women in Australia. *J Reprod Infant Psychol* **20**: 7–24.

Walters, L. (2004). Human embryonic stem cell research: an intercultural perspective. *Kennedy Inst Ethics J* **14**: 3–38.

Wong, M. L., Chia, K. S., Wee, S., *et al.* (2004). Concerns over participation in genetic research among Malay-Muslims, Chinese and Indians in Singapore: a focus group study. *Community Genet* **7**: 44–54.

Yaseen, M. N. (1995). The rulings for the donation of human organs in the light of Shar'i rules and medical facts. In *Health Policy, Ethics and Human Values: Islamic Perspective*, ed. A. R. El-Gindy. Kuwait: Islamic Organization of Medical Sciences, pp. 303–67.

Related websites

BBC World Service guide to Islam: www.bbc.co.uk/worldservice/people/features/world_religions/islam.shtml

Canadian Council of Muslim Women: http://www.ccmw.com/

Islamic studies: www.arches.uga.edu/~godlas

Islam Top Sites: www.islamtopsites.com

52

Jehovah's Witness bioethics

Osamu Muramoto

A 65-year-old Jehovah's Witness (JW) elder was admitted for a three-day history of dizziness, weakness, shortness of breath, and hematochezia. His hemoglobin level on admission was 70 g/l. He was mentally competent and fully committed to the religion. He refused any blood products under any circumstances. Colonic diverticular bleeding was diagnosed. Despite maximum conservative treatment, the bleeding continued. A decision was made to perform a subtotal colectomy without blood products.

A 17-year-old JW female was brought to an emergency department after a suicide attempt by self-inflicting multiple cuts to her left medial elbow. The wound reached the main artery. By the time she was found in her bed, she had lost a large amount of blood and was hypotensive and lethargic. The first words the JW parents gave to the emergency personnel were that she must not receive blood transfusion. When confronted with the emergency physician who advised them that blood transfusion was inevitable, the parents threatened lawsuit against him and the hospital if he gave her blood. They called in a congregation elder, who handed out the list of "no-blood alternatives" published by their organization and insisted on using them, but not blood. She did not carry an advance directive. Despite a large volume fluid resuscitation, hemorrhagic shock ensued.

What is Jehovah's Witness bioethics?

What is Jehovah's Witnesses?

Jehovah's Witnesses (JW) is a bible-based religion founded in the late nineteenth century in Pennsylvania, USA (Penton, 1998). Although the new religion then had a strong influence from the Second Adventist movement, the current JWs do not consider themselves as a Christian denomination. There are fundamental differences in theology from traditional Christian faiths. The central organization of JWs is the Watchtower Bible and Tract Society (WTS), which grew out of a small religious sect in the USA in the early and mid twentieth century to a worldwide publishing giant producing their religious magazines and books today. It has an extensive network of branches, printing factories, and congregations in 235 lands with total 6.5 million baptized followers (WTS, 2006). The religious life of JWs is centered around five religious meetings every week and door-to-door preaching. Important religious activities include weekly studies and discussion of the magazines, books, and the Bible published by the WTS. Preaching or "field service" is another important activity, and each JW is required to report monthly the time spent for preaching activity and the amount of literature distributed. Many unique religious rules govern their personal lives. The following are strictly prohibited: participation in politics and the military, association with other religions, celebration of holidays and birthday, pledging allegiance to a national flag, singing a national anthem, smoking, and medical use of certain blood products. JWs also must shun excommunicated ("disfellowshipped") members including those who willfully accepted forbidden blood products, and opposing former members ("apostates").

The JWs believe the Bible as the ultimate source of their religious doctrines, which are often based on strict literal interpretations that are not shared by Christian denominations. The blood doctrine is the best example. One of the most important doctrines of JWs is that this world is currently in the "Last Days," awaiting imminent Armageddon or cataclysmic destruction of the present system. According to their doctrine, the Last Days started in 1914, and the WTS has predicted different years as the starting year of Armageddon, including 1918, 1920, 1925, and 1975. In 1995, they finally abandoned the previous practice of predicting specific years. Nonetheless, the WTS maintains that Armageddon is still imminent in the near future, a literal destruction of this system is inevitable, and only the faithful JWs will survive and live forever in paradise on earth. This sense of urgency, constant preparation for Armageddon, and repeated postponements of paradise, are very important in understanding JWs' psychology and worldview.

Views on life

The JW's views on life are key to understanding their unique attitudes toward medical care. Unlike most other Bible-based religions, JWs do not believe in immortal souls. Instead, their future hope is their physical survival of Armageddon (or if they die before Armageddon arrives, resurrection in fresh bodies) to enter paradise on earth. Their current life in this world is only a temporary period of preparation for Armageddon and life in paradise. Since their entry into paradise depends on their conduct in this world, the most important concern in JWs' lives is to work hard to fulfill Jehovah's requirements, which include strict adherence to teachings of the WTS and dedication to preaching activity. Violations of the religious rules are one of the worst offences, which disqualify JWs from survival in paradise. Their eventual goals are not in this present system of the world, but in the future paradise. Many JWs even postpone childbearing until after Armageddon (WTS, 1988).

Views on health and disease

JWs believe in the literal presence of Satan, who is ruling in the Last Days and is the ultimate cause of all social injustice, disasters, epidemics, and death that increasingly plague this system (WTS, 1988). Diseases and suffering are the results of the original sin that has been inherited through the genetic system. Since Satan will not be destroyed until after Armageddon, they believe that no cure is available to human diseases and suffering in this system. They have no expectation or trust in human efforts to solve these evils (WTS, 2001). This is the main reason that JWs are not interested in social improvement or charitable contribution through traditional means, as are other religions.

JW's eventual "health" lies in survival or resurrection in paradise on earth. While they seek the best medical care in ordinary circumstances, when the decision comes to the point where they have to choose between a violation of the Jehovah's law and their own health and preservation of life in this system, they would readily forgo their own health.

Views on blood and blood transfusion

The most well-known and frequently encountered bioethical issue involving JWs is their refusal of blood products. The doctrine had not existed until 1945, when the WTS decided that the prohibition of eating blood in the Bible also prohibited blood transfusions. In 1951, the doctrine was firmly established based on three biblical passages, Genesis 9:4, Leviticus 17:12, and Acts 15:28,39 (WTS, 1951). For many years, they prohibited all the constituents of blood, including serum, and vaccination until 1952. Various medical and surgical procedures that take out blood and return it to circulation, such as heart–lung machine and hemodilution were also prohibited. In the 1960s and 1970s, owing to increasing demand and availability of blood component treatments and new technologies, the WTS gradually introduced exceptions to the rules, allowing use of serum and hemophiliac clotting factors. In 1981, a WTS physician wrote to the

Journal of the American Medical Association on the blood policy, which became a standard for the treatment of JWs in 1980s and 1990s (Dixon and Smalley, 1981). This 1981 article established that autologous blood could not be used, and hemodilution was objectionable, whereas hemodialysis, heart–lung machine, and intraoperative salvage were acceptable. All plasma fractions were now permitted as a result of this article.

The most recent policy change involves the use of hemoglobin. In 2000, as hemoglobin-based blood substitutes were being tested in clinical use, the WTS announced that hemoglobin products were now permissible (WTS, 2000a), retracting their long-standing prohibition against the medical use of human or animal hemoglobin, a policy that had been restated as recently as 1998 (Bailey and Ariga, 1998). Another change involves transfusion of autologous blood. Prior to 2000, the WTS prohibited transfusion of autologous blood that had been removed from a JW's circulatory system. As of 2000, the WTS permits JWs to accept autologous transfusions of blood so long as the collection and re-infusion is part of what its policy calls "current therapy" (WTS, 2000b). In practical terms, this policy change permits hemodilution, blood cell tagging, and blood patch, which all require removal of own blood, temporary storage outside the patient's circulatory system, and infusion. However, the WTS still prohibits preoperative autologous blood donation (WTS, 2000b). The only difference between now permitted hemodilution and still prohibited autologous transfusion is whether the infused blood is collected intraoperatively or preoperatively.

As of this writing, the WTS seems to try to streamline the blood policy that has become so technical and incomprehensible to medically uneducated JWs. The way to understand the current policy is to prohibit the whole blood and "primary" components (red blood cells [RBCs], white blood cells, platelets, and plasma), whereas "fractions" derived from the primary components are now all acceptable (WTS, 2004). However, such a distinction between "primary" component and "fraction"

is not universally defined, and the usage of such vague terms does not help in the comprehension of the rationale behind such a distinction. For example, RBCs, a fraction of the whole blood, are still prohibited, but hemoglobin, a primary component (98% of dry weight) of the RBC, is now permitted. Another example of a lack of rationale is that the removal and return of own blood for "current therapy" is permitted, but the same procedure for future therapy is prohibited, as mentioned above. JWs are unable to articulate why one is acceptable and the other unacceptable, other than saying "the Society (WTS) said so." As one JW elder wrote to the WTS (2000) such distinctions are beyond what JWs can explain based on their scriptural reasoning, or are simply beyond their common sense reasoning.

Originated in 1945 as a simple doctrine of refusal of whole blood transfusion, the current policy has become an extremely complicated technological protocol. The WTS first prohibited every component of blood, but then later progressively permitted various parts of blood and certain selected technologies. The most difficult predicament of the bioethics of JWs is found in this very fact that the religious doctrine has become intricately woven into the most advanced technological specifications in medicine, which is constantly changing through rapid technological advancement. When a life and death decision relies on the religious doctrine that is published by the medically untrained religious authority in religious publications, yet involves highly technical and evolving details of medical, rather than religious, information, neither the patient nor the clinicians can have a solid foundation of their informed decisions.

Views on mental health

JWs traditionally have unique views on mental health. Instead of recognizing mental disorders as diseases, they often attribute these conditions to "spiritual weakness." The WTS also interpreted the nature of certain mental illnesses as a possession of Satan, who dominates this system in the

"Last Days." This is consistent with their literal interpretation of the Bible concerning human illnesses (e.g., James 5:13–16). The advice given by the WTS to congregations has been to treat mentally ill members with spiritual advice of elders, rather than to take them to psychiatrists (WTS, 1963). The JWs have mistrusted psychiatrists and psychologists for many years because their advice is not consistent with the teaching of the Bible (WTS, 1975). In recent years, the WTS does not prohibit members from seeking advice from these professionals, but many JWs still follow the traditional advice to treat mental illnesses within the religious context (Bergman, 1992). It is noteworthy that JWs' religious doctrines, such as imminent cataclysmic disaster with a "narrow gate" to survive in paradise on earth, repeated postponements of paradise for almost one century since the foundation of the religion, many strict rules of conducts, and shunning of former members including their own family, have provided fertile soil for mental disorders. Yet the issue of JWs' mental health has been mostly unnoticed in medical literature (Spencer, 1975; Weishaupt and Stensland, 1997).

Views on other health and medical issues

There are several other medical and health issues which are unique to JWs, and clinicians should be aware of. Their lifestyle is generally healthy: they strictly avoid smoking and illicit drugs, though use of alcohol is permitted. JWs also prohibit potentially risky behaviors such as sexual promiscuity, martial arts, and contact sports. Regarding reproductive ethics, they strictly prohibit abortion and oppose to the use of intrauterine devices and morning-after pills because they are considered "abortive" (WTS, 1979), but they permit sterilization and birth control pills. Although the WTS has prohibited vaccination for the same reasons as they currently prohibit blood transfusions, and also prohibit organ transplantation as "cannibalism" (WTS, 1967), they now accept both vaccination and transplantation, including bone marrow

transplantations (Ballen *et al.*, 2000). Apparently, the WTS is not concerned about the fact that bone marrow transplants contain numerous immature as well as some mature blood cells. Rather, they justify bone marrow transplants based on a biblical passage that ancient Israelites ate bone marrow (Isaiah 25:6; WTS, 1984).

Why is Jehovah's Witness bioethics important?

There are several important points that are unique to JWs bioethics. Firstly, JW's refusal of blood products is one of the most frequent and universal cases of refusal of treatment, affecting more than 16 million people worldwide (including sympathizers and former members who attend the annual Memorial), which leads to life or death situations that could be easily reversed but which the clinician is constrained from doing so. It has often been considered a "paradigm case" of bioethics for refusal of treatment in relation to autonomy, informed consent, and advance directives. Historically, JW cases have contributed to the development of the concept and practice of informed consent and advance directives for healthcare.

Secondly, the ethical issues involving JWs have become increasingly complicated today because of the technical complexity and the wavering of the blood policy. Most JWs simply cannot comprehend it sufficiently enough to make a truly informed consent. Moreover, the internal information promulgated to the general membership tends to delay, overestimate the danger of blood transfusions, and underestimate the risk of alternative treatments. Such a misrepresentation on the part of the WTS might be morally disturbing (Louderback-Wood, 2005).

Thirdly, there is an increasing diversity among JWs toward the blood policy. Some JWs, particularly those who are well educated, can see obvious contradictions and inconsistencies inside the technical web of the blood policy. Since the late

1990s, an increasing number of dissident JWs who have different views on the blood policy have become vocal (Muramoto, 1998a; Elder, 2000). This has raised an important moral issue of personal identity of the members of a religious organization. Clinicians tend to treat JWs uniformly according to the policy of the WTS. While such a treatment may be respecting their uniform religious identity, their diverse personal identity may be ignored. Such a "standard" treatment is also problematic when a refusal of blood is made by non-JWs; their wishes may not be respected as much as those of JWs because they lack a religious identity.

How should I approach Jehovah's Witness bioethics in practice?

The fundamental moral principle I propose when clinicians approach JW patients is to respect autonomous wishes of the individual person, but not necessarily her religion (Muramoto, 2001). Put in other words, respect the patient as a person, but not necessarily as a member of her religious organization. If the doctrines and policies of her religion are identical with her autonomous wishes at any given time and in any particular situation, then these two are inseparable. However, such is almost impossible, given ever-changing human cognition and individuality of each medical and surgical condition. Moreover, as discussed above, there are very few JWs who actually understand the entirety of the technical details of the policy. Chances are that your JW patient has never seriously thought about such technical details until the issue becomes her own. It is likely that the commitment to the blood policy of your next JW patient is quite different from your last JW patient. It is critical to maintain an open-minded attitude and discuss the patient's personal conviction regarding blood first, rather than obediently following the guidelines published by the WTS. Misinformation and biased information circulated inside the JW community are quite common (Muramoto, 1998a; Louderback-wood, 2005). It is critical to discuss

such misinformation in order to ensure a chance for the JW patient to be fully informed (Muramoto, 1998b). If possible, such an inquiry should be done with strict confidentiality to relieve the peer pressure from her family and religious friends (Muramoto, 1999, 2000).

Faced with the need for blood products, JW patients have shown many different reactions depending on individual personality, social environment, educational level, and the degree of commitment to the religion. One reaction is to decline every possible treatment that has anything to do with blood, even if some of them are recently permitted by the WTS. Their reaction might be based on misinformation but could be uniquely personal. Another reaction is to leave their decisions to the congregational officials. Many JW patients call in special elders of their congregation or "the hospital liaison committee," who have special training to deal with the blood issue. Many JW patients delegate their decisions to those officials who function as a judge to decide which treatment is acceptable or unacceptable according to the then current WTS policy. Other JW patients are willing to accept some of the prohibited blood products based on their own interpretation. For example, some educated JWs may know that platelets are, in fact, a very small fraction, much smaller than the permitted albumin, and may conscientiously accept it. Others may have been skeptical about the blood policy all along but have not had a chance to seriously consider the issue. Such JWs might be willing to accept prohibited products under strict confidentiality. In any of those cases of deviation from the official policy, it is critical to maintain the strict confidentiality of the clinician–patient communications, and the specifics of the treatment (Muramoto, 1999, 2000).

When the patient expresses unequivocal conviction that she refuses any treatment that the WTS teaches as unacceptable, the clinician should accede to her request to the extent his own moral conviction can accommodate. Whenever alternative treatments are available without a substantial increase in risk, such treatments should be provided, and the refusal of objectionable blood products should be honored. When the clinician feels that it is impossible or uncomfortable to accede to the patient's demand, he should refer the patient promptly to a willing clinician after stabilization.

In an emergency when there is no current advance directive available and the patient cannot express her own wishes, it is legally defensible to use whatever is necessary to stabilize the patient's life-threatening condition first based on implicit consent (American College of Emergency Physicians, 2001). While the Canadian court ruled that the "no-blood card" carried by an exsanguinating and unconscious JW could not be overridden even in emergency (*Malette* v. *Shulman*, 1990), this ruling has been criticized because the card was signed but not dated nor witnessed (Noble, 1991). The emergency physician had no way of knowing her contemporaneous wishes or her status of being adequately informed of the risks (Migden and Braen, 1998). In recent years, the WTS is using more formal advance directive forms compliant with each jurisdiction, which the WTS requires each JW to execute and carry, in addition to the "no-blood card." If a valid and adequately executed advance directive is made available, it is legally indefensible to override it even in an emergency.

In any case, the best legal defense in cases of refusal of treatment is based on thorough communication with the patient, complete documentation of the patient's directives, and strict protection of medical confidentiality.

Finally, minors of JW parents should be treated separately from the parent's religion. Courts have repeatedly ruled that minors cannot become a martyr of the parent's religious beliefs in healthcare. Beauchamp (2003) argued that it is morally required, not merely permitted, to overrule the parental refusal of treatment. Decisions regarding "mature minors" or adolescent children are more problematic. The maturity of each child is different, and so is the child's understanding and commitment to the blood policy. If there is any unsolved

ethical or legal issue regarding JW minors, it is most appropriate to obtain a court order after necessary stabilization. (For more information on this topic, see Ch. 17.)

The cases

The first case is a straightforward case of competent and fully committed adult JW who unequivocally refuses any blood products. As an elder, he is also well informed of the blood policy, even though it is still unclear how biased his internal information was. There was no morally justifiable reason to override his autonomous and informed decision. Postoperatively, his hemoglobin level fell to 39 g/l, requiring neuromuscular blockade and full ventilatory support. His recovery was protracted, with several complications including pneumonia and cardiac failure secondary to severe anemia, requiring a total of 21 days of stay in intensive care and several weeks of hospital admission with incomplete recovery. If there was any ethical issue involved in this case, it is the excessive cost of care that would probably have been avoided if pre- and postoperative blood transfusions had been given. The issue is distributive justice of finite resources (Wooding, 1999).

The second case is more complicated. The patient was admitted to the intensive care unit where she received four units of packed red blood cells to stabilize her life-threatening condition. Her wound was repaired and then she was transferred to a psychiatric unit. Subsequent interviews by a psychiatrist revealed that she was born and raised in a JW family, but she was recently "disfellowshipped" because of a forbidden sexual activity and smoking. She still lived with her JW family, but the stress of guilt and being treated as the "spiritually weak" made her depression worse. Apparently she had not been committed to the religion for several months, though her parents were hopeful that she would return to the religion soon. She had a chance of being reinstated to the congregation if she repented her previous sins and led a "godly" life by adhering to all the standards set forth by the WTS. For her parents, it was critical that their daughter be in good standing from JW standards. Naturally, their concern was primarily her "spiritual health," which was to be defiled by consenting to blood transfusion, rather than her impending physical death.

She was not resentful nor did she feel defiled by receiving blood, yet she was fearful of the consequences, including the repercussions from her family and friends, and punishment from Jehovah, which is a painful death at the upcoming Armageddon. A week later, she was released under the custody of her parents. Antidepressants were prescribed, and a follow-up visit to the psychiatrist was arranged. However, the family never brought her back to the psychiatrist. Six weeks later, she committed suicide by hanging herself.

This case highlights several difficult issues involving JWs' healthcare. Firstly, the patient was 17 years old and legally a minor. Secondly, the patient was suicidal and most likely mentally ill, and her autonomy and competency could be compromised. Thirdly, at the moment of life-threatening emergency, it was highly unlikely that any of the "no-blood alternatives" the JW congregation elder offered would work. Fourthly, although she was presented as a JW by her family, she was in fact disfellowshipped and at that time she was in probationary status, which became known to the clinician only after the life-saving treatment. The judgement and decision by the team of clinicians were extremely difficult, but they were fully justified morally and legally based on the overriding emergency, her minor status, and mental illness.

Finally the other important point this case highlights is the mistrust of mental health services by JWs. While her mental disorder was deeply rooted in her religion, the "spiritual" treatment by the parents and the congregation officials eventually failed. Culturally sensitive psychiatric care of JWs is badly needed to gain trust from the JW community in order to provide better mental health services to this vulnerable population.

REFERENCES

American College of Emergency Physicians (2001). *Code of Ethics for Emergency Physicians.* [Policy 400188, 1997; reaffirmed October 2001.] Dallas, TX: American College of Emergency Physicians (http://www.acep.org/webportal/PracticeResources/PolicyStatements/ethics/codeethics.htm) accessed 14 August 2006.

Bailey, R. and Ariga, T. (1998). The view of Jehovah's Witnesses on blood substitutes. *Artif Cells Blood Substit Immobil Biotechnol* **26**: 571–6.

Ballen, K. K., Ford, P. A., Waitkus, H., *et al.* (2000). Successful autologous bone marrow transplant without the use of blood product support. *Bone Marrow Transpl* **26**: 227–9.

Beauchamp, T. L. (2003). Methods and principles in biomedical ethics. *J Med Ethics* **29**: 269–74.

Bergman, J. R. (1992). *Jehovah's Witnesses and the Problem of Mental Illness.* Clayton, CA: Witness.

Dixon, J. L. and Smalley, M. G. (1981). Jehovah's Witnesses. The surgical/ethical challenge. *JAMA* **246**: 2471–2.

Elder, L. (2000). Why some Jehovah's Witnesses accept blood and conscientiously reject official Watchtower Society blood policy. *J Med Ethics* **26**: 375–80.

JW elder (2000). Blood and upholding righteous standards. [A personal letter addressed to the Watchtower Bible and Tract Society by a Jehovah's Witness elder] (http://ajwrb.org/watchtower/2000.03.01Jensen.pdf) accessed 14 August 2006.

Louderback-Wood, K. (2005). Jehovah's Witnesses, blood transfusions, and the tort of misrepresentation. *J Church State* **47**: 783–822.

Malette v. *Shulman* (1990) 72 O.R. (2d) 417 (Ontario Court of Appeal).

Migden, D. R. and Braen, G. R. (1998). The Jehovah's Witness blood refusal card: ethical and medicolegal considerations for emergency physicians. *Acad Emerg Med* **5**: 815–24.

Muramoto, O. (1998a). Bioethics of the refusal of blood by Jehovah's Witnesses: part 1. Should bioethical deliberation consider dissidents' views? *J Med Ethics* **24**: 223–30.

Muramoto, O. (1998b). Bioethics of the refusal of blood by Jehovah's Witnesses: part 2. A novel approach based on rational non-interventional paternalism. *J Med Ethics* **24**: 295–301.

Muramoto, O. (1999). Bioethics of the refusal of blood by Jehovah's Witnesses: part 3. A proposal for a don't-ask-don't-tell policy. *J Med Ethics* **25**: 463–8.

Muramoto, O. (2000). Medical confidentiality and the protection of Jehovah's Witnesses' autonomous refusal of blood. *J Med Ethics* **26**: 381–6.

Muramoto, O. (2001). Bioethical aspects of the recent changes in the policy of refusal of blood by Jehovah's Witnesses. *BMJ* **322**: 37–9.

Noble, W. H. (1991). CMPA and Jehovah's Witness. *Can J Anesthesiol* **38**: 262–3.

Penton, M. J. (1998). *Apocalypse Delayed: The Story of Jehovah's Witnesses*, 2nd edn. Toronto: University of Toronto Press.

Spencer, J. (1975). The mental health of Jehovah's Witnesses. *Br J Psychiat* **126**: 556–9.

Weishaupt, K. J. and Stensland, M. D. (1997). Wifely subjection: mental health issues in Jehovah's Witness women. *Cultic Studies J* **14**: 106–44.

Wooding, N. (1999). Costs incurred by one severely ill Jehovah's Witness could run one unit in Africa for one year. *BMJ* **318**: 873.

WTS (1951). Question from readers. *The Watchtower*, 1 July, 414–16.

WTS (1963). Where to turn for counsel. *The Watchtower*, 15 January, 37–9.

WTS (1967). Question from readers. *The Watchtower*, 15 November, 702–4.

WTS (1975). Question from readers. *The Watchtower*, 15 April, 255–6.

WTS (1979). Questions from readers. *The Watchtower*, 15 May, 30–1.

WTS (1983). Disease: sign of the last days? *The Watchtower*, 1 May, 3–4.

WTS (1984). Questions from readers. *The Watchtower*, 15 May, 30.

WTS (1988). Childbearing among God's people. *The Watchtower*, 1 March, 18–22.

WTS (2000a). Questions from readers. *The Watchtower*, 15 June, 29–31.

WTS (2000b). Questions from readers. *The Watchtower*, 15 October, 30–1.

WTS (2001). God's permission of suffering nears its end. *The Watchtower*, 15 May, 4–8.

WTS (2004). Be guided by the living God. *The Watchtower*, 15 June, 19–24.

WTS (2006). 2005 service year report of Jehovah's Witnesses worldwide. *The Watchtower*, 1 February, 27–30.

53

Jewish bioethics

Gary Goldsand, Zahava R. S. Rosenberg-Yunger, and Michael Gordon

Mrs. G is an 85-year-old resident of a Jewish long-term care facility who has vascular dementia, controlled heart failure, and diabetes mellitus. She is bed bound and occasionally recognizes her daughter with a slight smile. The gastrostomy feeding tube she received two years ago has begun leaking and needs to be replaced. Her daughter, who has become her surrogate since the recent death of Mrs. G's husband, has indicated that if the tube were to come out, she would not consent to the insertion of a new tube: a decision she feels would be in accord with her mother's wishes. She would not, however, request that the tube be deliberately removed. The staff are concerned that, by not replacing the tube, they would be failing to maintain the current level of treatment, and she would starve. They feel that this would amount to taking the mother's life, without any substantial decline in her clinical condition. The daughter acknowledges the concern and devotion of the staff and her mother's unchanged clinical status, but reiterates her belief that her mother would prefer to be allowed to die rather than be force fed through a gastrostomy tube.

What is Jewish bioethics?

Judaism

Judaism is the religion of the Jewish People. Judaism is a 3500-year-old tradition based on foundational stories in the Pentateuch – the five books that make up the Torah. In the first book, Genesis, the Jewish people become defined as the descendents of the

monotheists Abraham and his wife Sarah. The Torah chronicles the people's covenant with God, deliverance to the holy land, exile and slavery in Egypt, acceptance of the laws of Moses at Sinai, and ends as the people are delivered back to the promised land of Israel. The rest of the Hebrew Bible (Tanach/Old Testament) tells of many centuries of prophets and kings, tribal rivalries, and conflicts with neighbors, as well as the temple in Jerusalem and the priests who kept the holy books. It ends with another story of exile and return, this time from Babylonia. In the ensuing centuries, from 500 BCE on, temple ritual and sacrifice evolved into synagogue-based communal prayer and study. With the temple's final destruction in 70 CE, ancient oral traditions became written in the Talmud. The practice of seeking wisdom through ongoing study of the holy books became a central feature of Jewish existence that persists and thrives today. In the past century, the Jewish people have suffered the trauma of losing six million people to Nazi genocide, and the joy of returning to full nationhood once again when the State of Israel was established in 1948.

Jewish bioethics

Although discussions of medical ethics have been recounted in Jewish writings since ancient times, modern medical technologies have placed new challenges before interpreters of Jewish tradition

An earlier version of this chapter has appeared: Goldsand, G., Rosenberg-Yunger, Z. R. S., and Gordon, M. (2001). Jewish bioethics. *CMAJ* **164**: 219–22.

(Green, 1985; Feldman, 1986; Rosner, 1986; Rosner and Bleich, 1987; Novak, 1990; Meier, 1991). The zeal with which these questions have been addressed has given rise to the field of Jewish medical ethics, which has developed since the 1960s. In keeping with Jewish ethics generally, Jewish bioethical inquiry appeals to the principles found in Jewish scriptures and commentaries and applies them to clinical decision making. In doing so, it takes a duty-based approach rather than the predominantly rights-based approach characteristic of some contemporary secular bioethical approaches. As the late Benjamin Freedman (1999) pointed out, ethical deliberations that are focused on rights often help in solving the procedural question of who gets to make a decision, but they do not necessarily offer guidance as to what that decision ought to be. Framing a dilemma in terms of the duties owed to those involved can clarify the issues and suggest a satisfactory course of action.

Interpersonal behavior in Judaism is traditionally conceived as the execution of duties within the context of one's relationships with other humans and with God. Accordingly, a preoccupation with rights implies, firstly, the relative isolation of individuals making claims upon one another and, secondly, an implicitly or overtly adversarial relationship. In a "regime of duty," participants seek to enable each other to satisfy the obligations inherent within relationships (Freedman, 1999), including professional relationships. Judaism urges one to perform mitzvoth (good deeds); that is, to act in accordance with one's duties, and this applies in the healthcare setting no less than anywhere else. The clinic thereby provides a relatively new arena in which mutual obligations between patients, healthcare providers, and families can be explored. Such explorations inevitably begin with the established norms of Jewish law and behavior, collectively known as Halacha (literally, "the way").

A variety of approaches

Traditional Jewish legal and ethical thinking is based on reading and interpreting three main sources, each of which is vast, varied, and complex. The oldest and most authoritative is the Hebrew Bible, which includes the five books of Moses (the Torah), the Prophets, and the Writings. The second source is the Talmud, which is composed of multi-layered commentaries on biblical texts and oral traditions by learned rabbis of the second to fifth centuries CE. To make the voluminous Talmud more accessible, several great codifications of Jewish law emerged that attempted to summarize the Talmud's primary teachings (Karo, 1965; Asher, 2000). One of the most notable, the Mishne Torah, comes from Maimonides (1962), the noted twelfth century physician and scholar. The third main source of Jewish legal authority is the *Responsa* literature, in which prominent Jewish scholars through the centuries have given opinions on contemporary matters as interpreted through the Hebrew Bible and Talmud (e.g., Waldenberg, 1990; Feinstein, 1994). *Responsa* are the continuation of a 2000-year-old interpretative tradition, which creates an intellectual link to the past, helping to keep the law relevant and vital to the present. (Descriptions of codes and *Responsa* can be found in Freedman [1999] and Rakover [1994], or in any general guide to the sources of Jewish law.)

Bioethical questions are treated by Jewish scholars in a variety of ways, which reflect different orientations toward Judaism and degrees of strictness in the interpretation of Talmudic texts and cases. Pioneering work in contemporary Jewish medical ethics in the 1960s and 1970s came primarily from Orthodox Judaism, in which the authority of God, as expressed through the Torah and Talmud, underlies the deliberative process (Jakobovits, 1959). Much Jewish bioethics literature comes from this perspective, which assumes that, through the proper interpretation of Talmudic texts and commentaries, answers to the most difficult questions can be discovered. In practice, the rabbi whose opinion is sought for an ethical answer serves as an "expert counselor" to physician and patient, interpreting Halachic law for the situation in question. A local rabbi or chaplain may, in turn, consult more learned Halachic authorities in difficult cases.

Inspired by these Orthodox sources, Jews from the more liberal Reform and Conservative movements have also made contributions to contemporary bioethics (Feldman, 1974; Borowitz, 1984; Maibaum, 1986; Dorff, 1990). The interpretative method and texts used are basically the same, but their rulings are often more flexible than those provided by Orthodox rabbis. Even within Orthodox Judaism, there exist multiple interpretations of most texts, with a resultant variability of rulings. Jews of the Reform movement are often more open to "extra-Halachic Jewish ethical analysis" (Grodin, 1995), in which Halacha becomes only one of several sources of moral authority.

Common principles

Although traditional Jewish scripture expresses many principles worthy of ethical consideration, there are a few foundational tenets that ground much of the Jewish bioethical tradition. One commentator identified three main principles: "human life has infinite value; aging, illness and death are a natural part of life; and improvement of the patient's quality of life is a constant commitment" (Meier, 1991, p. 60). Other important concepts are that human beings are to act as responsible stewards (Freedman, 1999) in preserving their bodies, which actually belong to God (Davis, 1994), and that they are duty bound to violate any other law in order to save human life (short of committing murder, incest/adultery or idolatry). Compared with secular values, these principles suggest a diminished role for patient autonomy. When a treatment is efficacious (*refuah bedukah*) there exists a duty to seek or preserve health, which overrides any presumed right to refuse/withhold treatment or to commit suicide. However, when the efficacy of the treatment is uncertain (*refuah she'einah bedukah*), then the individual is permitted to decide and possibly refuse (Flancbaum, 2001).

The problem faced by Jews in end of life decisions is not usually in determining the appropriate Halacha; a greater challenge is determining the

moment when hope for continued life is lost and the process of death has begun. Jewish law is relatively clear that life is not to be taken before its time. It is equally clear that one is not to impede or hinder the dying process once it has begun (Feldman, 1986). Lenient rulings in such cases may be based on the same texts as strict rulings; one authority may see continued treatment as prolonging life, where another may see it as prolonging death. Working through this dilemma is a common feature of Jewish end of life decision making. Both the duty to treat and the duty not to prolong death must be considered in light of the more general duty to care for one's parents in old age or ill health.

Why is Jewish bioethics important?

Today approximately 13 million Jews live in many parts of the world. Israel's population of more than six million is over 80% Jewish, and a similar number live in the USA. Russia and France have large Jewish populations, followed closely by Argentina, Canada, and the UK. While the majority of Jewish people have secularized to varying degrees and adopted the language and customs of their local countrymen, a significant minority remain committed to upholding the laws of the Torah through prayer, study, adherence to tradition, and commitment to the covenant with God.

To traditionally minded Jews, Jewish bioethics is a subset of Halacha, which guides all of their activities. To more secular Jews seeking guidance in difficult decisions about their health, Jewish bioethics offers helpful lessons and considered opinions from the sages. Many non-religious Jews welcome traditional views to help to ease the uncertainty inherent in difficult ethical decisions, even though they may not live according to traditional religious practice.

An understanding of Jewish bioethics can help anyone, Jewish or not, who wishes to explore the many ways people think about difficult ethical issues. Even without accepting the authority of the Hebrew Bible and the Talmud, healthcare professionals may benefit from seeing how principles or norms can be derived from authoritative texts, how minority opinions can be incorporated into such deliberations (the Talmud consistently records these), and how grappling with tough questions in this structured way can increase sensitivity to ethical and decisional nuance. Perhaps the most important lesson to be learned is that there are few easy answers to complex problems. Jews do not have a guidebook that explicitly tells them what to do in every situation. Rather, their guidebook is cryptic and requires them to consider thoroughly the range of possible answers to ethical dilemmas. It is a tradition of continued and ongoing questioning rather than one of absolute theological law passed down from above (Fasching, 1992). Furthermore, familiarity with Jewish bioethics would give the practitioner the perspective to consider ethical dilemmas through the lens of duty rather than of rights, asking the question, "What are the obligations of each of the parties involved in this discussion?" Although the rabbis of the Talmud would have appreciated the procedural question of who gets to decide, they were more concerned with finding the best course of action for the particular case at hand, irrespective of the participants' wishes.

How should I approach Jewish bioethics in practice?

Both Jewish and non-Jewish healthcare professionals can benefit from being acquainted with Jewish bioethics in caring for patients and their families when issues related to Judaism are raised. Table 53.1 summarizes essential points to keep in mind when providing care to Jewish patients.

The patient's life history might have some bearing on the type of treatment approaches he or she requires. Older Jews not born in Western nations might be more likely to appreciate a rabbi's input, as they are often more traditional than their children. Also, there are still a significant number of Holocaust survivors in most Western cities, some of

whom have significant psychological associations stemming from traumatic experiences.

Patients who are religious may doubly appreciate hospital attire that preserves modesty. Some Jewish patients may also appreciate brief periods set aside for prayer or other ritual obligations.

A practitioner treating a Jewish patient should not make assumptions about the extent to which the patient would like his or her care to be guided by Jewish tradition. It would be perfectly appropriate to ask a patient whether Jewish opinions are considered in the decision-making processes, and to consult with a rabbi – a specific one if so requested – when the patient wishes to explore the tradition's wisdom on a particular matter.

In general, traditional Judaism prohibits suicide, euthanasia, withholding or withdrawal of potentially beneficial treatment, abortion when the mother's life or health is not at risk, and many of the traditional "rights" associated with a strong concept of autonomy. For example, an observant Jew would not consider it his or her right to seek physician-assisted suicide as a way to avoid present or future suffering from metastatic carcinoma. Exceptions to these prohibitions are sometimes made in extreme circumstances.

The case

Mrs. G's daughter is undoubtedly trying to respect her mother in not consenting to the insertion of a new gastrostomy feeding tube, but she will find it difficult to get rabbinical support for reducing or withdrawing treatment that would result in her mother's death without a prior serious decline in Mrs. G's overall condition. How best to respect her parent is not easy to determine, but usually Judaism teaches that prolonging life is more respectful than assuming an incompetent patient wishes to end her suffering prematurely.

There is a clear duty to "cause to eat" (Freedman, 1999) in the Jewish tradition, which her daughter should not, according to the Halacha, violate unless Mrs. G is deemed to be a *goses* (a person in

Table 53.1. Essential qualities of ethical approaches to communication and caregiving involving Jewish patients

Religious observance	Try to determine the patient's degree of orthodoxy (observance). This information may help to determine the degree of adherence to Jewish laws, including dietary laws. Orthodox men will usually wear a head covering (yarmulke) at all times. Explore the needs for prayer and, whenever possible, facilitate such participation. During special "high holidays" (Rosh Hashanah and Yom Kippur), Jewish patients may want to have access to special religious services. Orthodox Jews should not "work" on the Sabbath (Saturday); however, necessary medical activities can be performed on the Sabbath. During Passover, special foods (unleavened bread) may be required. The patient may want to consult a rabbi when medical recommendations are made that affect dietary restrictions
Diet	Many Jews, particularly Orthodox Jews, adhere to a strict diet of kosher food. If it is unavailable in hospital, patients may choose to bring kosher food from home. Some of the dietary principles include not eating pork or seafood and not mixing dairy and meat products. Three or six hours (customs vary) must pass before an Orthodox Jew can eat meat after a dairy meal. Usual dietary restrictions may be waived if necessary for medical reasons. Feeding is considered important, even in the late stages of disease, and therefore families may be reluctant to agree to the withholding of food unless the patient is in the dying process
Privacy and modesty	Whenever possible, very personal care should be provided by a healthcare professional of the same sex, especially for female patients. Married, divorced, or widowed Orthodox women may wear a wig or hair covering in public as part of their adherence to the principle of modesty
Consent	In general, the process of consent used in Western countries is also applicable to Jewish patients. Orthodox Judaism requires that a patient follow medical directions, but it is also expected that the best information be disclosed before the patient agrees to a procedure or treatment. Judaism promotes a strong commitment to the sanctity of life; as a result, there may be some difficulties when discussions take place about the withdrawal or withholding of treatments
Rabbinical advice	Jewish people have a long tradition of asking a rabbi for advice when faced with difficult decisions. Families may present physicians with the results of rabbinical deliberations, which must be taken into account when decisions are made. It is always best to ask the patient or family if they would like the advice of a rabbi
Life history	Many older Jewish patients may be Holocaust survivors. It is important to know this because such a history may affect their response to proposed treatments and their relationships with family members

the throes of dying), in which case treatment or feeding that would hinder the dying process would not normally be allowed. Even as death approaches, performing duties as articulated by Jewish law is the essence of traditional Jewish life, a source of joy and fulfillment for both patients and families, and Jewish bioethics suggests that the articulation and performance of such duties be the focus of clinical decision making. The daughter agrees to have the gastrostomy tube replaced. She and the healthcare team determine conjointly the basis for future care within a palliative care framework. Mrs. G succumbs comfortably to pneumonia some months later.

REFERENCES

Ben Asher, J. (2000). *Tur Shulkhan Aruch.* (No English translation available but explanation at www.shamash. org/lists/scj–faq/HTML/faq/03–38.html) accessed August 2006.

Borowitz, E. (1984). The autonomous self and the commanding community. *Theol Stud* **45**: 34–56.

Davis, D.S. (1994). Method in Jewish bioethics. In *Religious Methods and Resources in bioethics* ed. P.F. Camenisch. Dordrecht: Kluwer Academic, pp. 109–26.

Dorff, E. (1990). A Jewish approach to end-stage medical care. *Conserv Judaism* **43**: 3–51.

Fasching, D. (1992). *Narrative Theology after Auschwitz.* Minneapolis, MN: Fortress Press.

Feldman, D.M. (1974). *Marital Relations, Birth Control, and Abortion in Jewish Law.* New York: Schocken Books.

Feldman, D.M. (1986). *Health and Medicine in the Jewish Tradition.* New York: Crossroad.

Feinstein, M. (1994). *Darash Moshe I: A Selection of Rabbi Moshe Feinstein's Choice Comments on the Torah.* Brooklyn, NY: Mesorah.

Flancbaum, L. (2001). *... And you Shall Live By Them: Contemporary Jewish Approaches to Medical Ethics.* Pennsylvania: Mirkov.

Freedman, B. (1999). *Duty and Healing: Foundations of a Jewish Bioethic.* New York: Routledge.

Green, R.M. (1985). Contemporary Jewish bioethics: a critical assessment. In *Theology and Bioethics: Exploring the Foundations and Frontiers*, ed. E.E. Shelp. Dordrecht: Reidel, pp. 245–66.

Grodin, M.A. (1995). Halakhic dilemmas in modern medicine. *J Clin Ethics* **3**: 218–21.

Jakobovits, I. (1959). *Jewish Medical Ethics.* New York: Bloch.

Karo, J. (1965). *Shulkhan Arukh.* New York: MP Press.

Maibaum, M. (1986). A "progressive" Jewish medical ethics: notes for an agenda. *J Reform Judaism* **33**: 27–33.

Maimonides, M. (1962). *Mishne Torah.* New York: MP Press.

Meier, L. (ed.) (1991). *Jewish Values in Health and Medicine.* New York: University Press of America.

Novak, D. (1990). Bioethics and the contemporary Jewish community. *Hastings Cent Rep* **20**: 14–17.

Rakover, N. (1994). *Guide to the Sources of Jewish Law.* Jerusalem: Library of Jewish Law.

Rosner, F. (1986). *Modern Medicine and Jewish Ethics.* New York: Yeshiva University Press.

Rosner, F. and Bleich, J.D. (eds.) (1987). *Jewish Bioethics.* Brooklyn, NY: Hebrew Publishing.

Waldenberg, E.Y. (1990). *Responsa Tzitz Eliezer.* [Contemporary rabbinic responsa covering the corpus of Jewish law.] Jerusalem: Rabbi Elizer Y. Waldenberg. [No English translation available.]

Related websites

The Gemara (Talmud): www.acs.ucalgary.ca/~elsegal/TalmudMap/Gemara.html

Jewish Law: www.jlaw.com

Judaism 101: www.jewfaq.org/toc.htm

Page from the Babylonian Talmud: www.acs.ucalgary.ca/~elsegal/TalmudPage.html

Physician-assisted suicide: www.jlaw.com/Articles/phys-suicide.html and www.jlaw.com/Articles/suicide.html

The right to die: a Halachic approach: www.jlaw.com/Articles/right.html

Risk: Principles of Judgment in HealthCare Decisions: www.thebody.com/iapac/freedman.html

Shulchan Aruch: www.torah.org/advanced/shulchan-aruch

Jewish populations world wide: www.jewishvirtuallibrary.org/jsource/Judaism/jewpop.html#top

The Thirteen Principles of Jewish Medical Ethics: http://members.aol.com/Sauromalus/index.html

54

Protestant bioethics

Merril Pauls and Roger C. Hutchinson

Mr. H is 82 years old and has many serious medical problems, including ischemic heart disease, hypertension, and diabetes mellitus. He has had a series of debilitating strokes that have left him severely disabled and unable to communicate his wishes. His healthcare providers feel that he would not benefit from resuscitation attempts if he were to suffer a cardiac arrest and suggest to his family that a do-not-resuscitate (DNR) order be placed on his chart. The devoutly Baptist family are quite upset and reject this suggestion. They believe that God could still heal their husband and father, and they accuse the healthcare providers of trying to "play God."

What is Protestant bioethics?

Origins of Protestantism

"Protestant" is a term applied to many different Christian denominations, with a wide range of beliefs, who trace their common origin to the Reformation of the sixteenth century. Protestant ideas have profoundly influenced modern bioethics, and most Protestants would see mainstream bioethics as compatible with their personal beliefs. This makes it difficult to define a uniquely Protestant approach to bioethics.

When Martin Luther first challenged the teachings of the Christian church in the early sixteenth century, few could have predicted the tumultuous consequences. The Reformation was founded on the idea that salvation could not be earned through human effort or bought through indulgences, concepts that were prevalent in the church at the time. The reformers preached that it is by God's grace alone that people are saved. They challenged the authority of the Pope and encouraged their followers to read and interpret the scriptures for themselves.

Today almost 30% of the world's Christians belong to a Protestant church. From their European origins, Protestants churches have spread throughout the globe: approximately 30% of Protestants live in North America, 25% in Africa, 20% in Europe, and 10% in Asia (Barrett *et al.*, 2001, p. 12). A wide variety of Protestant denominations have grown out of the common roots of the Reformation (Eliade, 1987), and while divisions and new visions have created many new branches, there have also been notable unions and reunification. Some of the larger and better-known denominations include the Anglican and Episcopalian, the United Church and United Church of Christ, Lutheran, Presbyterian, Baptist, Pentecostal, and Charismatic.

Describing a distinct "Protestant bioethic" is difficult, for a number of reasons. Much of the contribution that Protestant thinkers have made to modern bioethics has occurred subtly, over hundreds of years, as part of the larger Protestant influence on Western culture. The value of autonomy is a good example of this. Protestants have

An earlier version of this chapter has appeared: Pauls, M. and Hutchinson, R. C. (2002). Protestant bioethics. *CMAJ* **166**: 339–43.

played an important historical role in articulating and promoting this concept, but it is now so widely accepted that it would not be considered a unique feature of a Protestant bioethic.

A second important factor is the secularization of Protestant thought and behavior (Bruce, 1990). Mainstream Western values and institutions reflect the culture-building role of Protestant churches. Most Protestants would see mainstream bioethics as compatible with their personal values and beliefs.

At the same time, there is tremendous diversity within Protestant thought and theology. Some Anglican churches are very close theologically to the Catholic Church, while others have adopted different positions on a variety of issues. Many smaller Protestant denominations are notable for their contributions to society, attention to social inequities (the Salvation Army), or their unique culture (the Mennonites). The full spectrum of beliefs and practices can be demonstrated by the positions different Canadian Protestant groups have adopted on a variety of issues. The United Church of Canada (a member of the World Council of Churches) is at the liberal end, as evidenced by their ordination of women and their acceptance of homosexual clergy. By comparison, many Baptist and Pentecostal churches, and advocacy groups such as the Evangelical Fellowship of Canada (a member of the World Evangelical Alliance), generally hold conservative positions on such issues as abortion and homosexuality.

Sectarian Protestantism describes groups with Protestant origins that have developed distinct theology or practices (Reich, 1995). Some have grown to be so different from other Protestant groups that they may question or even reject the label of Protestant; examples include Jehovah's Witnesses, the Church of Jesus Christ of Latter-Day Saints, Seventh-Day Adventists, and the Church of Christ, Scientist. Many of these groups have specific doctrines or beliefs related to illness and medical care.

Because it is so difficult to define a "typical" Protestant approach to bioethics, we will instead identify common Protestant beliefs and highlight

concepts that have emerged from the Protestant tradition that are particularly relevant to bioethics.

Beliefs

Protestants share some fundamental beliefs with other Christians, and most Protestant denominations have common features that reflect their shared origins. Protestants have traditionally believed in an omnipotent, omniscient God, as described in the Bible. They believe that every person has been "made in the image of God" but has been tainted by sin. Protestant theology places a particular emphasis on Jesus Christ, the human incarnation of God's love. Through faith in Jesus Christ, believers establish a personal relationship with God that transforms them. Jesus' death on the cross and his resurrection provide a way for people's sinful nature to be forgiven and for believers to be reconciled to a Holy God. When believers die, they will spend eternity with God in heaven.

Protestants particularly emphasize that it is through grace that believers are reconciled with God. It is not something they deserve or earn. This does not mean that they do not concern themselves with good deeds or acts of charity. One of the key assertions made by the early Protestant reformers was that all believers are to be ministers or servants to one another and that their beliefs should find an outward expression. A true faith in Christ will give rise to virtues such as love, joy, peace, and patience in the lives of believers (Galatians 5:22–3).

Protestants have traditionally viewed the Bible as their primary source of direction and guidance (Eliade, 1987). New Testament writings are particularly emphasized, and Jesus Christ is considered the ultimate role model. Biblical principles are understood and applied to daily living through prayer and through discussion with fellow believers.

Concepts relevant to bioethics

Some Protestant themes or ideas are particularly relevant to the practice of medicine and the field of bioethics (Reich, 1995). A key Protestant belief is that God is sovereign and that believers can trust in God's goodness and faithfulness. This is an idea associated particularly with John Calvin, one of the early reformers. When faced with illness and pain, many people question God's existence and benevolence. A Protestant perspective asserts that God is in control and that there is a greater meaning or purpose in illness of which we may not be aware. Even in death, families may take comfort in their belief that God has "conquered death" and their loved one is with God in heaven (Lammers and Verhey, 1987). Some Protestants pray for miraculous cures as a sign of God's authority. Most believe a miracle could occur but also believe that God works through human ingenuity and technology to cure illness and relieve suffering. Believers are cautioned against a form of idolatry that invests physicians and medical interventions with more power than they have. Ultimately it is God who is in control (Reich, 1995).

A second Protestant theme is the value of individual freedom. One of the foundational ideas of the Reformation was that earthly authorities are fallible and that believers should read and understand the scriptures themselves. This historical Protestant emphasis on personal freedom has contributed to the establishment of respect for persons or autonomy as a foundational concept in modern bioethics (Veatch, 1997). However, significant differences exist between secular and Protestant conceptions of autonomy. Many secular formulations emphasize personal freedom and argue that autonomy is best served by minimizing restrictions on individual choice. Protestants would argue that autonomy can be fully expressed only in the context of a relationship with God, and that individuals must account for their personal relationships and their responsibilities to the larger community (Gustafson, 1981).

Protestant ideas about work and vocation have important implications for how the physician–patient relationship is viewed. In rejecting the traditional church structure, early Protestants asserted that all believers should be "ministers" to one another. God's love and compassion are revealed in many different jobs, not just the work of the priest. Medicine is seen as a calling, and the language of covenant is used to describe the relationship between doctor and patient (Ramsey, 1970). Physicians are to be more than "hired guns" or technical experts. They are called to empathize with their patient's suffering and to establish relationships of care and respect that allow them to enter into their patient's world (May, 1983).

Many religious traditions rely on historical precedence or guidelines to encourage uniformity of belief and practice. In the Jewish tradition, it is the Torah, Talmud, Codes, and *Responsa*. Casuistry helps serve this purpose in the Catholic Church. These practices shape the way followers of these religions approach bioethical concerns and dilemmas. In contrast to these highly articulated procedures, one finds a diversity of methods used in Protestant churches.

Why is Protestant bioethics important?

The influence of Protestant scholars on modern bioethical thought is pervasive. Twentieth century ethicists Paul Ramsey, Joseph Fletcher, and James Gustafson have been particularly influential (Jonsen, 1998). Ramsey (1970) described a deontological approach to bioethics in which he articulated "unexceptionable moral principles." He wrote on a variety of topics, and his ideas on the value of the individual and the "canon of loyalty" that exists between physician and patient have had a significant impact on subsequent work in the field. Fletcher (1966) advocated a situation ethic that closely resembles act-utilitarianism, in which the consequences of an action are used to assess whether the action is morally right or wrong. Fletcher (1960) was an Episcopalian who emphasized the need to understand moral issues from the patient's perspective and felt that human freedom and choice were of the utmost importance. Ramsey and Fletcher represented the opposite ends of the polarities of principles versus situation, deontological versus consequentialist, and norms versus context. Gustafson (1965) helped to move the debate forward. He focused on the agent and emphasized the web of human relationships in which the actors are situated. The starting place for his ethical reflections was ordinary human existence rather than church doctrines or scriptural passages. After describing a situation in terms that do not presuppose distinctive religious teachings or authority, Gustafson (1974) then asked how religious beliefs and presumptions might influence how a situation is being described, and what weight should be assigned to different values and consequences. Gustafson provides useful guidance for understanding the thought patterns of many Protestants in the clinical setting.

How should I approach Protestant bioethics in practice?

Patients want their physicians to respect their spiritual beliefs, and they feel better cared for when this important part of their life is recognized (Daalman and Nease, 1994; King and Bushwick, 1994; Ehman *et al.*, 1999). Including a spiritual history is particularly important when assessing a serious or terminal illness or when making significant treatment decisions.

Because of the influence that Protestant thought has had on Western culture, and the secularization of Protestantism, most physicians (religious or not) will find that they share many values and beliefs with the majority of their Protestant patients. Examples include the importance of respecting patient's wishes and the value of a caring, empathic relationship between physician and patient.

Physicians should be particularly sensitive to their Protestant patients' beliefs when dealing with end of life issues, concerns about consent and refusal of care, and beginning of life issues such as abortion, genetic testing, and the use of assisted reproductive technologies. Physicians should also recognize that certain Protestant groups and denominations, particularly those with conservative beliefs, might have different approaches to making decisions and unique treatment wishes. Understanding how to identify these wishes and to respond appropriately will enhance patient care and minimize conflict. In these cases, the physician should inquire about the patient's personal beliefs and their relationship to their faith community. This discussion will help physicians to identify the particular needs or desires of the patient that the physician may not have anticipated. It also will identify areas of potential conflict that physicians can address before they arise. A withdrawal of treatment may be more easily negotiated if a family's views are understood beforehand. Great care must be taken not to stereotype or generalize. There is a great diversity of Protestant beliefs and a variety of expression of these beliefs. A chaplain from the same denomination as the patient may be an invaluable resource.

End of life care

Most Protestants are comfortable with a wide variety of life-sustaining treatments and will want them when indicated. Faced with little hope of recovery, most Protestant patients and families understand why healthcare providers suggest a withdrawal of aggressive interventions and often are in agreement. Many Protestants draw strength from their belief that their loved one will go to Heaven when he or she dies. At the same time, Protestant beliefs have played a role in cases in which families have been reluctant to withhold or withdraw treatment (Cranford, 1991; *Sawatzky* v. *Riverview Health Center Inc.*, 1998). The families in these situations argued that healthcare providers should not be "playing God." In one case, the family was hoping that a miracle might occur and that their loved one would be healed (Cranford, 1991). Although the reluctance to withhold or withdraw treatment may be the exception rather than the rule, physicians should listen carefully to the family's wishes and proceed cautiously (Weijer, 1998). In cases that have gone before the courts, judgments have consistently stated that the wishes of the substitute decision maker be respected.

Consent and refusal of care

When faced with important decisions, many devout Protestants seek to determine God's "will" for their lives through prayer, reading the Bible, and consulting with other believers. Healthcare providers who do not understand this decision-making process may question their patient's capacity to make decisions or feel that friends or church leaders are coercing their patients.

Physicians should not assume, however, that such a process is invalid or inappropriate when it leads to what they see as negative consequences. In an often-cited Canadian case, *Malette* v. *Shulman* (1990), a physician caring for a woman severely injured in a motor vehicle collision felt that she required a blood transfusion to save her life. He knew she had a signed card asking that no blood products be given because of her religious beliefs, but chose to give the blood anyway. He was sued for battery, and the judge found in the plaintiff's favor.

Although physicians must respect a competent adult's informed decision, this is not the case with dependent minors. An important rationale for respecting adult's religious beliefs is that they may be carefully considered and deeply held. Young children are not seen as capable of this same kind of careful consideration and should not suffer harmful consequences as a result of their parents' beliefs. Courts have affirmed this in many cases. In cases involving older children and teenagers, courts may decide that they are mature enough to make their own decisions and allow them to reject care on the basis of their own beliefs (Rozovsky and Rozovsky, 1992).

Abortion, genetic testing, and new reproductive technologies

Protestant views and practice are particularly diverse when it comes to the issue of abortion. Conservative groups are among the most active in the pro-life movement, as many believe that life begins at conception. Some liberal denominations are pro-choice: they believe that principles such as the right to life and the freedom to choose must be applied and weighed by taking into account the particular circumstances, and that, during the first trimester, the decision to have an abortion should be between a woman and her doctor.

Protestant attitudes toward postconception genetic testing are similarly diverse and often linked to the individual's views on abortion. If there is no situation in which a person would consider an abortion, they may refuse this type of testing. Although some Protestants may object to in vitro fertilization because of the potential for embryo wastage, many would consider this an option if they were infertile.

The case

In response to the family's objections, the physician does not write the do-not-resuscitate (DNR) order for Mr. H. She arranges a family conference, and the family's pastor is invited to attend. It becomes apparent that the family is not really expecting a miracle to happen. They are concerned that their father is not receiving enough rehabilitation services. They feel that the healthcare team is giving up on their father and that the suggested DNR order is evidence of this. The family is reassured that the healthcare providers are committed to their father's rehabilitation and that the DNR order would not affect the level of care he receives. A discussion about the resuscitation process helps the family to understand that the healthcare providers may be "playing God" just as much by trying to resuscitate Mr. H as by letting him die. The family is able to reaffirm their belief that it is God who will determine when their father dies, not the resuscitation team. They subsequently agreed to a DNR order.

REFERENCES

Barrett, D. B., Kurian, G. T., and Johnson, T. M. (2001). *World Christian Encyclopedia*, 2nd edn, New York: Oxford University Press.

Bruce, S. (1990). *A House Divided: Protestantism, Schism, and Secularization*. New York: Routledge.

Cranford, R. E. (1991). Helga Wanglie's ventilator. *Hastings Cent Rep* **21**: 23–4.

Daaleman, T. P. and Nease, D. E., Jr. (1994). Patient attitudes regarding physician inquiry into spiritual and religious issues. *J Fam Pract* **39**: 564–8.

Ehman, J. W., Ott, B. B., Short, T. H., Ciampa, R. C., and Hansen-Flaschen, J. (1999). Do patients want physicians to inquire about their spiritual or religious beliefs if they become gravely ill? *Arch Intern Med* **159**: 1803–6.

Eliade, M. (ed.) (1987). *The Encyclopedia of Religion*, Vol. 12. New York: McMillan.

Fletcher, J. (1960). *Morals and Medicine. The Moral Problems of the Patient's Right to Know the Truth, Contraception, Artificial Insemination, Sterilization, Euthanasia*. Boston, MA: Beacon Press.

Fletcher, J. (1966). *Situation Ethics: The New Morality*. Philadelphia, PA: Westminster Press.

Gustafson, J. M. (1965). Context vs. principles: a misplaced debate in Christian ethics. *Harr Theol Rev* **58**: 171–202.

Gustafson, J. M. (1974). Moral discernment in the Christian life. *Theology and Christian Ethics*. Philadelphia, PA: United Church Press, pp. 99–120.

Gustafson, J. M. (1981). *Theology and Ethics*, Vol. 1. Chicago, IL: University of Chicago Press.

Jonsen, A. R. (1998). *The Birth of Bioethics*. New York: Oxford University Press.

King, D. E. and Bushwick, B. (1994). Beliefs and attitudes of hospital inpatients about faith healing and prayer. *J Fam Pract* **39**: 349–52.

Lammers, S. E. and Verhey, A. (eds.) (1987). *On Moral Medicine: Theological Perspectives in Medical Ethics*. Grand Rapids, MI: William B. Eerdmans.

Malette v. *Shulman* (1990). [Ontario 67 DLR (4th) 321 (Ont CA)].

May, W. F. (1983). *The Physician's Covenant: Images of the Healer in Medical Ethics*. Philadelphia, PA: Westminster.

Ramsey, P. (1970). *The Patient as Person: Explorations in Medical Ethics*. New Haven, CT: Yale University Press.

Reich, W. T. (ed.) (1995). *Encyclopedia of Bioethics*, Vol. 4. New York: Simon and Schuster Macmillan.

Rozovsky, L. E. and Rozovsky, F. A. (1992). *The Canadian Law of Consent to Treatment*. Toronto: Butterworths.

Sawatzky v. *Riverview Health Center Inc.* (1998) [Manitoba] 167 DLR (4th) 359, 132 ManR (2d) 222 (QB).

Veatch, R. M. (1997). *Medical Ethics*, 2nd edn, Boston, MA: Jones and Bartlett.

Weijer, C. (1998). Cardiopulmonary resuscitation for patients in a persistent vegetative state: Futile or acceptable? *CMAJ* **158**: 491–3.

Related websites

Evangelical Fellowship of Canada: www.efc-canada.com

Salvation Army, Sally Anne Center for Bioethics: http://ethics.salvationarmy.ca

Christian Medical and Dental Associations: www.cmds.org

Christian Medical Fellowship: www.cmf.org.uk

Center for Bioethics and Human Dignity: www.bioethix.org/index.html

The Church of Christ, Scientist: www.tfccs.com

The Church of Jesus Christ of Latter-Day Saints: www.lds.org

55

Roman Catholic bioethics

Hazel J. Markwell and Barry F. Brown

Mrs. I is 25 years old and is about 10 weeks' pregnant. She has tuberculous meningitis. Her disease was in an advanced stage when she was admitted to hospital and underwent surgery to relieve the pressure on her brain. She is now clinically brain dead. Her husband – like the patient, a devout Catholic – requests that her body be maintained on life support in the intensive care unit to save her fetus. Other family members concur that she is "pro-life" and would want to carry the fetus to term if possible. (Although far from typical, this is an actual case. All of the details included in this discussion are taken from the public record [Fox 1999; Priest and Slaughter 1999]).

What is Catholic bioethics?

There is a long tradition of bioethical reasoning within the Roman Catholic faith, a tradition that extends from Augustine's writings on suicide in the early Middle Ages to recent papal teachings on euthanasia and reproductive technologies. Roman Catholic bioethics (which we refer to in this article simply as Catholic bioethics) comprises a complex set of positions that have their origins in scripture, the writings of the doctors of the Church, papal encyclicals, and reflections by contemporary Catholic theologians and philosophers. Informed by scriptural exegesis and by philosophical argument, Catholic bioethics is rooted in both faith and in reason. During Vatican II (a reformational council held in the early 1960s), Catholics were directed to read the "signs of the times" in applying the teachings of the Church to the contemporary situation (Flannery, 1988): in other words, to remain attuned to the progressive revelation of Christ through history.

Fundamental to Catholic bioethics is a belief in the sanctity of life: the value of a human life, as a creation of God and a gift in trust, is beyond human evaluation and authority. God maintains dominion over it. In this view, we are stewards, not owners, of our own bodies and are accountable to God for the life that has been given to us (Wildes and Mitchell, 1997). Life, however, is not an absolute value, for the Catholic understanding of its meaning and purpose is founded in a belief in the resurrection of Christ and the hope of an afterlife.

The doctrine of natural law, as articulated by Thomas Aquinas in the thirteenth century, views human life as a basic good that cannot be made subject to utilitarian estimation. Life is the basis and necessary condition of other goods, and human beings have an innate desire to seek these goods, such as sexual reproduction, social life, and knowledge. Our inborn human tendencies provide the basis for our moral obligations and for fundamental human rights. The Catholic tradition also holds that human life and personhood begin prenatally. Therefore, although the criminal law in many jurisdictions takes birth as the point at which a legal person comes into existence, Catholic ethics

An earlier version of this chapter has appeared: Markwell, H. J. and Brown, B. F. (2001). Catholic bioethics. *CMAJ* **165**: 189–92.

presumes a human fetus to be, at every stage, a person possessing a right to life.

Underlying the Catholic stance on specific bioethical questions is a metaphysical conception of the person as a composite of body and soul. As long as there is a living body, even if mental capacities are reduced or absent, there is still a person present. A human being is considered to be a person from conception to the death of the whole. In contrast, modern society sometimes tends to take a developmental or "gradualist" view, such that personhood begins some time later than conception and can be lost (for example, in the extreme stages of dementia or in a persistent vegetative state) well before the physical death of the individual. The difference between these stances is of profound ethical significance for both beginning of life and end of life decisions.

Although bioethical principles such as beneficence, non-maleficence, autonomy, and justice are compatible with Catholic beliefs, some patients will be guided by the theological requirements of faith, hope, love, and fidelity and by more specific religious requirements that are not completely captured in the principles of secular bioethics. Catholic patients may appreciate various kinds of spiritual aid and support at the end of life, be it psychological support or the offering of Holy Communion, the Sacrament of Reconciliation, or the Sacrament of the Sick (last rites). It is appropriate to call a priest on behalf of Catholic patients when death is imminent.

Contemporary Catholic bioethics is concerned with a broad range of issues, including sexuality, marriage, reproduction, birth control, sterilization, and abortion. In recent years, Catholic bioethicists have registered opposition to some emerging reproductive technologies, including artificial donor insemination, in vitro fertilization, surrogacy, and cloning. Also of concern are end of life issues, including advance directives, palliative care and pain control, suicide, euthanasia and the refusal or cessation of futile treatments, organ donation, and the definition of death. Catholic bioethicists have contributed to the debate on the right to healthcare, conceived as a community and governmental responsibility. In general, they have applied principles of social justice to this debate.

Why is Catholic bioethics important?

Patients and their families expect that their religious beliefs and values will be respected whatever the faith of the healthcare professionals responsible for their care. A large number of individuals in Western cultures profess to be Catholic. For instance, there were 12.2 million Roman Catholics in Canada at the time of the 1991 census (Statistics Canada, 1999). Many hospitals and institutions in that country have a Catholic orientation and mission statement. It is important for clinicians who work in such settings to be aware of the policies that flow from such a mission. Clinicians should be aware of the religious convictions of their patients and the possibility that some procedures they might suggest could seriously violate the patient's beliefs and lead to problems of conscience. So too, patients should not expect physicians to engage in practices that they consider to be morally unacceptable.

How should I approach Catholic bioethics in practice?

A basic understanding of Catholic bioethics can help physicians to understand the needs and aspirations of their Catholic patients. It is also helpful to appreciate that some issues, such as matters concerning reproduction, are controversial even within Catholic bioethics. For example, certain actions that, from a natural-law perspective, would be viewed as intrinsically evil might be regarded, from a "proportionalist" perspective (McCormick, 1981), as justifiable, if they bring about a good that is proportionate to or greater than the associated evil. Proportionalism has been a point of some contention in recent Catholic bioethical debate (Grisez, 1983; Pope John Paul II, 1993).

Reproduction

Catholic teaching on birth control and abortion derives from a view of marital sexuality and responsible parenthood in which the sexual expression of love between the spouses is integrated with the procreative implications of that union. By this standard, contraception and contraceptive sterilization are not permissible, although those who take a proportionalist approach have expressed some dissent on these matters.

The Catholic tradition rejects "direct" abortion on the grounds that it takes an innocent human life. Although there is some discussion as to what counts as a direct abortion, the generally accepted view is that any intentional termination of a pregnancy is a direct abortion, whereas an "indirect" abortion occurs when a tubal pregnancy or a cancerous uterus is removed. In such a case, the death of the fetus would be viewed as the unintended consequence of an action intended to save the mother's life.

The Catholic position on new reproductive technologies has been generally cautious. The use of in vitro fertilization that does not preserve the integrity of the unitive and procreative aspects of marital sex puts a couple at odds with the official position of the Church, which asserts the right of the child to be born to parents united in the exclusive commitment that is marriage. The same is true of any procedure involving donated gametes or embryos.

Genetic testing

To the extent that genetic screening and counseling, as well as prenatal genetic diagnosis, may precipitate deliberation about birth control and abortion, an effort should be made to explore the convictions of the parties involved before genetic tests are carried out. Some Catholic couples may seek prenatal diagnosis solely for the sake of knowing the results and being prepared. Open access to genetic testing and non-directive counseling respect this purpose.

Organ donation

The Catholic Church has no objection to cadaveric organ donation and transplantation; indeed, it views such gifts as a demonstration of Christian love. Some Catholics, however, may have folk beliefs that make them disinclined to donate organs; that is, they may think that a lack of bodily integrity postmortem may preclude the resurrection of the body after death. Church doctrine does not support these beliefs.

Proposals to change the criterion of death from whole brain death to persistent vegetative state (Veatch, 1975; Wikler, 1988) will meet with much resistance from the Catholic community, which sees the body as an essential aspect of the human person. Catholics also share in the general reluctance to offer payment of any kind for organ donations on the grounds that it runs contrary to the idea of the "gift of life" and treats human remains as a commodity.

Hospitalization for episodes of acute mental illness

Although the duty to preserve one's health extends to all types of illness, in cases of mental illness a clash between the principles of autonomy and of beneficence can become sharply evident. The Catholic position on a person's right to refuse treatment unless he or she is a potential harm to themself or others may be less liberal than the requirements of the civil law in many countries. Within Catholicism, the individual has a duty to promote his or her own health, and thus may be seen as having a moral obligation to seek treatment even if he or she does not meet legal criteria for involuntary commitment and treatment.

Research involving human subjects

Given the Catholic view that a person does not have the moral right to take serious risks to health, the likelihood of harm will set limits to participation in clinical trials. The deliberate use of deception in psychological or behavioral experiments is also problematic for those who take the view that deception is inherently wrong and cannot be justified by the beneficial results of a study. With respect to genetic research, the generally accepted principles that protect confidentiality, privacy, self-determination, justice and ultimately, the dignity of the human person are compatible with Catholic healthcare ethics.

Life support

The monotheistic religions of Judaism, Islam, and Christianity maintain that we have a duty to protect the life given to us by God; accordingly, these faiths have always rejected suicide. Early authorities in the Catholic Church, including Augustine and Aquinas, condemned rational suicide, holding it to be outside the authority of the individual to take his or her own life. Failure to use ordinary measures to preserve life is regarded as morally equivalent to suicide within the Catholic tradition. What is less clear is whether this position commits the Church to an absolute duty to prolong life in all circumstances, regardless of the condition of the patient.

Since at least the sixteenth century, Catholic theologians have made a distinction between ordinary and extraordinary measures, holding that a person is obligated to use ordinary measures but has the choice whether to accept extraordinary measures (Cronin, 1958). Gerald Kelly's definition (1958, p. 129) of these terms was used for many years in Catholic hospitals in the United States and Canada:

Ordinary means of preserving life are all medicines, treatments, and operations which offer a reasonable hope of benefit for the patient and which can be obtained and used without excessive expense, pain or other inconvenience … *Extraordinary* means of preserving life … mean all medicines, treatments, and operations, which cannot be obtained without excessive expense, pain or other inconvenience, or which, if used, would not offer a reasonable hope of benefit.

It seems that these terms were originally used within a common-sensical understanding of what is medically customary. The issue was primarily the patient's obligations, and only secondarily the physician's duties. Patients were obligated to use measures within their financial means; they were not obligated to reduce their family to poverty in an effort to stay alive. The level of pain that patients could endure, and the distances they would have to travel to obtain care were relevant. Some authorities stressed the aspect of burden; others, including Kelly, included the notion of medical futility in the calculation.

Two points are in order here. Firstly, in recent medical practice, many extreme measures to preserve life have become customary. It is now necessary to ask which means of preserving life *should* be medically routine and which should be a matter of choice. Use of a procedure should be determined not by whether or not it is routine but by factors such as financial burden to the family and to society, pain, disfigurement, and perhaps most significant, medical futility.

Secondly, it is also clear that one cannot think in terms of an A list of ordinary procedures and a B list of extraordinary ones (Ramsey, 1978). The use of a ventilator, for example, may be ordinary or extraordinary, depending on the condition of the patient, his or her prognosis, the stage of the illness, and so forth. Although the physician has the right and the duty to inform the patient about treatment possibilities and their potential benefits and risks, it is primarily the patient and his or her family who have the right to determine what is ordinary or extraordinary from an ethical point of view.

The case

Because Mrs. I has suffered whole brain death, the complete death of the person has occurred even though respiration and pulse are being artificially maintained. Although we may speak loosely of "sustaining her life for the sake of her child," it is really a matter of sustaining vital functions in a deceased person for the same purpose.

The first question, then, concerns medical capability. Is it medically possible to carry her 10-week pregnancy to term? If not, the question is moot. If it *is* possible, then the question for Catholic ethics is two-fold. Firstly, is it obligatory to sustain her body to save the fetus? Secondly, if it is not obligatory, is it nevertheless morally permissible?

There have been a handful of cases worldwide in which an early pregnancy in a woman who had suffered brain death was carried close to term or to the point of viability (Bernstein *et al.*, 1989). Given these cases, there appears to be at least a possibility that the fetus would survive. However, given the necessity of using large doses of drugs to control the tuberculous meningitis and to sustain vital functions, and the lack of a healthy nutritional environment for the fetus, the process could impose an excessive burden on the unborn child. Because of the very early stage of development of the fetus, the likelihood of sustaining the mother's body long enough to bring the child to the point of viability is slight. It seems that there is both excessive burden and only a tenuous hope of benefit. The process thus constitutes extraordinary means and, therefore, there is no moral obligation to sustain Mrs. I's body for the sake of her unborn child.

It is a different story when we ask what is *permissible*. The issues that determine permissibility are three-fold. Can we justify the use of medical resources from a financial perspective? What would Mrs. I have wanted? Are we harming the fetus?

With regard to the financial question, it could be argued that a decision to designate a procedure as extraordinary on financial grounds implies that there is no entitlement to costly treatment in the context of a publicly funded healthcare system. However, unless and until society identifies certain procedures as being too expensive to be supported, we cannot make a financial case to deny this family the opportunity to try to bring the baby to term.

The second question relates to protecting the autonomy of the patient after death. Is this what Mrs. I would have wanted? Does her ''pro-life'' stance allow us to assume that she would wish to be used as a human incubator? Such an assumption may be an illogical leap and an affront to the dignity of the human person (Purdy, 1994). However, Mrs. I's family feels that she would want the fetus to live and, therefore, would want her body to be used in this way. Although it is difficult to make this assumption, it is perhaps more problematic to assume that we *cannot* make this particular leap in this *particular* case. From the perspective of preserving the patient's autonomy after death, it seems that it is permissible to provide the care that the family is requesting.

Thirdly, can we justify the possibility of causing harm to the fetus? The physicians have a Hippocratic duty to ''do no harm.'' However, we must be careful to draw a distinction between causing disability and causing harm. One's humanity does not depend on freedom from disability; therefore, the possibility of disability should not be decisive. Whether the drugs to which the fetus is exposed will have harmful effects is highly uncertain; it is possible that the drugs will not harm the fetus. From this perspective, it is morally permissible to provide the care requested.

In conclusion, although not obligatory, it is morally permissible to maintain Mrs. I's body in order to attempt to preserve the life of her fetus. As a result, her husband, in consultation with the physicians, may make this decision.

REFERENCES

Bernstein, I. M., Watson, M., Simmons, G. M., *et al.* (1989). Maternal brain death and prolonged fetal survival. *Obstet Gynecol* **74**: 334–7.

Cronin, D. A. (1958). *The Moral Law in Regard to the Ordinary and Extraordinary Means of Conserving Life*. Rome: Gregorian University, pp. 47–87.

Flannery, A. (ed.) (1988). *Vatican Council II: The Conciliar and Post Conciliar Documents*, rev edn, Northport, NY: Costello.

Fox, K. (1999). Faith, ethics and science collide. *Globe and Mail* [Toronto], 3 December, A18.

Grisez, G. (1983). *The Way of the Lord Jesus*, Vol. 1. Chicago, IL: Franciscan Herald Press, pp. 141–72.

Kelly, G. (1958). *Medico Moral Problems*. St. Louis, MO: Catholic Hospital Association.

McCormick, R. A. (1981). *Notes on Moral Theology: 1965–1980*. Washington, DC: University Press of America, pp. 709–11.

Pope John Paul II (1993). *Veritatis Splendor*. Rome: The Vatican, pp. 74–6

Priest, L. and Slaughter, M. (1999). Family of brain dead mother fights to save her fetus. *Toronto Star*, 2 December, A1.

Purdy, L. (1994). Commentary on "The baby in the body." *Hastings Cent Rep* **24**: 31–2.

Ramsey, P. (1978). *Ethics at the Edges of Life*. New Haven, CT: Yale University Press.

Statistics Canada (1999). *Canada Yearbook*. Ottawa: Statistics Canada.

Veatch, R. M. (1975). The whole-brain-oriented concept of death: an outmoded philosophical foundation. *J Thanatol* **3**: 13–30.

Wikler, D. (1988). The definition of death and persistent vegetative state. *Hastings Cent Rep* **18**: 44–77.

Wildes, K. M. and Mitchell, A. C. (eds.) (1997). *Choosing Life: A Dialogue on Evangelium Vitae*. Washington: Georgetown University Press.

Related websites

National Catholic Bioethics Center (formerly the Pope John Center): www.ncbcenter.org/home.html

Guild of Catholic Doctors (and related links): www.catholicdoctors.org.uk

Catholic Resources for Medical Ethics: www.usc.edu/hsc/info/newman/resources/ethics.html

Linacre Center for Healthcare Ethics (United Kingdom): www.linacre.org

SECTION X

Speciality bioethics

Introduction

A. M. Viens

While there are no doubt ethical principles and concepts that extend across all aspects of bioethics, it is now becoming common to find separate treatments of specialty fields emerging in the bioethics literature and in clinical ethics areas of specialization. In most academic fields and interdisciplinary areas of study, it is not uncommon to find scholars and practitioners focusing on developing particular areas of specialty. What is fairly unique about bioethics, however, is that we find that its speciality areas are not just reconceiving central disciplinary questions or using different ways of looking at issues but are bringing to light the importance of examining the ethical issues specific to their areas of clinical and research practice.

It will always be the case that considerations such as informed consent, confidentiality, minimizing harm, and priority setting, among other considerations, will be central ethical issues that clinicians will confront in all areas of practice. Nevertheless, the development and study of various speciality fields of bioethics places us in a better position to be able to give a more nuanced and pertinent analysis of the distinctive ethical issues faced by particular clinical areas of practice, especially where the traditional application of overarching ethical theory or bioethical methodologies may have been found to be limiting.

The chapters in this section provide an overview of the most pressing and relevant ethical issues unique to their clinical speciality. For instance, in Ch. 57, Gail Van Norman examines the distinctive ethical issues that arise because anesthesia routinely alters the patient's consciousness, sometimes affecting a patient's competence and autonomy, and that there are instances where anesthesiologists can be expected to use their knowledge and skills to abolish patient resistance. These issues are made stark in her examination of the special role of anesthesiologists in participating in state executions (in jurisdictions where it is required by law) and in upholding do-not-resuscitate orders in the operating room. Similarly, in Ch. 64, Margaret Eaton examines the singularity of ethical issues faced in pharmacy practice by virtue of several facts. For example, pharmacists are one step removed from the diagnostic aspect of the therapeutic encounter and are usually the last healthcare professional the patient has contact with before drug treatment commences. Numerous issues also arise from the fact that pharmacists often control the drug formulary in healthcare institutions.

Some areas of specialization within bioethics will be driven by scientific progress and technological advancement. For example, the specialty area of neuroethics has recently exploded and we find the ethical issues surrounding the brain, mind, and consciousness becoming one of the predominant areas in bioethics literature and ethical issues that are discussed more widely outside of clinical medicine. In Ch. 63, Eric Racine and Judy Illes discuss the importance of the ethical issues surrounding clinicians acting as gatekeepers in the marketing of neuroimaging and therapeutic products to treat neurological and psychiatric diseases.

Other areas of specialization within bioethics are driven by immediate societal threats that require prompt and effective responses. For instance, with the increase threat of pandemics and bioterrorism, we have seen rapid development of treatment and institutional structures related to infectious diseases. In Ch. 61, Jay Jacobsen examines the distinctive ethical tension that arises in the practice of infectious disease medicine between respecting patient preferences and preventing harm to others in society.

There will also be times where the development of different areas of bioethics specialization will depend on factors surrounding the expanding scope of what constitutes medical care. For instance, in Ch. 65, Michael Cohen examines how the integration of therapies such as acupuncture, chiropractic, herbal medicine, massage therapy, and so on concurrent to conventional medical therapies presents new ethical challenges with respect to whether and how clinicians should acknowledge a pluralistic foundation of healthcare that contains multiple modes of legitimate therapeutic interventions.

We additionally have chapters on emergency and trauma medicine (Ch. 59), critical and intensive care medicine (Ch. 58), surgery (Ch. 56), psychiatry (Ch. 62), and primary care (Ch. 60). All these provide both a basis from which to explore further developments in specialty fields of bioethics and, for clinicians who work with colleagues in these specialties, a better understanding of how the clinical issues specific to their area of practice presents and informs the ethical issues they must deal with on a daily basis.

56

Surgical ethics

James Andrews and Larry Zaroff

Mrs. A is a 72-year-old woman suffering from coronary artery disease. Upon angiography, the medical team diagnoses triple vessel involvement and determines that Mrs. A requires surgical management. She then meets with her surgeon, Dr. B, to discuss treatment options, and together they decide upon triple bypass surgery. Aware of the associated risks, Mrs. A does not relish the thought of surgery, but she desperately wishes to "put these heart troubles behind her." In the operating room the following week, when Dr. B exposes the heart he discovers an obvious dissection of the ascending aorta. The lesion must be repaired, but the risks are much greater than those discussed with the patient and family.

What is surgical ethics?

The truly defining institution of surgical medicine is the operation itself. Ultimately, that which distinguishes surgery, in practice and in ethics, from the other medical specialties arises in the operating room. Whether referred to as a simple "room," or more grandly as a "suite" or "theater," mystery has always enshrouded this sacred ground where surgeons practice their art. Here, amidst secrecy and sterility, surgeons confront fundamental ethical quandaries unique to their practice. Surgical ethics, thus, captures the unique ethical dilemmas that arise in the operating room.

Why is surgical ethics important?

The surgeon, unlike other clinicians, confronts first and foremost the ethical dilemma that any operation performed harms before healing. Postoperative side effects, such as pain, a wound, and scarring, represent not an undesirable possibility for the patient but rather a near certainty. Consequently, by striving to minimize this necessary temporary injury to the patient while maximizing the therapy's curative potential, surgeons have forever engaged in ethical deliberations. Once in the operating theater, the patient literally surrenders his or her body to the surgeon's expertise. The surgeon serves as the patient's advocate in the purest sense, responsible for protecting not only the patient's physical well-being but also his or her values and beliefs.

Our discussion of surgical ethics begins with the patient–surgeon relationship, then deals with issues associated with the preoperative conference – informed consent and disclosure – and finally ends with decisions involving patients presenting as emergencies.

Patient–surgeon relationship

Certain ethical considerations distinguish the patient–surgeon relationship from interactions between patients and clinicians in non-surgical specialties. An ultimate trust exists on the part of patients when they confide their entire beings to a surgeon during the operation. Indeed, Palmer (1982, p. 2) in the *Bulletin of the American College of Surgeons* characterized this special rapport as a:

... physical interaction, including the act of making an intentional, permanent "wound," in which the therapy produces measurable pathophysiologic change and mixes with the disease process ... creat[ing] unique bonds. This extraordinary contact cannot but influence how you feel about the patient and how he or she feels about you.

The ultimate trust that surgeons must cultivate with their patients comes to the fore in the operating room. For, here patient's immediate control ends. The balance of power shifts such that now essentially all authority resides with the surgeon. This increased authority naturally engenders increased responsibility and liability.

Reduced to its essence, the patient–clinician relationship is a fiduciary contract, founded on both trust and loyalty (Beauchamp and Childress, 2001a). The physician pledges, either implicitly or explicitly, to protect the patient's rights. A complete discussion of these rights is beyond the scope of this chapter. However, to differentiate between positive and negative rights is useful. Traditionally, liberal individualist societies more readily justify negative rights (Beauchamp and Childress, 2001b). For example, few North Americans would argue against the patient's negative right to refuse surgery, but they would be more reluctant to grant that patient the positive right to demand a given operation.

To respect the patient's autonomy, the surgeon should always disclose who will perform each step of the operation and who will be responsible (McCullough et al., 1998a). For surgeons practicing in universities and teaching hospitals, disclosing the role of trainees, residents, and medical students is essential. The surgeon in academia balances two responsibilities: to provide trainees the practice they require, and to offer patients optimal care. When properly informed of the students' involvement, patients often report a positive benefit (York et al., 1995). Furthermore, the American Medical Association Council on Ethical and Judical Affairs (1994a) condemned the substitution of the surgeon without the patient's consent claiming: "A surgeon who allows a substitute to operate on his or her patient without the patient's knowledge and consent is deceitful. The patient is entitled to choose his or her own physician and should be permitted to acquiesce or to refuse the substitution." The

patient specifically agrees to allow the surgeon to whom consent was granted to perform the operation. To betray that agreement undermines the patient–surgeon relationship and is both deceptive and unprofessional.

Informed consent

The preoperative conference affords the patient and the surgeon the opportunity to discuss viable treatment options and to decide together which option best suits the needs, both medical and practical, of the patient. The patient's values, beliefs, and preferences factor prominently in this discussion. Principles that form the basis of a successful conference include effective communication, assessment of competence, and sufficient disclosure. Many of these issues fall under the more general heading of informed consent, a pivotal topic in surgical ethics. Hébert et al. (1997) rightly argued that "[t]he candid disclosure and discussion of information not only helps patients to understand and deal with what is happening to them but also fosters and helps to maintain trust." Indeed, informed consent is the basis for the therapeutic patient–surgeon relationship, fostering mutual trust and promoting shared responsibility for decision making.

Disclosure, another pivotal component of adequate informed consent, dictates that during the preoperative conference the surgeon discusses with the patient the available treatment options, the expected outcomes, and the risks and benefits of each. Each option should be evaluated as to how well the choice aligns with the patient's medical needs, lifestyle preferences, and values. For example, during a preoperative meeting with an orthodox Jew needing heart valve replacement therapy, the authors had to determine whether or not he was comfortable receiving the recommended porcine valve (Zaroff, 2005a). After discussing the viable options, the surgeon may then document the conversation in the patient's medical record.

In addition to evaluating treatment options within the context of patient preferences, surgeons also encounter patients who insist that treatment be carried out in a manner that entails increased risk. A commonly cited example is the Jehovah's Witness patient who refuses to receive a blood transfusion during surgery (Zaroff, 2005b). Such requests place the surgeon in an ethical position where a decision must be made whether or not the risk to the patient is too great to justify operating as the patient wishes.

Conflicts of interest

The surgeon also needs to disclose any potential conflicts of interest. These conflicts of interest are often financial, as George Bernard Shaw (1946) lamented in the following oft-quoted passage from *The Doctor's Dilemma: A Tragedy*: "That any sane nation having observed that you could provide for the supply of bread by giving bakers a pecuniary interest in baking for you, should go on to give a surgeon a pecuniary interest in cutting off your leg, is enough to make one despair of political humanity."

However, we wish to highlight conflicts of interest arising in the context of surgical innovation. The quest to further knowledge through scientific research creates a troubling ethical dilemma for the surgeon–scientist. The surgeon has the primary obligation to do whatever is best for the patient's health (Frader and Caniano, 1998). But history has demonstrated, at times quite tragically, that deciding whether this fiduciary contract is violated by an experiment can prove anything but straightforward (Lefall, 1997). Moreover, as no centralized body exists for evaluating new surgical procedures, new operations are sometimes implemented without prior proof of their efficacy. McKneally (1999, p. 786) offered the following pessimistic condemnation of surgical innovation: "When innovative surgeons who take unaccredited courses return with uncertified skills to introduce non-validated treatments in trusting patients, we have a recipe for disaster."

Lastly, one should remember that the control procedure in surgical trials is often quite invasive to the patient. The use of so-called "sham surgeries"

as controls, for example, continues to provoke heated ethical debates (Macklin, 1999; Albin, 2005). One recent example debated in the literature involves the drilling of burr holes in the skull as a control treatment for the evaluation of new Parkinson's disease therapies (Albin, 2002; Kim *et al.*, 2005).

Emergency patients

Many of the most compelling ethical dilemmas that surgeons face come to the fore while treating the urgently ill patient. The preoperative conference becomes an irrelevant luxury, and disclosure and informed consent are often partially overlooked. When faced with a patient in urgent need of treatment, the surgeon must assume not only great authority, but a great deal more as well. Firstly, he or she assumes that the immediacy of care is important and will benefit the patient. Secondly, the literature refers to three classic assumptions used to justify treating emergency patients before obtaining their informed consent: the life-preserving goal of medicine, the premise that most patients would want their life saved, and the condition that the benefits outweigh the risks (Mattox and Engelhardt, 1998).

Finally, surgeons, despite the breadth of their craft, are limited in their ability to heal. They deal with emotionally and morally wrenching decisions about when to forgo further surgical treatment. Selzer's "Sarcophagus," part of his anecdotal anthology *The Doctor Stories* (1998), insightfully portrays the emotional trials of an operating team accepting the futility of further intervention. In many cases, patients have decided in advance how they would like their surgeon to proceed in given dire situations. The main challenge for the surgeon then becomes deciding whether or not the patient's advance directive applies to the current situation. Many resources exist to assist the surgeon in deciding, but if there is any doubt and the benefits of treatment outweigh the risks, then the surgeon is best advised to treat (Emanuel *et al.*, 1994; King, 1996).

How should I approach surgical ethics in practice?

The preoperative conference

McCullough *et al.* (1998b) have proposed a schema, which we adapt here, for facilitating the patient–surgeon conference and subsequent decision making. Firstly, the surgeon must identify the relevant facts, particularly the viable treatment options and what is important to the patient. Then, the ethical analysis is undertaken, wherein one must consider the fiduciary responsibilities of the surgeon towards the patient, the relative benefits and risks of each option, the patient's rights and values, and the obligation to allocate limited resources with justice and equality. The final step asks the surgeon to arrive at and justify a conclusion within the context of the above considerations.

Secondly, and early in the preoperative interview, the surgeon should determine the degree to which the patient wishes to participate in this decision-making process. While the actual degree to which the patient desires to participate may vary, encouraging the patient's comfortable involvement has been shown to improve not only patient–surgeon rapport but also the overall health outcome (Siegler, 1996). The patient may choose to participate more or less in the decision-making process, but the presentation of options always occurs. In addition to the degree of desired participation, the surgeon must also determine whether the patient is competent to make decisions regarding treatment. We simply point out that surgeons, in particular, must remember that as the cost to the patient of refusing treatment increases, so too does the burden to prove competence (Mattox and Engelhardt, 1998).

Lastly, the surgeon has both an ethical and a legal obligation to ensure that the patient understands the information that has been discussed. Often the emotional impact of the information compromises the patient's ability to register what has been discussed. Having a family member or close friend of the patient present during the conference facilitates an effective conversation. The complexity of medical terminology can also be the source of great frustration and confusion for patients, and the surgeon is obligated to help the patient to overcome these difficulties. As an example of one such misunderstanding taken from the authors' experience, consider a devoutly Catholic patient, a nun, who greatly feared that when her Jewish surgeon spoke of "cardioversion" and "converting" her irregular heartbeat, she was in grave danger of having her religious faith converted against her will (Zaroff, 2005c). Clearly, effective communication can alleviate great potential for misinterpretation and can engender a more effective patient–surgeon relationship.

For patients to make the best decision possible, the surgeon is also ethically obliged to provide information on the expected outcomes of each treatment option. Most surgeons openly disclose statistics on the industry-wide outcomes of a procedure, whereas our experience suggests that few surgeons routinely present their personal outcome statistics. In the USA, many national medical associations, such as the American College of Surgeons and the American Medical Association, sidestep this question of complete disclosure with non-specific statements such as: "Eligibility to perform surgical procedures as the responsible surgeon must be based on an individual's adequate education and training, continued experience, and demonstrated proficiency,"(American College of Surgeons, 1997) and "Only through full disclosure is a patient able to make informed decisions regarding future medical care" (American Medical Association, Council on Ethical and Judicial Affairs, 1994b).

Many have criticized the medical establishment's continued quiet ambivalence on this matter. Bosk, over 25 years ago, insightfully studied perceptions and repercussions surrounding error in surgical practice in his *Forgive and Remember: Managing Medical Error* (Bosk, 1979). More recently, Clarke and Oakley (2004) cogently championed increased patient access to surgeons' comparative clinical performance. Furthermore, this reluctance on the part of surgeons to disclose individual outcome statistics has ultimately led many patients and health professionals to call for the creation of public databases of surgeon-specific outcomes as a means of achieving greater transparency. However, as Lo (2000) pointed out, making such information available raises additional ethical debates about how most accurately to represent the data and who should have access. Until a more widespread consensus is reached, the individual surgeon will continue to be responsible for adequately disclosing personal outcome information.

Emergency patients

When making assumptions regarding the treatment of emergency patients, the surgeon risks arriving at an ethically unjustifiable decision. Among the determinations to be made, the surgeon must first decide whether the chosen course of action best benefits the patient and aligns with the patient's wishes. Moreover, if the surgeon concludes that the patient cannot be helped by the available treatment options, then ethical reasoning does not justify proposing an operation (Halevy and Brody, 1996). Lest the surgeon appear alone in making these weighty ethical decisions, various surgeons and ethicists have devised patient classification schemes based on the degree of urgency to facilitate decisions regarding when to treat (Mattox and Engelhardt, 1998). Finally, many authors concur that surgeons should consult their peers often and regularly. However, doing so does presuppose a willingness to seek help from others.

The inability to engage the urgently ill in the consent process poses yet another dilemma. In situations of the utmost urgency, the surgeon may opt to treat the patient without consent or may assume the patient's consent. This scenario, borne of necessity, occurs regularly. Yet clinicians must recognize one important limitation to this assumption: clinicians may not administer emergency treatment without consent if they believe that the patient would refuse such treatment if he or she were capable (Etchells *et al.*, 1996). Alternatively,

for patients with limited competence or in situations where time is exceedingly precious, surgeons may apply a truncated version of the consent process. In the ideal situation, when time permits, the surgeon identifies a surrogate to stand in the patient's stead during the consent process. In the majority of cases, this solution offers the best means of honoring the patient's autonomy. The two chief concerns in surrogate decision making are identifying the most appropriate surrogate and determining how the decision should be made (Buchanan and Brock, 1989; Lazar *et al.*, 1996). Finally, when complications arise during the operation, the surgeon has to decide, and oftentimes rather precipitously, whether or not to step away from the operating table to consult with the patient's loved ones regarding the patient's wishes.

The case

Faced with an unexpected finding, the aortic aneurysm, Dr. B must decide how to proceed. Should he perform a less risky but incomplete repair of the aortic tear, or a more invasive and complete repair in which the ascending aorta is replaced with a graft and the ostia of the diseased coronary vessels are incorporated into the graft? Dr. B should first consult the referring physician and cardiologist. Then, if possible, the surrogate-decision maker should be informed of the reasons to proceed despite the increased risks. By helping this individual understand the risks and benefits of each option, he or she is better equipped to offer advice as to what Mrs. A would prefer.

Inasmuch as possible, foreseeable scenarios should be discussed with patients in advance. When unanticipated complications arise intraoperatively, however, the ultimate trust that the patient has granted the surgeon guides all decision making. Dr. B must take into consideration the opinions of his peers and determine which option best aligns with Mrs. A's wishes. But finally the problem is surgical, and the surgeon makes the decision. Emily Dickinson (1924) captures beautifully the delicate line that surgeons tread:

> Surgeons must be very careful
> When they take the knife!
> Underneath their fine incisions
> Stirs the culprit, –Life!

REFERENCES

Albin, R.L. (2002). Sham surgery controls: intracerebral grafting of fetal tissue for Parkinson's disease and proposed criteria for use of sham surgery controls. *J Med Ethics* **28**: 322–5.

Albin, R.L. (2005). Sham surgery controls are mitigated trolleys. *J Med Ethics* **31**: 149–52.

American College of Surgeons (1997). *Statements on Principles*. Washington, DC: American College of Surgeons (http://www.facs.org).

American Medical Association Council on Ethical and Judicial Affairs (1994a). Substituting of surgeon without patient's knowledge or consent. In *Code of Medical Ethics: Current Opinion with Annotations*. Chicago, IL: American Medical Association.

American Medical Association Council on Ethical and Judicial Affairs (1994b). Patient information. In *Code of Medical Ethics: Current Opinion with Annotations*. Chicago, IL: American Medical Association.

Beauchamp, T. and Childress, J. (2001a). Professional–patient relationships. In *Principles of Bioethics*, 5th edn, New York: Oxford University Press, pp. 283–336.

Beauchamp, T. and Childress, J. (2001b). Moral theories. In *Principles of Bioethics*, 5th edn, New York: Oxford University Press, pp. 358–9.

Bosk, C.L. (1979). *Forgive and Remember: Managing Medical Error*. Chicago, IL: University of Chicago Press.

Buchanan, A. and Brock, D. (1989). *Deciding for Others: the Ethics of Surrogate Decision Making*. New York: Cambridge University Press.

Clarke, S. and Oakley, J. (2004). Informed consent and surgeons' performance. *J Med Philos* **29**: 11–35.

Dickinson, E. (1924). *The Complete Poems of Emily Dickinson*. Boston: Little, Brown.

Emanuel, L.L., Emanuel, E.J., Stoeckle, J.D., Hummel, L.R., and Barry, M.J. (1994). Advance directives: stability of patients' treatment choices. *Arch Intern Med* **154**: 209–17.

Etchells, E., Sharpe, G., Walsh, P., Williams, J.R., and Singer, P.A. (1996). Bioethics for clinicians: 1. consent. *CMAJ* **155**: 177–80.

Frader, J.F. and Caniano, D.A. (1998). Research and innovation in surgery. In *Surgical Ethics*, ed. L. McCullough, J. Jones, and B. Brody. New York: Oxford University Press, pp. 216–41.

Halevy, A. and Brody, B.A. (1996). A multi-institution collaborative policy on medical futility. *JAMA* **276**: 571–4.

Hébert, P.C., Hoffmaster, B., Kathleen, C., and Singer, P.A. (1997). Bioethics for clinicians: 7. truth-telling. *CMAJ* **156**: 225–8.

Kim, S.Y., Frank, S., Holloway, R., *et al.* (2005). Science and ethics of sham surgery: a survey of Parkinson disease clinical researchers. *Arch Neurol* **62**: 1357–60.

King, N. (1996). *Making Sense of Advance Directives*, rev edn. Washington, DC: Georgetown University Press.

Lazar, N.M., Greiner, G.G., Robertson, G., and Singer, P.A. (1996). Bioethics for clinicians: 5. substitute decision-making. *CMAJ* **155**: 1435–7.

Lefall, L.-S.D. (1997). Ethics in research and surgical practice. *Am J Surg* **174**: 589–91.

Lo, B. (2000). *Resolving Ethical Dilemma: A Guide for Clinicians*, 2nd edn, Philadelphia, PA: Lippincott, Williams and Wilkins, pp. 294–301.

Macklin, R. (1999). Ethical problems with sham surgery. *N Engl J Med* **341**: 992–6.

Mattox, K.L. and Engelhardt, H.T. (1998). Emergency patients: serious moral choices with limited time, information, and patient participation. In *Surgical Ethics*, ed. L. McCullough, J. Jones, and B. Brody. New York: Oxford University Press, pp. 78–96.

McCullough L., Jones J., and Brody B. (1998a). Informed consent: autonomous decision making of the surgical patient. In *Surgical Ethics*, ed. L. McCullough, J. Jones, and B. Brody. New York: Oxford University Press, pp. 15–37.

McCullough L., Jones J., and Brody B. (1998b). Principles and ethics of surgery. In *Surgical Ethics*, ed. L. McCullough, J. Jones, and B. Brody. New York: Oxford University Press, pp. 3–14.

McKneally, M.F. (1999). Ethical problems in surgery: innovation leading to unforeseen complications. *World J Surg* **23**: 786–8.

Palmer, M. (1982). Ethics of a professional surgeon. *Bull Am Coll Surg* **67**: 2–5.

Selzer, R. (1998). Sarcophagus. In *The Doctor Stories*. New York: Picador.

Shaw, G. B. (1946). *The Doctor's Dilemma: A Tragedy.* Baltimore, MD: Penguin Books.

Siegler, M. (1996). Identifying the ethical aspects of clinical practice. *Bull Am Coll Surg* **81**: 23–5.

York, N. L., DaRosa, D. A., Markwell, S. J., Niehaus, A. H., and Folse, R. (1995). Patients' attitudes towards the involvement of medical students in their care. *Am J Surg* **169**: 421–3.

Zaroff, L. (2005a). Two worlds of rituals are joined in the operating room. *New York Times*, 11 October (late edn), F5.

Zaroff, L. (2005b). A physician's challenge: cancer surgery, but "no blood". *New York Times*. 8 November (late edn), F5.

Zaroff, L. (2005c). In the operating room, matters of heart and mind. *New York Times*, 21 June (late edn), F5.

57

Anesthesiology ethics

Gail A. Van Norman

Mrs. C is an 86-year-old woman with metastatic colon cancer, scheduled for surgery for bowel obstruction. She is hypotensive and tachycardic. She agrees to invasive monitoring but does not want to be resuscitated if her heart stops in the operating room. Her surgeon argues not to place invasive monitors because she is a "no code."

Mr. D is scheduled to be executed for the rape and murder of a child in the state of Missouri. He appeals his sentence on the grounds that lethal injection subjects the prisoner to potential prolonged suffering during the execution process. A court rules that an anesthesiologist must be present to assure unconsciousness before administration of the paralytic agent and potassium. The ruling states that the anesthesiologist must personally mix the drugs and administer them, or directly supervise their administration.

What is anesthesiology ethics?

Conflicts concerning patient choices and autonomy are particularly challenging in anesthesiology, in part because anesthesia care routinely alters patient consciousness, interferes with patient competence, and restricts or abolishes physical autonomy. Anesthesiologists are at times expected to use their knowledge and skills for the very purpose of abolishing patient resistance. Such expectations present conflicts with core values in the ethical practice of anesthesiology, and of medicine itself. Navigating the complicated course among ethical principles governing patient choice, fulfillment of beneficent intentions, and preservation of professional integrity requires understanding of ethical values and principles such as respect for patient

autonomy, beneficence, non-maleficence, preservation of human dignity, promotion of patient safety, and safeguarding of professional integrity. When patients refuse resuscitation in the operating room (OR), anesthesiologists may experience conflicts between the ethical principle of respect for patient autonomy and choice, and professional imperatives to act beneficently. In the matter of executions, anesthesiologists must answer the question of whether they should engage in acts that superficially resemble medical care but require a personal moral transformation embodying the very antithesis of the medical profession's philosophies of valuing human life, respecting individuals, and taking moral responsibility for their actions.

Why is anesthesiology ethics important?

Ethics

The competent patient with intact autonomy

Requesting a patient's permission for a medical procedure implies that the patient can and will sometimes deny that permission. Physicians are obliged to honor informed and competent refusals, lest the "consent" process be devoid of actual choice or autonomy. The tension between "informed consent" and "informed refusal" is especially great when one course of action would likely sustain life, and another would likely lead to death.

Physicians often argue that "benefits" outweigh "harms" of cardiopulmonary resuscitation (CPR) in the OR. In-hospital CPR is associated with low overall survival rates of 10–15% (Brindley *et al.*, 2002; Myrianthefs *et al.*, 2003; Abella *et al.*, 2005) and devastating neurological injuries (Zandbergen *et al.*, 2003). In contrast, survival rates for CPR in the operating room approach 90% (Reis *et al.*, 2002). The difference reflects underlying causes of cardiac arrest; in-hospital arrests are often caused by severe underlying disease. When an arrest occurs in an unmonitored situation, resuscitation may be delayed, contributing to poor outcomes. In the OR, underlying causes of cardiac arrest are often identifiable and reversible, and intervention occurs immediately (Olsson and Hallen, 1988; Sprung *et al.*, 2003).

Allowing a patient to die in the OR from a cardiac arrest that is highly treatable does not appear to many OR physicians to uphold the principle of beneficence. But patients may not believe that resuscitation from cardiac arrest is "beneficial" if they are left with significant physical impairments or are merely revived to die in a short time of a preexisting terminal illness. In weighing the beliefs of the patient and their physicians, physicians are ethically obliged to give priority to patients' perception of benefits and harms over their own (Clemency and Thompson, 1993, 1994; SUPPORT Principle Investigators, 1995; Wenger *et al.*, 1997).

Some anesthesiologists claim that anesthesia is "ongoing resuscitation," and that the two cannot be separated from one another. This unfortunate statement implies that anesthesia is riskier than it actually is, and that cardiac arrest is more likely to occur in the OR than other hospital settings, when in fact the opposite is true. Although anesthetic care and CPR share some common techniques, they are almost always easily distinguishable from one another. Would any anesthesiologist seriously argue that a patient undergoing mechanical ventilation during an elective laparoscopy is being "resuscitated?" Or that CPR is a routine part of anesthesia care? Although some life-sustaining procedures, such as assisted ventilation, are necessary during some surgeries, CPR is not integral to surgery, is rarely needed in the OR, and only then to treat

rare complications which OR physicians strive to avoid.

Many physicians feel that it may be appropriate to allow a patient with a do-not-resuscitate (DNR) order to die from a terminal disease, but that they are ethically obliged to "rescue" a patient whose cardiac arrest is a consequence of the physician's actions (Casarett and Ross, 1997; Casarett *et al.*, 1999). Examples include arrests caused by drug reactions, hemorrhage, or arrhythmia provoked by surgical manipulation. Often, however, complications are not attributable to only one action or cause, nor are they usually the result of negligent care. Primary therapies and treatments for the complications of primary therapies both have their origins in the problem for which the patient sought medical care, and it is difficult to reason that the patient may refuse one but not the other (Ross, 2003).

Finally, withholding surgery that a patient desires, such as surgery to relieve a bowel obstruction, unless the patient also agrees to submit to unwanted procedures that are not integral to the surgery, such as CPR, is coercive and, therefore, unethical. As Walker (1991) stated: "Surgery may provide palliative treatment for otherwise untreatable disease. Suspension of DNR orders in the perioperative period places the patients in the unfair position of having to weigh the benefits of palliative treatment against the risks of unwanted resuscitation."

The competent "patient" with compromised autonomy

Founding principles of the medical profession prohibited killing, but those principles must now be reconciled in modern cultures that accept physician participation in pregnancy terminations, physician-assisted suicide, and euthanasia. Arguments favoring physician involvement in executions often cite the principle of respect for "autonomy" by helping a prisoner to have their "desired" mode of death (Baum, 2001; Clark, 2006). Prisoners, however, are among the most vulnerable of society's constituents. This is reflected in efforts to regulate how the state or medical researchers can treat prisoners. The Nuremburg Code (1949) restricting the use of human subjects in medical experimentation arose out of experiments on prisoners during the second, World War. The United Nations (UN) Third Geneva Convention mandated humane treatment of prisoners of war, and protections against violence, intimidation, public curiosity or insults, torture, or coercion (UN, 1949).

A state of imprisonment is one of severely restricted autonomy. But execution represents the ultimate *destruction* of autonomy. Prisoners do not usually seek capital punishment of their own free will, and when they do, mental incapacity is cited as a defense against their execution (Blume, 2005). With regard to autonomy and rights, a prisoner's situation is less like that of an autonomous adult than that of a vulnerable older child, who possesses intellectual capacity, without many legal rights. Arguments seeking to justify physician participation in execution could theoretically cite the ethical value of preserving a prisoner's dignity, but not respect for non-existent autonomy.

Beneficence-based arguments that physician executioners are needed and best qualified to relieve suffering are based on flawed concepts of "suffering," as those physical sensations experienced by the prisoner during execution, and a limited concept of beneficence as being measured by only one aspect of the execution process. Capital punishment causes suffering in many persons, including victims' families, convicts' families, and prison staff (Osofsky and Osofsky, 2002), none of which is resolvable by medical means. There are also no data to support contentions that competent technicians are less capable of efficient, painless, or "humane" executions than physicians. Forensic examination reveals that all execution methods are fraught with complications, even when physicians are involved. The most frequent problems associated with lethal injection are difficulties obtaining vascular access, and painful subcutaneous infiltration of medications, delaying onset of unconsciousness (Khan and Leventhal, 2002). A recent study suggests that blood levels of hypnotics

administered during lethal injections are inadequate to assure unconsciousness in almost half of cases (Koniaris *et al.*, 2005). There is no evidence that these problems would be significantly lessened in the hands of physician–executioners, when complications with intravenous access and awareness during anesthesia also occur during the course of routine medical care.

Arguments invoking the principle of beneficence to justify physician involvement in criminal executions have historically been associated with subsequent "slippery slope" justifications for physician involvement in the killing of persons who have never faced an accuser or had a fair hearing, including those with physically or mentally handicaps or other social "flaws" (Hinman, 1944; Jonsen, 1993; Pelligrino and Thomasma, 2000). If physicians accept a role in executions based on beneficence arguments, it becomes harder to draw the line at participation in other state-sponsored activities, such as torture, coercion, and "medical incarceration," because they too are often defended as being "beneficial" to society (Silver, 1986; van Es, 1992; Pelligrino, 1993; Pelligrino and Thomasma, 2000).

Physician participation in executions produces many harms and is, therefore, not "non-maleficent." It causes harm through the "medicalization" of a non-medical and distasteful act in order to defuse moral objections and render it more acceptable to an increasingly skeptical public. In this regard, it parallels historical misuse of psychiatric diagnoses and mental illness-based incarcerations to manage non-medical social or political problems (Rood, 1979; Gluzman, 1991; Adler *et al.*, 1992). Agreeing to participate in executions transforms the physician into a deceptive "double agent," who is acting on behalf of the state while appearing to act on behalf of the "patient" (Silver, 1986; van Es, 1992; Pelligrino, 1993). It erodes public respect and trust (Sikora and Fleischman, 1999). It also sometimes undoubtedly engages the physician in the killing of innocent persons (Hinman, 1944; Dieter, 2004; Gross *et al.*, 2005).

Physicians have typically tried to divorce the issue of physician participation in executions from the question of whether capital punishment itself is moral. But the morality of engaging in an activity simply cannot be completely separated from moral aspects of the activity itself (Thorburn, 1987; Hastings Center, 1996). The practice of medicine involves consideration of the principle of justice, and the extent to which capital punishment intrinsically fulfills that principle is relevant to whether physician participation in executions is consistent with professional integrity.

DNA technology has proven that innocent people are wrongly convicted of capital crimes and sentenced to die, and that innocent people almost certainly have actually been executed (Langer, 2001; Dieter, 2004; Gross *et al.*, 2005). Capital punishment for comparable crimes is applied unequally across racial and socioeconomic groups (Baldus and Woodworth, 1997). Studies consistently demonstrate that it does not deter violent crime (Sorensen *et al.*, 1999; US Department of Justice, 2003; Rosenfeld, 2004; Berk, 2005). It unfairly consumes economic resources, because it is much more expensive than lifelong incarceration (Cook *et al.*, 1992; Dieter, 1992; Forsberg, 2005). It fuels ethically objectionable proposals to curtail existing "safeguards" – the appeals process – in order to cut costs (US Senate, 2005). It does not appear to provide the closure that victims' families seek (Lithwick, 2006; Schieber, 2006).

There is disturbing evidence that executioners undergo a process of "moral disengagement," or a kind of moral degradation (Osofsky *et al.*, 2005). Executioners avoid self-condemnation by dehumanizing the convict, devaluing his or her life, and deflecting personal moral responsibility away from themselves by blaming juries, judges, governors, and "the law" for the prisoner's execution, and not themselves.

Law

Do-not-resuscitate in the operating room

The courts unambiguously support the rights of competent patients to refuse life-sustaining interventions and to have treatment refusals honored while they are unconscious (*In the Matter of Quinlan*, 1976; *Barber* v. *Superior Court*, 1983; *Cruzan* v. *Director MDH*, 1990). Because anesthetic care usually interferes with a patient's ability to make and express decisions, courts have found that anesthesiologists have legal obligations to protect the patient in the OR from unwanted intrusions (*Schloendorff* v. *Society of New York Hospital*, 1914; Kroll, 1992). Recently, physicians have been found liable when an unwanted resuscitation resulted in survival but significant morbidity (*Anderson* v. *St. Francis–St. George Hospital, Inc.*, 1996; *Osgood* v. *Genesys Regional Medical Center*, 1997).

Physician participation in executions

In the USA, persons who participate in legally sanctioned executions are protected from criminal charges or civil penalties. In almost all cases, anonymity is promised to participants, making it difficult to know exactly how many executions are carried out with the help of physicians. Although lethal injection was developed as a "humane" method of execution, reports of complications and undue suffering of prisoners has called the constitutionality of lethal injection into question. Several state courts have recently ruled that lethal injection must be carried out under the supervision of a physician. In the state of Missouri, a court has ruled that an anesthesiologist must mix and personally administer the drugs, or supervise their administration (*Michael Anthony Taylor* v. *Larry Crawford et al.*, 2006). Physicians are not legally compelled, however, to participate in the execution of prisoners.

Policy

Do-not-resuscitate in the operating room

Automatic suspension of DNR orders in the OR does not appropriately recognize patient rights to refuse medical therapies during the perioperative period. Guidelines established by the American Society of Anesthesiologists (1993), the American

College of Surgeons (1994), the Association of Operating Room Nurses (Murphy, 1993), and the Joint Commission on Accreditation of Health Care Organizations (1996) require that DNR orders be rediscussed in the setting of surgery and anesthesia and state that automatic suspension of DNR orders in the perioperative setting is unethical. Discussion of DNR orders in patients undergoing anesthesia and surgery should include an explanation of the risks and benefits, including the more favorable outcomes for CPR in the OR, and the medical staff should document either the patient's goals for treatment or specific treatments the patient refuses or accepts.

Physician participation in executions

In the USA, physician organizations have consistently held that physician participation in executions is unethical (American Medical Association, 2000; American Psychiatric Association, 2003). However, there are no reported cases of disciplinary action against a physician or expulsion from a professional society for such involvement. In part, anonymity provided to executioners prevents many professional organizations from even being able to identify which, or how many, of their members aid in executions.

Physician involvement in euthanasia and executions concerns anesthesiologists in particular; to the uninformed, their skills appear to make them ideal candidates for duties that involve killing (Jonsen, 1993; Truog and Berde, 1993). The American Society of Anesthesiologists (ASA) has, therefore, addressed the issue in several ways. The ethical guidelines of the society specifically support those of the American Medical Association, which prohibit physician involvement in executions (American Medical Association, 2000; American Society of Anesthesiologists, 2003). A statement by the President of the American Society of Anesthesiologists in 2006 (Guidry, 2006) concluded that, "physicians should not participate in executions, either by direct action or by performing ancillary functions. This includes making recommendations about drugs to

be used. Physicians are healers, not executioners. The doctor–patient relationship depends upon the inviolate principle that a doctor uses his or her medical expertise only for the benefit of patients."

How should I approach anesthesiology ethics in practice?

Do-not-resuscitate in the operating room

The favorable prognosis for resuscitation in the OR obligates anesthesiologists to revisit DNR orders with patients in the perioperative period, because the patient may make a different decision in the specific setting of surgery. Presenting a patient with an exhaustive "consent check list" of possible invasive or resuscitation measures, however, can be intimidating, confusing, and coercive at a time of significant stress. Some authors have, therefore, suggested a "goals-directed" approach to DNR in the OR that focuses on patient desires regarding outcomes rather than on specific techniques to try to meet those desires (Jackson and Van Norman, 1999; Truog et al., 1999). The patient may agree to have obvious, reversible problems addressed in a medically appropriate fashion but wish withdrawal of life support after surgery if other complications arise.

There is probably no single "best" way of approaching the patients with DNR orders who are scheduled for surgery. The process of informed consent and refusal depends on individual patient–provider relationships and conversations (Jackson and Van Norman, 1999). By the same token, DNR orders do not constitute permission to stop "caring" for the patient in other ways. Invasive monitoring, for example, may help the anesthesiologist to prevent the cardiac arrest that cannot subsequently be treated.

Physician participation in executions

Current ethical standards of most medical professional organizations either explicitly prohibit or discourage the involvement of physicians in the execution process, although such standards are often vague as to what constitutes "participation." Most organizations appear to define participation as being present during executions, directing medical procedures involved in the execution, and prescribing further measures when the prisoner does not immediately die. The appropriateness of physician participation in declaring death (which may indirectly lead the physician to "prescribe" further measures if death has not resulted), or formulating methods of execution or recipes for lethal injection, remains controversial. In recent statements from the American Society of Anesthesiologists, however, involvement in such "ancillary" aspects of lethal injection is also discouraged (Guidry, 2006).

Although it is tempting to believe that physician participation in executions is somehow "merciful" or "beneficial," such activities nevertheless cause tremendous harms, both to persons involved and to the medical profession at large. Physicians should, therefore, not participate in executions.

The cases

The first case considers a do not resuscitate order in the operating room. Mrs. C was competent to refuse life-saving therapy. She was at moderate risk for cardiac arrest in the OR. It became obvious through discussion that she hoped to survive her surgery, obtain relief from pain caused by the bowel obstruction, and rejoin her family. She wished to avoid prolonged mechanical ventilation, particularly if things appeared "hopeless." She did not see any purpose in resuscitation if her heart stopped beating during surgery, but expected medications to be administered to "prevent it from stopping," if possible. Despite her surgeon's objections, the anesthesiologist placed invasive monitoring lines to facilitate hemodynamic management and reduce the risks of cardiac arrest in the OR. He also planned placement of the patient in the intensive care unit postoperatively. During the surgery, dopamine was initiated to support

blood pressure and cardiac output. She remained mechanically ventilated postoperatively. Dopamine was gradually weaned and she was extubated on the third postoperative day. After 10 days in the hospital, she was discharged to a nursing facility, and returned home to her family two weeks later. She died at home after four months from the effects of metastatic cancer.

The second case deals with an execution. Despite a court order that lethal injection could only be carried out if a physician was present to supervise the execution, no physician could be found who agreed to participate. In February of 2006, executions by lethal injection in the state of Missouri were placed on an indeterminate "stay" until the issues could be resolved. Mr. D remains on death row awaiting execution.

REFERENCES

Abella, B. S., Alverado, J. P., Myklebust, H., *et al.* (2005). Quality of cardiopulmonary resuscitation during in-hospital cardiac arrest. *JAMA* **293**: 305–10.

Adler, N. and Mueller, G. O. (1992). Psychiatry under tyranny: a report on the political abuse of Romanian psychiatry during the Ceausescu years. *Curr Psychol* **12**: 3–17.

American College of Surgeons (1994). Statement of the American College of Surgeons on Advance Directives by Patients. "Do not resuscitate" in the operating room. *Bull Am Coll Surg* **79**: 29.

American Medical Association (2000). *AMA Opinion 2.06 Capital Punishment.* Chicago, IL: American Medical Association.

American Psychiatric Association (2003). *The Principles of Medical Ethics with Annotations Especially Applicable to Psychiatry,* Section 1, No. 4. Arlington, VA: American Psychiatric Press.

American Society of Anesthesiologists (1993). *Ethical Guidelines for the Anesthesia Care of Patients with Do-Not-Resuscitate Orders,* Park Ridge, IL: American Society of Anesthesiologists [amended 2001].

American Society of Anesthesiologists (2003). *Guidelines for the Ethical Practices of Anesthesiology.* Park Ridge, IL: American Society of Anesthesiologists.

Anderson v. *St. Francis–St. George Hospital, Inc.* (1996) 617 N.E. 2nd 225 Ohio.

Baldus, D. and Woodworth, G. (1997). *Race Discrimination in America's Capital Punishment System since Furman v. Georgia (1972): The Evidence of Race Disparities and the Record of our Courts and Legislatures in Addressing this Issue*. Chicago, IL: American Bar Association.

Barber v. *Superior Court* (1983) 147 Cal App 3d 1006, 195 Cal Rptr 484, 491.

Baum, K. (2001). "To comfort always": physician participation in executions. *J Legisl Pub Policy* **5**: 47–82.

Berk, R. (2005). *New Claims about Executions and General Deterrence: Deja Vu All Over Again?* Los Angeles, CA: University of California Press.

Blume, J. (2005). Killing the willing: "volunteers," suicide and competency. *Michigan Law Rev* **103**: 939–71.

Brindley, P. G., Markland, D. M., Mayers, F., and Kutsogiannis, D. J. (2002). Predictors of survival following in-hospital adult cardiopulmonary resuscitation. *CMAJ* **167**: 343–8.

Casarett, D. and Ross, L. F. (1997). Overriding a patient's refusal of treatment after an iatrogenic complication. *N Engl J Med* **336**: 1908–10.

Casarett, D. J., Stocking, C. B., and Siegler, M. (1999). Would physicians override a do-not-resuscitate order when a cardiac arrest is iatrogenic? *J Gen Intern Med* **14**: 35–8.

Clark, P. A. (2006). Physician participation in executions: care giver or executioner? *J Law Med Ethics* **34**: 95–104.

Clemency, M. V. and Thompson, N. J. (1993). "Do not resuscitate" (DNR) orders and the anesthesiologist: a survey. *Anesth Analg* **76**: 394–401.

Clemency, M. V. and Thompson, N. J. (1994). "Do not resuscitate" (DNR) orders in the perioperative period: a comparison of the perspectives of anesthesiologists, internists, and surgeons. *Anesth Analg* **78**: 651–8.

Cook, P. J. and Slawson, D. B. (1992). *The Costs of Processing Murder Cases in North Carolina*. Durham, NC: Terry Sanford Institute of Public Policy, Duke University.

Cruzan v. *Director, MDH* (1990) 497 US 261 US Supreme Court.

Dieter, R. C. (1992). *Millions Misspent: What Politicians Don't Say About the High Costs of the Death Penalty*, Washington, DC: Death Penalty Information Center.

Dieter, R. C. (2004). *Innocence: A Death Penalty Information Center Report*. Washington, DC: Death Penalty Information Center.

Forsberg, M. (2005). *Money for Nothing? The Financial Cost of New Jersey's Death Penalty*, Trenton, NM: New Jersey Policy Perspective.

Gluzman, S. F. (1991). Abuse of psychiatry: analysis of the guilt of medical personnel. *J Med Ethics* **17**: 19–20.

Gross, S., Jacoby, K., Matheson, D. J., Montgomery, N., and Patil, S. (2005). Exonerations in the United States 1989 through 2003. *J Crim Law Criminol* **95**: 523–37.

Guidry, O. F. (2006). *Message from the President; Observations Regarding Lethal Injection*. Highland, Park, IL: American Society of Anesthesiologists.

Hastings Center (1996). The goals of medicine. Setting new priorities: mistaken medical goals and the misuse of medical knowledge. *Hastings Cent Rep* **26**: S1–27.

Hinman, F. (1944). Euthanasia. *J Nerv Ment Dis* **99**: 640.

In the Matter of Quinlan (1976) 70 NJ 10, 355 A.2d.647 Supreme Court of New Jersey.

Jackson, S. H. and Van Norman, G. A. (1999). Goals- and values-directed approach to informed consent in the "DNR" patient presenting for surgery: more demanding of the anesthesiologist? *Anesthesiology* **90**: 3–6.

Joint Commission on Accreditation of Health Care Organizations (1996). *Comprehensive Accreditation Manual for Hospitals*: Advanced Directives. Oakbrook Terrace, IL: Joint Commission on Accreditation of Health Care Organizations.

Jonsen, A. R. (1993). To help the dying die: a new duty for anesthesiologists? *Anesthesiology* **78**: 225–8.

Khan, A. and Leventhal, R. M. (2002). Medical aspects of capital punishment executions. *J Forensic Sci* **47**: 847–51.

Koniaris, L. G., Zimmers, T. A., Lubarsky, D. A., and Sheldon, J. P. (2005). Inadequate anaesthesia in lethal injection for execution. *Lancet* **365**: 1412–14.

Kroll, D. A. (1992). *Professional Liability and the Anesthesiologist*. Park Ridge, IL: American Society of Anesthesiologists.

Langer, G. (2001). *Death Penalty Ambivalence; Polls Point to Support for Execution Moratorium in US*. Philadelphia, PA: International Communications Research, Media.

Lithwick, D. (2006). Does killing really give closure? Washington Post. 24 March, Bo3.

Michael Anthony Taylor v. *Larry Crawford et al.* (2006). United States District Court Western District of Missouri, Central Division 2:05–cv–04173–FJG, June 26.

Murphy, E. K. (1993). Do-not-resuscitate orders in the OR. *AORN J* **58**: 399–401.

Myrianthefs, P., Kalafati, M., Lemonidou, C., *et al.*, (2003). Efficacy of CPR in a general, adult ICU. *Resuscitation* **57**: 43–8.

Nuremberg Code (1949). *Trials of War Criminals before the Nuremberg Military Tribunals under Control Council Law No. 10*, Vol. 2, Washington, DC: US Government Printing Office, pp. 181–2 (http://www.hhs.gov/ohrp/references/nurcode.htm).

Olsson, G. and Hallen, B. (1988). Cardiac arrest during anaesthesia. A computer-aided study in 250543 anesthetics. *Acta Anaesthesiol Scand* **32**: 653.

Osgood v. *Genesys Regional Medical Center* (1997), No. 94–267331–NH Circuit Court for Genesee County.

Osofsky, M. J. and Osofsky, H. J. (2002). The psychological experience of security officers who work with executions. *Psychiatry* **65**: 358–70.

Osofsky, M. J., Bandura, A., and Zimbardo, P. G. (2005). The role of moral disengagement in the execution process. *Law Hum Behav* **29**: 371–93.

Pellegrino, E. D. (1993). Societal duty and moral complicity: the physician's dilemma of divided loyalty. *Int J Law Psychiatry* **16**: 371–91.

Pellegrino, E. D. and Thomasma, D. C. (2000). Dubious premises – evil conclusions: moral reasoning at the Nuremberg trials. *Camb Q Healthc Ethics* **9**: 261–274.

Reis, A. G., Nadkarni, V., Perondi, M. B., Grist, S., and Berg, R. A. (2002). A prospective investigation into the epidemiology of in-hospital pediatric cardiopulmonary resuscitation using the international Utstein reporting style. *Pediatrics* **109**: 200–9.

Rood V. (1979). Soviet abuse of psychiatric commitment: an international human rights issue. *Calif West Int Law J* **9**: 629–53.

Rosenfeld, R. (2004). The case of the unsolved crime decline. *Sci Am.*

Ross, L. F. (2003). Do not resuscitate orders and iatrogenic arrest during dialysis: should "no" mean "no"? *Semin Dial* **16**: 395–8.

Schieber, V. (2006). *Testimony to the Subcommittee on the Constitution, Civil Rights and Property Rights*. Washington, DC: US Senate Committee on the Judiciary.

Schloendorff v. *Society of New York Hospital* (1914) 211 NY 125; 105 N.E. 92 Court of Appeals of New York.

Sikora, A. and Fleischman, A. R. (1999). Physician participation in capital punishment: a question of professional integrity. *J Urban Health* **76**: 400–8.

Silver, G. (1986). Whom do we serve? *Lancet* **i**: 315–16.

Sorensen, J., Wrinkle, R., Brewer, V., and Marquart, J. (1999). Capital punishment and deterrence: examining the effect of executions on murder in Texas. *Crime Delinquency* **45**: 481–93.

Sprung, J., Warner, M. E., Contreras, M. G., *et al.*, (2003). Predictors of survival following cardiac arrest in patients undergoing noncardiac surgery: a study of 518294 patients at a tertiary referral center. *Anesthesiology* **99**: 259–69.

SUPPORT Principle Investigators (1995). A controlled trial to improve care for seriously ill hospitalized patients. The Study to Understand Prognoses and Preferences for Outcomes and Risks of Treatments (SUPPORT). *JAMA* **274**: 1591–8.

Thorburn, K. M. (1987). Physicians and the death penalty. *W J Med* **146**: 638–40.

Truog, R. D. and Berde, C. B. (1993). Pain, euthanasia, and anesthesiologists. *Anesthesiology* **78**: 353–60.

Truog, R. D., Waisel, D., and Burns, J. P. (1999). DNR in the OR: a goal–directed approach. *Anesthesiology* **90**: 289–95.

UN (1949). *Geneva Convention Relative to the Treatment of Prisoners of War*. [Adopted on 12 August 1949 by the Diplomatic Conference for the Establishment of International Conventions for the Protection of Victims of War, held in Geneva from 21 April to 12 August, 1949. Entry into force 21 October 1950.] Geneva: Office of the United Nations High Commissioner for Human Rights, pp. 1997–2002.

US Department of Justice (2003). *Uniform Crime Reports; January to December, 2002. Washington*, US Department of Justice, Federal Bureau of Investigation.

US Senate (2005). The Streamlined Procedures Act of 2005, S.1088. United States Senate, 109th Cong., 1st Session.

van Es, A. (1992). Medicine and torture. *BMJ* **305**: 380–1.

Walker, R. M. (1991). DNR in the OR. Resuscitation as an operative risk. *JAMA* **266**: 2407–12.

Wenger, N. S., Greengold, N. L., Oye, R. K., (1997). Patients with DNR orders in the operating room: surgery, resuscitation, and outcomes. SUPPORT Investigators. *J Clin Ethics* **8**: 250–7.

Zandbergen, E. G., de Haan, R. J., Reitsma, J. B., and Hijdra, A. (2003). Survival and recovery of consciousness in anoxic–ischemic coma after cardiopulmonary resuscitation. *Intens Care Med* **29**: 1911–15.

58

Critical and intensive care ethics

Phillip D. Levin and Charles L. Sprung

A 70-year-old male patient (Patient E) is admitted to the intensive care unit (ICU) following a road traffic accident in which he suffered severe head and abdominal injuries. After four weeks in the ICU, the patient's neurological condition has stabilized with minimal function (the patient does not communicate but withdraws all four limbs to painful stimuli). Following numerous bouts of sepsis, the patient is developing renal failure. He is anuric, hyperkalemic, and acidotic. He is also ventilator dependent and on high doses of inotropes. The patient's family states that in their culture, life continues until the heart stops beating. The family (that includes a physician) requests that all resuscitative efforts be continued, including dialysis.

In parallel, a second patient (Patient F) with similar injuries, but with metastatic prostate cancer, is admitted to the emergency room and requires an ICU bed. In addition to his traumatic injuries, however, he is wheel-chair bound as a result of dementia. No beds are currently available. According to the assessment of the ICU physician attending, the trauma patient described in case one has the least to benefit from ICU therapy and should be assessed for withdrawal of ventilation, to which the family strenuously objects.

What is critical and intensive care ethics?

Many aspects of medical care practiced today would not be feasible without the support of an intensive care unit (ICU). Critical and intensive care ethics concerns the moral issues related to, amongst other things, major surgery performed in an increasingly older and sicker population, interventional radiology procedures, such as those required in the therapy of acute stroke, and the ever-present population of those injured in traffic accidents.

There are three predominant aspects of ICU care that make up the majority of ethical dilemmas encountered by clinicians working in critical and intensive medical care: cost, availability of resources, and outcome. The requirement for ICU beds has increased over recent years, while the number of beds has increased at a slower rate. This has led to a situation of limited ICU bed availability in many countries (Vincent, 1999). Care in ICU is both very expensive (accounting for up to 20% of all inpatient costs and 0.8% of the US gross national product in 1986 [Jacobs and Noseworthy, 1990]) and not guaranteed to lead to a successful outcome. Indeed, the definition of a successful ICU outcome has become blurred. While survival is a measure of ICU outcome, it is no longer considered as a marker of success of ICU therapy. For many patients, survival to a state of ICU dependence or survival with marked physical or mental impairment is considered as a fate worse than death. Many of these patients (or their families) choose death over survival with low quality of life and define this as an acceptable outcome of ICU care.

We will not investigate the significance of macrofinancial allocation decisions made at the national level. While these decisions undoubtedly have ethical implications (whether money be used for ICUs that may save lives or for schools that may educate the future generation), the ICU physician has very limited, if any, influence over them. In contrast, the assumption that ICU care saves or prolongs lives in the presence of multiple organ failure makes deciding which are the best patients to admit to the ICU when resources are limited (e.g., bed availability) and ICU care providing uncertain benefits (e.g., outcome) everyday problems faced by clinicians working in this area.

This chapter attempts to portray the two most common ethical dilemmas facing the ICU physician: the difficult decisions regarding whom to admit to the ICU in the face of limited resources and how to manage the patient who has not recovered despite ICU care. While these difficulties occur daily, the following must be emphasized. Firstly, ICU care succeeds in facilitating patient recovery in the large majority of patients admitted. Secondly, while ICU care may undoubtedly be stressful, after one year, 78% of patients who were ventilated had no recall of pain or discomfort, and 86% were willing to undergo ventilation again (Mendelsohn et al., 2002). Finally, despite all the difficulties associated with ICU care, satisfaction amongst ICU survivors able to express an opinion is very high: 81% of them were extremely pleased that resuscitative equipment had been used and 80% were willing to undergo ICU care again if required under any circumstances (Russell, 1999), even if for only one month of post-ICU survival (Danis et al., 1988).

Why is critical and intensive care ethics important and how do I approach them in practice?

Triage

When faced with a new referral, the ICU physician has to weigh three main issues. (i) Does the patient's acute condition warrant ICU admission: that is, is the patient sick enough that they will require and potentially benefit from ICU care or can they receive adequate care on a regular ward? (ii) Is there a preexisting medical problem (such as severe dementia) that might make ICU care inappropriate, or is the patient so sick that ICU care will be of no benefit? (iii) Is there a bed available in the ICU for this patient, or can an existing ICU patient be discharged safely to make room for the new patient?

While these issues may at first sight seem easy to resolve, they are not. Firstly, there are no existing objective criteria determining who will benefit from ICU admission, and no universally accepted exclusion criteria. Secondly, the consequences of triage decisions may be very significant as patients requiring ICU but refused admission have a higher morbidity or death compared with those admitted (odds ratio for mortality, 3.04; 95% confidence interval, 1.49–6.17) (Sinuff et al., 2004). Thirdly, there is significant post-ICU discharge mortality (estimated to occur following up to approximately 30% of ICU discharges), part of which is thought to result from premature ICU discharge (Daly et al., 2001; Moreno et al., 2001).

Current studies shed light on the process of triage but have not determined any means of deciding whether a specific patient should be accepted or not. Amongst patients refused ICU admission, the reasons for refusal can be divided into two groups: medical and administrative. Medical reasons include those described above, for example the patient was too well or too sick to benefit from ICU admission and had a preexisting illness or condition that was considered to make ICU admission inappropriate. Unfortunately, our ability to categorize patients into these medical groups is not particularly successful. One triage study showed that patients refused ICU admission as they were considered to be too well had a mortality of 9%, while 18% of those refused ICU admission as they were considered to be too sick to benefit survived with ward care alone (Garrouste-Org et al., 2005). Further, deciding which preexisting medical conditions should preclude ICU admission is entirely subjective. For example, advanced age, a criterion frequently cited as a reason not to admit patients to ICU, does not inevitably determine a poor ICU outcome (Chelluri et al., 1993; Demoule et al., 2005), nor does disseminated malignant disease or hematological malignancies. Finally regardless of the long-term prognosis, patients are willing to undergo ICU care to achieve as little as one month of post-ICU survival (Danis *et al.*, 1988).

Triage decisions are also influenced by factors unrelated to the patient and their illness. The simplest example of these administrative factors is bed availability. If no ICU bed is available, then the patient cannot be admitted to ICU regardless of their medical problems or prognosis. There may, however, be more complexity to administrative issues, as patients examined by a physician (rather than referred by phone) and patients examined by junior rather than senior physicians are refused ICU admission more frequently, as are patients from medical units and those referred at night (Garrouste-Org *et al.*, 2005).

How then should decisions be made about how to use the scarce resource of ICU beds? The professional societies have published guidelines to help to direct triage decisions for ICU care. The Task Force of the American College of Critical Care Medicine and the Society of Critical Care Medicine (1999) emphasized benefit as a priority, while the American Thoracic Society(1997) suggested that patients should be admitted on a first come first served basis, provided there is an expected minimal benefit to ICU admission. Unfortunately, as described above, medical benefit, is not well assessed by physicians while benefit, as determined by patients and their family, is not measurable. In an attempt to improve medical benefit assessments, scoring systems have been suggested. The APACHE and SAPS systems are inappropriate for this task as they are dependent on data accumulated during the first 24 hours of ICU care, which are not available at the time of triage. Recently, a large multicenter trial including more than 7000 patients referred for ICU care has been completed, aiming to provide a triage scoring system to assist in ICU admission and discharge decision making. The preliminary results will be published shortly in abstract form (C. L. Sprung, personal communication).

In conclusion, at present no clear evidence-based guidelines are available to assist the physician in deciding which patients should be admitted to

the ICU when bed supply is limited. While many medical and administrative factors have been identified that influence the triage process, most of these factors, unfortunately, have been identified in a negative context – meaning perhaps that they represent biases rather than valid independent criteria. For more on issues related to resource allocation and triage, see Ch. 33.

End of life care

For many patients dying in the ICU, there comes a point where further medical intervention will not result in a cure but rather will either leave the patient chronically ICU dependent or prolong the dying process. Beyond this point, while medical interventions may have physiological effects, they will not alter the final outcome, and they are considered by many (but not all) to be non-beneficial. Defining the point beyond which further therapy is non-beneficial is, however, by no means straightforward, as the decision has physiological, functional, psychological, and ethical elements. For example, for some patients or families, while the heart is beating, the patient is alive, even if there is extensive damage to other organs or even if the patient is defined as brain dead. For such patients or their families, the no-benefit point may only be reached after prolonged resuscitation. In contrast, for a patient who believes that life has no meaning without functional independence, quality of life determines the no-benefit point and that point might be reached soon after a head injury, despite the fact that a full physical recovery, albeit with reduced mental ability, can be achieved. In any event, there comes a point where therapeutic interventions change to interventions designed to manage the end of life.

Similar to other hospital areas, the objectives of end of life care in the ICU are to prevent suffering and to ensure death with dignity. However, in contrast to other hospital areas, ICU interventions (such as ventilation, inotropes, and dialysis) are able to maintain or support organ function for long periods of time. Consequently, while on an oncology ward, it might be sufficient to refrain from life-support interventions while nature takes its course, in the ICU environment, measures that are sustaining life might already be in place. These measures, while not contributing to the patient's recovery, can delay death. Once the no-benefit point has been reached, consideration must be given to the management of life-supporting interventions.

In the ICU, end of life care exists as a continuum beginning with full care and ending with euthanasia. While different categories can be recognized on the continuum, and are described below, the borders between them are often blurred. It should be noted, however, that in most jurisdictions euthanasia is illegal.

The first limitation often applied is the do-not-resuscitate (DNR) order (or the do-not-attempt-resuscitation order). Such an order may have been determined in advance in a ''living will,'' or may be applied on ICU admission or at any stage during ICU care. While the patient is stable and does not require active intervention to prolong life, the care that a patient with a DNR order receives may be identical to that of any other patient. A DNR order represents a specific type of decision to ''withhold'' therapy. Withholding therapy means not beginning a therapy that might be required to prolong life. Such a decision might include not starting ino-tropes despite a decrease in blood pressure, or not beginning dialysis for acute renal failure.

Further along the spectrum of end of life care is withdrawal. Withdrawal means the cessation of a therapy required to prolong life. An example is the cessation of mechanical ventilation, or extubation of a patient despite the prediction that the patient will not be able to sustain spontaneous ventilation and is, therefore, almost certain to die.

Finally, the most ''aggressive'' form of end of life care includes steps taken to shorten the dying process, or active euthanasia. In this circumstance, interventions (such as the administration of drugs) are performed with the specific intent of causing death. The administration of opiates at very high dosage together with muscle relaxants to a spon-taneously breathing patient might be an example.

It has been claimed there is no ethical difference between withholding and withdrawing therapy (American Thoracic Society, 1991; American Medical Association, 2006; UK General Medical Council, 2006); as both may ultimately result in the patient's demise. Despite this, there is a clear rec-ognition that in practice these two options are not the same. For example, the UK General Medical Council has stated (2006): ''it may be emotionally more difficult ... to withdraw a treatment ... than to decide not to provide a treatment in the first place.'' Physician questionnaires have also revealed that 66% of physicians and nurses do not see withholding and withdrawing as equivalent in Eur-ope (Vincent, 1999), while 26% of North American physicians felt more disturbed by withdrawing therapy than withholding (Society of Critical Care Medicine Ethics Committee, 1992). The outcomes of these decisions are also different. A DNR order placed in a living will may be followed by many years of good life. However, a recent study of the events surrounding end of life decisions for 4248 patients in European ICUs (Sprung et al., 2003), showed that 89% of patients for whom therapy was withheld died, compared with 99% of patients for whom therapy was withdrawn, with a median time to death being 14 hours following withholding and four hours following withdrawal of therapy. The difference between withholding and withdrawing therapy has also been noted in a new law intended to regulate end of life care in Israel. This law accepts and permits cessation of intermittent therapies in terminally ill patients but does not allow withdrawal of continuous therapies (Eidelman et al., 1998).

Decisions regarding the type of end of life care appropriate for a specific patient do not seem to be objective. For example, using questionnaire responses from 1361 Canadian physicians and nurses to 12 case vignettes (Cook et al., 1995), in only one example tested was there greater than 50% agreement regarding the limitation strategy to be employed. Further, in an observational study of 5910 ICU deaths in North America (Prendergast et al., 1998), the proportion of deaths preceded by withdrawal of therapy ranged from 0 to 79% across different centers, with a range of 0 to 67% for withholding therapy. In Europe, similar variability has been described, with 47% of ICU deaths in northern Europe being preceded by withdrawal compared with 18% of deaths in southern Europe (Sprung *et al.*, 2003).

The most relevant factor determining the end of life strategy employed by clinicians and patients seems to be cultural. For example, more religious physicians tend to be more conservative in their end of life practices (38% of ''religious'' physicians felt uncomfortable withdrawing care as opposed to 21% of non-religious physicians [Vincent, 1999]), as are physicians who are in non-academic practice (Society of Critical Care Medicine Ethics Committee, 1994) or who are older (Alemayehu *et al.*, 1991). Ethnic differences may be equally important. Limitation of life support seems to be less common in Japan and Hong Kong, for example (Ip *et al.*, 1998; Nakata *et al.*, 1998; Sirio *et al.*, 2002; Yaguchi *et al.*, 2005), while even within the USA, different ethnic subgroups view end of life care very differently (Blackhall *et al.*, 1999).

Given that many patients are treated in multicultural urban societies, it can be expected that significant differences in approach to end of life care will be found between patients and healthcare providers. Therefore, the question arises as to who should decide on the most appropriate end of life care for a given patient. In the USA, autonomy is the preeminent value in decision making; however, 95% of ICU patients may lack decision-making capacity at the time end of life decisions have to be made, and only 20% will have previously expressed their views (Cohen *et al.*, 2005). Consensus seems to exist that the patient's natural proxy is their family and in the USA, family involvement in end of life decision making is the rule, with 93–100% family involvement (Smedira *et al.*, 1990; Prendergast and Luce 1997; Cohen *et al.*, 2005). In Europe, family involvement in end of life decision making is variable, ranging from 84% involvement in northern European countries to 47% in southern European countries. It must be noted, however, that family involvement may not mean a sharing of

decision making, as 88% of families in Europe were told of the end of life policy being enacted, while only 38% were asked for their views (with some discussions including both telling and asking) (Cohen *et al.*, 2005).

Further, even when involved in the end of life decision-making process, family members do not accurately represent the wishes of their loved ones, with agreement concerning end of life care preferences between the patient and their family members ranging from 50 to 88% (Seckler *et al.*, 1991; Sonnenblick *et al.*, 1993; Marbella *et al.*, 1998). Also, even when known, only 46% of children are willing to abide by their parents wishes (Sonnenblick *et al.*, 1993). Finally, despite the espoused importance of patient autonomy in North America, 23% of 879 US physicians had withdrawn therapy without the patient or their family's consent, 12% without their knowledge, and 3% despite their objections (Asch *et al.*, 1995). It seems, therefore, that although autonomy is a sought-after value, it is both hard to determine and difficult to respect.

Perhaps because of the vast differences in approach to end of life care expressed by different cultural groups, or the inherent difficulties in dealing with death, conflict between families and the ICU staff at the end of life is not uncommon. In one study, 44% of all conflicts between the ICU team and family members originated in differences of opinion regarding end of life care (Studdert *et al.*, 2003). Resolution of these conflicts can usually be achieved with sensitive negotiation; however, when these measures fail, external arbiters may have to be considered. These might include an ethics consultant (Fletcher and Siegler, 1996) (a third party not involved in the ICU care of the specific patients, and indeed not necessarily a physician), an ethics committee, or the courts (Gostin, 1997).

For more on issues related to end of life issues, see Section II.

The cases

The situation described at the beginning of this chapter illustrates a number of points. Firstly, a triage decision has to be made regarding Patient F. Does he have an indication for ICU admission, or is he too well or too sick? The patient does have an indication for ICU admission (traumatic head injury); however, his chances of surviving to hospital discharge may be reduced by his limited functional capacity (the patient is wheel-chair bound). In addition, the history of dementia may indicate a low post-ICU quality of life. To be meaningful, however, this diagnosis needs to be fully explored with family members and the family physician. In our experience emergency room diagnoses of dementia range from mild benign senile forgetfulness to full blown organomental syndrome. In our institution, this patient would certainly be accepted to the ICU at least for a trial of therapy.

As no beds are currently available, the next decision required relates to how to provide a bed. One option would be to transfer or withdraw ventilation from Patient E. Is this decision ethical? Should Patient F, whose chances of survival are also poor, act as a lever to limit the therapy given to Patient E? Or should a first-come-first-served approach be taken, and Patient F left in the emergency room?

Patient E is deteriorating and unlikely to recover; however, his family, for cultural reasons, rejects the possibility of withdrawal of therapy. In practice, in family meetings our main objective would be to avoid conflict. We would state that the patient is dying and that no therapy will stop this process. The family, however, is requesting that dialysis be performed, raising the question to what extent patients and their families can determine patient care when it is contradictory to physician recommendations. We would maintain that dialysis could potentially cause more harm than good in this hemodynamically unstable patient, and that as such we should not take steps that may cause harm. We would then attempt to negotiate with the family agreement to transfer the patient to the regular floor. If this failed, we have the fortunate prerogative of admitting ICU patients to the anesthetic recovery room, and this is what we would do.

REFERENCES

Alemayehu, E., Molloy, D. W., Guyatt, G. H., *et al.* (1991). "Variability in physicians" decisions on caring for chronically ill elderly patients: an international study. *CMAJ* **144**: 1133–8.

American Medical Association (2006). *Code of Medical Ethics*. Chicago, IL: American Medical Association.

American Thoracic Society (1991). Withholding and withdrawing life-sustaining therapy. This Official Statement of the American Thoracic Society was adopted by the ATS Board of Directors, March 1991. *Am Rev Respir Dis* **144**: 726–31.

American Thoracic Society (1997). Fair allocation of intensive care unit resources. *Am J Respir Crit Care Med* **156**: 1282–1301.

Asch, D. A., Hansen-Flaschen, J., and Lanken, P. N. (1995). Decisions to limit or continue life-sustaining treatment by critical care physicians in the United States: conflicts between physicians' practices and patients' wishes *Am J Respir Crit Care Med* **151**: 288–92.

Blackhall, L. J., Frank, G., Murphy, S. T., *et al.* (1999). Ethnicity and attitudes towards life sustaining technology. *Soc Sci Med* **48**: 1779–89.

Chelluri, L., Pinsky, M. R., Donahoe, M. P., and Grenvik, A. (1993). Long-term outcome of critically ill elderly patients requiring intensive care. *JAMA* **269**: 3119–23.

Cohen, S., Sprung, C., Sjokvist, P., *et al.* (2005). Communication of end of life decisions in European intensive care units. *Intensive Care Med* **31**: 1215–21.

Cook, D. J., Guyatt, G. H., Jaeschke, R., *et al.* (1995). Determinants in Canadian health care workers of the decision to withdraw life support from the critically ill. Canadian Critical Care Trials Group. *JAMA* **273**: 703–8.

Daly, K., Beale, R., and Chang, R. W. (2001). Reduction in mortality after inappropriate early discharge from intensive care unit: logistic regression triage model. *BMJ* **322**: 1274–6.

Danis, M., Patrick, D. L., Southerland, L. I., and Green, M. L. (1988). Patients' and families' preferences for medical intensive care. *JAMA* **260**: 797–802.

Demoule, A., Cracco, C., Lefort, Y., *et al.* (2005). Patients aged 90 years or older in the intensive care unit. *J Gerontol A Biol Sci Med Sci* **60**: 129–32.

Eidelman, L. A., Jakobson, D. J., Pizov, R., *et al.* (1998). Foregoing life-sustaining treatment in an Israeli ICU. *Intensive Care Med* **24**: 162–6.

Fletcher, J. C. and Siegler, M. (1996). What are the goals of ethics consultation? A consensus statement. *J Clin Ethics* **7**: 122–6.

Garrouste-Org, M., Montuclard, L., Timsit, J. F., *et al.* (2005). Predictors of intensive care unit refusal in French intensive care units: a multiple-center study. *Crit Care Med* **33**: 750–5.

Gostin, L. O. (1997). Deciding life and death in the courtroom. From Quinlan to Cruzan, Glucksberg, and Vacco: a brief history and analysis of constitutional protection of the "right to die." *JAMA* **278**: 1523–8.

Ip, M., Gilligan, T., Koenig, B., and Raffin, T. A. (1998). Ethical decision-making in critical care in Hong Kong. *Crit Care Med* **26**: 447–51.

Jacobs, P. and Noseworthy, T. W. (1990). National estimates of intensive care utilization and costs: Canada and the United States. *Crit Care Med* **18**: 1282–6.

Marbella, A. M., Desbiens, N. A., Mueller-Rizner, N., and Layde, P. M. (1998). Surrogates' agreement with patients' resuscitation preferences: effect of age, relationship, and SUPPORT intervention. Study to Understand Prognoses and Preferences for Outcomes and Risks of Treatment. *J Crit Care* **13**: 140–5.

Mendelsohn, A. B., Belle, S. H., Fischhoff, B., *et al.* (2002). How patients feel about prolonged mechanical ventilation 1 year later. *Crit Care Med* **30**: 1439–45.

Moreno, R., Miranda, D. R., Matos, R., and Fevereiro, T. (2001). Mortality after discharge from intensive care: the impact of organ system failure and nursing workload use at discharge. *Intensive Care Med* **27**: 999–1004.

Nakata, Y., Goto, T., and Morita, S. (1998). Serving the emperor without asking: critical care ethics in Japan. *J Med Philos* **23**: 601–15.

Prendergast, T. J. and Luce, J. M. (1997). Increasing incidence of withholding and withdrawal of life support from the critically ill. *Am J Respir Crit Care Med* **155**: 15–20.

Prendergast, T. J., Claessens, M. T., and Luce, J. M. (1998). A national survey of end of life care for critically ill patients. *Am J Respir Crit Care Med* **158**: 1163–7.

Russell, S. (1999). An exploratory study of patients' perceptions, memories and experiences of an intensive care unit. *J Adv Nurs* **29**: 783–91.

Seckler, A. B., Meier, D. E., Mulvihill, M., and Paris, B. E. (1991). Substituted judgment: how accurate are proxy predictions? *Ann Intern Med* **115**: 92–8.

Sinuff, T., Kahnamoui, K., Cook, D. J., Luce, J. M., and Levy, M. M. (2004). Rationing critical care beds: a systematic review. *Crit Care Med* **32**: 1588–97.

Sirio, C. A., Tajimi, K., Taenaka, N., *et al.* (2002). A cross-cultural comparison of critical care delivery: Japan and the United States. *Chest* **121**: 539–48.

Smedira, N. G., Evans, B. H., Grais, L. S., *et al.* (1990). Withholding and withdrawal of life support from the critically ill. *N Engl J Med* **322**: 309–15.

Society of Critical Care Medicine Ethics Committee (1992). Attitudes of critical care medicine professionals concerning forgoing life-sustaining treatments. *Crit Care Med* **20**: 320–6.

Society of Critical Care Medicine Ethics Committee (1994). Attitudes of critical care medicine professionals concerning distribution of intensive care resources. *Crit Care Med* **22**: 358–62.

Sonnenblick, M., Friedlander, Y., and Steinberg, A. (1993). Dissociation between the wishes of terminally ill parents and decisions by their offspring. *J Am Geriatr Soc* **41**: 599–604.

Sprung, C. L., Cohen, S. L., Sjokvist, P., *et al.* (2003). End-of-life practices in European intensive care units: the Ethicus Study. *JAMA* **290**: 790–7.

Studdert, D. M., Mello, M. M., Burns, J. P., *et al.* (2003). Conflict in the care of patients with prolonged stay in the ICU: types, sources, and predictors. *Intensive Care Med* **29**: 1489–97.

Task Force of the American College of Critical Care Medicine, Society of Critical Care Medicine (1999). Guidelines for intensive care unit admission, discharge, and triage. *Crit Care Med* **27**: 633–8.

UK General Medical Counil (2006). *Good Medical Pratice*. London: General Medical Council.

Vincent, J. L. (1999). Forgoing life support in western European intensive care units: the results of an ethical questionnaire. *Crit Care Med* **27**: 1626–33.

Yaguchi, A., Truog, R. D., Curtis, J. R., *et al.* (2005). International differences in end-of-life attitudes in the intensive care unit: results of a survey. *Arch Intern Med* **165**: 1970–75.

59

Emergency and trauma medicine ethics

Arthur B. Sanders

A 25-year-old male is brought to the emergency department by medics at midnight on Saturday night after being assaulted outside a downtown bar. The medics report that he was hit on the head and unconscious for a few minutes. When they arrived at the scene, the patient was confused but talking. He has a 4-inch laceration in his left parietal scalp and alcohol on his breath. When the patient arrives in the emergency department, he is slurring his speech and reports drinking several beers at the bar before being assaulted. He refuses any diagnostic tests or thera- peutic interventions. He does not let the nurse start an intravenous line or draw blood, nor let the physician examine his laceration or do an adequate neurological examination. He demands to leave. He says he has been assaulted before and will be OK. He becomes increasing abusive to the staff and repeats his demands to leave.

The paramedics are called to a skilled nursing facility for an 80-year-old woman who is in cardiac arrest. The patient was last seen four hours previously by a healthcare aide and later found in her room unresponsive. When the medics arrive, the patient is unresponsive with no pulse or blood pressure. They call their base station asking to declare the patient dead. They say that it is futile to resuscitate elderly patients in nursing homs because such patients never survive. In addition, since she has been down a long time she will have severe neurological dysfunction. The patient has no advance directive. She has been in the nursing facility for three weeks for rehabilitation after a hip replacement.

What is emergency and trauma ethics?

Ethical dilemmas are common in the emergency medical care system. In this chapter, we will discuss how the emergency department is different than other environments in medicine. These differences create unique ethical issues that are dealt with on a daily basis by emergency healthcare professionals (Iserson *et al.*, 1995; Sanders, 1995; Adams *et al.*, 1998; Larkin for the SAEM Ethics Committee, 1999; American College of Emergency Physicians, 2004; Girod and Beckman, 2005). Patients presenting to an emergency department (ED) are inherently different from those in primary care or specialty practices. Some of the differences include the following con- siderations, which may influence ethical decision making in emergency and trauma medicine.

1. Patients come to the ED with an actual or perceived acute medical or surgical emergency. A fundamental principle of emergency medicine is primarily to assess patients for serious diseases with threats to life or limb. When serious diseases are ruled out, the patient is assessed for common diseases. This focus on life-threatening condi- tions means that time pressures are key to completing diagnostic tests to rule out life- threatening conditions (Sanders, 1995; American College of Emergency Physicians, 2004).

2. Patients seeking care in the ED do not choose their doctor. In clinic practice, the patients usually choose their doctor and develop a rapport and trust relationship over many years. Physicians in clinic practices have the time to get to know the patient and understand his/her values. Without knowing the patient and their lifestyle and values, it is much more difficult for emergency physicians to address ethical dilemmas (Sanders, 1995).

3. Many patients seen in EDs with trauma or acute medical conditions have altered mental status. Alcohol, drugs, head trauma, pain, psychiatric conditions, and anxiety over the acute change in health status are common among such patients and can influence decision making and informed consent (Sanders, 1995; American College of Emergency Physicians, 2004). Sometimes these conditions are suspected but unknown at the time of treatment.

4. Diagnostic and therapeutic decisions must be made quickly for patients in ED, often with incomplete data. In a clinic or inpatient hospital environment, physicians can take time to consult with experts, search the literature, and discuss options before specific decisions are made. In contrast, the patient who presents to the ED with an acute myocardial infarction, a dislocated shoulder, or a ruptured spleen presents with an emergency condition that must be promptly addressed (Sanders, 1995).

5. The ED is an open and less controlled environment compared with clinics. Police, paramedics (often from the local fire department), and others are often present. This leads to potential issues with confidential information. There can also be potential ethical conflicts regarding obligations to patients and responsibilities to society. The inebriated patient involved in a motor vehicle crash and the patient who presents with a drug overdose are examples of patients that present potential conflicts of interest. Should the ED report these patients to the police or confidentially treat their medical conditions? Emergency healthcare providers often balance obligations to the patients with obligations to society (Sanders, 1995; Knopp and Satterlee, 1999; American College of Emergency Physicians, 2004).

6. The emergency medical care system is an essential part of emergency and trauma medicine. Medics and emergency medical technicians operate under the license and orders of the emergency physician. They face potential ethical dilemmas with conflicting responsibilities to patients, base station physicians, law enforcement agencies, employers, and society. Medics often face angry, hostile patients, many of whom are under the influence of alcohol or drugs or have psychiatric conditions. They balance respect for patient autonomy with trying to deliver optimal care for patients in the community (Sanders, 1995; American College of Emergency Physicians, 2004).

Why is emergency and trauma ethics important?

Ethics

Many of the traditional ethical dilemmas exempt emergency conditions. For example, fundamental ethical considerations such as informed consent, confidentiality, and patient autonomy may not apply for patients having emergency conditions. The patient who suffers multisystem trauma, who is unconscious, or who is in cardiac arrest is immediately treated with standard medical or surgical treatment including surgery and other invasive treatments. Standards of confidentiality may not be met as emergency healthcare professionals may request medical records from other hospitals without informed consent of the patient (Knopp and Satterlee, 1999). If many traditional ethical considerations do not apply to emergency conditions, do they apply when there is a potential for an emergency condition? This can only be determined after a thorough ED work-up.

Law

It is important that emergency healthcare professionals be aware of legal precedents that affect the practice of emergency medicine. In the USA, for example, the Emergency Medicine Treatment and Labor Act (EMTALA) is a federal law that requires that each patient presenting to an ED receives a screening examination and be medically stabilized. Prior to the EMTALA law, hospital emergency departments could refuse to care for patients who did not have the ability to pay and were referring them to government hospitals, with resultant delays in care. This was termed "patient dumping." Since the EMTALA laws were enacted in 1986 and updated in 1994 and 2003, patients must be stabilized and an accepting physician contacted before patients are transferred to another hospital for specialized care not available at the initial hospital (Capron, 1995; Derse, 1999).

Some traditional legal precedents such as the need for informed consent and confidentiality have exceptions when a patient presents in a true emergency condition. Under this exception, the patient must be unconscious or incapacitated with no immediate family available, time is critical for diagnostic or therapeutic procedures, and a reasonable person would consent to the procedure or request for medical information (Derse, 1999).

Policy

Ethics in emergency and trauma medicine is thus more complex than ethical issues in a primary care setting. The special circumstances and nuances of emergency medical care is addressed in the subspecialty *Codes of Ethics* developed for emergency physicians (Larkin, 1999; American College of Emergency Physicians, 2004). This emphasizes the unique duties of emergency physicians, including the "social role and responsibility to act as healthcare providers of last resort for patients who have no other ready access to healthcare." The basic principles of the emergency physician–patient relationship includes beneficence, respect for patient autonomy, fairness, respect for privacy, and non-maleficence. Informed consent by patients is important provided they have decision-making capacity.

How should I approach emergency and trauma ethics in practice?

It is important to understand that ethical issues are common in the ED. Each patient encounter is unique and clinicians cannot follow definitive rules for all cases.

In emergency medicine and trauma care, evaluating decision-making capacity is the key element of informed consent. The patient may be suspected to have taken alcohol, drugs, or have unknown medical conditions that affect their decision-making capacity. Their clinical picture, as well as mental status, may fluctuate in the same ED visit. Even more confusing is the fact that decision-making capacity is decision specific and depends on the consequences of the decision. An inebriated patient with a laceration may be released if they refuse sutures, with the consequences of a scar or wound infection. However, the same inebriated patient may be restrained and forced to stay in the ED after a serious motor vehicle crash if they refuse medical care. The consequences of refusing trauma care after a motor vehicle crash can be immediate death (Iserson *et al.*, 1995; Derse, 1999).

Although emergency healthcare providers respect and value patient autonomy, exceptions to informed consent also exist. Patients in true life-and-death situations must be treated appropriately even if there is no time to obtain informed consent. Implied consent is assumed, as a reasonable person would want standard medical treatment to save his/her life. A trauma patient who is acutely bleeding from his/her ruptured spleen is promptly taken to the operating room. The unconscious patient with a drug overdose is treated as an emergency regardless of consent. In addition, patients who do not have decision-making capacity are treated with standard medical care until their capacity to make decisions is restored. The most common example is the inebriated patient, who sobers up in the ED and is then able to make rational decisions about healthcare. Finally, there may be public health and societal benefits that overrides an individual's consent to treatment. For example, a patient with an infectious disease such as tuberculosis may not have a choice about treatment options (Iserson *et al.*, 1995; Palmer and Iserson, 1997; Moskop, 1999; Naess *et al.*, 2001; American College of Emergency Physicians, 2004).

Emergency healthcare professionals operate under the assumption that patients want full resuscitation for medical or traumatic emergencies (Moskop, 1999; Marco and Larkin, 2000; Naess *et al.*, 2001; American Heart Association, 2005). The clinical teaching is to "err on the side of life." Patients facing life- or limb-threatening conditions receive full resuscitation efforts with the following exceptions: (i) the patient has a valid advance directive saying they do not want resuscitation, and (ii) resuscitation attempts would be futile (American Heart Association, 2005).

Cardiopulmonary resuscitation (CPR) is one of the few procedures that is begun unless a limitation of medical care order is in effect. The default CPR order is appropriate since cardiac arrest is the ultimate medical emergency where a delay of even minutes drastically reduces the chances for successful resuscitation. Patients with valid advance directives will have these honored by emergency and prehospital care professionals. Many communities have a standardized prehospital do-not-resuscitate (DNR) form that the medics will look for when they find a patient in cardiac arrest. It is important that primary care physicians be aware of the community standards for DNR (Marco, 1999; Sanders, 1999; Marco and Larkin, 2000; American Heart Association, 2005). Patients with terminal diseases who do not have DNR forms available will have resuscitation procedures instituted when they call for medics. From an ethical standpoint, there is no issue in stopping resuscitation efforts if valid information is presented that the patient or their surrogate decision maker does not want resuscitation. It must be pointed out, however, that medics are trained to resuscitate, to "err on the side of life," unless there is a valid DNR form. It is also important to remember that not all advance directives ask to limit care. Some advance directives ask that everything be done to save a person's life.

If a resuscitation attempt is considered futile, emergency healthcare professionals are under no obligation to provide it. There is controversy about exactly what the circumstances are when resuscitation attempts should be considered futile.

A number of factors influence the prognosis for patients in cardiac arrest. These include patient factors such as comorbid diseases and etiology of the arrest, and systems factors such as down time before CPR, time to defibrillation, and initial rhythm (American Heart Association, 2005). None of these factors is, in itself, predictive of medical futility. Some factors can also be subjected to bias of the individual treating physician. Therefore, emergency healthcare providers should follow standard guidelines for when to withhold resuscitation efforts. Guidelines are developed and updated by the International Resuscitation Liaison Council on Resuscitation and local resuscitation councils. The American Heart Association (2005) gives the following criteria for withholding CPR efforts.

(a) The patient has a valid Do Not Attempt Resuscitation (DNAR) order
(b) The patient has signs of irreversible death (e.g., rigor mortis, decapitation, or dependent lividity)
(c) No physiological benefit can be expected because vital functions have deteriorated despite maximal therapy (e.g., progressive septic or cardiogenic shock).

Physicians can stop resuscitation efforts when the patient is unresponsive to advanced cardiac life-support efforts. This is a clinical decision the emergency physician makes based on known prognostic factors such as time in arrest, setting, response to treatment, comorbid diseases, etc. The vast majority of patients who survive an out-of-hospital arrest will have return of spontaneous circulation with the treatment of paramedics. There is no advantage in transporting a patient in cardiac arrest to a hospital as long as the emergency medical services system has a protocol for pronouncing a patient dead (American Heart Association, 2005).

The cases

The first case illustrates that emergency healthcare providers try to respect the patient's autonomy and in this case, the patient requested not to be treated. However, in order to respect the patient's request, he must have the decision-making capacity to understand the consequences of his decision. In this case, there are a number of factors that may impair his judgement. Firstly, the patient admits to drinking several beers. His breath smells of alcohol and he is slurring his speech. Could the alcohol be clouding his judgement to refuse treatment? If he were sober, would he still refuse medical care? Secondly, the extent of his trauma is unknown. He was hit on the head, has a laceration, and was reported to be unconscious for a few minutes. Is his decision about refusing medical care influenced by his recent head trauma? Are there other unknown medical conditions involved? Did the patient also ingest drugs, such as cocaine or amphetamines, which also may affect his judgement? The patient is refusing diagnostic tests and there is no immediate way to sort out these factors. The patient does not cooperate with a formal mental status examination. The emergency physician must make an immediate decision and there is not time to get consultations. If the patient is getting aggressive, then he must either be restrained or allowed to leave. Because the consequences to the patient for a bad decision are significant, including a cerebral bleed that can cause death, the emergency physician decides the patient does not have adequate decision-making capacity and restrains him until diagnostic tests are complete and his alcohol wears off.

The second case, an 80-year-old woman in a skilled nursing facility who suffers a cardiac arrest, raises the question of the futility of resuscitation efforts. Patients who suffer cardiac arrest are assumed to want resuscitation (implied consent) unless they clearly indicate otherwise through a DNR order presented to the medics. The absence of such an order in the nursing home indicates that the patient wishes everything be done to save her life. However, healthcare professionals are under no obligation to provide care that does not have

proven benefit even if the patient requests such care. In the experience of the medics, it is rare for older patients in a nursing home to resuscitate from cardiac arrest, especially if they have been down a long time. Do we respect the patient's autonomy or withhold resuscitation on the basis of futility? The medical literature on the success of cardiac arrest shows that there are poor prognostic factors such as down time before CPR and comorbid diseases. In this case, we actually do not know what the true down time to CPR was. It could have been as long as four hours or as short as one minute prior to being found unconscious. We are also uncertain of the patient's comorbid diseases. For instance, many nursing home patients are severely disabled. However, the patient in this case was temporarily in the nursing home to help with rehabilitation. There is also no way to determine a neurological outcome until 48–72 hours after the arrest. Emergency healthcare professionals should always err on the side of life. There are published international guidelines for when to withhold resuscitation efforts. The patient does not have a DNR, clear signs of death (rigor mortis or dependent lividity), and there is no indication of deteriorating physiological functions. Therefore, the emergency physician orders the medics to immediately begin CPR and advanced cardiac life support protocols.

REFERENCES

Adams, J., Schmidt, T., Sanders, A., Larkin, G. L., and Knopp, R. (1998). Professionalism in emergency medicine. *Acad Emerg Med* **5**: 1193–9.

American College of Emergency Physicians (2004). Code of ethics for emergency medicine. *Ann Emerg Med* **43**: 686–94.

American Heart Association (2005). Guidelines for cardiopulmonary resuscitation and emergency cardiovascular care, Part II: ethical issues. *Circulation* **112**: 6–11.

Capron, A. M. (1995). Legal setting of emergency medicine. In *Ethics in Emergency Medicine*, 2nd edn, ed.

K. V. Iserson, A. B. Sanders, and D. Mathieu. Tucson, AZ: Galen Press, pp. 11–30.

Derse, A. R. (1999). Law and ethics in emergency medicine. *Emerg Med Clin* **17**: 307–25.

Girod, J. and Beckman, A. W. (2005). Just allocation and team loyalty: a new virtue ethic for emergency medicine. *J Med Ethics* **31**: 567–70.

Iserson, K. V., Sanders, A. B., and Mathieu, D. (eds.) (1995). *Ethics in Emergency Medicine*, 2nd edn, Tucson, AZ: Galen Press, pp. 51–105.

Knopp, R. K. and Satterlee, P. A. (1999). Confidentiality in the emergency department. *Emerg Med Clin* **17**: 385–96.

Larkin, G. L. for the SAEM Ethics Committee (1999). A code of conduct for academic emergency medicine. *Acad Emerg Med* **6**: 45.

Marco, C. A. (1999). Ethical issues of resuscitation. *Emerg Med Clin* **17**: 527–38.

Marco, C. A. and Larkin, G. L. (2000). Ethics seminars; case studies in futility: challenges for academic medicine. *Acad Emerg Med* **7**: 1147–51.

Moskop, J. C. (1999). Informed consent in the emergency department. *Emerg Med Clin* **17**: 327–40.

Naess, A. C., Foerde, R., and Steen, P. A. (2001). Patient autonomy in emergency medicine. *Med Healthc Philos* **4**: 71–7.

Palmer, R. B. and Iserson, K. V. (1997). The critical patient who refuses treatment: an ethical dilemma. *J Emerg Med* **15**: 729–33.

Sanders, A. B. (1995). Unique aspects of ethics in emergency medicine. In *Ethics in Emergency Medicine*, 2nd edn, ed. K. V. Iserson, A. B. Sanders, and D. Mathieu. Tucson, AZ: Galen Press, pp. 7–10.

Sanders, A. B. (1999). Advance directives. *Emerg Med Clin* **17**: 519–26.

60

Primary care ethics

Margaret Moon, Mark Hughes, and Jeremy Sugarman

Ms. G is 17 years old and needs a physical examination prior to participating in high school sports. Her physician, Dr. M, has been the primary care clinician for Ms. G and her parents for the last 10 years. During Ms. G's last annual visit, Dr. M engaged her in a routine discussion about sex, birth control, abstinence, and safety. Ms. G asked questions but denied any sexual activity. Dr. M counseled Ms. G to continue the discussion with her mother. At today's clinic visit, Ms. G reports that she has been sexually active for a few months and would like to start birth control. Additionally, she is worried because her menstrual period is a little late and she complains of some abdominal discomfort and a vaginal discharge. Ms. G is adamant that Dr. M does not reveal her sexual activity to her parents.

Mr. H is 47 years old and has hypertension and high cholesterol, despite an active exercise regimen and healthy eating habits. He has a strong family history of hypertension. His mother had a stroke at age 57 and is disabled. Mr. H supports his mother as well as his wife and their three young children. He refuses to take medication, either for his blood pressure or for his elevated cholesterol. He mentions that he has "no faith in medications" and that his mother was taking appropriate medication when she had a stroke.

What is primary care ethics?

To understand the ethics of primary care, it is important to delineate the unique characteristics of primary care. Some view primary care as the cornerstone of the healthcare system, providing "most care for most people, for most conditions, most of the time." Primary care is, ideally, accessible, patient-centered, continuous and comprehensive (Starfield, 1998). Each of these characteristics has a moral dimension.

Accessibility suggests that primary care clinicians are readily available to serve as the usual point of initial contact with the healthcare system. Depending upon the setting in which they work, they may be faced with a tremendous range of patients. Accessibility often implies that the primary care clinics are physically in the local community, giving clinicians insight into patients' life experiences.

Patient-centered care incorporates patients' values, goals, preferences, and needs. It "sees patients first as people, with hopes, fears, lives, jobs, families, and relationships, over and above any health problems that may be presented" (Rogers and Braunack-Meyer, 2004). Primary care that involves patients as partners in decision making is likely to be more effective. The challenge for clinicians is to manage values and goals that may be contrary to good health or to the clinician's own values.

Continuous care may provide an opportunity for clinicians and patients to know one another both in sickness and in health, but it also includes the challenges of maintaining a therapeutic relationship. This can contribute to making the clinician–patient relationship ethically complex.

Comprehensive care requires that clinicians address any number of presenting physical, social, or psychological problems, in addition to providing preventive care. When referral to specialty care is necessary, the primary care clinician may need to manage conflicting recommendations while keeping an eye on the "big picture" with the patient.

Primary care clinicians encounter ethical issues on a regular basis in their routine care of patients. However, traditional bioethics scholarship and teaching has highlighted specific high-intensity ethics topics usually encountered in hospital and tertiary care settings. Tertiary care is characterized by subspecialized and highly technical "rescue" medicine. There has been much less emphasis on the ethically significant nature of primary care practice. This chapter examines ethics in the particular setting of primary care, focusing on the ethical content of primary care practice and offering some guidance when such issues are encountered.

Why is primary care ethics important?

Ethical issues in primary care are important both because they are frequent and because they can affect the quality of care. Although precise estimates are unavailable, the prevalence of ethical issues is high in the primary care setting, in part because that is where most patients receive most of their healthcare. The overwhelming majority of healthcare encounters take place in clinicians' offices. For patients aged 65 and older, office visits occur 20 times more frequently than hospitalizations; in childhood, there are 40 to 60 office visits per hospitalization (Fryer *et al.*, 2003).

Moreover, ethical issues are commonplace in primary care office visits. While there are few studies on the nature and prevalence of ethical issues in the outpatient clinic, Connelly and Dalle Mura (1988) reported that, in one outpatient office practice, ethical problems were present for 30% of the patients and in 21% of the office visits. The most common ethical problems for the patients were costs of care (11.1%), psychological factors that influence preferences (9.6%), competence and capacity to choose (7.1%), refusal of treatment (6.4%), informed consent (5.7%), and confidentiality (3.2%). Ethical problems were more common in patients over 60 years of age.

Consequently, primary care clinicians face a multitude of ethical issues every day. While many of the ethical issues raised in tertiary care may involve intense and dramatic choices, there is usually a structure, such as a hospital ethics committee, to assist the clinician in analyzing and resolving issues. However, in the outpatient setting, such structures are unlikely to be available and clinicians may be more isolated. Therefore, in order to meet the overriding ethical obligation to deliver appropriate care to patients, it is essential for clinicians to understand the ethical issues that arise in this setting and to develop a sensible approach to addressing them.

How should clinicians approach primary care ethics in practice?

Towards preventive ethics in primary care

Preventive ethics necessitates anticipating the ethical issues common in primary care and promoting clinic practices and standards that help to minimize avoidable problems (Forrow *et al.*, 1993; McCullough, 1998). The defining characteristics of primary care (accessible, comprehensive, patient-centered, and continuous) suggest opportunities for preventive ethics. In many instances, policy and legal structures exist in this regard. For example, while primary care clinicians strive to offer patient-centered care that reflects patients' desires and values, patients sometimes make requests that are inappropriate. Professional standards and clinical guidelines help guide the clinician in properly responding to many requests for unreasonable care (Brett, 2000).

In addition, continuity of care stresses the importance of maintaining a therapeutic clinician–patient relationship. There are circumstances, however, in which this relationship becomes ineffective or detrimental and the clinician must find a means to end the relationship. The ethical guidelines for ending a doctor–patient relationship usually center on avoiding abandonment and ensuring continuity of care with another provider (American College of Physicians, 2005). Professional societies may offer specific legal guidelines (American

Medical Association, 2003; College of Physicians and Surgeons of Ontario, 2000).

When legal or policy guidelines are not clear or specific enough to provide a preventive approach, clinicians can work to establish relevant clinic policies and practices. Some target areas that may benefit from such an approach are listed in Table 60.1.

Table 60.1. Preventive ethics

Qualities of primary care	Nature of conflict	Examples	Methods of prevention
Accessible care	Preserving openness to all patients when some requests for treatment may not fit within the clinician's own moral boundaries	Abortion; confidential services for adolescents	Describe clinic and clinicians' availability, expertise, and limits on the provision of care. Make services and limits clear to affected patients and families early in the relationship. Identify alternative sources of care and provide this information when appropriate
Patient-centered care	Keeping the patient's values and goals at the center of treatment decisions when the patient's goals or preferences are unknown and are not ascertainable (necessitating the need for a proxy), seem contrary to physical or psychological well-being, or results in conflicts	Requests for futile care, non-standard therapies, or inappropriate care; non-adherence with care plans; identifying an appropriate proxy	Define and help patients to understand the focus and limits of the clinician's duty to provide care. Identify appropriate surrogates early in the course of care
Comprehensive care	Simultaneous roles as patient advocate and gatekeeper for limited resources (societal, health system, or practice)	Inappropriate requests; requests for excessive care; conflicts of interest related to billing and referrals	Establish a policy of honest communication with both patients and insurers. Deny requests to falsify reports. Advocate politically for necessary care. Use the model of informed decision making to help patients to understand economic constraints related to managed care. Develop and maintain ethically defensible business practices
Continuous care	Balancing the benefits and risks of maintaining a long-term clinician–patient relationship	Non-therapeutic clinician–patient relationships; problems with respect for boundaries between clinician and patient; unreasonable demands on clinician	Develop relationships with other local practices should patients need to be transferred. Make boundaries clear and keep them. Discuss problems with patients and enlist their help in resolving the conflicts

Responding to ethical issues in primary care

Despite the best preventive efforts, ethical issues will arise and a systematic approach to responding to them is necessary. The complex nature of primary care can make it difficult to define a clear and consistent process for managing ethical conflicts. In many situations, using the systematic approach proposed by Jonsen *et al.* (2002) provides a reasonable structure for analysis. Specifically, they suggest that complex ethics cases be analyzed in terms of four key questions. What are the medical facts affecting the dilemma? What are the patient's preferences? What impact will a decision have on the patient's quality of life? What are the other contextual features (including patients' values, family issues, legal issues) that affect the decision?

Establishing the medical facts around a case that involves difficult ethical issues is very effective in helping to identify the range of reasonable ethical options. Making sure that all parties involved share an understanding of the relevant medical features can often resolve or at least minimize the extent of the conflict. Once the medical aspects of an issue are clear, the patients' preferences are explored. The clinician can bring the ethical issue to the patient, explain the nature of the conflict, and ask the patient for guidance on the range of possibilities. When primary care has been comprehensive and continuous, the clinician is in an excellent position to understand the multiple dimensions of patients' preferences, including the influence of personal history, family, and community. Although always valid, family and community influences can be overwhelming and the clinician may have to work to protect patients' autonomous decisions about preferences.

This combination of clarifying the medical facts and helping the patient to define preferences is the key to resolving most conflicts. The next step is to identify the impact of possible choices on the patient's quality of life. Primary care clinicians often have unique insight into the quality of life for their patients, addressing both long-term knowledge of the patient's life circumstances and awareness of the patient's social and physical environment. Finally, other external factors that affect an ethical conflict should be considered. These include legal questions, family needs and values that may be different from the patient's values, community standards and constraints, resource issues, and other issues that may limit or influence the feasibility of morally acceptable options.

This method works well as a means to structure the necessary information about an ethical issue in a logical and consistent manner. Many cases can be resolved just by sorting and arranging the relevant ideas and working with the patient to share understanding. For persistent problems, clinicians can seek advice from neutral colleagues or local professional organizations.

The cases

Ms. G presents a good example of the value of preventive ethics. Most jurisdictions allow a sexually active teen to request and receive confidential care for sexually transmitted diseases, pregnancy, as well as psychiatric services. Adolescent access to confidential contraceptive services is also common. At the same time, there is substantial variation in rules regarding a clinician's option to inform parents when it is deemed to be in the best interest of the adolescent. Furthermore, clinicians are not always bound to provide confidential care to adolescents, even when legally available. Regardless, it would be prudent for the clinic to develop and present a very clear policy about confidential adolescent visits. A clinician who is not comfortable providing confidential care to teens can make that clear and redirect teen patients to a local free clinic or some other provider. In Ms. G's case, the medical facts are clear. The patient's preferences are likewise clearly stated, although the clinician can revisit the patient's request for confidential care, particularly to identify her concerns. Why is she afraid to discuss this with her parents? Is there any history of violence or abuse from a parent, sibling, relative, neighbor, or other person?

Was the sexual experience consensual? Are there older siblings or other adults who can help? Would it be helpful if the clinician presented the problem to her parents? Quality of life issues are also important. If the patient is pregnant, what are her goals and to whom can she turn for help and support? The contextual factors at play may involve the position of this teen in her family and community, the physician's own values with regard to contraception and adolescent sexuality, and the legal issues around providing care to minors. If the clinic offers confidential care to teens, it seems fair to make sure that parents are apprised of this policy early in the course of care. In this case, there is no explicit information regarding whether the clinic had a prior policy regarding these issues. If it did not have, and make available, a policy directing sexually active teens elsewhere for family planning care, the patient can reasonably expect to receive care at this clinic. It follows that the clinician is bound to respond personally to the current crisis even if he is uncomfortable providing confidential care. Assuming this is the case, if the clinician is unsuccessful in counseling Ms. G to share her problems with her family, it may be necessary for him to provide confidential care initially while continuing counseling. If necessary, the clinician may need to find another local clinic that has an established practice of confidential family planning services.

The case of Mr. H, involving non-adherence to medical therapy, is a common and perplexing ethical issue that may pit the ethical principle of respect for autonomy against beneficence. There are no simple methods to avoid the ethical challenges of non-adherence, nor are there simple responses. The medical facts are reasonably clear; Mr. H has a significant history that puts him at risk for stroke, a condition that he wants to avoid. Medications are generally helpful, although cannot guarantee favorable results, as Mr. H has established. The clinician should ensure that the patient understands the potential benefits of medication as well as the risks of stroke given his history. Careful discussion of side effects that may be troubling

Mr. H should be part of the discussion with him. There may be other concerns that Mr. H has not raised, such as the cost of the medications or his use of complementary medications. Alternatively, he may still be coming to terms with his mother's illness and needs an opportunity to reflect on her disability and what caused it. The clinician may need to revisit this discussion repeatedly to elicit all relevant issues, since the patient's preferences are not very clear in this picture. Mr. H refuses medications but works hard to stay healthy. He has important experience with the aftermath of a stroke. His non-adherence seems in conflict with his other behaviors. It is likely that there are other factors affecting his behavior. There may be important quality of life concerns related to medication use. Contextual factors are notable; Mr. H's family responsibilities are weighty and may be causing anxiety. One of the most well-recognized benefits of primary care is its focus on a long-term relationship between clinician and patient. The clinician can revisit Mr. H's non-adherence over time, supporting his efforts at maintaining health while continuing to look for acceptable medical therapies.

REFERENCES

American College of Physicians (2005). *Ethics Manual*, 5th edn. Philadelphia, PA: American College of Physicians (www.acponline.org/ethics/ethicman.htm#init) accessed 29 April 2006.

American Medical Association (2003). *Policy E-8.115: Termination of the Physician Patient Relationship*. Chicago, IL: American Medical Association (www.ama–assn.org/ama/pub/category/8496.html) accessed 29 April 2006.

Brett, A. (2000). Inappropriate requests for treatment and tests. In *20 Common Problems: Ethics in Primary Care*, ed. J. Sugarman. New York: McGraw-Hill Press, pp. 3–11.

College of Physicians and Surgeons of Ontario (2000). *Policy 4–0: Ending the Physician Patient Relationship*. Ontario: College of Physicians and Surgeons (www.cpso.on.ca/Policies/ending.htm) accessed 29 April 2006.

Connelly, J. and Dalle Mura, S. (1988). Ethical problems in the medical office. *JAMA* **260**: 812–15.

Forrow, L., Arnold, R., and Parker, L. (1993). Preventive ethics: expanding the horizons of clinical ethics. *J Clin Ethics* **4**: 287–94.

Fryer, G. E., Green, L. A., Dovey, S. M., Yean, B. P., and Phillips, L. D. (2003). Variation in the ecology of medical care. *Ann Family Med* **1**:81–9.

Jonsen, A. R., Siegler, M., and Winslade, W. (2002). *Clinical Ethics: A Practical Approach to Ethical Decisions in Clinical Medicine*, 5th edn. New York: McGraw-Hill.

McCullough, L. (1998). Preventive ethics, managed practice and the hospital ethics committee as a resource for physician executives. *HEC Forum* **10**: 136–51.

Rogers, W. and Braunack-Mayer, A. (2004). *Practical Ethics for General Practice*. New York: Oxford University Press, p. 3.

Starfield, B. (1998). *Primary Care: Balancing Health Needs, Services, and Technology*, 2nd edn, New York: Oxford University Press.

61

Infectious diseases ethics

Jay A. Jacobson

Dr. I was vaguely disturbed by something about the slim, handsome young man who was in his examining room because of an unstable knee. The knee, however, had unequivocal indications for surgical repair of three ligaments. It could probably be done by arthroscopy but might require an open procedure. The patient agreed to the procedure and it was scheduled. Dr. I asked him to provide a blood sample for routine laboratory tests. He also scheduled a preoperative chest X-ray. After the patient left, Dr. I added an HIV test to the laboratory request. Dr. I was anxious about blood-borne infections and was glad he had gotten his hepatitis B shots. He knew one colleague who had been very ill from that viral infection and another one who was a hepatitis B antigen carrier but had been afraid to reveal that at his hospital or clinic for fear of losing his privileges. The day before the planned surgery, the patient's laboratory and radiology reports came back. His blood cell count showed reduced lymphocytes. His clotting studies were normal. The HIV test was positive. To make matters even more perplexing, the radiologist reported a lung infiltrate that suggested tuberculosis. Dr. I wondered about what to tell his patient and what to do about the surgery.

What is infectious diseases ethics?

Infections are important because they are major causes of disease, death, and disability. Paradoxically, most are curable and many are preventable. They are unique in that they can be knowingly or unintentionally transmitted from person to person. They cause serious epidemics and devastating pandemics. Finally, despite remarkable technical progress that has radically diminished the incidence of childhood infections in developed countries and entirely eliminated smallpox, new infectious diseases such as Ebola virus infections, severe acute respiratory distress syndrome (SARS) and Avian influenza continue to emerge, evolve, and kill significant numbers of people and frighten and threaten many more. Infectious diseases entail some unique ethical features that are often encountered by public health officials. The fact that nearly all infectious diseases are caused by microorganisms and that many are relatively easily transmissible, diagnosable, treatable, curable, and preventable leads to the characteristic ethical problems that arise in the context of this class of diseases (Smith *et al.*, 2004). Patients often bring these problems directly to physicians when they present for diagnosis, treatment, or preventive care. Ethical problems arise from conflicts between values, principles, and interests. Infectious diseases ethics examines how features of infection shape these problems, especially the tension between honoring patients' preferences and preventing harm to others (Francis *et al.*, 2005).

Why is infectious diseases ethics important?

Ethics

The transmissibility of an infection, such as tuberculosis or gonorrhea, places a physician's duty of confidentiality to the patient in conflict with a duty to society and an obligation to obey the law (Fox, 1986). This may entail reporting the infected patient to public health authorities so that they can investigate an epidemic, alert contacts, and arrange diagnostic testing and treatment. Such mandatory reporting may be inconsistent with the patient's expectation of confidentiality. Disclosure of this requirement prior to diagnosis may change the expectation and avoid this potential conflict. However, it may make the patient reluctant to proceed with proper diagnosis and treatment. In that event, to ensure best possible care of his patient, the physician can correct any misunderstandings and explain other options. Physicians can assure patients that public health practitioners will respect their privacy insofar as possible. The doctor can remind the patient that he, himself, can alert his contact(s) to their exposure and reduce the shock of a public health visit.

Because diagnostic tests for infection in symptomatic and even asymptomatic individuals have value to others, the usual calculus of benefit and risk to the patient may be expanded to include those benefits. The standard practice of voluntary informed consent may be modified to accommodate strong recommendations, presumed consent, or required testing. It was common practice in the USA, for instance, to test all hospitalized patients for syphilis without their informed consent when this infection was more prevalent (Nakashima *et al.*, 1996). Screening of refugees for the human immunodeficiency virus (HIV) and hepatitis B is currently carried out (Barnett, 2004).

The generally safe, effective, brief, and relatively inexpensive treatment and cure of infectious diseases make it unusual for patients to refuse treatment and more difficult for doctors to understand and accept such refusals. If the patient's infection is likely to be transmitted to others, as tuberculosis would be, his/her refusal is even more problematic. Here, too, considerations of third parties may lead to respectful efforts to persuade patients or to even stronger measures that would seem to abrogate the principle of voluntary informed consent.

Because so many infectious diseases can be prevented, physicians have opportunities and perhaps a duty to recommend measures to prevent them. Sometimes this could help patients to avoid a serious, difficult to treat infectious disease such as tetanus. In many cases, like measles or hepatitis B, disease prevention for the patient, such as immunization, also provides protection for the community. Therefore, the physician may not always be able to offer the patient the usual option to refuse an intervention since some immunizations, such as polio and yellow fever, may be required for school entry or travel to another country.

Because some infectious diseases, such as meningitis, occur suddenly, advance rapidly, and impair cognitive function, there may be only a brief time during which patients can participate in medical decision making. Although most patients acquiesce quickly to diagnostic tests and antibiotic treatment, refusals of either can be very disconcerting. It is important to investigate the patient's reasons for refusing a diagnostic test and correct any misunderstandings that contribute to the refusal. While a diagnostic test such as a lumbar puncture is desirable and helpful, a sustained refusal does not preclude effective treatment. Fortunately, there are ethical options that do not absolutely depend on a laboratory-confirmed diagnosis. Because probabilistic selection of antimicrobial agents is virtually the norm in infectious disease management, a clinician can proceed to use one or more agents to address the most likely causes of meningitis in that patient.

The person-to-person transmissibility of infectious disease in the context of a medical encounter makes this category of diseases unique and raises special ethical issues. The problem was first recognized by transmission of group A streptococci on doctors' hands to obstetric patients, who developed puerperal fever. Recent concerns have focused on the possible, but rare, transmission of hepatitis B and HIV between patient and doctor or dentist. Does the doctor have an obligation to accept some level of personal risk to care for a patient with a communicable disease? Does a doctor with a transmissible infection have a duty to avoid or anticipate the risk of transmission and, if the risk is not eliminated, to disclose it to patients (Hoey, 1998)?

To treat infections, doctors usually prescribe antimicrobial drugs. The widespread use of a particular antibiotic may induce microbial resistance to that agent and possibly the entire class to which it belongs. Examples include vancomycin, penicillins, and cephalosporins. The benefit of using an especially potent or specifically targeted antibiotic for a current patient conflicts with the possible loss of benefit to future patients. A situation commonly encountered in infectious diseases, the empiric use of a new, broadly active antibiotic before the identity and sensitivity of the pathogen is known confounds this problem. We may provide no added benefit to the present patient and increase the risk of antimicrobial resistance and therapeutic failure for future patients (Metlay *et al.*, 2002; Foster and Grundmann, 2006).

Law

Although most laws address medical treatment in general, there are some that pertain to certain categories of disease. Some infectious diseases, because they can be transmitted and prevented, have evoked laws intended to reduce transmission and protect individuals and the public (Colgrove and Bayer, 2005). Laws mandate immunizations, such as those for measles, diphtheria, polio, rubella, tetanus, and *Haemophilus influenzae*, for children by a certain age or upon school entry. They may require yellow fever vaccination as a condition of entry to certain countries. While not often used, there are laws that permit quarantine of exposed and potentially infected and contagious persons. Historic examples include streptococcal scarlet fever and smallpox. The most well-known recent example is SARS. An avian influenza pandemic might provoke this response (Gostin, 2006).

Other laws facilitate surveillance and epidemiological investigation. Many government entities require reporting of cases of particular infectious diseases to track disease incidence and the contact of exposed individuals for testing, treatment, or prevention (Chorba *et al.*, 1989). For some infectious diseases, such as syphilis and tuberculosis, laws require screening and treatment if infected. These laws are responsive to the incidence of these diseases. Laws about the manner of testing also respond to the social and political environment. Early in the HIV epidemic in the USA, some states had laws that permitted anonymous, hence, not individually reported, testing. Some required counseling and informed consent before testing (Frith, 2005).

Because of fear and stigma associated with some infectious diseases, most recently HIV/AIDS, some laws have addressed discrimination against infected persons in schools or the workplace. In the USA, HIV/AIDS (acquired immunodeficiency syndrome) is legally regarded as a disability and patients with it acquire the protections afforded by the Americans with Disabilities Act (Webber and Gostin, 2000). Also, in the USA, some infectious diseases, because of their risk to others, qualify patients for free treatment, testing, and prevention at public health clinics.

Policy

Just as there are laws focused on infectious diseases, there are policies about them that address behaviors and practices of health professionals. Like laws, policies are written at many levels: professional organizations, healthcare organizations, hospitals, and clinics. Again, transmissibility and prevention are common themes. Hospital policies that address when and how to gown, glove, mask, and wash hands are familiar examples. They may require employees and staff to be immunized against hepatitis B to protect themselves and patients. Hospitals may require annual or post-exposure testing for tuberculosis to identify, treat, and prevent transmission. There may be policies about when and for how long susceptible staff exposed to an infection such as varicella must stay away from work.

Other policies may address which staff may be excused from caring for certain infected patients.

On the one hand, policies may require staff to care for HIV-infected patients and to use appropriate infection control measures. On the other hand, some policies may excuse susceptible pregnant healthcare professionals from caring for patients with cytomegalovirus infection or varicella.

Policies for doctors infected with a transmissible agent such as hepatitis B or HIV are usually crafted to protect patients and permit physicians to practice safely. They take into account infectivity, type of practice, and associated risk and usually involve monitoring of the physician's health status and patient outcomes (Reitsma *et al.*, 2005). Hospital policies also address what can and should be done for employees or staff exposed to potentially infectious material.

Professional organizations such as the American Medical Association, Canadian Medical Association, and British Medical Association have policies that apply to doctors who encounter patients with infections. General policies prohibit discrimination and require that doctors obey the law. This means that a doctor may not exercise personal discretion in deciding whether to treat and/or complete a required report on a patient with an infectious disease. Recent policies have addressed the specific obligation to treat HIV-infected patients within one's scope of practice (American Medical Association, 1988; Canadian Medical Association, 1989) and to take precautions against the transmission of hepatitis B.

How should doctors approach ethical problems of infectious disease in practice?

Patients may realize that details of their illness may be accessible to others with a "need to know." They may not be aware of the need to report their name and particular infectious disease to public health officials. Clinicians should inform patients who may have a reportable infectious disease that the law requires reporting of a clinical or laboratory diagnosis. This disclosure should include the benefits to the patient of proceeding with diagnosis

and treatment, the potential benefit to others if contacts are elicited and investigated, and the practice of public health officials to protect confidentiality insofar as possible. Doctors should know the law with respect to infectious diseases, because in some jurisdictions, the laboratory must report positive results.

Because treatment for infectious disease is relatively simple, safe, and effective, patients accept it almost routinely. However, because all drugs have potential adverse effects, doctors should advise all patients of the risks as well as the benefits of treatment.

When a competent patient refuses therapy for a specific communicable and reportable disease such as tuberculosis, doctors should strive assiduously to determine what the patient understands about the disease, its natural history with and without treatment, and the risk and consequences of transmission to others. Often when clinicians recognize knowledge gaps and misunderstandings, they can explain things well enough to secure understanding and consent to treatment. If that fails, doctors should remind their patient about the necessity of reporting and the likelihood that public health officials will be concerned about adherence to required treatment and take steps to achieve it, monitor it, or restrict the patient's movements to minimize risk to others. The doctor should not use steps beyond information and sound argument to persuade the patient. The doctor should personally comply with reporting requirements to the health department.

The duty to do good for the patient and provide competent medical care is not obviated by an exaggerated fear of personal risk. Doctors with no likely exposure to a patient's blood or bodily fluids have no basis for avoiding their duty to care for their patient with an infection transmitted via these fluids. Clinicians who risk such accidental exposure in the course of surgery or procedures have an understandable concern about personal risk. An appropriate way to address it is to use prevention when possible, such as personal immunization against hepatitis B, universal precautions, safe needle use, and masks and gowns when appropriate to minimize transmission of blood- and fluid-borne pathogens.

It is not appropriate to test patients for infections like HIV surreptitiously and/or decline to provide medically necessary treatment to them because of a known or suspected infection (Beecham, 1987; British Medical Association, 1987). If medical treatment is withheld for that reason and the doctor offers an alternative but untrue explanation for the refusal, it is even more ethically inappropriate.

If a doctor has likely been exposed to a transmissible pathogen, he/she has two reasons to determine if an infection has occurred. The first is their personal health, since many infectious diseases such as HIV, hepatitis B, and syphilis can be averted or effectively treated if suspected or diagnosed at a very early stage. The second is to prevent inadvertent transmission to a patient. If a doctor discovers that he or she has an infectious disease transmissible in the context of their practice, the doctor should comply with the policy that governs such situations in that institution. In the absence of a policy, doctors should seek advice from an infectious disease specialist, preferably the hospital's infection control officer and also determine whether any overriding public health policies apply (Reitsma et al., 2005).

Because overuse and unnecessary use of certain antibiotics contribute predictably to the emergence of microbes resistant to them, doctors should choose antibiotics thoughtfully. While it is generally desirable to optimize care for the present patient, if that treatment compromises or even precludes effective treatment for many other future infected patients then considerations of justice should weigh significantly in decision making. It is appropriate to use a drug when it is the only or far superior choice for a specific proven infectious agent. Even if this may contribute to resistance, the predictable benefit, lack of an equally effective alternative, and the low likelihood of induced resistance in this particular case argue for the principle of optimizing patient benefit. Quite commonly a patient has an infection of uncertain etiology,

possibly but not probably requiring the antibiotic of concern. One could use the newer, broader antibiotic "just in case." However, the patient benefit here seems diminished compared with the possible harm to others if resistance emerges. As doctors make these difficult choices, they should consider the probability of infection with the pathogen of interest and the rapidity and severity of the infection that would occur if that pathogen were not effectively treated. A thoughtful balance of all these considerations is all that we can expect of clinicians, but we should expect nothing less (Metlay et al., 2002; Foster and Grundmann, 2006).

The case

Dr. I erred when he obtained a potentially life-changing test and did not inform his patient and obtain consent. He probably realized this when the result returned. At that point, the ethical imperatives for Dr. I are to ascertain whether the patient knows his HIV status, to explain why the patient was tested for HIV, to disclose the results of that test and the chest radiograph, to defer the scheduled operation until it is safe and desirable for the patient to proceed, to determine whether the patient has another doctor who can capably address his infectious diseases, and to find out if he has an obligation to report the HIV result to health officials and, if so, disclose that to the patient and report it. If and when the knee surgery is likely to be safe and beneficial for the patient, it should be performed using universal precautions and sterile technique. Dr. I should learn what preventive measures are available for him if he sustains an exposure to infectious material in the course of surgery.

For future cases, Dr. I can prevent ethical problems if he candidly addresses his concerns about blood-borne pathogens with his patients, discloses what steps he prefers to take to assess and prevent the risk of transmission, discloses the reporting requirements for positive tests, and reaches a mutually agreeable decision about how to proceed. He should become knowledgeable about the actual risk of infection from surgery on HIV-infected patients especially those on effective antiretroviral therapy. He should be clear about whether his reluctance to operate on these cases reflects an evidence-based fear of infection, a misperception of the risk, or other common but professionally inappropriate responses to some of the individuals at greatest risk of infection.

REFERENCES

American Medical Association [Council on Ethical and Judicial Affairs] (1988). Ethical issues in the growing AIDS crisis. *JAMA* **259**: 1360–1.

Barnett, E. D. (2004). Infectious disease screening for refugees in the United States. *Clin Infect Dis* **39**: 833–41.

Beecham, L. (1987). No HIV testing without consent, say lawyers. *BMJ* **295**: 936–7.

British Medical Association (1987). HIV antibody testing: summary of BMA guidance. *BMJ* **295**: 940.

Canadian Medical Association (1989). A CMA position: acquired immunodeficiency syndrome. *CMAJ* **140**: 64A–D.

Chorba, T. L., Berkelman, R. L., Safford, S. K., Gibbs, N. P., and Hull, H. F. (1989). Mandatory reporting of infectious diseases by clinicians. *JAMA* **262**: 3018–26.

Colgrove, J. and Bayer, R. (2005). Manifold restraints: liberty, public health, and the legacy of Jacobson v. Massachusetts. *Am J Public Health* **95**: 571–6.

Foster, K. R. and Grundmann, H. (2006). Do we need to put society first? The potential for tragedy in antimicrobial resisitance. *PloS Med* **3**: e29.

Fox, D. N. (1986). From TB to AIDS: value conflicts in reporting disease. *Hastings Cent Rep* **11**: L11–L16.

Francis, L. P., Battin, M. P., Jacobson, J. A., Smith, C. B., and Botkin, J. R. (2005). How infectious diseases got left out: and what this omission may have meant for bioethics. *Bioethics* **19**: 307–22.

Frith, L. (2005). HIV testing and informed consent. *J Med Ethics* **31**: 699–700.

Gostin, L. (2006). Public health strategies for pandemic influenza: ethics and the law. *JAMA* **295**: 1700–4.

Hoey, J. (1998). When the physician is the vector. *CMAJ* **159**: 45–6.

Metlay, J. P., Shea, J. A., Crossette, L. B., and Asch, D. A. (2002). Tensions in antibiotic prescribing: pitting social concerns against the interests of individual patients. *J Gen Intern Med* **17**: 87–94.

Nakashima, A. K., Rolfs, R. T., Flock, M. L., Kilmarx, P., and Greenspan, J. R. (1996). Epidemiology of syphilis in the United States, 1941–1993. *Sexu Transm Dis* **23**: 16–23.

Reitsma, A. M., Closen, M. L., Cunningham, M., *et al.* (2005). Infected physicians and invasive procedures: safe practice management. *Clin Infect Dis* **40**: 1665–72.

Smith, C. B., Battin, M. P., Jacobson, J. A., *et al.* (2004). Are there characteristics of infectious diseases that raise special ethical issues? *Devel W Bioethics* **4**: 1–16.

Webber, D. W. and Gostin, L. (2000). Discrimination based on HIV/AIDS and other health conditions: "disability" as defined under federal and state law. *J Healthc Law Policy* **3**: 266–329.

62

Psychiatric ethics

Sidney Bloch and Stephen A. Green

Mrs. J, a 22-year-old secretary, began to exhibit restlessness, perplexity, and remoteness from her husband, Mr. K, following the birth of her first baby 10 weeks earlier. A psychiatrist was summoned after she had visited several neighbors without obvious purpose. He found a reticent, detached woman complaining that, "They have been out to get me from the beginning," and alluding to "world famine and starving children." Mental status examination revealed vague, paranoid thinking but firm denial of suicidal and homicidal impulses; she was not obviously delirious. Mrs. J resisted the psychiatrist's recommendation that she be admitted to the local psychiatric hospital. Mr. K supported her in this, insisting that he did not regard his wife as mentally ill and feared she would deteriorate if placed alongside genuinely disturbed patients.

What is psychiatric ethics?

Psychiatric ethics is concerned with the application of moral rules to situations and relationships specific to the field of psychiatry. Resolution of ethical dilemmas confronting psychiatrists, as illustrated by the above case, requires deliberation grounded in a moral theoretical framework that provides methods and justifications for clinical decision making. An outline of such theories is covered in the introductory chapter of the book. We will focus exclusively on ethical aspects of clinical practice that are especially challenging to psychiatrists and briefly offer a preferred theoretical framework to deal with them.

Why is psychiatric ethics important?

Ethical aspects of diagnosis

Conferring a diagnosis of mental illness on a person has significant ethical sequelae since the act may embody profound adverse effects, notably stigmatization, prejudice, and discrimination (e.g., limited job prospects, inequitable insurance cover). Furthermore, those deemed at risk to harm themselves or others may have their civil rights abridged. These consequences justify Reich's (1999) call for the most thorough ethical examination of what he terms the clinician's "prerogative to diagnose."

Psychiatrists strive to diagnose by using as objective criteria as possible and information gained from previous clinical encounters. The process is relatively uncomplicated when findings, such as gross defective memory and life-threatening social withdrawal, strongly suggest severe depression. Other situations are not so obvious. For instance, the distress experienced by a bereaved person may incline one clinician towards diagnosing clinical depression whereas another may attribute the picture to normal grief. Expertise, peer review, and benevolence help to protect against arbitrariness and idiosyncrasy. Notwithstanding, psychiatrists must, to some extent, employ what might be termed "reasoned subjectivism." Consequently, specified criteria in the American Psychiatric Association's (1994) *Diagnosis and Statistical Manual (DSM) IV* and the World Health Organization's (1992) *International Statistical Classification of Diseases and*

Related Health Problems (ICD) *10* do not preclude debate about the preciseness or legitimacy of certain syndromes like attention deficit hyperactivity disorder (ADHD) and sexual orientation disturbance. Concern about the intrusion of value judgements into contemporary classifications has led to the contention that some diagnoses reflect pejorative labeling rather than scientific decisions (Green and Bloch, 2006). For example, charges of sexism were leveled against *DSM-III* (Kaplan, 1983) on the grounds that masculine-based assumptions shaped criteria, resulting in women receiving unwarranted diagnoses like premenstrual dysphoria (Chesler, 1972).

The issue central to this debate is whether certain mental states are grounded in fact or value judgements. Szasz (1960) took a radical position, arguing that disorders of thinking and behavior result from objective abnormalities of the brain whereas mental illness per se is a ''myth'' created by society in tandem with the medical profession for the purpose of exerting social control. The ''anti-psychiatrist movement'' (Scheff, 1966; Laing, 1969, 1970) asserted that mental illnesses are social constructions reflecting deviations from societal norms. This argument is supported by the role of values in both defining homosexuality as a psychiatric disorder and then reversing that position through a ballot among members of the American Psychiatric Association in 1973 (Stoller *et al.*, 1973). Legitimate diagnoses necessarily combine aspects of fact and value, as Wakefield (1992) contended in his conception of ''harmful dysfunction.'' He viewed ''dysfunction'' as a scientific and factual term based in biology that refers to the failure of an internal evolutionary mechanism to perform a natural function for which it is designed, and ''harmful'' as a value-oriented term which refers to the consequences of the dysfunction for the person that are deemed detrimental in terms of sociocultural norms. Applying this notion to mental functioning, Wakefield (1992) described the beneficial effects of natural mechanisms, like those mediating cognition and emotional regulation, and

judged their dysfunction harmful when it yielded consequences disvalued by society (e.g., aphasia or self-destructive acts). Diagnosable conditions exist when the inability of an internal mechanism to perform its natural function causes harm to the person.

Consequences of these sorts of disputes can be considerable (e.g., exposing children erroneously labeled as having ADHD to long-term dexamphetamine medication with its attendant risks) (Halasz, 2002). A related issue, so-called ''cosmetic psychopharmacology,'' involves the use of medication to enhance psychological functioning. As Kramer (1993) noted, fluoxetine may modulate emotions such as anxiety, guilt, and shame, raising ethical questions as to a person's capacity to possess ''two senses of self.'' Psychiatric diagnosis may also mitigate legal and personal consequences of one's actions (e.g., interpreting excessive sexual activity or kleptomania as variants of obsessive–compulsive disorder rather than wilful, chosen behaviors).

Ethical aspects of psychiatric treatment

Assessing and treating patients require a working alliance and informed consent. Many psychiatric patients are in a position to understand and appreciate the nuances of treatment options, to express an informed preference, and to feel comfortably allied with a therapist in their collaborative work. When the process of informed consent is responsibly handled, particularly with reference to benefits and risks of therapeutic options, patients undergoing psychiatric treatment are in a comparable position to their counterparts in general medicine. This comparability is grounded in two concepts: competence (Lidz *et al.*, 1984) and voluntarism (Roberts, 2002). The former covers the required criterion that the person facing choices in treatment enjoys the ''critical faculties'' to appreciate the implications of each course of action. Voluntarism refers to a condition whereby the process of consent is devoid of coercion and suggestion. Obviously, given that the organ of decision making is the same one that is impaired in many psychiatric conditions, profound ethical complications may ensue when seeking informed consent.

How should I approach psychiatric ethics in practice?

Ethical issues in the therapeutic process

Ethical issues arise once therapist and patient embark on treatment. At the outset, the patient is bewildered, vulnerable, and distressed, while the therapist is ostensibly omniscient. Dependency bolsters the authority already vested in the therapist and may be reinforced by his divulging little about the nature of treatment, believing this would undermine the transference (irrational feelings and attitudes patients develop towards therapists), regarded by dynamically oriented schools as central to the process.

As noted above, informed consent (Beahrs and Gutheil, 2001) is one means to dispel this air of mystery. Carl Goldberg's (1977) admirably clear model invoked the concept of "therapeutic partnership," its cornerstone a "mutually agreed upon and explicitly articulated working plan" subject to regular review. Among its elements are identifying goals and methods to reach them, monitoring efficacy, and permitting either partner to voice dissatisfaction. Moreover, respective roles, tasks, and responsibilities are examined as necessary. The partnership does not imply an equal share of power but rather an agreement about how power will be allocated. Thus, total autonomy in the patient, whereby the patient enjoys the capacity to reflect, to decide, and to act freely, may not always be apt. A patient in the throes of an intense crisis, for instance, may lack the wherewithal to appreciate what is in her best interests. In collaboration with the therapist, she may agree to a redistribution of responsibility, assigning the latter a more paternalistic role. As the crisis wanes, so restoration of the patient's state of autonomy occurs. The key feature of such shifts is their determination by both protagonists.

In reviewing models pertinent to informed consent in the therapeutic relationship, Dyer and Bloch (1987) proposed a fiduciary approach given its emphasis on trust and time. The therapist works to earn the patient's trust which occurs over time and is not a one-off negotiation at the outset. The fiduciary-based relationship also enhances a sense of responsibility in the therapist, who responds to patients' particular needs. Although autonomy in the patient is always a preeminent goal, it is not the therapist's sole preoccupation.

Values and psychotherapy

Permeation of treatment by values is another ethically based feature that must be addressed since the problems for which patients seek help are bound up with the question of how they should live their lives, and therapists may impose values intentionally or unwittingly (Holmes, 1996).

Engelhardt (1973) posited that psychotherapy is about meta-ethics in that it paves the way for ethical decision making by patients; the aim is not for them to adopt a particular set of values. Indeed, the therapist avoids recommending how patients should live their lives. Instead, they are helped to reach a point where they can make their own choices, unhindered by psychological conflict and unconscious influences. Freud (1924, p. 118), also intent on promoting value-free treatment, argued that a therapist "should be opaque to his patients and, like a mirror, should show them nothing but what is shown to him." He insisted that therapy was limited to "freeing someone from his neurotic symptoms, inhibitions and abnormalities of character" through making conscious the unconscious. However, he also pointed out an educative role, suggesting that the analyst "possess some kind of superiority, so that in certain analytic situations he can act as a model for his patient and in others as a teacher" (Freud, 1937, p. 248).

It is difficult to conceive of this hybrid role of mirror, model, and teacher as value free, even if the ultimate goal in analysis is to achieve autonomy, free of the influence of irrational forces. Therefore, if therapy amounts to ethical intervention, the question arises as to how the therapist should handle this? He or she could make every effort to minimize the ethical role, but the likelihood of succeeding is slim since unavowed values will be manifest non-verbally.

Another option is to accept the ethical intervention function but recognize this as the therapist's "problem," not the patient's. The former must be aware of a potential role as moral agent and regard personal values as a factor in the encounter. The therapist should be sensitive to his or her own values and monitor any unconsciously derived impulses to influence the patient. A process of "value-testing" ensures that their intrusion is never ignored and imposition thus obviated.

A third option has the therapist declaring his or her values as a value in itself. The argument runs as follows: psychotherapy is a form of social influence; the therapist influences patients; the therapist acknowledges this state of affairs; and the therapist is "transparent" regarding the values personally espoused.

Some homosexual therapists, for example, have aligned themselves with the "gay movement" when treating homosexual patients. A distinguished psychotherapist and committed Christian, Alan Bergin (1980), has evolved a school of "theistic realism" in which the therapist shares values derived from a Judeo-Christian tradition, including forgiveness, reconciliation, spiritual belief, and love. A group of therapists who functioned in the context of apartheid South Africa not only declared their repudiation of racism but also demonstrated their support for traumatized Blacks, especially those who had been victims of detention and torture (Steere and Dowdall, 1990). Particular constituencies are being served in these three illustrations. Avowal of values can also be applied generally. A therapist may adopt an approach with *all* his patients in which he will strive to be transparent about his ethical attitudes on the premise that values are central in selecting therapeutic options. The corollary is unambiguous: "Therapists do not have a choice about whether

they need to deal with their values in therapy, only how well" (Aponte, 1985).

The right to treatment

The emphasis on society providing adequate resources brings us to the right to treatment where liberty is restricted. The asylum has been marked by tragic neglect of patients' interests (Bloch and Pargiter, 2002). The overcrowded institution became little more than a warehouse. Its custodial nature persisted even after the advent of psychotropic drugs and psychosocial therapies. It took a plaintiff (*Donaldson* v. *O'Connor*, 1974; *O'Connor* v. *Donaldson*, 1975) to determine that a person committed involuntarily had the "right to receive treatment that would offer him a reasonable opportunity to be cured or to improve his mental condition." Diagnosed with schizophrenia in 1957, Kenneth Donaldson received minimal treatment for the next decade and a half. The US Supreme Court concluded in 1975 that a patient who does not pose a danger to himself or to others and who is not receiving treatment should be released if able to live safely in the community.

The right to effective treatment

The right to treatment has been revisited in subsequent judgments, predominantly in the USA (*Wyatt* v. *Stickney*, 1971, 1972). However, the right has lacked a guarantee that patients will receive *effective* treatment. This opens up a Pandora's box, reflected vividly in *Osheroff* v. *Chestnut Lodge* (Klerman, 1990). The plaintiff sued a private psychiatric hospital for failure to provide antidepressants in the face of his deteriorating depression. Klerman (1990) subsequently argued that the clinician is duty-bound to use only "treatments for which there is substantial evidence" or seek a second opinion in the absence of a clinical response. Stone (1990) countered this position, which he proposed was tantamount to "... promulgating more uniformed scientific standards of treatment in psychiatry, based on ... opinion about science and clinical practice." Moreover, legal standards of care should not be established by one "school" for the whole profession, even if enveloped in science. Instead, we should depend on "the collective sense" of psychiatry, as well as use the "respectable minority rule," namely that a relatively small group within psychiatry can legitimately develop new therapies (Stone, 1990).

The right to refuse treatment

As a voluntary patient, Osheroff could have refused treatment of any type as part of informed consent. His lawsuit pinpointed the institution's alleged failure to offer him an alternative treatment in the face of his deterioration with the therapy offered. If principles of informed consent had been applied correctly, his freedom to choose one treatment over others, and to withdraw consent at any stage thereafter, should have prevailed.

The situation differs radically when the patient is committed involuntarily to hospital or community treatment. The right to refuse treatment then looms large (Appelbaum, 1988). A key event was another US legal judgment when a court ruled that detained patients had a constitutional right to refuse treatment (*Rogers* v. *Okin,* 1979; *Rogers* v. *Commissioner of the Department of Mental Health,* 1983). This coincided with changing commitment laws in many jurisdictions from criteria linked to need for treatment to those highlighting the danger posed to oneself and/or others. The ethical repercussions are profound. If psychiatrists are empowered to detain patients, is it not a contradiction if they are then powerless to offer them treatment should they refuse? The argument rests on the premise that a person sufficiently disturbed to warrant involuntary admission is axiomatically entitled to treatment, and the consulting psychiatrist suitably placed to provide it. Without this arrangement, the psychiatrist's functions are reduced to custodial.

A countervailing argument is grounded in constitutional rights. Merely because people are committed does not mean they are incapable of participating in the process of informed consent. In the event they cannot understand or appreciate the

rationale for a course of action, a form of substituted judgement should be employed thereby ensuring that rights remain prominent.

An assortment of legal remedies has emerged in response to this ethical quandary, ranging from a full adversarial process to reliance on a guardian's decision. Appelbaum (1988) has offered a lucid account of the options and his predilection for a treatment-driven model in which patients are committed because their capacity to decide about treatment is lacking as part of a disturbed mental state. His own research demonstrates that most refusing patients voluntarily accept treatment within 24 hours (Appelbaum and Gutheil, 1979).

In another pragmatically oriented account, Stone (1981) proposed that presumption of competence is dealt with *before* hospitalization. Dealing with commitment and competence would obviate the problem of compulsory admission without treatment. The difficulty is the fluidity of one's mental state. What patients think about treatment during the maelstrom of being detained may well change once they are admitted and suitably cared for.

Involuntary treatment

A consensus has prevailed for generations that a proportion of psychiatric patients loses the capacity for self-determination. They become vulnerable to harming themselves and/or others, acting in ways they will later regret (e.g., a manic patient's sexual indiscretions) and suffer from self-neglect (e.g., schizophrenic patients who are homeless, malnourished, and physically ill). What is not universally agreed is how best to deal with such vulnerable people. Society has, generally, assigned the law to serve as the vehicle to respond to the thorny issue of when and how to protect this group. However, variations in legislation and its application are legion, reflecting, in part, the ethical underpinnings of the process. Psychiatrists and society need coherent arguments concerning the moral principles we should heed. A good start is J. S. Mill's contention, in his essay *On Liberty* in the 1850s, that the "only purpose for which power can be rightfully exercised over any member of a civilised community, against his will, is to prevent harm to others. His own good, either physical or moral, is not a sufficient warrant" (Gray, 1976) Mill's caveat that an exception must be made in children and mentally disturbed people (i.e., "delirious" or in a "state of excitement or absorption incompatible with the full use of the reflecting faculty") suggests they can legitimately be assisted.

Paul Chodoff (1984) has addressed the awesome question of compulsory treatment on the grounds of mental illness. He found utilitarian and deontological theories wanting and, therefore, proposed a "chastened and self-critical" paternalism, one "willing to commit to strong safeguards against abuse." This humanism is epitomized in a concluding sentiment: involuntary treatment is not a conflict of right versus wrong but one over the right to remain at liberty against the right "to be free from dehumanising disease." This notion of being imprisoned by illness would resonate with all psychiatrists who have treated psychotic patients.

Our account hitherto has referred to patients as a homogeneous group. Loss of critical faculties may be a unifying feature but ethical factors will vary according to particulars of the clinical state. One obvious example is suicidal behavior.

Szasz (1986) saw suicide as the act of a moral agent. The state should, therefore, not assume power to prevent self-killing although it may opt to advise for or against. This argument is libertarian, with the corollary that everyone should have the right to end their life. Szasz had, however, neglected Mill's point that, when respecting a person's right to liberty, a possible exception is the loss of critical faculties. This is not to aver that all suicidal behavior is the product of a disordered mind. Suicide in the wake of chronic, debilitating illness, and a long-standing commitment to euthanasia, seems rational and coherent. For example, the renowned author, Arthur Koestler, left a suicide note demonstrating that he arrived at his decision authentically and with his critical faculties intact (Cesarani, 1998).

The suicidal patient epitomizes the psychiatrist's dilemma in having no choice but to impose

treatment in various circumstances and having to declare a person's incapacity, by dint of mental illness, to make rational judgements about what is in their best interests. Van Staden and Kruger (2003) covered this topic by highlighting its dimensions, namely the failure to understand relevant information, choose decisively between options, and accept that the need for treatment prevails. They refer to the utility of a "functional approach" in determining capacity, especially the temporal factor, so that a patient incapable of consenting at one point in their illness may well become capable at another. Ethical arguments to justify detention in a hospital can be extrapolated into the community setting. Similar restrictions on liberty lie at the heart of the moral dilemma, and the psychiatrist again has to consider patients' competence. Munetz and his colleagues (2003) applied three ethical arguments – utilitarian, communitarian, and beneficence – concluding that all three support the application of compulsory community treatment. For more on issues related to consent and capacity, see Section I.

The case

If we return to the family described at the beginning of this chapter, we can readily note how ethical challenges exist at several levels, both diagnostically and therapeutically. A combination of two ethical approaches, principlism (Beauchamp and Childress, 2001) and care ethics (Baier, 1985, 2004), can be gainfully adopted in wrestling with these challenges. Principlism (or principle-based ethics) relies on a set of well-recognized moral principles to identify and analyze ethical problems: respect for autonomy, non-maleficence (avoidance of causing harm), beneficence, and justice. The essence of care ethics is a reliance on the natural inclination of a health professional to extend care to dependent and vulnerable people and to react sensitively to such "moral" feelings as compassion, love, and trustworthiness. The approach fits well with psychiatry since its practitioners rely significantly on empathy in order to understand the wishes and needs of patients and their families.

We conclude by applying the interplay of care and principle ethics in relation to the family in the case opening this chapter. Buffeted by frightening internal forces, Mrs. J's withdrawal and bizarre behavior since her baby's birth point to the question of whether or not she is competent to appreciate her circumstances. Above all, can she protect her infant? Extending care to a deeply distressed woman who has lost her anchorage (as well as to her anxious husband and the vulnerable baby) directs the psychiatrist to the option of responding in accordance with the tenets of care ethics, particularly the goal of promoting trust. It remains an open question whether this means advising Mrs. J (in tandem with gaining Mr. K's support) to enter hospital, committing her to involuntary treatment, or arranging for her rigorous supervision by family and friends. What is vital is that the psychiatrist adopts a caring posture. However, his options must be considered in the context of basic bioethical principles; for example, is respect for Mrs. J's autonomy possible or must the psychiatrist necessarily act *in loco parentis*, in accordance with the principle of beneficence? And given the entitlements owing to the three participants in the scenario, what role does justice play?

A synthesis of care ethics and principlism permits sound moral reflection within an environment of emotionally based connectedness between patients and therapist. We believe this approach acknowledges and best exploits the importance of moral emotions when clinicians are presented with the varied, nuanced ethical conundrums of psychiatric practice.

REFERENCES

American Psychiatric Association (1994). *Diagnostic and Statistical Manual of Mental Disorders*, 4th edn. Washington DC: American Psychiatric Press.

Aponte, H. J. (1985). The negotiation of values in therapy. *Fam Process* **24**: 323–38.

Appelbaum, P. (1988). The right to refuse treatment with antipsychotic medications: retrospect and prospect. *Am J Psychiatry* **145**: 413–19.

Appelbaum, P. and Gutheil, T. (1979). ''Rotting with their rights on'': constitutional theory and clinical reality in drug refusal by psychiatric patients. *Bull Am Acad Psychiatry Law* **7**: 308–17.

Baier, A. (1985). *Postures of the Mind*. Minneapolis, MN: University of Minnesota Press.

Baier, A. (2004). Demoralization, trust and the virtues. In *Setting the Moral Compass*, ed. C. Calhoun. New York: Oxford University Press, pp. 176–88.

Beahrs, J. and Gutheil, T. (2001). Informed consent in psychotherapy. *Am J Psychiatry* **158**: 4–10.

Beauchamp, T. and Childress, J. (2001). *Principles of Biomedical Ethics*, 5th edn. New York: Oxford University Press.

Bergin, A. (1980). Psychotherapy and religious values. *J Consult Clin Psychol* **48**: 95–105.

Bloch S. and Pargiter, R. (2002). A history of psychiatric ethics. *Psychiatr Clin North Am* **25**: 509–24.

Cesarani, D. (1998). *Arthur Koestler: The Homeless Mind*. London: William Heineman.

Chesler, P. (1972). *Women and Madness*. New York: Avon Books.

Chodoff, P. (1984). Involuntary hospitalisation of the mentally ill as a moral issue. *Am J Psychiatry* **141**: 384–9.

Donaldson v. *O'Connor F.* (1974). 2d 5th Cir, decided April 26.

Dyer, A. and Bloch, S. (1987). Informed consent and the psychiatric patient. *Journal of Medical Ethics* **13**: 12–16.

Engelhardt, H. T. (1973) Psychotherapy as meta-ethics. *Psychiatry* **36**: 440–5.

Freud, S. (1924). *Recommendations to Physicians Practising Psychoanalysis*, standard edn 12. London : Hogarth Press, pp. 111–20.

Freud, S. (1937). *Analysis Terminable and Interminable*, standard edn 23. London: Hogarth Press, pp. 211–53.

Goldberg, C. (1977). *Therapeutic Partnership: Ethical Concerns in Psychotherapy*. New York: Springer.

Gray, J. (ed.) (1976). *John Stuart Mill on Liberty*. Oxford: Oxford University Press.

Green, S. and Bloch, S. (eds.) (2006). *An Anthology of Psychiatri Ethics*. Oxford: Oxford University Press, pp. 93–8.

Halasz, G. (2002). A symposium of attention deficit hyperactivity disorder (ADHD): an ethical perspective. *Aust NZ J Psychiatry* **36**: 472–5.

Holmes, J. (1996). Values in psychotherapy. *Am J Psychother* **50**: 259–73.

Kaplan, M. (1983). A woman's view of DSM-III. *Am Psychol* **38**: 786–92.

Klerman, G. (1990). The psychiatric patient's right to effective treatment: implications of *Osheroff* v. *Chestnut Lodge*. *Am J Psychiatry* **147**: 419–27.

Kramer, P. (1993). *Listening to Prozac.* New York: Viking.

Laing, R. (1969). *The Divided Self.* New York: Pantheon Books.

Laing, R. (1970). *Sanity, Madness and the Family.* New York: Penguin Books.

Lidz, C. W., Meisel, A., Zerubavel, E., *et al.* (1984). *Informed Consent: A Study of Decision Making in Psychiatry.* New York: Guilford.

Munetz, M., Galon, P., and Frese, F. (2003). The ethics of mandatory community treatment. *J Am Acad Psychiatry Law* **31**: 173–83.

O'Connor v. *Donaldson* (1975). 422US. 563.

Reich, W. (1999) Psychiatric diagnosis as an ethical problem. In *Psychiatric Ethics*, 3rd edn, ed. S. Bloch, P. Chodoff, and S. Green. Oxford: Oxford University Press, pp. 193–224.

Roberts, L. (2002). Informed consent and the capacity for voluntarism. *Am J Psychiatry* **159**: 705–12.

Rogers v. *Okin* (1979) 478 F Supp 1342 (D Mass).

Rogers v. *Commissioner of the Department of Mental Health* (1983) 458NE 2d 308 (Mass Sup Jud Ct).

Scheff, T. (1966). *Being Mentally Ill: A Sociological Theory.* Chicago, IL: Aldine.

Steere, J. and Dowdall, T. (1990). On being ethical in unethical places: the dilemma of South African clinical psychologists. *Hastings Cent Rep* **20**: 11–15.

Stoller, R., Marmor, J., Beiber, I., *et al.* (1973). A symposium: should homosexuality be in the APA nomenclature. *Am J Psychiatry* **130**: 1207–16.

Stone, A. (1981). The right to refuse treatment: why psychiatrists should and can make it work. *Arch Gen Psychiatry* **38**: 358–62.

Stone, A. (1990). Law, science, and psychiatric malpractice: a response to Klerman's indictment on psychoanalytic psychiatry. *Am J Psychiatry* **147**: 419–27.

Szasz, T. (1960). The myth of mental illness. *Am Psychol* **15**: 113–18.

Szasz, T. (1986). The case against suicide prevention. *Am Psychol* **41**: 806–12.

Van Staden, C. and Kruger, C. (2003). Incapacity to give informed consent owing to mental disorder. *Journal of Medical Ethics* **29**: 41–3.

Wakefield, J. (1992). The concept of mental disorder: on the boundary between biological facts and social values. *Am Psychol* **47**: 373–88.

World Health Organization (1992). *International Statistical Classification of Diseases and Related Health Problems, 1989 Revision.* Geneva: World Health Organization.

Wyatt v. *Stickney* (1971) 325 F Supp 781.

Wyatt v. *Stickney* (1972) 344 F Supp 373, 376, 379–385.

63

Neuroethics

Eric Racine and Judy Illes

Mr. L is a 65-year-old man who has entered early retirement after a long and successful career as a business executive. Having had little time to keep up with current political events, let alone scientific events for which he always had particular curiosity while making his fortune, he has begun to devour a number of major newspapers each day and listen to medical talk shows. He even recently bought a subscription to a high-quality science news publication geared for the educated lay public, and goes on the Internet daily to read news alerts he has signed up for about major scientific advances. His interest in having a brain scan is piqued by Internet and print media advertisements for a computed tomographic scan of the whole body, which includes a free head scan, and by announcements from a nearby university known to be doing cutting-edge Alzheimer' research recruiting for subjects in his age group. He is puzzled by some claims made that preventive brain scans find serious conditions before the manifestations of symptoms. He asks his physician if he should purchase the scan service and if the research opportunity he is offered could serve the same purpose.

What is neuroethics?

Neuroethics is a new field at the intersection of bioethics and neuroscience that focuses on the ethics of neuroscience research and the ethical issues that emerge in the translation of neuroscience research to the clinical and public domain (Marcus, 2002; Illes and Racine, 2007). Although there are lively discussions on the nature of this new field (Doucet, 2005; Illes and Racine, 2005; Vries, 2005), the single most important factor

supporting it is the opportunity for an increased focus and integration of the ethics of medical specialties (neurology, psychiatry, and neurosurgery) and of the ethics of related research to improve patient care. Research on medical neurostimulation techniques (e.g., deep brain stimulation) is a good example to illustrate why there is an important need for integrated interdisciplinary ethical approaches. Neurology and psychiatry separated more than a century ago, and surgical procedures for psychiatric illness (psychosurgery) such as leucotomies and lobotomies have left a history of abuse and unethical behaviors (Gostin, 1980). However, recent techniques for deep brain stimulation that are now widely applied to neurological disorders such as epilepsy and Parkinson disease are being introduced in psychiatry (Abbott, 2005; Chittenden, 2005; Mashour *et al.*, 2005; Mayberg *et al.*, 2005). Discussion has even been initiated on the potential for these techniques to enhance mood and cognitive function in normal individuals (Wolpe, 2002; Farah *et al.*, 2004). Given the scope of the issues and the nature of the challenges found in this example of technology transfer (e.g., informed consent), we can no longer approach the ethics of different medical specialties in an isolated manner. Neuroethics is, therefore, an effort to bring together neuroscientists, physicians, ethicists, and other scholars to address the ethical challenges brought about by the diseases of the mind and brain.

Other important issues discussed in neuroethics span the breadth of scholarship in bioethics and include topics in neuroscience research, healthcare, and policy. The alteration of cognition and mood in normal individuals ("cognitive enhancement") with neuropharmaceuticals is one major area in which physicians will play an increasingly important role. For example, lifestyle uses of the stimulant methylphenidate to augment memory and concentration (Babcock and Byrne, 2000; Kroutil *et al.*, 2006) and the sleep medication modafinil to enhance alertness (Vastag, 2004) are emerging with unknown social and public health consequences. Another important area of neuro-ethics concerns the ethical use of neuroimaging technology outside the medical setting. There are social and economic pressures for rapid availability of applications such as lie detection. They raise fundamental issues of privacy and autonomy (Editorial, 2006), especially given sometimes over-stated promises and threats disseminated through the media (Racine *et al.*, 2005a). These are a few examples of the major issues that have led to the emergence of neuroethics. In addition to these, others are shown in Table 63.1. Physicians and allied healthcare providers must tackle them with an eye to serving as gatekeepers between biomed-ical science and society. In this chapter, we focus on direct-to-consumer advertising (DTCA) of neuro-imaging services and specifically discuss the role of physicians in this currently evolving environment. We have chosen this topic given its overall rele-vance to and immediacy for physicians.

Why is neuroethics important?

Physicians have long acted as the gatekeepers to medical technology and healthcare. Polls indicate that trust in physicians is high (British Medical Association, 2005; Gallup Poll, 2005) and phys-icians, with their knowledge, expertise, and the patient's best interests in mind, are best placed to help and inform their patients in health-related decisions (Pellegrino and Thomasma, 1988). Accordingly, and conforming to fiduciary obliga-tions to the patient (American Medical Association,

2001), physicians must promote patient autonomy while avoiding risks (non-maleficence) and maxi-mizing the possible beneficial outcomes (benefi-cence) of healthcare products and information (Beauchamp and Childress, 2001). However, the physician's role of gatekeeper is currently put to the test by patient information seeking and by aggressive commercial campaigns that market not only traditional health products (e.g., pharma-ceuticals) but also health services (e.g., neuroim-aging) and alternative medicines (e.g., "natural" products to treat neurological and psychiatric diseases) (Racine *et al.*, 2007). The commitment of physicians to evidence-based practice and the patient's welfare is, therefore, complicated in the context of a rapid explosion of attractive health claims for DTCA products and services. In this chapter, we suggest that proactive mitigation of risks and informed approaches to ethical challenges are the best route to high-quality patient information and sound patient–provider relationships.

Ethics

The DTCA of healthcare products refers to a spectrum of marketing practices based on a com-bination of information and promotion strategies and directed at consumers through different media (e.g., newspapers, the Internet; Illes *et al.*, 2003a, 2004a; Caulfield, 2004; Hollon, 2004). The situation specifically discussed here is the DTCA of self-referred imaging services. Self-referral to health-care products and services in the USA has risen steadily since the mid 1980s when the US Food and Drug Administration (FDA) moratorium on DTCA of pharmaceuticals was lifted. Since the late 1990s, self-referral to whole-body computed tomography (CT) and magnetic resonance imaging (MRI) for early screening of cancer, cardiovascular disease, and other disorders has followed this trend.

There has been some discussion in the medical and scientific community concerning whether CT and MRI scans are advertised in the media for unwarranted uses (O'Malley and Taylor, 2004).

Table 63.1. Emerging challenges in neuroethics

Neurotechnology	Description	Therapeutic potential	Emerging challenges
Neuropharmacology	Development of target-specific molecules based on increased understanding of neurobiological mechanisms and systems neuroscience	Improve outcome in acute neurological disease; improve treatment and compliance in psychiatric illnesses; slow neurodegeneration	Identify conditions for consent in patients with acute neurological disorder for emergency neuroprotection trials; tackle proactively enhancement of normal cognition and mood and the emergence of a cosmetic neurology with major social implications; conduct global analysis of costs and benefits for cognitive enhancers in the treatment of neurodegenerative diseases
Neuroengineering	Development of functional brain–computer interfaces and neurostimulation techniques based on advances in neurophysiology, neuroengineering and neurosurgery	Restore motor function; relieve major psychiatric illnesses	Determine requirements of safety and reliability for experimental neurosurgical treatments; establish conditions for consent of vulnerable psychiatric patients for deep-brain stimulation; develop fair and just approaches to improve access to expensive neurosurgical procedures and devices
Neurogenetics	Development of neurogenetic knowledge and tests based on advances in genetic research and bioinformatics	Make lifestyle choices to delay pathological processes; make reproductive choices based on patient autonomy	Provide patient and family genetic counseling; mitigate possible stigma and discrimination based on contemporary knowledge of illness and complexity of genetic information; regulate tests offer in non-conventional settings
Neuroimaging	Advances in structural and functional imaging based on advances in research design and increased resolution of imaging devices	Improve diagnosis of neurological and psychiatric diseases; plan and monitor neurosurgical interventions	Manage incidental findings in research; ensure appropriate knowledge transfer in clinical applications such as presurgical mapping and promote public understanding outside the healthcare system; protect privacy and confidentiality of data in imaging banks

Studies of DTCA of neuroimaging services have found that risks were not consistently reported in advertisements and that a strong emphasis was put on patient success stories (Illes *et al.*, 2004a; Racine *et al.*, 2007). Consequently, the most widely discussed ethical topic related to DTCA concerns the quality of healthcare and scientific information offered to patients and the public through advertisements. Are these advertisements empowering patient autonomy and improving health information or hindering them by conflating information with promotion (Wolfe, 2002; Hasman and Soren, 2006)? Aware of the current challenges, the American Medical Association (1999) has asked physicians to "take an active role in ensuring that proper advertising guidelines are enforced and that the care patients receive is not compromised as a result of direct-to-consumer advertising." The proper ethical role of physicians interacting directly or indirectly with private sector facilities offering such products is another area of debate (Cho, 2002).

The case outlined at the start of this chapter also features an opportunity for a layperson to participate in neuroimaging research. There is now a growing interest in the science and challenges related to the healthcare and public uses of neuroimaging. Examples of ethical issues include confidentiality of brain scans that can reveal patient identity (Olson, 2005), hasty social uses of neuroimaging as a lie-detection device (Wolpe *et al.*, 2005), and ethical use of predictive neuroimaging (akin to genetic testing) (Rosen *et al.*, 2002). One of the most compelling and concrete research ethics issues is the unexpected discovery of abnormal findings in the context of research (i.e., incidental findings; Illes *et al.*, 2004b, c, 2006).

Law

The legal and regulatory context of DTCA is complex. Only in the USA and New Zealand is it legal to advertise directly prescription drugs to consumers. Other healthcare products such as medical devices and dietary supplements are not as strictly regulated

and monitored for safety and marketing (New York State Task Force on Life and the Law, 2005).

Regarding neuroimaging research, we know that physicians acting as investigators must respect all applicable research guidelines, such as the *Helsinki Declaration*. How the current guidelines would apply to advising volunteers to participate in a research study (in which the physician is not involved) is less clear, but physicians should not recommend participation in a study not approved by an institutional oversight committee. We are unaware of neuroimaging researchers being held liable for the disclosure or non-disclosure of abnormal neuroimaging findings. However, some legal precedents point to the possible existence of fiduciary obligations of researchers conducting non-clinical research to disclose clinically relevant information (*Grimes* v. *Kennedy Krieger Institute, Inc.*, 2001).

Policy

In matters of DTCA of healthcare products in the USA, there is evidence of a policy gap in the regulation of healthcare products, neuropharmaceuticals being more tightly regulated and monitored by the FDA than neuroimaging services and natural neuroproducts (Racine *et al.*, 2007). Health authorities and many professional societies have specifically warned against self-referred whole-body imaging since it is currently not indicated for any medical condition (Health Canada, 2004).

No formal and specific policies currently exist for handling the ethics of neuroimaging research, but all relevant general ethics regulations and guidelines remain applicable. An important step in that direction is the results of a workshop sponsored by several institutes of the US National Institutes of Health and Stanford University. Certain fundamental principles to incidental findings achieved broad consensus (Illes *et al.*, 2006). Among these principles was that researchers must respect the subject's right to privacy – the right to know and not to know – and, therefore, anticipate the possibility of detecting brain anomalies in their research. The methods for dealing with this possibility must be clearly articulated in institutional review protocols and consent forms (Illes *et al.*, 2006).

Empirical studies

Direct-to-consumer advertising and public understanding of neuroscience

There is evidence of growing commercialization of imaging services. In the USA, there is a widespread distribution of centers offering self-referred whole-body imaging, with a concentration on the east and west coasts (Figure 63.1). Despite calls for clinical trials, better regulation of these services and even closure of several privately held and academically based centers, the resilience of the industry suggests that in the USA innovative medical technology is rapidly equated with better care because of the support for market-based approaches to a range of services emphasizing consumer choice and responsibility (Fuchs, 1968; Illes *et al.*, 2003a). In Canada, the number of CT and MRI imaging

scanners in free-standing facilities has steadily increased from 1998 to 2004 (Figure 63.2).

Marketing of imaging services, like marketing of prescription pharmaceuticals, is accomplished through print and broadcast media and generally capitalizes on a range of consumer emotions and potential motivations, from fear about disease to promises of health (Shiv *et al.*, 1997; Terzian, 1999; Duke *et al.*, 2001; Wolfe, 2002; Arthur and Wuester, 2003). Several studies have reported that, when commercial interests are at stake, print advertisements, printed information for providers and consumers, and self-accessible web-based materials all fail to provide truly balanced information in terms of completeness and quality for frontier health products and services (Cho *et al.*, 1997; Gollust *et al.*, 2002, 2003; Risk and Petersen, 2002). For imaging services, consumers may not be made aware, for example, of the possibility or rate of false-positive findings and the procedures needed to follow up ambiguous test results, or of the absence of clinical trials validating the benefit of screening asymptomatic individuals. References to the potential risk of radiation associated with CT scans are also

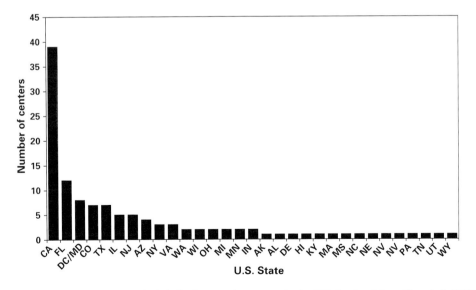

Figure 63.1. Geographic distribution of whole-body screening centers in the USA (updated from Illes *et al.*, 2003a).

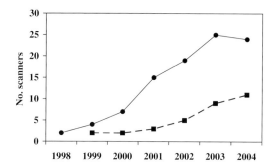

Figure 63.2. Number of magnetic resonance imaging (●) and computed tomographic (■) scanners in free-standing imaging facilities in Canada. (Data from the Canadian Institute for Health Information, 2004.)

notably missing. In contrast, advertisements for MRI services by the same companies make explicit reference to the non-invasive character of this non-radiation modality. These strategies may have an adverse impact on patient views about well-substantiated primary care disease-screening practices. In one series of studies relevant to imaging services, DTCA for genetic screening in print media and on the Internet was heavily criticized for the inadequate presentation of the complexity and probabilistic nature of the information being advertised, the exaggerated promises, and the lack of scientific evidence for the clinical value of the product (Gollust *et al.*, 2002, 2003).

Further evidence suggests that psychiatric and neurological patients are targets of current DTCA practices. Findings from the literature show that the multibillion marketing investments are geared toward the newer pharmaceuticals for chronic conditions with huge market potentials such as psychiatric and neurological illnesses (Gahart *et al.*, 2003; Hollon, 2004; Styra, 2004). In a study on "DTCA visits" (i.e., visits where the patient initiated discussion about a prescription drug advertised on broadcast media), anxiety, depression, and pain were found to be prevalent target conditions (Weissman *et al.*, 2004). Moreover, its has been shown that the Internet per se is more often used by patients with self-reported stigmatized conditions

(e.g., anxiety, herpes, or urinary incontinence) than by patients with non-stigmatized conditions (e.g., cancer, heart problems) to get health information, communicate with healthcare professionals, and utilize healthcare based on Internet information (Berger *et al.*, 2005).

Data on public and patient understanding of neuroscience also suggest that information available through print media is an inadequate source of healthcare information and that it creates high or false expectations about benefits and risks. For example, a recent study that examined press coverage (1995–2004) of frontier neurotechnology (e.g., electroencephalography, positron emission tomography, neurostimulation techniques, neurogenetic testing) for ethical content and reporting practices found that coverage in major newspapers in the USA and UK (more than 1000 articles) was overwhelmingly optimistic except for neurogenetic testing, where almost half of articles featured the "pros and cons" of neurogenetic testing technology. Most technologies went unexplained when they were mentioned in articles (Racine *et al.*, 2005b). Various other studies of medical technologies such as prescription pharmaceuticals (Cassels *et al.*, 2003), neuroimaging (Racine *et al.*, 2005a), and genetics research and technologies (Conrad, 2001; Bubela and Caulfield, 2004; Kua *et al.*, 2004; Racine *et al.*, 2006) have consistently shown that the benefits are hyped and that the risks are underdiscussed.

Risks of neuroimaging research and incidental findings

Like all research, neuroimaging carries risks, such as the potential for breach of confidentiality and physical risks. One of the challenges of neuroimaging research ethics is the occurrence of incidental findings of clinical consequence in non-clinical neuroimaging research. With tens, if not hundreds of thousands of volunteers and patients in Canada, the USA, and Europe participating in research, this is no surprise (Illes *et al.*, 2003b). Although population statistics vary from study to study, even a

1–2% rate of findings yields a high number of people who may then face difficult life decisions about follow-up, and accompanying psychological and financial costs, as indicated in some self-reported cases (Anon., 2005; Hilgenberg, 2005). Current data suggest that approximately 15% of the asymptomatic population of research subjects have unusual variations in their brain structure and in 2–8% of these the findings are clinically significant (Katzman, 1999; Kim *et al.*, 2002; Illes *et al.*, 2004c). These data reflect higher rates than some population studies (Central Brain Tumor Registry of the United States, 2004; Weber and Knopf, 2006) but seem to vary consistently with age, gender, and even with the geography of the data taken. Procedures for handling these findings in the research environment vary substantially, and range from strict protocols to ad hoc procedures (Illes *et al.*, 2004b). Subjects have reported that they expect that if an abnormality is present it will be discovered and disclosed to them (Kirschen *et al.*, 2006). Accordingly, benefits could be expected from simple participation in research, creating potential therapeutic misconceptions (Appelbaum *et al.*, 1987).

How should I approach neuroethics in practice?

We can expect that growing numbers of patients will bring to the clinic information found through the Internet and other media regarding prescription drugs, natural products, genetics tests, and whole-body and brain scans (Gollust *et al.*, 2002; Illes *et al.*, 2003a, 2004a; Check, 2005; Racine *et al.*, 2007). For patients suffering from neurological and psychiatric disorders, the increasing targets of such technology in the open marketplace, vulnerability and compromised decisional capacity are critical factors. Physicians must be aware of the type of claims backing the products patients can learn about and purchase. Physicians should approach patient information on frontier technologies such as neuroimaging with the patient's needs in mind. In cases of conflicting interests, the patient's

interest must come first and, if the physician cannot achieve this, the patient's care should be conferred to a colleague. Knowledge of the current trends and literature is vital for guiding patients who seek counseling on these matters. Akin to encouraging physician consultation for prescription drugs, consumers interested in self-referred imaging services would benefit considerably from involvement of personal physicians in procedure selection and follow-up.

The case

This case presents some of the topics discussed in the neuroethics literature today and that clinicians may face as frontier neurotechnology is translated into healthcare products and services. The two parts of the case introduce many issues in patient information and physician counseling. Our immediate analysis and discussion focuses, first, on public understanding of neuroscience in a context of DTCA for healthcare products and services such as neuroimaging, and, second, on informing patients about research participation in neuroimaging research. More broadly, we hope that this case will also spark discussion on technology transfer and patient information in areas other than neuroscience, such as prenatal genetic testing for a broad range of disabling conditions (Check, 2005).

Self-referred imaging and direct-to-consumer advertising

The physician should inform the patient that self-referred whole-body imaging is not medically indicated for any condition, and the overall value of such screening is still open to debate. Further, the patient should be informed that imaging findings may lead to follow-up testing with a certain degree of morbidity and risks to future insurability. The patient could have tacit expectations about neurotechnology that should be discussed in the light of current scientific and medical evidence. Given that some misconceptions of neuroimaging may be acquired from the media, and that practices of DTCA are still emergent, advance consultation should be encouraged. Patients' questions provide an ideal opportunity for clarifying the pitfalls of unregulated healthcare services and products.

Neuroimaging research

The physician should inform patients that imaging modalities have varying risks even for non-invasive procedures with low-risk profiles. For example, discovery of abnormal findings and other consequences are possible. Participation in any research project should be based on consent and patients may expect to be fully informed about their rights as research subjects. It is essential that physicians dispel therapeutic misconceptions and assist patients, as needed, in differentiating between expectations that are reasonable and appropriate for medical care versus those for medical research.

Advising and counseling patients on healthcare and research uses of frontier neurotechnology

The following advice can be used when counseling patients.
- Inform patients that current sources of scientific and healthcare information transmitted in the media do not provide a substitute for physician counsel and advice.
- Inform patients that medical use of whole-body screening is not currently supported by scientific evidence.
- Inform patients that participation in research may result in unexpected findings that may need follow-up.
- Be prepared to address therapeutic misconceptions and the value of alternative medicine.
- As suggested by the American Medical Association, communicate to the FDA or other relevant authorities wrongful and misleading health messages found in media advertising.
- Promote both patient autonomy and trust in the patient–physician relationship.

REFERENCES

Abbott, A. (2005). Deep in thought. *Nature* **436**: 18–19.

American Medical Association (1999). *Policy E-5.015: Direct-to-Consumer Advertisements of Prescription Drugs*. Chicago, IL: American Medical Association (http://www.ama-assn.org/ama/pub/category/print/8347.html) accessed 23 March 2006.

American Medical Association (2001). *AMA Code of Ethics*. Chicago, IL: American Medical Association (www.ama-assn.org/ama/pub/category/2498.html) accessed 23 March 2006.

Anon. (2005). How volunteering for an MRI scan changed my life. *Nature* **434**: 17.

Appelbaum, P. S., Roth, L. H., Lidz, C. W., Benson, P., and Winslade, W. (1987). False hopes and best data: consent to research and the therapeutic misconception. *Hastings Cent Rep* **17**: 20–4.

Arthur, D. and Wuester, P. (2003). The ethicality of using fear for social advertising. *Aust Market J* **11**: 12–27.

Babcock, Q. and Byrne, T. (2000). Student perceptions of methylphenidate abuse at a public liberal arts college. *J Am Coll Health* **49**: 143–5.

Beauchamp, T. and Childress, J. (2001). *Principles of Biomedical Ethics*, 5th edn. Oxford: Oxford University Press.

Berger, M., Wagner, T. H., and Baker, L. C. (2005). Internet use and stigmatized illness. *Soc Sci Med* **61**: 1821–7.

British Medical Association (2005). *Trust in Doctors*. London: British Medical Association (www.bma.org.uk/ap.nsf/Content/MORI05) accessed 23 March 2006.

Bubela, T. M. and Caulfield, T. (2004). Do the print media "hype" genetic research? A comparison of newspaper stories and peer-reviewed research papers. *CMAJ* **170**: 1399–1407.

Canadian Institute for Health Information (2004). *Medical Imaging in Canada*. Ottawa: Canadian Institute for Health Information.

Cassels, A., Hughes, M. A., Cole, C., *et al.* (2003). Drugs in the news: an analysis of Canadian newspaper coverage of new prescription drugs. *CMAJ* **168**: 1133–7.

Caulfield, T. (2004). The commercialisation of medical and scientific reporting. *PLoS Med* **1**: e38.

Central Brain Tumor Registry of the United States (2004). *Statistical Report: Primary Brain Tumors in the United States, 1997–2001*. Hinsdale, NJ: Central Brain Tumor Registry of the United States.

Check, E. (2005). Fetal genetic testing: screen test. *Nature* **438**: 733–4.

Chittenden, M. (2005). Brain 'pacemaker' can lift depression. *Sunday Times*, 7 February, 4.

Cho, M. K. (2002). Conflicts of interest in magnetic resonance imaging: issues in clinical practice and research. *Top Magn Reson Imaging* **13**: 73–8.

Cho, M. K., Arruda, M., and Holtzman, N. A. (1997). Educational material about genetic tests: does it provide key information for patients and practitioners? *Am J Med Genet* **73**: 314–20.

Conrad, P. (2001). Genetic optimism: framing genes and mental illness in the news. *Cult Med Psychiatry* **25**: 225–47.

Doucet, H. (2005). Imagining a neuroethics which would go further than genetics. *Am J Bioethics* **5**: 29–31.

Duke, C., Pickett, G. M., Carlson, L., and Groe, S. J. (2001). A method for evaluating the ethics of fear appeals. *J Public Policy Market* **12**: 120–9.

Editorial (2006). Neuroethics needed. *Nature* **441**: 907.

Farah, M. J., Illes, J., Cook-Deegan, R., *et al.* (2004). Neurocognitive enhancement: what can we do and what should we do? *Nat Rev Neurosci* **5**: 421–5.

Fuchs, V. R. (1968). The growing demand for medical care. *N Engl J Med* **279**: 190–5.

Gahart, M. T., Duhamel, L. M., Dievler, A., and Price, R. (2003). Examining the FDA's oversight of direct-to-consumer advertising. *Health Aff (Millwood) Suppl Web Exclusives*, W3-120-3.

Gallup Poll (2005). *Nurses Remain Atop Honesty and Ethics List*. Princeton: Gallup Poll (http://poll.gallup.com/content/?ci=20254) accessed 23 March 2006.

Gollust, S. E., Hull, S. C., and Wilfond, B. S. (2002). Limitations of direct-to-consumer advertising for clinical genetic testing. *JAMA* **288**: 1762–7.

Gollust, S. E., Wilfond, B. S., and Hull, S. C. (2003). Direct-to-consumer sales of genetic services on the Internet. *Genet Med* **5**: 332–7.

Gostin, L. O. (1980). Ethical considerations of psychosurgery: the unhappy legacy of the prefrontal lobotomy. *J Med Ethics* **6**: 149–56.

Grimes v. *Kennedy Krieger Institute, Inc.* (2001). *West's Atl Rep* **782**: 807–62.

Hasman, A. and Soren, H. (2006). Direct-to-consumer advertising: should there be a free market in healthcare information. *Camb Q Healthc Ethics* **15**: 42–9.

Health Canada (2004). *Whole Body Screening Using MRI or CT Technology*. Ottawa: Health Canada (www.hc-sc.gc.ca/iyh-vsv/med/mri-irm_e.html) accessed 23 March 2006.

Hilgenberg, S. (2005). Formation, malformation, and transformation: my experience as medical student and patient. *Stanford Med Stud Clin J* **9**: 22–5.

Hollon, M. F. (2004). Direct-to-consumer marketing of prescription drugs: a current perspective for neurologists and psychiatrists. *CNS Drugs* **18**: 69–77.

Illes, J. and Racine, E. (2005). Neuroethics: a dialogue on a continuum from tradition to innovation. *Am J Bioethics* **5**: 5–18.

Illes, J. and Racine, E. (2007). Neuroethics: From neurotechnology to healthcare. *Camb Q Healthc Ethics* **16**: 125–8.

Illes, J., Fan, E., Koenig, B., *et al.* (2003a). Self-referred whole-body CT imaging: current implications for health care consumers. *Radiology* **228**: 346–51.

Illes, J., Kirschen, M. P., and Gabrieli, J. D. (2003b). From neuroimaging to neuroethics. *Nat Neurosci* **6**: 205.

Illes, J., Kann, D., Karetsky, K., *et al.* (2004a). Advertising, patient decision making, and self-referral for computed tomographic and magnetic resonance imaging. *Arch Intern Med* **164**: 2415–19.

Illes, J., Kirschen, M. P., Karetsky, K., *et al.* (2004b). Discovery and disclosure of incidental findings in neuroimaging research. *J Magn Reson Imaging* **20**: 743–7.

Illes, J., Rosen, A. C., Huang, L., *et al.* (2004c). Ethical consideration of incidental findings on adult brain MRI in research. *Neurology* **62**: 888–90.

Illes, J., Kirschen, M. P., Edwards, E., for the Working Group on Incidental Findings in Brain Imaging Research (2006). Incidental findings in brain imaging research. *Science* **311**: 783–4.

Katzman, G. L., Dagher, A. P., and Patronas, N. J. (1999). Incidental findings on brain magnetic resonance imaging from 1000 asymptomatic volunteers. *JAMA* **281**: 36–9.

Kim, B. S., Illes, J., Kaplan, R. T., Reiss, A., and Atlas, S. W. (2002). Incidental findings on pediatric MR images of the brain. *Am J Neuroradiol* **23**: 1674–7.

Kirschen, M. P., Jaworska, A., and Illes, J. (2006). Subjects' expectations in neuroimaging research. *J Magn Reson Imaging* **23**: 205–9.

Kroutil, L. A., Van Brunt, D. L., Herman–Stahl, M. A., *et al.* (2006). Nonmedical use of prescription stimulants in the United States. *Drug Alc Depend* **84**: 135–43.

Kua, E., Reder, M., and Grossel, M. J. (2004). Science in the news: a study of reporting genomics. *Public Underst Sci* **13**: 309–22.

Marcus, S. J. (ed.) (2002). *Neuroethics: Mapping the Field, Conference Proceedings.* New York: Dana Foundation.

Mashour, G. A., Walker, E. E., and Martuza, R. L. (2005). Psychosurgery: past, present, and future. *Brain Res Rev* **48**: 409–19.

Mayberg, H. S., Lozano, A. M., Voon, V., *et al.* (2005). Deep brain stimulation for treatment-resistant depression. *Neuron* **45**: 651–60.

New York State Task Force on Life and the Law (2005). *Dietary Supplements: Balancing Consumer Choice and Safety.* Albany, NY: Department of Health.

Olson, S. (2005). Brain scans raise privacy concerns. *Science* **307**: 1548–50.

O'Malley, P. G. and Taylor, A. J. (2004). Unregulated direct-to-consumer marketing and self-referral for screening imaging services. *Arch Intern Med* **164**: 2406–8.

Pellegrino, E. D. and Thomasma, D. C. (1988). *For the Patient's Good: The Restoration of Beneficence in Health Care.* New York: Oxford University Press.

Racine, E., Bar-Ilan, O., and Illes, J. (2005a). fMRI in the public eye. *Nat Rev Neurosci* **6**: 159–64.

Racine, E., Waldman, S., and Illes, J. (2005b). Ethics and scientific accuracy in print media coverage of modern neurotechnology. In *Proceedings of the 2005 Annual Meeting of the Society for Neuroscience*, Washington.

Racine, E., Gareau, I., Doucet, H., *et al.* (2006). Hyped biomedical science or uncritical reporting? Press coverage of genomics (1992–2001) in Québec. *Soc Sci Med* **62**: 1278–90.

Racine, E., Van der Loos, H. Z. A., and Illes, J. (2007). Internet marketing of neuroproducts: New practices and healthcare policy challenges. *Camb Q Healthc Ethics* **16**: 181–94.

Risk, A. and Petersen, C. (2002). Health information on the Internet: Quality issues and international initiatives. *JAMA* **287**: 2713–15.

Rosen, A. C., Bodke, A. L. W., Pearl, A., and Yesavage, J. A. (2002). Ethical, and practical issues in applying functional imaging to the clinical management of Alzheimer's disease. *Brain Cogn* **50**: 498–519.

Shiv, B., Edell, J. A., and Payne, J. W. (1997). Factors affecting the impact of negatively and positively framed ad messages. *J Consum Res* **24**: 285–94.

Styra, R. (2004). The Internet's impact on the practice of psychiatry. *Can J Psychiatry* **49**: 5–11.

Terzian, T. V. (1999). Direct-to-consumer prescription drug advertising. *Am J Law Med* **25**: 149–67.

Vastag, B. (2004). Poised to challenge need for sleep, "wakefulness enhancer" rouses concerns. *JAMA* **291**: 167–70.

Vries, R. D. (2005). Framing neuroethics: a sociological assessment of the neuroethical imagination. *Am J Bioethics* **5**: 25–7.

Weber, F. and Knopf, H. (2006). Incidental findings in magnetic resonance imaging of the brains of healthy young men. *J Neurol Sci* **210**: 81–4.

Weissman, J. S., Blumenthal, D., Silk, A. J., *et al.* (2004). Physicians report on patient encounters involving direct-to-consumer advertising. *Health Aff (Millwood), Suppl Web Exclusives*, W4-19-33.

Wolfe, S. M. (2002). Direct-to-consumer advertising: education or emotion promotion. *N Engl J Med* **346**: 524–6.

Wolpe, P. R. (2002). Treatment, enhancement, and the ethics of neurotherapeutics. *Brain Cogn* **50**: 387–95.

Wolpe, P. R., Foster, K. R., and Langleben, D. D. (2005). Emerging neurotechnologies for lie-detection: promises and perils. *Am J Bioethics* **5**: 39–49.

64

Pharmacy ethics

Margaret L. Eaton

A pharmacist at a drug store has been presented with prescriptions for two drugs that the pharmacist knows are being prescribed "off-label" or "off-list" (meaning, for a non-approved use) for obesity. The patient presenting the prescription appears to be somewhat overweight but not obese. The pharmacist knows that the medical literature has recently contained reports that patients on this drug combination have developed severe cardiac problems and some have died from the condition. Since the reports are anecdotal in nature and not supported by scientifically controlled research studies, the consensus opinion among healthcare providers is that there is no proof that the drugs cause cardiac problems but there is cause to be alarmed about the risk. For this reason, some physicians have stopped prescribing the combination for their overweight patients. When the pharmacist asks the patient about the prescriptions, he learns that the patient has been on the drugs for months and has lost a considerable amount of weight, a fact that he says has "turned his life around." He reports, improved blood lipid chemistries, better mobility, and a tremendous boost in his self-esteem. The patient also discloses that his usual physician has stopped prescribing the drugs because of the side effect reports, forcing the patient to locate another willing prescriber. In the midst of this prescription intake session with the patient, the pharmacy supervisor calls the pharmacist aside and tells him that there is a backlog of prescriptions that need filling immediately.

What is pharmacy ethics?

With regard to the basic biomedical ethical responsibilities – benefiting the patient, supporting a patient's right to self-determination/autonomy, refraining from harming the patient, assisting and advocating on behalf of the patient to ensure effective and safe healthcare, protecting the patient's medical privacy, and maintaining professional competency and knowledge – pharmacists are no different to any other healthcare professional. However, the role that pharmacists play in healthcare creates unique situations in which these ethical duties occur. This singularity arises from four aspects of pharmacy practice: a pharmacist is expected to dispense medications but also now has responsibilities to provide clinical services; a pharmacist is at least one step removed from a patient's primary encounter with a physician, who diagnoses illness and prescribes treatment; in the outpatient setting, the pharmacist is the last healthcare professional encountered by a patient before drug treatment commences; and pharmacists often control the drug formulary at healthcare institutions. These four features of the profession generate most of the ethical conflicts in pharmacy practice. These are in the areas of (i) allocation of time between dispensing and clinical services; (ii) patient advocacy responsibilities; (iii) social, moral, or religious objections to certain drug uses; (iv) conflicts of interest with pharmaceutical companies; (v) drug diversion and abuse; and (vi) healthcare resource stewardship. This chapter discusses these ethical issues in pharmacy ethics in practice.

Why is pharmacy ethics important?

Pharmacy ethics is important to the same degree that drug therapy is important to a patient's health and well-being. That is, they are both often fundamental. A pharmacist's primary responsibility is to benefit patients and prevent harm by dispensing the right drug in the right amount and with complete use information. Failure to fulfill these responsibilities can lead to loss of disease control, disability, and/or death. Adherence to both professional standards and a code of ethics is imperative if these problems are to be avoided. According to the American Hospital Association and the US Food and Drug Administration, the most common medication errors stem from incomplete patient information (such as allergies to drugs or use of other medications), unavailable drug information (such as up-to-date warnings), miscommunication of drug orders (such as misuse of zeros or decimal points), lack of appropriate labeling, environmental factors that degrade drugs (such as temperature), and distractions that lead to dispensing errors. Medication errors such as these cause at least one death every day and injure approximately 1.3 million people annually in the USA (US Food and Drug Administration, 2006). Many of these kinds of error were involved recently when patients died from a 20-fold overdose of morphine when a certain concentrated oral solution was prescribed in milliliters (ml) instead of milligrams (mg) (US Food and Drug Administration, 2003). This and the other causes of medication error can be avoided by the careful intervention of a pharmacist.

How do I approach pharmacy ethics in practice?

This section contains brief discussions of the most common ethical dilemmas faced by pharmacists.

Conflicts between dispensing and clinical services

A primary source of ethical tension in pharmacy practice stems from the current transition of professional focus from the drug product to the patient. So-called dispensing pharmacists spend much of their professional time interpreting, filling, and dispensing prescriptions. These functions require that the pharmacist reviews the prescription for proper drug use and dosage. Either because it is required by law or because it is considered standard professional practice, some pharmacists also review the list of the other drugs dispensed to a patient to ensure that no dangerous contraindications or interactions exist. For instance, a pharmacist who receives a propranolol prescription for a patient who is already using an inhaled β_2-adrenoceptor agonist would be alert to the fact that the beta blocker could trigger an asthma attack. Prescription problems such as this are rectified by contacting the physician, who can then modify the drug order if needed. For all of these dispensing services, pharmacists receive a fee, and the number of prescriptions filled becomes the primary measure of the pharmacist's income, especially in a chain drug store setting.

Other pharmacists spend a significant part of their time focusing on patient health. These so-called clinical pharmacists perform a number of non-dispensing functions: obtaining drug histories from patients so that drug duplication and interactions are avoided and to determine if any current medical problem has been caused by an untoward drug effect; monitoring for drug compliance, side effects, and interactions between drugs; and counseling patients about proper and safe drug use. More advanced clinical pharmacists also monitor for drug effects (taking blood pressure, testing blood glucose levels, monitoring drug levels) and advise physicians on drug choice, dosing, and toxicity. A clinically oriented pharmacist such as this is most often found in a hospital setting. Since there is usually no reimbursement for clinical pharmacy services, this group must secure a non-traditional source of income for their clinical services and so are often paid as faculty at medical and pharmacy teaching hospitals.

In the middle of the pharmacy practice spectrum is the largest group of pharmacists, who both dispense and provide some limited clinical service, usually counseling patients about a new prescription medicine. This group is often challenged by a situational pressure since time spent counseling interferes with the income-producing dispensing function. The time pressures can, in turn, impinge on the quality of the services provided. The conflict has both legal and ethical dimensions. Some pharmacists are legally required to offer counseling to all patients (Scott and Wessels, 1997). However, even with no legal obligation, many pharmacists believe that patient counseling is ethically required since, especially for complicated drug regimens, counseling can reduce drug administration mistakes and patient morbidity.

This kind of income versus dispensing versus patient health conflict can be resolved with advance planning, triage systems, and staffing adjustments. The planning should identify the priority of obligations that are owed to patients. For instance, a group of pharmacists can determine that counseling services are almost always a priority unless a patient is in acute medical need of a prescription (for pain, asthma, infection, etc.). Communication systems can be developed to alert pharmacists when service priorities need to shift, and staffing adjustments can be made to accommodate the priorities. Notices in the waiting areas that educate patients about professional service priorities can lessen patient stress when delays occur. When patients perceive a benefit from medication counseling, they can more easily tolerate disruptions in dispensing services.

Patient advocacy

It can be difficult to decide how far the scope of a pharmacist's duty to serve patient interests should extend. For instance, most pharmacists acknowledge a duty to recommend generic substitution – when available and if the generic is well formulated – in the interest in benefiting patients (some of whom cannot afford the cost of branded prescription drugs and might go without) and in the interest of rational healthcare resource allocation. However, other situations are not so clear. Pharmacists are not simply a conduit through which a patient receives a prescription drug. Training and specialized knowledge should be put to use to determine if the prescription is valid, beneficial, and safe. Yet pharmacists, especially those in retail settings, are limited by several circumstances in their ability to make these determinations. If, for example, a physician has written a prescription for one medication but a similar drug for the same indication has a better efficacy:safety profile, should the pharmacist attempt to intervene in the interest of rational prescribing and patient safety? As an example, a growing number of cases of violent agitation in the elderly treated with triazolam (Halcion) led pharmacists and medical payors to reject prescriptions for the drug in aged patients (Hensley, 2006). Also, some drugs (propoxyphene [Darvon] is one) come to be recognized as lacking a reliable risk–benefit profile, leading pharmacists to contact prescribers with a request that another drug be selected. The difficulty in questioning a physician's drug choice stems from the fact that the medical data may not be clear about the attributes of various medicines. A pharmacist also lacks the medical information that the physician has about the patient, and pharmacists often cannot take the time to inquire about the prescribing choices of a busy physician who may, in turn, resent the interference. Circumstances can also influence what choice to make. Is the physician known to be prescribing outside of his or her specialty, so prescribing advice may be welcome? Is there credible medical evidence that the prescription drug is inferior to the alternative? Two guiding principles may help the pharmacist in cases such as this: (i) the more severe the potential harm to the patient, the more the pharmacist should be motivated to intervene, and (ii) informing patients of any concern and advising them to seek further advice from their physician is always advisable.

Pharmacists are also always better positioned to promote rational drug use when they have kept abreast of the clinical pharmacology literature.

Refusal to fill a prescription on the basis of social, moral, or religious objections

Pharmacists can have moral objections to the use of medications in many circumstances. The use of drugs for physician-assisted suicide is one such circumstance, and debates exist about whether pharmacists should fill these prescriptions, both in jurisdictions where the practice is legal and those in which it is not (Veatch, 1989; Canadian National Association of Pharmacy Regulatory Authorities, 1999; Catholic News Agency, 2005). Some pharmacists who deplore drug abuse do not wish to participate in the treatment of addicts by dispensing drugs such as buprenorphine. Other pharmacists object to the use of medications to combat obesity. Use of medication, they believe, undermines personal responsibility for discipline, self-restraint, and healthy living. In other cases, pharmacists have objected on moral grounds to filling prescriptions for contraception for unwed women or medications that act as emergency contraception or abortifacients (McClain, 2005). Once having arrived at these conclusions, pharmacists must determine how their moral principles should be balanced against the rights of patients seeking access to medication. The laws and ethics guidelines can be divided on the issue (National Conference of State Legislatures, 2005). Some state that, despite personal objections, pharmacists have a duty to fill legal prescriptions and sometimes even to counsel patients on appropriate use. In other jurisdictions, pharmacists are legally allowed to refuse to fill morally objectionable prescriptions but some laws further require (so that the patient is not abandoned medically) that the pharmacist then refer patients to another willing dispenser. What is not condoned in most countries is a pharmacist refusing to return the prescription to the patient or telling a patient that it is morally forbidden to use the medication for the intended purpose.

Pharmacists have been known to do both (Greenberger and Vogelstein, 2005; Stein, 2005). As communities become increasingly pluralistic, these kinds of conflict are inevitable. They require accommodations (such as a timely referral) that recognize the legitimate personal beliefs of the pharmacist and preserves as much as possible the ethical underpinnings of the patient–pharmacist relationship: a patient's autonomy and right to treatment and the duty of the pharmacist to benefit the patient and to refrain from harming someone seeking medication.

Using prescription records to assist the marketing activity of pharmaceutical companies

Some large pharmaceutical companies pay US pharmacies to mail material or call patients about company drugs or competing products. The materials and messages urge patients to do such things as continue taking a currently prescribed drug, switch to a new form of the drug, or switch from a competitor's drug. Theses programs ostensibly do not invade a patient's medical privacy and are not illegal, since the company does not have access to the list of patients taking its drugs. Although viewed by many as promotional material directed to patients taking selected drugs, companies call such material "patient education," "patient compliance," or "disease management" programs. However they are characterized, these programs raise several troubling ethical questions (O'Harrow, 1998). Are such actions by a pharmacist an improper invasion of the privacy of patients' prescription records? Is there a conflict of interest when pharmacists are paid to urge patients to take a particular brand of drug? Is this interfering with the patient–physician relationship when the material advises a patient to take a drug other than one prescribed by the physician? These programs have been challenged in lawsuits brought by US pharmacy customers against major chain pharmacies for invasion of privacy, and in investigations by attorneys general in different states and the Federal Trade Commission for possible violations of laws prohibiting unfair and deceptive trade practices. The US Congress and the Department of Health and Human Services have also considered new privacy laws and regulations to stop the practice (Zimmerman and Armstrong, 2002). Leaving aside the merits of the claims against the companies and pharmacists, which have not been resolved, this is a classic example of how ethically questionable but legal activity can lead to censure, litigation, regulation, and loss of trust in the profession. Pharmacists who are approached to participate in these programs need to place primary emphasis on protecting patients' privacy interests and should only convey information clearly intended to promote health interests.

Drug diversion and abuse

Surveys indicate that prescription drug abuse has been rising over a number of years to what is now considered epidemic proportions (National Center on Addiction and Substance Abuse at Columbia University, 2005). Pharmacists increasingly suspect that when a patient presents a prescription for a controlled drug, it is for the purpose of diversion or abuse. Professional responsibilities in such a case often conflict. Pharmacists have a duty to dispense opioid analgesics when the drug has been legally prescribed and is therapeutically appropriate for the patient. Determining if both of these requirements have been met can be difficult, and errors in judgement can have dire consequences. Refusal to fill a legitimate prescription can withhold pain relief from a suffering patient, and pharmacists have been sued and disciplined for refusals to fill these prescriptions based on the mistaken belief that abuse or diversion was occurring (Simons-meier, 2005). Alternatively, filling a narcotic prescription that is used abusively increases the risk of harm to the patient and perpetuates a dangerous threat to the public health. Since most pharmacists will face this kind of challenge, all should receive training that focuses equally on decision-making

skills to detect drug abuse and diversion and also on the recognition of valid and appropriate prescriptions for controlled substances. Armed with these skills, pharmacist are less likely to err in either direction. The second task for the pharmacist is to recognize and avoid any tendency to make decisions in these cases based on racial or other biases, fear of liability or other personal harm, lack of reimbursement, or other extraneous considerations. Finally, when faced with an ambiguous situation and contacting the prescriber or questioning the patient and others, pharmacists must be diligent, appropriately timely, and considerate of the patient's need.

Medical resource stewardship

No system of healthcare is free of the burdens of cost and the fair and rational allocation of constrained resources. Pharmacists play a central role in these matters since they control or manage institutional drug formularies, which are systems designed to limit the choice of drugs that can be prescribed based on cost-effectiveness determinations. A typical drug formulary decision involves selecting the least expensive among a class of drugs that provide the same or similar therapeutic benefit and risk. At times, however, the decision can involve whether or not to stock a particularly expensive drug. Assessing the cost effectiveness of drugs in these cases often requires an economic analysis involving calculations based on factors such as cost per life year and cost per quality-adjusted life year. However important these numbers are to the economic viability of healthcare systems, they are considered unfair by patients in desperate need of treatment and by physicians who want to do everything possible for their patients. An example is drotrecogin alfa (Xigris), a drug approved in 2001 for the treatment of sepsis, a condition with a high risk of death and for which there is no consistently effective treatment. Some hospital pharmacies did not want to stock the drug, however, since it is not uniformly effective; costs it over $6800 per treatment in the USA (£5000 in the

UK); and, at least at first, was inadequately reimbursed by insurers or the government. This combination meant that pharmacy budgets could be depleted to save only a relatively few patients. Of the hospitals that did offer the drug, many limited patient eligibility to severe sepsis in an attempt to improve the cost–benefit ratio (Regalado, 2003; Green *et al.*, 2006). Rationing of scarce or expensive medical care raises very contentious issues especially when patients learn that they may not be offered (or cannot afford) the most advanced treatments. Hospital politics also enters the picture when the request to add the drug to the formulary comes from a highly valued physician who controls a department and/or admits a large number of patients. Institutional pharmacists often find themselves in the middle of these dilemmas and need to study carefully and objectively all the available drug and cost data and balance equality and fairness so that formulary decisions that limit access to treatments will be accepted by physicians, patients, and the community. Periodic reassessment and physician and patient education will reinforce the viability of these decisions (Bochner *et al.*, 1996). For more on issues related to resource allocation, see Ch. 33.

The case

The case at the beginning of this chapter is loosely based on the early reports of death and disability from pulmonary and cardiac disease attributed to the diet pill combination of fenfluramine and phentermine (called fen-phen; Connolly *et al.*, 1997). The case represents a conflict between a pharmacist's duty to act in the best interests of a patient's health and the duty to respect the autonomy rights of patients to make their own personal and medical decisions. In many Western countries particularly, respecting a patient's autonomy is a highly valued medical ethics obligation, supported by laws and medical ethics codes that require healthcare professionals to provide full information to patients about the benefits and risks of medical treatment options and otherwise assist patients in making their own medical decisions. Since ignorance undermines autonomy, the first duty of the pharmacist in this case is to ascertain whether the patient has been informed of the potential drug risks. If the answer is "yes," a second question for the patient is whether the physician intends to monitor for the cardiovascular risk. With a second affirmative response, the pharmacist has more assurance that both the physician and the patient understand the potential consequences of the choice to medicate. If either one of these conditions does not exist, the patient needs more information. The patient can be informed about the medical literature reports and then referred back to the prescribing physician to address questions about potential adverse effects and monitoring. Promoting patient safety may require that the pharmacist notifies the physician that the patient has been so advised and that continuing the drugs can be harmful. The patient should also be told to inform his primary care physician of the choice to continue taking the medication so that medical care can proceed in as safe a manner as possible. Some may disagree with these proposed courses of action as unwarranted intrusions into the physician–patient relationship but, when potentially lethal side effects are possible and when refraining from drug treatment presents no immediate risk, a pharmacist's advocacy duties should err on the side of preserving patient health.

The case also raises the issue of "off-label" or "off-list" prescribing and dispensing, that is, using a drug for a purpose other than its labeled indication. In most jurisdictions, physicians are not prevented from prescribing off-label; this is considered the practice of medicine and subject only to professional standards. Pharmacists are likewise not prevented from dispensing drugs intended for off-label use. The question here is whether physicians have the sole responsibility for determining what off-label uses are appropriate. Even if dispensing pharmacists are free from a legal duty to act, do they have an ethical obligation to intervene if they think that this prescribing is irresponsible? Again, pharmacists may not know the medical situation that prompted the off-label prescription. But sometimes this information is available to the pharmacist, either from patient disclosures or because the use is obvious. This situation existed with Genentech's recombinant human growth hormone, approved and labeled initially for use in children with a rare form of dwarfism caused by lack of natural growth hormone. After the product was launched, physicians began prescribing the drug to short healthy children to help them to grow taller, to adults to improve athletic performance, to obese patients for weight loss, and for other off-label uses. Little was known about the efficacy or safety of the product for these other uses, and concerns existed about the potential for harm, especially in children. Although off-label uses can be bring beneficial treatments to patients faster than if all new uses were first researched, the lack of prior data leaves both healthcare providers and patients in the dark about the consequences of this kind of drug use. It can also invite the kind of criticism that undermines trust in the healthcare system. In the recombinant human growth hormone situation, both Genentech and the prescribing physicians were said to be profiting from purposefully ignoring and/or engaging in irresponsible prescribing that could harm children (Veatch, 1983; Kolata, 1994). The same question could have been directed to pharmacists who dispensed this product. The guidelines stated above concerning the duty of advocacy can guide a pharmacist when dealing with off-label prescribing. It is advisable that physicians who prescribe drugs off-label in their medical practice (i.e., they are not collecting data in a research setting) should institute a monitoring program that would allow them to detect drug-related problems and then disseminate that information. Pharmacists can do likewise by asking patients about possible adverse effects during drug-refill counseling sessions and alerting the physician if indicated.

REFERENCES

Bochner, F., Burgess, N.G., and Martin, E.D. (1996). Approaches to rationing drugs in hospitals. An Australian perspective. *Pharmacoeconomics* **10**: 467–74.

Canadian National Association of Pharmacy Regulatory Authorities (1999). Model statement regarding refusal to provide products or services for moral or religious reasons. Ottawa: Canadian National Association of Pharmacy Regulation Authorities (http://www.napra.org/docs/0/95/157/165/179.asp).

Catholic News Agency (2005). Catholic pharmacists in Spain refuse to sell condoms. Rome: Catholic News Agency (http://www.catholicnewsagency.com/new.php?n=5187).

Connolly, H. M., Crary, J. L., McGoon, M. D., *et al.* (1997). Valvular heart disease associated with fenfluramine-phentermine. *N Engl J Med* **337**: 581–8.

Green, C., Dinnes, J., Takeda, A., *et al.* (2006). Evaluation of the cost-effectiveness of drotrecogin alfa (activated) for the treatment of severe sepsis in the United Kingdom. *Int J Technol Assess Healthc* **22**: 90–100.

Greenberger, M. D. and Vogelstein, R. (2005). Pharmacists' refusals: a threat to women's health. *Science* **308**: 1557–8.

Hensley, S. (2006). As drug bill soars, some doctors get an ''unsales'' pitch. *Wall Street Journal* 13 March, A1.

Kolata, G. (1994). Selling growth hormone for children: the legal and ethical questions. *New York Times*, 15 August, A2.

McClain, C. (2005). Rape victim: ''morning after'' pill denied. *Arizona Daily Star*, 23 October. (http://www.azstarnet.com/dailystar/dailystar/99156.php.) [This article cited a 2004 survey of more than 900 Arizona pharmacies that found less than half kept emergency contraception drugs in stock, with most citing low demand as a reason but some pharmacists cited moral reasons. The article also featured the story of a 20-year-old rape victim who spent three days attempting to find a Tucson pharmacy to dispense the medication, which is most effective the earlier it is taken.]

National Center on Addiction and Substance Abuse at Columbia University (2005). *Under the Counter: The*

Diversion and Abuse of Controlled Prescription Drugs in the US. New York: Columbia University Press (http://www.casacolumbia.org).

National Conference of State Legislatures (2005). *Pharmacist Conscience Clauses: Laws and Legislation.* Denver, CO: National Conference of State Legislatures (http://www.ncsl.org/programs/health/conscienceclauses.htm).

O'Harrow, R. (1998). Plan's access to pharmacy data raises privacy issue. *Washington Post,* 27 September, A1.

Regalado, A. (2003). To sell pricey drug, Lilly fuels a debate over rationing. *Wall Street Journal* 18 September, A1.

Scott, D. M. and Wessels, M. J. (1997). Impact of OBRA '90 on pharmacists patient counseling practices. *J Am Pharmaceut Assoc* **4**: 401–406. [OBRA '90 is the US Omnibus Budget Reconciliation Act of 1990. OBRA '90 also requires Medicaid pharmacy providers to offer prescription drug-use counseling to patients at the time that drugs are dispensed. However, laws are sometimes insufficient to change professional practice. The Scott and Wessels study showed that, six years after OBRA '90 passed, fewer than half of retail pharmacists reported that time devoted to patient counseling increased as a result of the law.]

Simonsmeier, L. M. (2005). False imprisonment alleged when patient is detained with suspicious Rx. *Pharmacy Times,* March, 96.

Stein, R. (2005). Pharmacists' rights at front of new debate. *Washington Post,* 28 March, A1.

US Food and Drug Administration (2003). *MedWatch; 2003 Safety Alert: Roxanol (morphine sulfate) Concentrated Oral Solution.* Washington, DC: Food and Drug Administration (http://www.fda.gov/medwatch/SAFETY/2003/roxanol.htm).

US Food and Drug Administration (2006). *Medication Errors.* Washington, DC: Food and Drug Administration (http://www.fda.gov/cder/drug/MedErrors/default.htm).

Veatch, R. M. (1983). Ethics of drugs for non-approved uses. *US Pharmacist* **8**: 69–72.

Veatch, R. M. (1989). Pharmacist's refusal to dispense diethylstilbestrol for contraceptive use. *Am J Hosp Pharm* **46**: 1413–16.

Zimmerman, A. and Armstrong, D. (2002). Use of pharmacies by drug makers to push pills raises privacy issues. *Wall Street Journal,* 1 May, A1.

Resources

Codes of ethics

American Pharmacists Association *Code of Ethics for Pharmacists.* http://www.aphanet.org/pharmcare/ethics.html

Model Standards of Practice for Canadian Pharmacists. http://www.napra.org/docs/0/95.asp

Royal Pharmaceutical Society of Great Britain *Code of Ethics and Standards.* http://www.rpsgb.org.uk/members/ethics/index.html

Smith, M., Strauss, S., Baldwin, J. H., and Alberts, K. T. (eds.) (1991). *Pharmacy Ethics.* Binghamton, NY: Haworth Press.

Veatch, R. M. and Haddad, A. (1999). *Case Studies in Pharmacy Ethics.* New York: Oxford University Press.

Wingfield, T. and Badcott, D. (2007). *Pharmacy Ethics and Decision Making.* London: Pharmaceutical Press.

65

Alternative and complementary care ethics

Michael H. Cohen

Ms. M, a patient with a rare skin condition who has failed all relevant conventional therapies, asks her dermatologist, Dr. N, about treatment options involving complementary and alternative medical (CAM) therapies. Dr. N mentions a homeopathic remedy commonly available in pharmacies and health food stores; Ms. M tries the remedy, and the skin condition quickly resolves. She is elated by this success and tells her best friend, a neurologist, who promptly files a complaint with the state medical board, noting that few, if any, physicians of any subspecialty in the state ever recommend homeopathy for any condition. The board holds a hearing at which there is no evidence that Dr. N has ever harmed a patient or acted unskillfully or incompetently in any way. Indeed, several dozen patients testify that Dr. N is a skilled, caring healthcare professional. The board nonetheless decides to revoke Dr. N's license based on a state statute defining professional misconduct as "any departure from acceptable and prevailing medical standards." Subsequently, Ms. M sues Dr. N for malpractice, alleging that he failed to adequately discuss the risks and benefits of a different CAM therapy – acupuncture – for her condition, and, in the alternative, that by inducing her to rely on homeopathy he neglected conventional dermatological treatment.

What are complementary and alternative medical therapies?

Complementary and alternative medical (CAM) therapies refer to those modalities and whole systems of healing that historically have not been part of the dominant system of medical practice in the West. These CAM therapies include acupuncture and traditional oriental medicine, chiropractic, herbal medicine, massage therapy, and "mind-body" therapies (such as hypnotherapy and guided imagery) (Institute of Medicine of the National Academies, 2005). Integrative healthcare refers to clinical practice that judiciously combines conventional medical therapies and evidence-based CAM therapies, focusing on patient-centered, relationship-driven care (Institute of Medicine of the National Academies, 2005).

This chapter discusses the ethical, legal, and policy aspects of clinical integration of CAM therapies. Legal and ethical rules suggest that inquiry into patient use of CAM therapies, disclosure and discussion of risks and benefits of potentially beneficial CAM therapies, and appropriate warnings as to possible contraindications, adverse reactions, and interference with conventional care, as applicable, should be standard practice. Such conversations will enhance shared decision making, help to balance non-maleficence and patient autonomy interests, and improve the therapeutic alliance, thus reducing the possibility of medical malpractice liability. Guidelines for liability risk management are explored.

Why are complementary and alternative medical therapies important?

Ethics

Like conventional care, clinical integration of CAM therapies implicates major ethical principles such as beneficence (the obligation to help the patient), non-maleficence (the obligation to "do no harm"), and autonomy (the obligation to honor a patient's freely made medical choices) (Institute of Medicine of the National Academies, 2005). In general, medical paternalism has tended to trump over patient autonomy interests in CAM therapies, whereas it may now be time to acknowledge the possibility for human transformation afforded by CAM therapies at the boundary of medicine and religion (Cohen, 2004a) alongside historical concerns for preventing healthcare fraud (Cohen, 2003).

To this end, ethical decision-making regarding clinical advice about CAM therapies consider the following factors: severity and acuteness of illness; curability with conventional treatment; invasiveness, toxicities, and side effects of conventional treatment; quality of evidence of safety and efficacy of the CAM treatment; degree of understanding of the risks and benefits of conventional and CAM treatments; knowing and voluntary acceptance of those risks by the patient; and persistence of patient's intention to utilize CAM treatment (Adams *et al.*, 2002).

Consequently in situations where an illness is not severe or acute, and is not easily curable with conventional treatment, and/or the conventional treatment is invasive and carries toxicities or side effects that are unacceptable to the patient, then, assuming the CAM therapy is not proven unsafe or ineffective, it may be ethically compelling to try the CAM approach for a limited period of time with monitoring conventionally (Adams *et al.*, 2002). The ethical posture is even further improved if the patient understands the risks and benefits, is willing to assume the risk of trying such an approach, and insists on this route. In this case, a monitored "wait-and-see" approach respects the patient's autonomy interest, while satisfying the clinician's obligation to do no harm (Adams *et al.*, 2002).

The Institute of Medicine report used this framework and also described two ethical values additional to beneficence, non-maleficence, and autonomy to enrich clinical decision making in integrative care. The two additional considerations are medical pluralism and public accountability. The report defined "medical pluralism" in terms of "acknowledgement of multiple valid modes of healing and a pluralistic foundation for healthcare," even if some CAM practices are "rooted, at least in part, in forms of evidence and logic other than used in biomedical sciences, often with long traditions and theoretical systems of interpretation divergent from those used in biomedicine" (Institute of Medicine of the National Academies, 2005, p. 169). The report defined "public accountability" in terms including attending to the "needs and desires of multiple constituents within the public sector (e.g., licensed clinicians and other healers, patients, professional organizations, regulatory boards, and other government authorities)," as well as the "heterogeneity of communities and interests within each set of constituents" (Institute of Medicine of the National Academies, 2005, p. 173).

Law

In general, basic principles of health law apply whether a therapy is labeled "conventional" or "CAM" (Cohen, 1998). The critical arenas of legal analysis are (i) licensure, (ii) scope of practice, (iii) malpractice liability, (iv) professional discipline, (v) access to treatments, (vi) third-party reimbursement, and (vii) healthcare fraud. These areas are broadly described with case examples by Cohen (1998), though it is worth briefly summarizing some of the major legal rules that would apply whether discussing integrative pediatrics (Cohen and Kemper, 2005), integrative oncology (Cohen, 2006), integrative cardiology (Schouten and Cohen, 2004), or any other medical specialty or healthcare practice.

This chapter focuses primarily on US law and regulation, although the issues cut across other common law nations, such as the UK (Stone and Matthews, 1996), Canada (Boon, 2002), and Australia (Cohen, 2004b). For example, the *Sixth Report*, entitled *Complementary and Alternative Medicine*, issued by the UK House of Lords Committee on Science and Technology (2002) made many regulatory recommendations that paralleled those made the same year in the *Final Report* by the US White House Commission on Complementary Medicine Policy (2002). Similarly, scholarly counterparts in the UK have argued that the highly individualized, more intuitive, whole-person approach of complementary medicine requires a more dynamic form of ethics-directed self-regulation that facilitates consumer choice while protecting against dangerous and abusive healthcare practices. In a similar vein, the Canadian federal government, like its counterpart in the USA, is deeply concerned with regulation of consumers' use of natural health products for nutritional purposes (Boon, 2003) (known in the USA as regulation of dietary supplements [Cohen, 2003]).

In the USA, licensure refers to the requirement in most states that healthcare providers maintain a current state license to practice their professional healing art. Historically, medical licensing statutes made the unlicensed practice of "medicine" a crime and defined the practice of "medicine" broadly in terms of "diagnosis" and "treatment" of "any human disease" or "condition" (Cohen, 1998). This put non-licensed practitioners of the healing arts at risk of prosecution for unlawful medical practice.

Over time, chiropractors, massage therapists, naturopathic physicians, practitioners of acupuncture and traditional oriental medicine, and other CAM therapy providers attempted to gain licensure on a state-by-state basis. Providers of CAM therapies may or may not be licensed depending on a particular state's licensing scheme. Chiropractors, for example, are licensed in every state, whereas massage therapists and acupuncturists are licensed in well over half the states, and naturopathic physicians in at least a dozen states. In most states, practitioners lacking any healthcare license are at risk of prosecution for practicing medicine without a license (Cohen, 1998).

State licensing statutes and regulations by the applicable professional board usually define a CAM provider's scope of practice, the legally authorized boundaries of care within the given profession (Cohen, 1998). For example, chiropractors can offer nutritional advice, acupuncture, or colonic irrigation in some states but not others (Cohen, 1998). Exceeding one's scope of practice can lead to charges of practicing other healing arts (such as, for example, medicine) without a license. Some institutions will further limit the practice boundaries of affiliated CAM providers beyond the existing limitations of the practitioner's legally authorized scope of practice: for example, restricting acupuncturists on hospital staff from offering patients herbal medicine even though the acupuncture licensing statute may consider herbal medicine within acupuncturists' scope of practice (Cohen and Ruggie, 2004).

Malpractice refers to negligence, which is defined as failure to use due care (or follow the standard of care) in treating a patient, and thereby injuring the patient. While medical standards of care specific to a specialty are applied in medicine, each CAM profession is judged by its own standard of care – for example, claims of chiropractic malpractice will be judged against standards of care applicable to chiropractic treatment (Cohen, 1998). In cases where the provider's clinical care overlaps with medical care – for example, the chiropractor who takes and reads a patient's radiograph – then the medical standard may be applied (Cohen, 1998).

Claims for healthcare malpractice resulting from inclusion of CAM therapy can involve allegations of misdiagnosis, failure to treat, failure of informed consent, fraud and misrepresentation, abandonment, vicarious liability, and breach of privacy and confidentiality (Schouten and Cohen, 2004). These are discussed more fully by these authors, but it is worth highlighting some common elements. Firstly, because the definition of malpractice includes both providing substandard care and thereby injuring the patient, adding complementary diagnostic systems (such as those of chiropractic or acupuncture, either by referral or by using modalities within the scope of one's clinical licensure) is not problematic in itself, so long as the conventional bases are not neglected (Cohen and Eisenberg, 2002). Conversely, a conventional provider who fails to employ conventional diagnostic methods where such methods could have averted unnecessary patient injury, or who substitutes CAM diagnostic methods for conventional ones and thereby causes patient injury, risks a malpractice verdict (Cohen and Eisenberg, 2002). Similarly, it is not malpractice for a CAM provider to use modalities within his or her legally authorized scope of practice, so long as the provider refers to medical care where necessary and appropriate.

Secondly, the legal obligation of informed consent (whether involving conventional medicine or CAM therapies) is to provide the patient with all the information material to a treatment decision – in other words, information that would make a difference in the patient's choice to undergo or forgo a given therapeutic protocol (Ernst and Cohen, 2001). Failure to provide adequate informed consent can constitute malpractice. The Institute of Medicine's *Report on Complementary and Alternative Medicine* (2005, p. x) stated: "The goal should be the provision of comprehensive medical care that is based on the best scientific evidence available regarding benefits and harm, that encourages patients to share in decision making about therapeutic options, and that promotes choices in care that can include CAM therapies, when appropriate."

Thirdly, while there are few judicial opinions setting precedent regarding referrals to CAM therapists, the general rule of conventional care – that there is no liability merely for referring to a specialist – should apply whether referral is to a practitioner labeled conventional or CAM (Studdert *et al.*, 1998). The major exceptions to this no-liability rule involve a negligent referral (one that delays necessary care and thereby causes harm to the patient, as in referral to a CAM provider that delays necessary conventional care), a referral to practitioner that the referring provider knew or should have known was "incompetent," and a referral involving "joint treatment," in which the referring clinician and the practitioner receiving the referral actively collaborate to develop a treatment plan and to monitor and treat the patient (Studdert *et al.*, 1998). "Integrative" care suggests a

sufficiently high degree of coordination between the referring provider and the one receiving the referral that a court conceivably could find that a "joint treatment" has occurred and, therefore, liability may be apportioned among conventional and CAM providers sharing diagnostic and therapeutic information (Studdert *et al.*, 1998; Cohen, 2000).

Professional discipline refers to the power of the relevant professional board to sanction a clinician, most seriously by revoking the clinician's license. The concern over inappropriate discipline, based on medical board antipathy to inclusion of CAM therapies, has led consumer groups in many states to lobby for "health freedom" statutes – laws providing that physicians may not be disciplined solely on the basis of incorporating CAM modalities. More recently, the Federation of State Medical Boards (2002) has issued *Model Guidelines for Physician Use of Complementary and Alternative Therapies* for: "(1) physicians who use CAM in their practices, and/or (2) those who co-manage patients with licensed or otherwise state-regulated CAM providers." These guidelines explicitly state that discipline should not be premised on inclusion of CAM therapies alone but should depend on whether the physician has delivered therapies lacking in safety and efficacy. The guidelines are not binding but rather offer a framework for individual state medical boards to regulate physicians integrating CAM therapies.

Third-party reimbursement typically involves a number of insurance policy provisions, and corresponding legal rules, designed to ensure that reimbursement is limited to "medically necessary" treatment; does not, in general, cover "experimental" treatments; and is not subject to fraud and abuse (Cohen, 1998). In general, insurers have been slow to offer CAM therapies as core benefits – largely because of insufficient evidence of safety, efficacy, and cost effectiveness – though a number of insurers have offered policy-holders discounted access to a network of CAM providers.

Finally, healthcare fraud refers to the legal concern for preventing intentional deception of patients. Overbroad claims regarding the potential success of a CAM therapy sometimes can lead to charges of common law fraud, and its related legal theory, misrepresentation (Cohen, 1998). Further, under Medicare and Medicaid fraud and abuse law, if the clinician or institution submits a reimbursement claim for care that the clinician knew or should have known was medically unnecessary, the practitioner could be liable for fraud under applicable federal law (Cohen, 1998).

Policy

The term "policy" often evokes government regulatory policy, though with respect to CAM therapies, policy can also refer to institutional policies and policy by professional medical associations and other actors.

Government policies run the gamut of issues such as which providers should be licensed (Cohen, 1998) to questions of regulating dietary supplements and other natural health products. Within the UK, questions of licensure have been particularly complex, as presently only the professions of osteopathy and chiropractic have statutory licensure, while others (such as acupuncture) rely on professional self-regulation (Stone, 2005).

Hospitals, free-standing clinics, nursing homes, and other healthcare institutions need to attend to institutional policy issues relating to CAM therapies, such as policies for confirming credentials, informed consent procedures, policies relating to limiting potential malpractice liability exposure, and institutional rules regarding continuance of patient use of dietary supplements (Cohen *et al.*, 2005a, b).

The policies of professional medical associations concerning CAM therapies have been shifting over time toward greater acceptance of the fact that many patients do use such therapies on their own and routinely request relevant information about CAM therapies from their physicians. Increasingly, it behooves the medical practitioner to become familiar with the evidence base regarding those CAM therapies commonly in use.

For example, the American Medical Association House of Delegates passed a resolution in May 2006 stating that it would "support the incorporation of complementary and alternative medicine (CAM) in medical education as well as continuing medical education curricula, covering CAM's benefits, risks, and efficacy." The British Medical Association (2004), in its Annual Representatives Meeting Policies, enacted a *Complementary Medicine Policy*, stating that: "complementary therapy should be regulated by statutory authority." As noted, some healthcare regulatory authorities outside of government have begun to enact more specific policies; a salient example would be the *Model Guidelines for Physician Use of Complementary and Alternative Therapies* issued by the US Federation of State Medical Boards (2002).

Empirical studies

The many empirical studies of CAM therapies have been reviewed by various panels of medical experts, most notably in the USA by the Institute of Medicine (Institute of Medicine of the National Academies, 2005) and in the UK by the Prince of Wales' Foundation for Integrated Health (2005).

The Institute of Medicine of the National Academies report (2005, Ch. 5 and Table 5-3) culled the best available evidence regarding CAM therapies as did the Cochrane review (Manheimer *et al.*, 2004). With some stated limitations, the former highlighted use of a number of therapies including acupuncture for headache, calcium for prevention of hypertensive disorders and related problems in pregnancy and for bone loss, calcium and vitamin D for corticosteroid-induced osteoporosis, cranberries for preventing urinary tract infection, echinacea for preventing and treating the common cold, electromagnetic fields for osteoarthritis, folic acid and folinic acid for reducing side effects in patients receiving methotrexate, inositol for respiratory distress syndrome in preterm infants, transcutaneous electrical nerve stimulation (TENS) for rheumatoid arthritis in the hand and osteoarthritis in the knee, and TENS and acupuncture for primary dysmenorrhoea.

To supplement the discussion of the Institute of Medicine of the National Academies, primary sources for literature reviews include PubMed (http://nccam.nih.gov/camonpubmed/[maintained by the US National Library of Medicine]), the Clinical Trials site for the National Institutes of Health (www.clinicaltrials.gov), and the Cochrane Collaboration reviews (Manheimer *et al.* [2004]) and (http://www.compmed.umm.edu/Cochrane/ cam_reviews.html). The US National Center for Complementary and Alternative Medicine also provides reviews by treatment or therapy (http:// nccam.nih.gov/health/bytreatment.htm).

Within the UK the Prince of Wales' Foundation for Integrated Health has conducted a number of detailed reviews regarding possible integration of CAM therapies in particular areas such as supportive and palliative care (Prince of Wales' Foundation, 2005). The Foundation has also produced a report entitled *Searching the Evidence: Complementary Therapies Research* (2006), which reviews evidence relating to women's health, pain management, and mental health.

How should I approach complementary and alternative medical therapies in practice?

In view of the above resources for empirical studies, clinicians can perform their own literature review to determine the relative liability risk pertaining to clinical integration of CAM therapies by assessing whether for a particular CAM therapy (i) the medical evidence supports both safety and efficacy; (ii) the medical evidence supports safety, but evidence regarding efficacy is inconclusive; (iii) the medical evidence supports efficacy, but evidence regarding safety is inconclusive; or (iv) the medical evidence indicates either serious risk or inefficacy (Cohen and Eisenberg, 2002).

In the first instance, clinicians can recommend the CAM therapy without undue fear of liability, as a therapy deemed both safe and effective could be recommended regardless of whether it is classified as conventional or CAM. In the last instance, a therapy that is either seriously risky or ineffective should be avoided and discouraged. Many CAM therapies will fall within the middle two groups, where liability is conceivable but probably unlikely; this would be particularly pertinent in (ii), where the product presumably is safe provided the clinician provides the patient with appropriate risk–benefit disclosure and warnings about possible contraindications and adverse reactions. In both (i) and (ii), clinicians can allow the patient to use the CAM therapy in question, while providing appropriate caution and continuing to monitor conventionally (Cohen and Eisenberg, 2002).

If the patient's condition deteriorates, then the physician should consider intervening conventionally (Cohen and Eisenberg, 2002). The clinician must remain alert to the medical evidence regarding CAM therapies, and particularly herbal therapies, which may contain previously unclassified hazards; the categorization of therapies over time into any given region of the framework may change according to new medical evidence (Cohen and Eisenberg, 2002). Further, since, as noted, injury to the patient is part of the definition of malpractice, the perception of injury – including a poor physician–patient relationship – can lead to litigation, while improving the therapeutic alliance tends to reduce liability risk (Schouten and Cohen, 2004).

In general, clinicians can attempt to limit liability risk through the following:
- Determine the clinical risk by assessing the medical evidence and thereby deciding whether to a recommend; allow, caution, and monitor; or avoid and discourage (Cohen and Eisenberg, 2002).
- Continue to monitor conventionally and intervene conventionally when medically necessary, so that the standard of care likely will be met and the possibility of patient injury minimized (Cohen and Eisenberg, 2002).
- Engage the patient in a robust informed consent and shared decision-making process, clearly laying out risks and benefits, and documenting the conversation in the medical record (Cohen and Eisenberg, 2002).

- When contemplating referral to a CAM provider, undertake reasonable investigation of the practitioner's credentials, practice style, malpractice and disciplinary history, and general competence in order to be satisfied that the referral is unlikely to increase the risk of patient injury and of vicarious or shared liability (Eisenberg *et al.*, 2002).
- Obtain consultation and document this in the patient's record to help to establish the standard of care in the community, and keep clear medical records that show how treatment options were discussed and decisions made with patients (Schouten and Cohen, 2004).
- Physicians also should familiarize themselves with documentation standards suggested by the Federation of State Medical Boards (2002) guidelines, and whether these are applicable in their state or home institution.

The legal doctrine of "assumption of risk" may, in some US states, be available as a defense to medical malpractice involving use of CAM therapies if the patient has knowingly, intelligently, and voluntarily make a choice to try such therapies in addition to or in lieu of conventional care (*Schneider* v. *Revici*, 1987). The few US cases on these issues so far have allowed both an express (*Boyle* v. *Revici*, 1992) and implied (*Charell* v. *Gonzales*, 1997) assumption of risk defense, suggesting that although courts generally tend to disfavor attempts to waive liability for medical malpractice (*Tunkl* v. *Regents of the University of California*, 1963) some courts may allow patients to make affirmative choices regarding use of CAM therapies, relieving physicians or some or all of liability.

The case

Dr. N's conversation with Ms. M concerning treatment options involving CAM therapies such as homeopathy should not, in itself, raise liability concerns. In fact, by describing the risks and benefits of the proposed approach, Dr. N can satisfy the obligation of informed consent and engage Ms. M in shared decision making. By monitoring and standing ready to intervene conventionally when medically necessary, Dr. N could further limit potential malpractice liability risk.

A state whose legislation allows medical board discipline for "any departure from prevailing and acceptable medical standards, irrespective of patient harm," could conceivably discipline Dr. N merely for discussing homeopathy in this case, though a number of states have "medical freedom" laws that would protect Dr. N from such unwarranted consequences. Furthermore, if Dr. N were to follow the Federation of State Medical Boards (2002) guidelines, disciplinary consequences would similarly be unlikely.

Once again, the above review and analysis are grounded in US law, and although an international, comparative law perspective is beyond the scope of this chapter, the salient issues and areas of controversy cut across nations, with particular resonance among common law countries, which will share basic definitions of practitioner licensure, informed consent, and medical malpractice.

REFERENCES

Adams, K. E., Cohen, M. H., Jonsen, A. R., and Eisenberg, D. M. (2002). Ethical considerations of complementary and alternative medical therapies in conventional medical settings. *Ann Intern Med* **137**: 660–4.

American Medical Association (2006). *House of Delegates, Resolution 3-06 (A-06)*. Chicago, IL: American Medical Association.

Boon, H. (2002). Regulation of complementary/alternative medicine: a Canadian perspective. *Complement Ther Med* **10**: 14–19.

Boon, H. (2003). Regulation of natural health products in Canada. *Clin Res Regul Aff* **20**: 299–312.

Boyle v. *Revici* (1992). 961 F.2d 1060 (2d Cir).

British Medical Association (2004). *Annual Representatives Meeting Policies: Complementary Medicine Policy*. London: British Medical Association.

Charell v. *Gonzales* (1997). 660 New York Supplement 2d 665, 668 (S.Ct., N.Y. County, 1997), affirmed and modified to vacate punitive damages award, 673 New York

Supplement 2d 685 (App Div., 1st Dept., 1998), reargument denied, appeal denied, 1998 New York Appellate Division LEXIS 10711 (App. Div., 1st Dept., 1998), appeal denied, 706 Northeastern Reporter 2d 1211 (1998).

Cohen, M. H. (1998). *Complementary and Alternative Medicine: Legal Boundaries and Regulatory Perspectives.* Baltimore, MD: Johns Hopkins University Press.

Cohen, M. H. (2000). *Beyond Complementary Medicine: Legal and Ethical Perspectives on HealthCare and Human Evolution.* Ann Arbor, MI: University of Michigan Press.

Cohen, M. H. (2003). *Future Medicine: Ethical Dilemmas, Regulatory Challenges, and Therapeutic Pathways to Health and Healing in Human Transformation.* Ann Arbor, MI: University of Michigan Press.

Cohen, M. H. (2004a). Healing at the borderland of medicine and religion: regulating potential abuse of authority by spiritual healers. *J Law Relig* **18**: 373–426.

Cohen, M. H. (2004b). Legal and ethical issues in complementary medicine: a US perspective. *Med J Aust* **181**: 168–9.

Cohen, M. H. (2006). Legal and ethical issues relating to use of complementary therapies in pediatric hematology/oncology. *J Ped Hematol Oncol.* **28**: 190–3.

Cohen, M. H. and Eisenberg, D. M. (2002). Potential physician malpractice liability associated with complementary/integrative medical therapies. *Ann Intern Med* **136**: 596–603.

Cohen, M. H. and Kemper, K. J. (2005). Complementary therapies in pediatrics: a legal perspective. *Pediatrics* **115**: 774–80.

Cohen, M. H. and Ruggie, M. (2004). Integrating complementary and alternative medical therapies in conventional medical settings: legal quandaries and potential policy models. *Cinn Law Rev* **72**: 671–729.

Cohen, M. H., Hrbek, A., Davis, R., *et al.* (2005a). Emerging credentialing practices, malpractice liability policies, and guidelines governing complementary and alternative medical practices and dietary supplements recommendations: a descriptive study of 19 integrative healthcare centers in the US. *Arch Int Med* **165**: 289–95.

Cohen, M. H., Sandler, L., Hrbek, A., *et al.* (2005b). Policies Pertaining to complementary and alternative medical therapies in a random sample of 39 academic health centers. *Alt Ther Health Med* **11**: 36–40.

Eisenberg, D. M., Cohen, M. H., Hrbek, A., *et al.* (2002). Credentialing complementary and alternative medical providers. *Ann Intern Med* **137**: 965–73.

Ernst, E. E. and Cohen, M. H. (2001). Informed consent in complementary and alternative medicine. *Arch Intern Med* **161**: 2288–92.

Federation of State Medical Boards (2002). *Model Guidelines for Physician Use of Complementary and Alternative Therapies in Medical Practice.* Washington, DC: Federation of State Medical Boards.

Institute of Medicine of the National Academies (2005). *Complementary and Alternative Medicine in the United States.* Washington, DC: National Academies Press.

Manheimer, E., Berman, B., Dubnick, H., Beckner, W. (2004). *Cochrane Reviews of Complementary and Alternative Therapies: Evaluating the Strength of the Evidence.* Ottawa: Cochrane Collaboration.

Prince of Wales' Foundation for Integrated Health (2005). *Evaluation of the National Guidelines for the Use of Complementary Therapies in Supportive and Palliative Care.* London: Prince of Wales' Foundation for Integrated Health.

Prince of Wales' Foundation for Integrated Health (2006). *Searching for Evidence: Complementary Therapies Research.* London: Prince of Wales' Foundation for Integrated Health.

Schneider v. *Revici* (1987) 817 Federal Reporter 2d 987 (2d Cir.).

Schouten, R. and Cohen, M. H. (2004). Legal issues in integration of complementary therapies into cardiology. In *Complementary and Integrative Therapies for Cardiovascular Disease*, ed. W. H. Frishman, M. I. Weintraub, and M. S. Micozzi. Edinburgh: Elsevier, pp. 20–55.

Stone, J. (2005). *Development of Proposals for a Future Voluntary Regulatory Structure for Complementary Health-Care Professions: A Report Commissioned by The Prince of Wales' Foundation for Integrated Health.* London: The Prince of Wales' Foundation for Integrated Health.

Stone, J. and Matthews, J. (1996). *Complementary Medicine and the Law.* Oxford: Oxford University Press.

Studdert, D. M., Ersenberg, D. M., Miller, F. H., *et al.* (1998). Medical malpractice implications of alternative medicine. *JAMA* **280**: 1620–5.

Tunkl v. *Regents of the University of California* (1963) 383 *Pacific Reporter* 2d 441.

UK House of Lords Committee on Science and Technology (2002). *Sixth Report: Complementary and Alternative Medicine.* London: Stationery Office.

US White House Commission on Complementary Medicine Policy (2002). *Final Report.* Washington, DC: Government Printing Office.

Index